Anatomy of the Eye and Orbit

THE CLINICAL ESSENTIALS

Anatomy of the Eye and Orbit

THE CLINICAL ESSENTIALS

Thomas F. Freddo, OD, PhD, FAAO
Professor of Ophthalmology, Pathology, Anatomy and Neurobiology (*Emeritus*)
Former Director of the Eye Pathology Laboratory
Boston University School of Medicine
Boston, Massachusetts
Adjunct Professor of Optometry
MCP Health Sciences University
Worcester, Massachusetts

Edward Chaum, MD, PhD
Plough Foundation Professor of Ophthalmology
Professor of Pediatrics, Anatomy and Neurobiology, and Biomedical Engineering
University of Tennessee Health Science Center
Memphis, Tennessee

Wolters Kluwer

Philadelphia • Baltimore • New York • London
Buenos Aires • Hong Kong • Sydney • Tokyo

Acquisitions Editor: Chris Teja
Product Development Editor: Ashley Fischer
Editorial Coordinator: Lindsay Ries
Editorial Assistant: Brian Convery
Marketing Manager: Rachel Mante Leung
Production Project Manager: David Saltzberg
Design Coordinator: Holly Reid McLaughlin
Artist/Illustrator: Jen Clements
Manufacturing Coordinator: Kel McGowan
Prepress Vendor: S4Carlisle Publishing Services

9 8 7 6 5 4 3 2 1

Printed in China

Library of Congress Cataloging-in-Publication Data

Names: Freddo, Thomas F., author. | Chaum, Edward, author.
Title: Anatomy of the eye and orbit : the clinical essentials / Thomas F.
   Freddo and Edward Chaum.
Description: First edition. | Philadelphia: Wolters Kluwer Health, [2018] |
   Includes bibliographical references.
Identifiers: LCCN 2017009025 | ISBN 9781469873282
Subjects: | MESH: Eye—anatomy & histology | Atlases
Classification: LCC QP475 | NLM WW 17 | DDC 612.8/4—dc23 LC record available at
   https://lccn.loc.gov/2017009025

This book is dedicated to my beloved son Matthew at whose bedside the earliest drafts of these chapters took form, as he fought the good fight against the cancer that would ultimately take him from us. This book is also dedicated to my wife Jan, daughter Catherine, our families, and our close friends, especially Ruth, Brian and Susan, Roger and Judy Kamm, and Melissa who supported us through that most difficult time.

Thomas F. Freddo

This book is dedicated to the memory of my colleague, mentor, and friend Dr. Barrett G. Haik, whose invitation to join him in building the Hamilton Eye Institute changed my life and academic career in so many profound and positive ways. And to Thom, an inspiring teacher from the first time I met him during my residency. Thank you for inviting me to make this journey with you.

Edward Chaum

Contributors

Igor I. Bussel, MD, MS, MHA
Resident Physician and Doris Duke Research Fellow
Department of Ophthalmology
University of Pittsburgh Medical Center, Eye Center
University of Pittsburgh
Pittsburgh, Pennsylvania
(Chapter 17)

Richard Hertle, MD, FAAO, FACS, FAAP
Director, Pediatric Ophthalmology
Department of Ophthalmology
Akron Children's Hospital
Akron, Ohio
(The Muscle Pulley System, Chapter 1)

Natalie Hutchings, BSc, PhD, MCOptom
Associate Professor
School of Optometry and Vision Science
University of Waterloo
Waterloo, ON Canada
(Axes of the Eye, Chapter 3)

Kelly N. Ma, MD, MPH
Glaucomatologist
Department of Ophthalmology
Northwest Permanente Physicians and Surgeons
Portland, Oregon
(The Surgical Limbus, Chapter 5)

John C. Morrison, MD
Weeks Professor of Ophthalmology
Casey Eye Institute
Oregon Health and Science University
Portland, Oregon
(The Surgical Limbus, Chapter 5)

Zach Nadler, BSc, MD candidate
Temple University School of Medicine
Philadelphia, Pennsylvania
(Chapter 17)

Joel Schuman, MD
Professor and Chair, Department of Ophthalmology
Professor, Departments of Neuroscience and Physiology
New York University School of Medicine
Chief of Service for Ophthalmology
NYU Langone Medical Center
New York, New York
(Chapter 17)

Ruth Trachimowicz, PhD, OD, FAAO
Associate Professor
Illinois College of Optometry
Chicago, Illinois
(Chapter 16)

Gadi Wollstein, MD
Associate Professor of Ophthalmology
Director, Ophthalmic Imaging Research Laboratories
University of Pittsburgh School of Medicine
Pittsburgh, Pennsylvania
(Chapter 17)

Preface

The eye is a truly remarkable and complex organ. One could wax forever about the wonders of seeing. But even viewed from the more mundane perspective of the array of specialized tissues it contains, the fact is that within a sphere, roughly 1 inch in diameter, one can find examples of virtually every major histologic tissue type found in the human body, except skeletal muscle, cardiac muscle, bone, and cartilage. And if, for a moment, we extend beyond the human eye to the eyes of birds, one can even find cartilage, skeletal muscle, and bone. As such, this book is written at a level that presumes the reader to be well-grounded in the histology of basic tissue types. A full appreciation of the variety of different tissue types within the eye should make it less surprising that the eye can be involved in such a large array of systemic diseases, each affecting these various tissue types.

The reasons for the contemporary clinician or clinician-in-training to understand the complexity of these tissues at the histologic and even the ultrastructural level are compelling. During a routine eye examination, using modern clinical imaging methods such as OCT, today's clinician can noninvasively examine most of the tissues of the eye at what amounts to histologic levels of detail.

Few other specialties provide this opportunity in everyday clinical practice. It is why we have chosen to add a chapter to this book on the anatomy of the eye as seen with OCT. But to take full advantage of this opportunity for the sake of their patients, the practitioner must have an everyday working knowledge of the microscopic anatomy of the eye, in greater detail than is required in almost any other specialty—with the obvious exception of pathology!

The goal of this book is to provide that clinical foundation in the anatomy of the eye in a way somewhat different from previous texts on this subject. In doing so, certain details of individual cells within the ocular tissues have been sacrificed in order to enhance the discussion of more clinical detail. More comprehensive, but less clinically oriented sources on the anatomy of the eye are available for the reader who wishes to extend their knowledge beyond the level of detail provided herein. There is always more to learn.

One of the most common refrains of clinical trainees is the question, "Why do I have to know this?" In each chapter, the reader will find several clinical correlates designated by the Eye of Horus symbol ( ) that will address this question by providing examples of abnormalities that illustrate why a given anatomic detail is essential to know. Seasoned clinicians may argue whether the authors have chosen the examples that they might have chosen to best make the case in each instance, but the hope in any clinical training program is that trainees reach the point where they can understand the pathobiology and envision the histopathology of an abnormality, as they are viewing its clinical presentation. Many clinicians never reach that point, but the path begins by learning *The Clinical Essentials*.

Thomas F. Freddo, OD, PhD, FAAO
Edward Chaum, MD, PhD
2017

Acknowledgments

The authors would like to acknowledge the contribution of images from the following institutions, organizations, and companies:

Jon Miles Research, Stroma Medical, Konan, Genoptic, EyeRounds Atlas of Ophthalmology at The University of Iowa, Accutome, Optos, Dr. Ben Glasgow and Mission for Vision (missionforvision.org), Tomey, RISC Software GmbH, EyePlastics, LLC, and the archives of the Eye Pathology Laboratory at Boston Medical Center. Many individual colleagues contributed images as well and they are credited in the legends of those images. Images not otherwise credited are those of the authors.

Special thanks to Robert Bert, MD, PhD, Associate Professor, Department of Radiology, University of Louisville School of Medicine, for his contribution of the series of orbital MRIs for the online supplement of this book. Special thanks as well to Paul Kaufman, MD, and Mary Ann Croft at The University of Wisconsin for their contribution of the in-vivo primate eye video clips of anatomical changes during accommodation.

The authors would like to thank the following colleagues, residents and students for reviewing various chapters or parts of chapters. Rand Allingham, Tyler Brown, Vincent Budac, Stephen Burns, James Chodosh, Ann Elsner, Amy Falk, Chris Fleming, Brian Fowler, Suzanne Freitag, Haiyan Gong, Andrew Hartwick, Richard Hertle, Dianna Johnson, Howard Leibowitz, Phillip Lewis, Joe Mastellone, William Morris, John Morrison, Stephen Moser, Daniel Roberts, Joel Schuman, Carol Toris, Andrew Williams, Matthew Wilson, Elizabeth Wyles, and Rebecca Zoltoski.

Special thanks to Drs. Ruth Trachimowicz and Janice Freddo who patiently read these chapters time and again. Additional thanks to Ryan Shaw of Wolters Kluwer for committing to the project. We would also like to thank our Editor, Ashley Fischer, and both David Saltzberg and Rebecca Gaertner at Wolters Kluwer, plus Shailaja Subramanian, Ann Francis, and the production team at S4Carlisle Publishing Services. Special thanks to our amazing Artistic Director Jennifer Clements for her magical treatment of the images. We are also grateful to Rob Flewell, CMI, who produced some exceptional new art for the book. Finally, sincere thanks to Peter Stirling at the Witer Learning Resource Center at the University of Waterloo, for his RefWorks expertise.

Contents

SECTION 6   OCULAR ANATOMY BY OPTICAL COHERENCE
TOMOGRAPHY   317

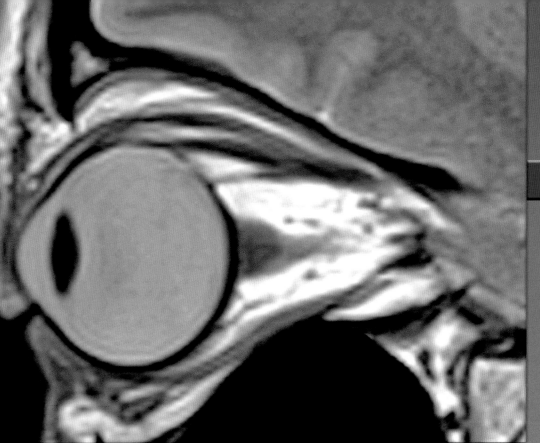

ORBITS, LIDS, AND ADNEXA

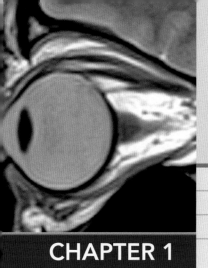

The Orbits

⬤ Overview

The eyes reside partially contained within the bony orbits. The orbits are roughly the shape of elongated pyramids, with their broad anterior bases represented by the orbital rims of the facial skeleton and their apices directed superomedially, being formed by the bones that separate the orbit from the cranial cavity.

The principal axes of the two orbits, from their apices to the midpoint of each orbital opening, commonly subtend an angle of approximately 45°, while the lateral walls of the two orbits commonly subtend an angle of 90° (**Fig. 1.1**). The midline nasal cavity and, lateral to the nasal cavity on each side, the compartments of the ethmoidal air cells (sinuses) separate the parallel medial walls of the orbits. The anterior to posterior axes

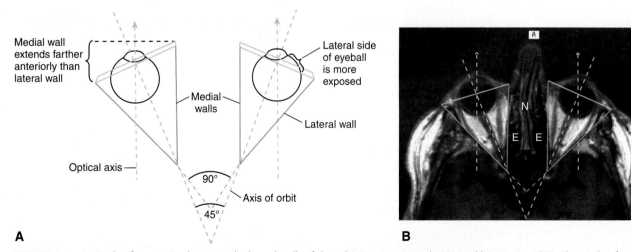

FIGURE 1.1   A: Angle of separation between the lateral walls of the orbit is approximately 90° (*red lines* in A and B). The angle of separation between the axes of the orbits is commonly 45° (*green lines* in A and B). **B:** Note that the optical axes of the eyes (dashed gold lines in A and B) and the axes of the orbits (*dashed green lines* in A and B) are not aligned. Also note how much of the lateral side of the eye is anterior to the lateral orbital rim. E, ethmoid air cells (sinuses); N, nasal cavity. A in white rectangle in Figure B indicates anterior. (Modified from Moore KL, Agur AMR, Dalley AF, eds. *Clinically Oriented Anatomy.* 7th ed. Philadelphia, PA: Wolters Kluwer; 2013.)

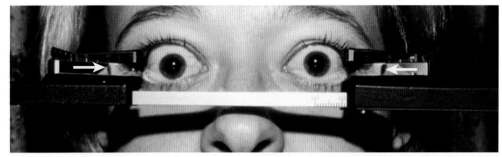

FIGURE 1.2 An exophthalmometer can be adjusted to align with the lateral orbital rims. Angled mirrors in the instrument permit a lateral view of the corneal apex from the front (*white arrows*). Above each mirror, the instrument contains a measurement scale that permits assessment of the amount of protrusion of each eye from the orbital rim. (Courtesy of Dr. Howard Leibowitz.)

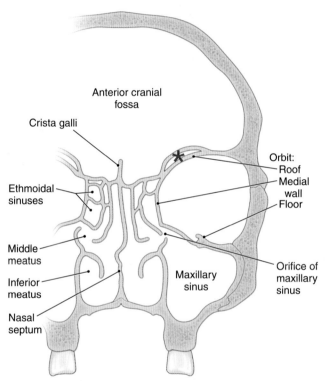

FIGURE 1.3 Coronal section through the skull showing relationship between orbit, paranasal sinuses, and anterior cranial fossa. The frontal sinus is indicated by an *asterisk*. (Modified from Detton AJ. *Grant's Dissector*. 16th ed. Philadelphia, PA: Wolters Kluwer; 2016.)

> *An instrument called an exophthalmometer is used to compare the positions of the corneal apices, relative to the orbital rims. In conditions that occupy space within the orbit and push the eye forward, this anterior displacement (proptosis/exophthalmos) can be measured (*Fig. 1.2*).*

by the frontal sinuses (**Fig. 1.3**). Inferiorly, each orbit is bordered by one of the paired, maxillary sinuses.

Medially, the orbits are bordered by the ethmoid sinuses (ethmoid air cells) anteriorly and, near the apex of the orbit, by the sphenoid sinus. Posteriorly, each orbit makes direct connections with the middle cranial fossa, via the optic canal and superior orbital fissure, and with the pterygopalatine fossa via the inferior orbital fissure (**Figs. 1.4** and **1.5**). Along the medial wall, just posterior to the inferomedial orbital rim, is a vertical channel that extends to the inferior meatus of the nasal cavity. This channel, called the nasolacrimal canal, houses the soft tissues of the nasolacrimal drainage system. The dilated, superior end of this canal houses the lacrimal sac and is termed the lacrimal fossa (**Figs. 1.4** and **1.5**).

Note that various texts use the term "lacrimal fossa" for the recess under the superolateral orbital rim that accommodates the presence of the lacrimal gland. We will use the term "lacrimal fossa" for the space provided for the lacrimal sac and the term "fossa for the lacrimal gland" to indicate the fossa posterior to the superolateral orbital rim that houses the lacrimal gland.

Bones of the Orbit

The bones that form the orbital rim include the frontal, maxillary, and zygomatic. The portions of the orbital bones forming the orbital rim are thicker than those portions that form the orbital walls. Despite this added thickness, approximately 40% to 60% of all facial fractures involve the orbital rims.

of the orbits do not align with the optical axes of the eyes (**Fig. 1.1**).

The eyes are positioned anteriorly within the orbit and slightly closer to the roof than to the floor. A normal horizontal (axial) magnetic resonance imaging (MRI) or computed tomography (CT) scan shows that the lateral rim of the orbit provides protection for only the posterior half of the globe on the temporal side so as not to interfere with the maximum traverse of the eyes and their maximal lateral visual field (**Fig. 1.1**).

The orbits are bordered superiorly by the anterior cranial fossa, and, along the medial half of the superior orbital rim,

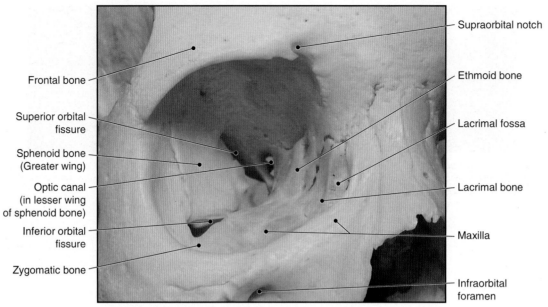

Frontal bone

Superior orbital fissure

Sphenoid bone (Greater wing)

Optic canal (in lesser wing of sphenoid bone)

Inferior orbital fissure

Zygomatic bone

Supraorbital notch

Ethmoid bone

Lacrimal fossa

Lacrimal bone

Maxilla

Infraorbital foramen

FIGURE 1.4   Anterior view of right orbit shows principal bones plus openings of the orbital apex including the optic canal, superior, and inferior orbital fissures. Also shown is the position of the lacrimal fossa that contains the lacrimal sac. (From Olinger AB. *Human Gross Anatomy*. 1st ed. Philadelphia, PA: Wolters Kluwer; 2015.)

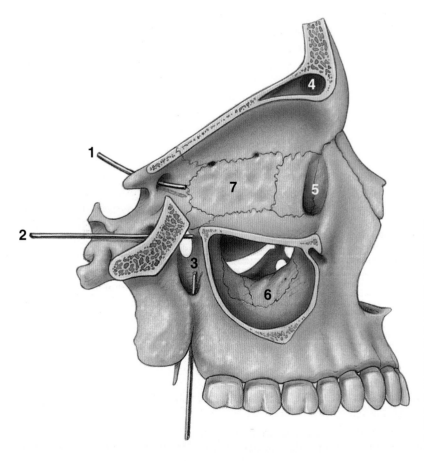

FIGURE 1.5   Sagittal section of skull showing medial wall of the right orbit. (*1*) Probe traverses optic canal between orbit and middle cranial fossa; (*2*), probe begins in the middle cranial fossa, passing through the foramen rotundum and across the roof of the pterygopalatine fossa (space labeled *3*) to nearly reach the floor of the orbit via the inferior orbital fissure (this is the path taken by the maxillary division of the trigeminal nerve). Probe extending from below traverses greater palatine canal to reach the pterygopalatine fossa (*3*) from posterior edge of the hard palate. (*4*) Frontal sinus; (*5*) lacrimal fossa for lacrimal sac; (*6*) maxillary sinus; (*7*) lamina papyracea of the ethmoid bone showing anterior and posterior ethmoidal foramina at superior margin. (Modified from the Anatomical Chart Company. *Eye Anatomical Chart*. Philadelphia, PA: Wolters Kluwer; 2000.)

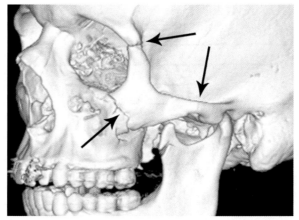

FIGURE 1.6   3D volume reconstructed CT scan showing locations of sutures that are damaged in tripod fractures (*arrows*). (Modified from Bittle MM, Gunn ML, Gross JA, et al, eds. *Trauma Radiology Companion.* 2nd ed. Philadelphia, PA: Wolters Kluwer; 2011.)

 Given its defensive position, forming the lateral rim of the orbit, it should not be surprising that the most common facial fracture is the zygomaticomaxillary or "tripod" fracture that disarticulates the zygomatic bone at its sutural connections to the maxilla inferiorly, the frontal bone superiorly, and the sphenoid and temporal bones laterally as seen in this 3D volume reconstructed CT scan (Fig. 1.6).

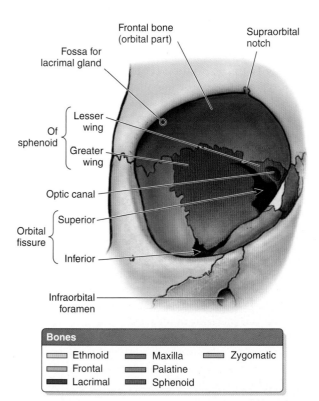

FIGURE 1.7   Drawing depicts the relationships between the seven bones that contribute to the orbit. Note position of fossa for the lacrimal gland. (Modified from Moore KL, Agur AM, Dalley AF. *Essential Clinical Anatomy.* 5th ed. Philadelphia, PA: Wolters Kluwer; 2014.)

The floor, roof, and medial and lateral walls of the orbit are formed by contributions from seven bones (**Figs. 1.4** and **1.7**).

The floor—is formed from the maxillary bone, the zygomatic bone, and a small contribution from the palatine bone. Although generally thicker than the medial wall, the floor of the orbit is most often damaged in blunt force injuries because of the long line of focal thinning present at the infraorbital groove that leads to the infraorbital foramen (**Fig. 1.7**).

Blunt force trauma to the soft tissues of the orbit momentarily increases the pressure of these tissues against the orbital walls. If the orbital floor is fractured (blow-out fracture), orbital tissues can be forced into the fracture by the increased tissue pressure. When the force of the impact is relieved, the fracture can partially close, trapping these orbital tissues. When such cases are imaged, one sees the "tear-drop sign" (arrows) representing a drop-like portion of orbital tissue (usually orbital fat) extending into the underlying maxillary sinus as shown in both coronal (A) and sagittal planes (B) in Figure 1.8. Note the relationship between the inferior rectus muscle and the fracture (arrowheads). In fractures that are more anterior than the one shown, the inferior oblique muscle (asterisk in B) can become incarcerated in the fracture, because it is the most inferior structure in the orbit at that location. In such cases, the patient will exhibit limited upward gaze until the muscle can be freed surgically.

The medial wall—is formed from the lesser wing of the sphenoid, the lamina papyracea of the ethmoid bone, the lacrimal bone, and the maxilla (**Figs. 1.5** and **1.7**). The medial wall is also vulnerable to fracture, from expanding orbital tissue in blunt trauma, due to the thinness of the translucent lamina papyracea.

The lateral wall—is formed from the greater wing of the sphenoid and the zygomatic bone (**Figs. 1.4** and **1.7**).

The roof—is formed from the lesser wing of the sphenoid and frontal bones. Just posterior to the superolateral orbital rim, the inner contour of the frontal bone rises sharply upward to provide space for the lacrimal gland within the superolateral portion of the orbit. As previously mentioned, this recess is termed the fossa for the lacrimal gland, to distinguish it from the lacrimal fossa that is posterior to the inferomedial rim of the orbit and accommodates the lacrimal sac (**Figs. 1.4** and **1.7**).

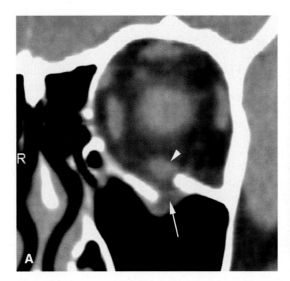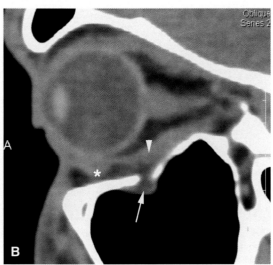

FIGURE 1.8   Coronal **(A)** and sagittal **(B)** CT scans of an orbit exhibiting soft tissues trapped in an orbital floor fracture ("*the tear-drop sign*" - *arrows*). Arrowhead identifies inferior rectus muscle. Asterisk **(B)** identifies position of inferior oblique muscle. (From Mancuso AA. *Head and Neck Radiology*. Philadelphia, PA: Wolters Kluwer; 2010.)

 Importantly, in children, the roof is also vulnerable to fracture because the orbital plate of the frontal bone has not reached its normal adult thickness. Such fractures in children can tear the meninges of the frontal lobe of the brain, giving rise to a cerebrospinal fluid (CSF) leak from the anterior cranial fossa into the orbital tissues or upper nasal cavity. In the latter case, the CSF leak may manifest itself as a "runny nose" of clear fluid.

Relationship between the Orbits and the Paranasal Sinuses

The orbits are surrounded by the paranasal sinuses. The frontal sinus resides within the medial half of the superior orbital rim (**Figs. 1.3** to **1.5**). The ethmoid sinuses (ethmoid air cells) are medial to the orbits, separated from them only by the thin, translucent lamina papyracea of the ethmoid bone (**Figs. 1.3** to **1.5**). The left and right ethmoid sinuses are separated from each other by the nasal cavity in the midline (**Fig. 1.3**). The floor of the orbit forms the roof of the maxillary sinus (**Figs. 1.3, 1.5, 1.8,** and **1.9**). The sphenoid sinus lies in close proximity to the medial wall at the orbital apex, adjacent to the optic canal (**Fig. 1.9**). These sinuses extend posteriorly and reside beneath the sella turcica (the fossa for the pituitary gland).

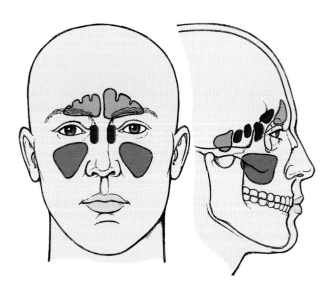

FIGURE 1.9   Anterior and lateral views of the head show the relationships between the paranasal sinuses and the orbit. *Gold*, frontal sinuses; *purple*, maxillary sinuses; *green*, sphenoid sinuses; *pink*, ethmoid air cells (sinuses). (Modified from an illustration by Neil O. Hardy, Westpoint, CT. In: Neil Hardy Art Collection. Philadelphia, PA: Wolters Kluwer; 2017.)

When patients complain of diffuse, dull aching pain in and around the eye, it is important to consider the possibility that this is referred pain from a sinusitis, even if no obvious swelling of the periorbital tissues is evident. In more severe cases, a sinusitis, especially one involving the ethmoid sinuses, can spread to the orbit, producing an orbital cellulitis (Fig. 1.10). Spread from the ethmoid sinus may occur through foramina or through the very thin lamina papyracea. But infections of any of the sinuses can, with time, erode through bone.

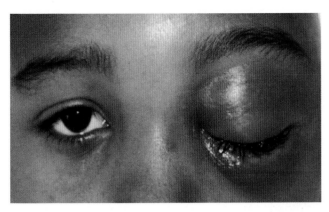

FIGURE 1.10 Orbital cellulitis. (Courtesy of Dr. Howard Leibowitz.)

 *The portion of the annulus of Zinn that extends between the origins of the superior and medial rectus muscles is also attached to the dura mater of the optic nerve, as it leaves the orbit via the optic canal (arrow in **Fig. 1.12**). Indeed some sources consider these attachments to be a second origin for these two muscles. When the optic nerve is inflamed, as in retrobulbar optic neuritis, the patient often complains of pain on movement of the eye. It is generally held that it is the traction put on the optic nerve, by movements of the extraocular muscles at this location, which provokes the pain occurring in these cases.[1]*

⊙ The Skeletal Muscles of the Orbit

Seven skeletal muscles are present in the orbit. Six of these, called the extraocular muscles, attach to and move the eye. The seventh skeletal muscle, the levator palpebrae superioris, vaults above the eye to enter and raise the upper eyelid.

THE EXTRAOCULAR MUSCLES

Four of the six extraocular muscles run a rectilinear course from their origins to their insertions. They are called the rectus muscles. These muscles are named for the surfaces of the eye to which they are attached. These are the superior, medial, lateral, and inferior rectus muscles. Two additional extraocular muscles approach the eye from above and below, at oblique angles of approximately 51°, and are thus named the superior and inferior oblique muscles (**Fig. 1.11**).

The complexities of extraocular movements are beyond the scope of this text but, in general, the six extraocular muscles commonly work as three antagonistic pairs (medial and lateral recti, superior and inferior recti, and superior and inferior obliques). In concert with a system of fascial pulleys, described later in this chapter, these muscles precisely position the eye toward the object of regard.

The four rectus muscles originate from a common tendinous ring (the annulus of Zinn) that is attached to the greater and lesser wing of the sphenoid at orbital apex (**Fig. 1.12**). The superior oblique originates separately, arising from the lesser wing of the sphenoid, above and medial to the annulus of Zinn. In sharp contrast to the other extraocular muscles, the origin of the inferior oblique muscle is just posterior to the inferomedial orbital rim and lateral to the lacrimal fossa. From its anterior origin on the maxilla, the inferior oblique runs posterolaterally, closer to the orbital floor than the inferior rectus, to reach the sclera at a point temporal to the optic nerve (**Figs. 1.11** and **1.12**).

The four rectus muscles and the inferior oblique are strap-shaped and run a direct course, from their origin to their insertion. The superior oblique is unique. The superior oblique muscle is more ovoid in shape (**Fig. 1.13**). From its origin, this muscle runs anteriorly, parallel to the medial orbital wall and above the medial rectus (**Fig. 1.11**). It gives rise to a long, slender tendon that runs through the pulley of the trochlea (**Figs. 1.11** and **1.12**). The trochlea is a cartilaginous loop that is fixed to the superomedial orbital rim (**Fig. 1.12**). After passing through the trochlea, the superior oblique tendon reverses course to insert onto the superior surface of the eye, sliding beneath the superior rectus muscle (**Figs. 1.11** and **1.12**).

LEVATOR PALPEBRAE SUPERIORIS

In addition to the extraocular muscles, another skeletal muscle extends anteriorly from the orbital apex. This muscle, called the levator palpebrae superioris, originates from the lesser wing of the sphenoid, lateral to the origin of the superior oblique. The muscle travels forward, above the eye and above the superior rectus, into the upper lid (**Fig. 1.13**). As its name implies, its function is to raise the upper lid. To ensure an even elevation of the upper lid as the muscle contracts, its tendon broadens dramatically as it passes the orbital rim. This allows the tendon to fan out and insert across the breadth of the tarsal plate. This expansion of the tendon of the levator palpebrae superioris is referred to as its aponeurosis (SEE CHAPTER 2: THE EYELIDS AND ADNEXA). On the lateral edge of the aponeurosis, its passage from the orbit into the upper lids deeply indents the lacrimal gland, which is just posterior to the lateral orbital rim, above and lateral to the eyeball. In this way, all but the most lateral portion of the gland is divided into an upper, orbital lobe and a lower palpebral lobe. The lower palpebral lobe is readily visible to the clinician, under the upper lid.

INNERVATION OF THE EXTRAOCULAR MUSCLES AND LEVATOR

Innervation of the extraocular muscles and the levator palpebrae superioris is from cranial nerves III, IV, and VI.

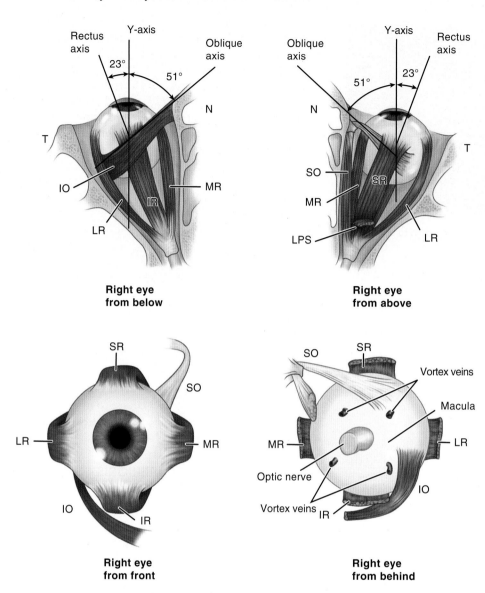

Right eye from below

Right eye from above

Right eye from front

Right eye from behind

FIGURE 1.11 Upper left image shows relations of extraocular muscles of a right eye from below, including origin of inferior oblique (IO) near the anterior orbital rim and its passage under the eye. Upper right image shows relations of extraocular muscles of a right eye from above, with levator palpebrae superioris (LPS) resected. Note the tendon of the superior oblique passes through the trochlea, changing direction to insert beneath the superior rectus (SR). Lower left image shows right eye from front and lower right image shows right eye from behind. IR, inferior rectus; LR, lateral rectus; MR, medial rectus; N, nasal; T, temporal. (From Chern KC, Saidel MA, eds. *Ophthalmology Review Manual.* 2nd ed. Philadelphia, PA: Wolters Kluwer; 2011.)

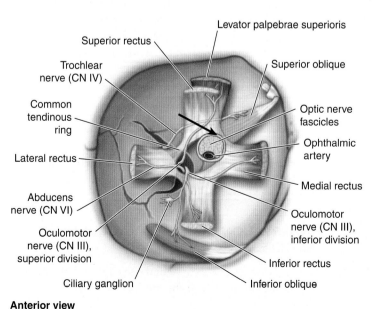

Anterior view

FIGURE 1.12 Diagrammatic representation of origins of the rectus muscles from the common tendinous ring (annulus of Zinn). Note attachment of superomedial aspect of the ring to the dural sheath of the optic nerve (*arrow*) and the pathways taken by branches of CN III, IV, and VI innervating the extraocular muscles and levator palpebrae superioris. Also note connection to ciliary ganglion from the nerve to the inferior oblique and passage of the tendon of the superior oblique through the pulley of the trochlea. (Modified from Moore KL, Dalley AF, Agur AM. *Clinically Oriented Anatomy.* 6th ed. Philadelphia, PA: Wolters Kluwer, 2009.)

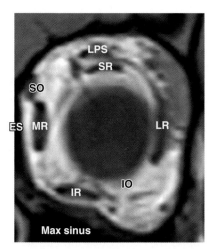

FIGURE 1.13 Coronal T1-weighted MRI of left orbit at the level of the vertical equator of the eye. Positions of the extraocular muscles and levator palpebrae superioris (LPS) are shown. Note the strap shape of the extraocular muscles, except for the superior oblique (SO), which is oval. Medial to the orbit the ethmoid air sinus (ES) is shown and below the orbit, the maxillary sinus is seen. IO, inferior oblique; IR, inferior rectus; LR, lateral rectus; MR, medial rectus; SR, superior rectus. (Courtesy of Dr. Robert Bert.)

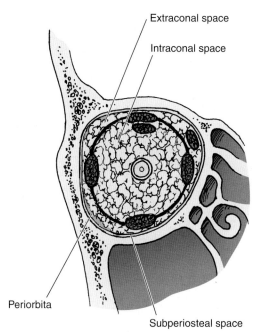

FIGURE 1.14 Simplified sketch of fascial extensions from free edges of rectus muscles enclosing the muscle cone (intraconal space) behind the eye and separating it from the surrounding extraconal fascial compartment of the orbit. The extraconal compartment continues anteriorly as far as the orbital septum. (From Urken ML, ed. *Multidisciplinary Head and Neck Reconstruction.* Philadelphia, PA: Wolters Kluwer; 2009.)

The pathways of these nerves are detailed later in this chapter, but they are shown in **Fig. 1.12**. Two of these, the trochlear nerve (CN IV) and the abducens nerve (CN VI) each innervate only a single extraocular muscle. CN IV innervates the superior oblique and CN VI innervates the lateral rectus. The remaining muscles, including the inferior oblique, medial, superior, and inferior rectus muscles and the levator palpebrae superioris are all innervated by the oculomotor nerve (CN III). As is generally the case with skeletal muscles, most of these muscles are innervated from their inner, more protected surfaces. In this regard, the superior oblique muscle is an exception. CN IV sometimes innervates the superior oblique from its upper surface.

Principal Fascial Compartments of the Orbit and Adnexa

The surfaces of the orbital bones are lined with periosteum, commonly referred to in the orbit as periorbita. The periorbita is loosely attached to the orbital bones, except at sutures and foramina, where firmer attachments occur. At the annulus of Zinn, the periorbita is continuous with the fascial epimysium that envelops each rectus muscle along its entire length. The obliques and levator are similarly invested with an epimysial fascial covering, which is continuous with the periorbita at their respective origins.

Where the extraocular muscles reach the surface of the eye, their tendons attach directly to the sclera. The fascia on their inner and outer surfaces blends with the fascial covering of the eye, termed the fascia bulbi or Tenon's capsule. The fascia of Tenon's capsule covers the exterior surface of the eye as far forward as the corneoscleral limbus and as far posteriorly as the dura mater surrounding the optic nerve (SEE CHAPTER 6: THE SCLERA, EPISCLERA AND TENON'S CAPSULE).

Importantly, the fascia surrounding the rectus muscles and levator palpebrae superioris does not simply cover these muscles. It also extends from the lateral edges of each rectus muscle to the edges of the adjacent rectus muscles. In this way, the space of the orbit is divided into two principal fascial compartments. The fascia connecting the lateral edges of the four rectus muscles circumscribes a conical space within the orbit that converges on the orbital apex. This fascial compartment within the orbit is commonly referred to as the "muscle cone" or intraconal space (**Fig. 1.14**). The portion of the orbital volume outside of the muscle cone is referred to as the extraconal orbital space (**Fig. 1.14**). The void volume of both of these spaces is filled with glistening adipose tissue set within a fibrovascular fascial interstitium that is denser in the anterior than in the posterior orbit. Some of these fascial connections have been shown to greatly influence the operation of the extraocular muscles as described later in this chapter.

The periorbital fascia covering the bones of the orbital rim also extends into the entire breadth of the eyelids, forming an anterior fascial wall for the extraconal orbital compartment. This wall, originating from the entire orbital rim, is referred to as the orbital septum (septum orbitale). Because this septum enters and divides the connective

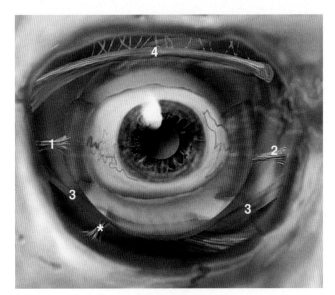

FIGURE 1.15   Depiction of major "check" ligaments and suspensory ligaments seen from an anterior view of the orbit. (*1*) Lateral check ligament; (*2*) medial check ligament; (*3*) ligament of Lockwood; (*4*) Whitnall's ligament; (*asterisk*) check ligament countering the pull of the superior oblique. The origin of the inferior oblique muscle is also shown near the inferomedial orbital rim. (Modified from Zide BM, ed. *Surgical Anatomy around the Orbit: The System of Zones.* Philadelphia, PA: Wolters Kluwer; 2005.)

tissue space of the eyelid, the portion of the lid anterior to the orbital septum is referred to as the preseptal space. The preseptal space and extraconal compartment of the orbit that is posterior to the orbital septum can be differentially involved in infectious diseases (cellulitis) of the lids and orbits. These are described in more detail in **CHAPTER 2: THE EYELIDS AND ADNEXA.**

In addition to covering the inner and outer surfaces of the muscles within the orbit, the fascia makes critical connections to the orbital walls, in part to limit the traverse of the eye beyond the limits of the orbital aperture and to modulate the pull of the extraocular muscles on the wall of the eye, preventing distortions of the wall of the eye during movement. These fascial connections are, by convention, referred to as "ligaments." The principal ligaments include the following:

- **Medial and lateral check ligaments**—connections from the external surfaces of both the lateral and medial recti attach to their respective orbital walls just posterior to the orbital rim (**Fig. 1.15**). Similar, but less readily identified fascial connections, from the remaining extraocular muscles and Tenon's capsule, serve to restrict the excursions of the other extraocular muscles. A recently described system of fascial pulleys and slings is described below.

  The check ligaments should not be thought of as static elements like a doorstop. Instead, they act more like springs that eventually reach their limit of elasticity. Acting in this manner, this complex system of fascial connections serves to dampen and

smooth the effects of abrupt muscular contractions and the effects of relaxation of the opposing muscles in movements of the eye.

- **Ligament of Lockwood**—Expansion of the intermingling fascia of the inferior rectus and inferior oblique, beneath the eye, extends medially and laterally to the orbital walls. Together with connections to Tenon's capsule on the surface of the eye, they form a structure like a hammock to support and bear the weight of the eye (**Fig. 1.15**). This support system, called the ligament of Lockwood, allows the extraocular muscles to more freely move the eye, as though it were in a gimbal system. This complex ligament also assists in holding the eye in a relatively fixed location within the orbit as the extraocular muscles act upon it. An inferolateral extension from this ligament to the orbital floor acts as a check ligament against the downward and outward directional vectors of the superior oblique muscle (**Fig. 1.15**, asterisk). Additional connections from this hammock extend forward into the lower lid, resisting posterior translocation of the eyeball when the extraocular muscles contract.[2]

- **Whitnall's ligament**—Whitnall's ligament runs an arcuate course across the upper lid, anterior to the aponeurosis of the levator palpebrae superioris and attaching the superior aspect of the aponeurosis to the orbital roof (**Figs. 1.15** and **1.16**). The classical description of this ligament was that it held up the aponeurosis of the levator palpebrae superioris across its breadth, as the aponeurosis transitioned from the orbit into the upper lid. More recent dissections have suggested that Whitnall's ligament may, instead, form a fascial sleeve around the aponeurosis, serving to both hold the ligament up, near the superior orbital rim, and create a glide path for muscle contraction to ensure stable elevation of the lid.[3] Whether operating as a sleeve or as a fixed line of attachment of the aponeurosis to the superior orbital wall, the result is to shift the functional origin of the levator anteriorly, to the location of the ligament. As a result, the directional vector of levator contraction is principally upward rather than posterior, thus optimizing elevation of the upper lid.

  Several of the fascial structures discussed, plus true ligaments from muscles in the lids, make connections to a single point, 4 to 5 mm posterior to the orbital rim on the lateral orbital wall. This point is termed Whitnall's tubercle (**Fig. 1.16**). Four principal structures share a common point of attachment at this location. From the list below, note that despite their shared name, Whitnall's ligament is not among the structures that attach to the tubercle of Whitnall. The structures attached to the orbital wall at Whitnall's tubercle include the:

- Lateral arm of the ligament of Lockwood
- Lateral edge of the aponeurosis of the levator palpebrae superioris
- Check ligament of the lateral rectus muscle

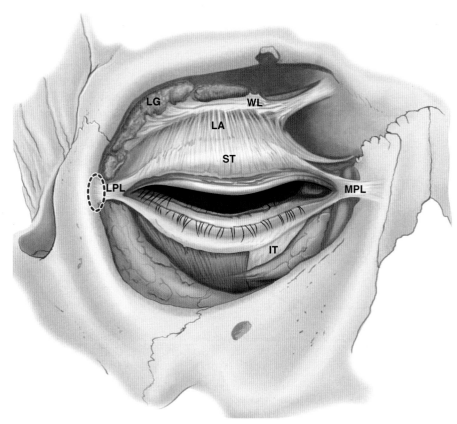

FIGURE 1.16 Sketch shows position of Whitnall's tubercle on the lateral orbital wall (*dashed red oval*). Note that the tubercle is posterior to the orbital rim. As such, the outline of the lateral palpebral ligament is not visible from the surface of the lids, whereas the outlines of the medial palpebral ligament, with its anterior insertion at the orbital rim, is visible just beneath the skin of the lids when examining the patient. Lacrimal gland (LG), orbital portion of lacrimal gland above the aponeurosis of the levator palpebrae superioris (LA). Whitnall's ligament (WL), which is *not* attached to Whitnall's tubercle. Note that the levator aponeurosis blends with the anterior surface of the superior tarsal (ST) plate. Also note how the lateral palpebral (canthal) ligament (LPL) and the medial palpebral (canthal) ligament (MPL) stabilize the edges of the ST and inferior tarsal (IT) plates. (Modified from Miller NR, Subramanian P, Patel V. *Walsh & Hoyt's Clinical Neuro-Ophthalmology: The Essentials.* 3rd ed. Philadelphia, PA: Wolters Kluwer; 2015.)

- The lateral palpebral (canthal) ligament

An additional, functionally important fascial connection is one that is between the superior surface of the superior rectus and the inferior surface of the levator palpebrae superioris. Because of this connection, when the superior rectus contracts and elevates the eye, the fascial connection to the levator helps to simultaneously elevate the lid beyond the point where contraction of the levator could elevate the lid on its own.[4]

cranial nerve inputs and constrained only at their two ends: each muscle always maintaining a straight path from its insertion to a point tangent with the globe, and then, a straight path to its origin at the orbital apex.[5] In other words, contraction of a rectus muscle pulled the insertion of the muscle toward the origin, with the muscle remaining straight along its course. The common understanding was that each rectus muscle's action was determined solely by its muscle plane, the plane containing the globe's center

*Fibrosis of orbital tissues, including fascia, can occur in thyroid disease. Among other things, this can prevent the lid from descending properly in inferior gaze. This gives rise to one of the cardinal findings of thyroid orbitopathy, termed "lid lag," (i.e. Von Graefe's sign) in which the eyelid does not follow the eye as well as it should in inferior gaze (**Fig. 1.17**).*

◉ The Muscle Pulley System Modulating Extraocular Muscle Movement

The "traditional" model of rectus muscle action was understood as muscles, controlled solely by their brain-directed

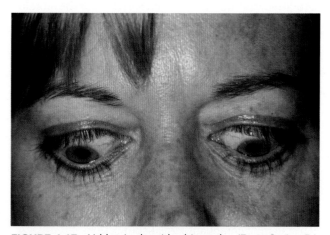

FIGURE 1.17 Lid lag in thyroid orbitopathy. (From Savino PJ, Danesh-Meyer HV. *Color Atlas and Synopsis of Clinical Ophthalmology—Wills Eye Institute—Neuro-Ophthalmology.* 2nd ed. Philadelphia, PA: Wolters Kluwer; 2012.)

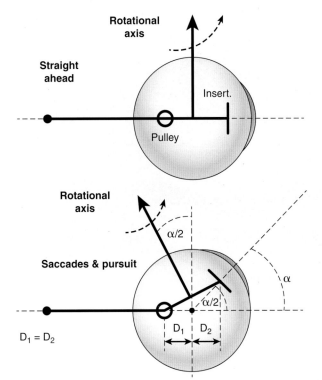

FIGURE 1.18   Anatomic effect of fascial pulleys on the rotational axis of horizontal rectus muscles. The orbit is viewed from a horizontal perspective (i.e., a view of the lateral or medial side of the eye). The rotational axes for these muscles is perpendicular to a line connecting the position of the fascial pulley of the muscle and the scleral insertion of that muscle. During saccade and pursuit movements, only the portion of the muscle anterior to its pulley rotates in the direction of the motion. The muscle does not remain straight along its entire length and simply allow the eye to rotate beneath it. Note that the amount of this movement ($\alpha/2$) is only half the amount of rotation of the eye, measured from its center of rotation (α). Note that in this case the distance between the pulley and the center of rotation of the eye (D_1) is equal to the distance from the center of rotation to the muscle insertion (D_2). (Modified from Demer JL, Oh SY, Poukens V. Evidence for active control of rectus extraocular muscle pulleys. *Invest Ophthalmol Vis Sci.* 2000;41:1280–1290.)

of rotation, the muscle's anatomic origin, and the muscle's point of insertion onto the globe. As such, if the eye moved upward, the lateral and medial rectus muscles remained straight and the eye slipped beneath them.

However, Miller and Robins[6] observed that this traditional model, if true, would allow the muscles to sideslip wildly about the globe, which would make eye rotation uncontrollable, at least with the precision that is routinely observed. As an alternative, they proposed that it was more likely that muscle paths were directionally stabilized by their fascial sheaths, which, through their connections to the orbital wall, functioned as pulleys. These connections were originally called "soft rectus muscle pulleys" to emphasize that they applied only to the rectus muscles and consisted of a system of compliant fascial connections.

Anatomic evidence for the existence of pulley structures is now compelling and includes extensive correlations between dissections and MRI, plus additional studies using computer modeling, histochemistry, innervational physiology, and electron microscopic studies in both human and nonhuman species.[7–9]

The pulleys form guiding sleeves that run through connective tissues rings and provide pivot points for the rectus muscles that are posterior to the muscle insertions onto the sclera (**Fig. 1.18**). By doing so, they alter muscle kinetics. The pulleys become the functional origins for these muscles. This is similar to, but anatomically less obvious than the way the trochlea redirects the vector of the contracting superior oblique muscle from its anatomic origin at the orbital apex, to its functional point of origin at the trochlea, near the superomedial orbital rim (**Fig. 1.11**).

The system of fascial connections that creates this complex matrix is not merely a passive, static system. The pulleys, instead, represent an active system in which the pulley sleeves, unlike the fixed trochlea, are moved somewhat by the muscles enveloped within them. Each pulley consists of a fascial sleeve, connecting to and passing through a pulley ring of collagen (**Figs. 1.18** and **1.19**), which is attached to Tenon's fascial capsule, on the eye, and to the adjacent orbital wall via fascial slings containing collagen, elastin, and some smooth muscle (**Fig. 1.19**). Collectively, these pulleys lie in a coronal plane, posterior to the vertical equator of the eye (**Fig. 1.19**).[10]

While remaining stabilized by their connections to the orbital wall, these active pulleys can shift slightly along the muscles they guide. It appears that the entire muscle contracts in a coordinated fashion, rotating the eye and moving the pulley. The muscles develop whatever force is necessary to rotate the eye against the counterforce of antagonistic muscles and elastic fascial tissues, including the pulley suspensions themselves. This system also serves to stabilize the eye in such a way as to provide a relatively unmoving center of rotation around which the eye rotates in any direction.[11] It has long been appreciated in the functional analyses of ocular motility that the eye moves from its primary position of gaze such that all three rotational axes lie within an imaginary fixed plane known as Listing's plane (**Fig. 1.20**).[12] The system of active pulleys that has now been described appears to provide an anatomic basis for this well-established functional concept.

These pulleys have been found to be comprised of a dense collagen matrix, with alternating bands of collagen fibers precisely arranged at right angles to one another, combined with a complement of parasympathetically driven smooth muscle cells[13] (**Fig. 1.19**).

MICROSCOPIC ANATOMY OF PULLEYS AND EXTRAOCULAR MUSCLES

The existence of pulleys is also consistent with findings regarding the microscopic structure of the rectus muscles themselves. It has long been recognized that mammalian rectus muscles consist of two microscopically discernable portions that are termed the global and orbital layers.

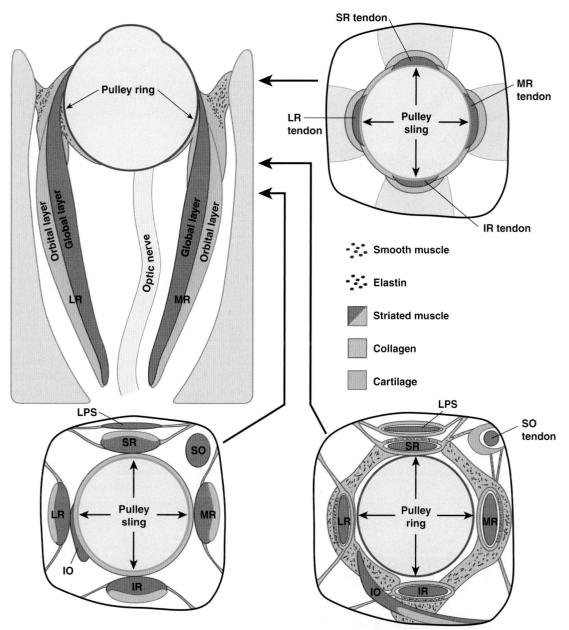

FIGURE 1.19 Structure of orbital connective tissues and their relationship with the fiber layers of the rectus muscles showing pulley rings of fascia surrounding the muscles that are attached to the fascial covering of the eye (Tenon's capsule) internally and to the adjacent orbital wall via fascial slings. These pulleys, surrounding the muscle, posterior to the muscle insertion, lie within a coronal plane. Three coronal views are shown at levels indicated by connecting arrows to horizontal section in upper left. Also seen is the relationship between the global layer of the muscle and the orbital layer. LR, lateral rectus; SR, superior rectus; MR, medial rectus; IR, inferior rectus; LPS, levator palpebrae superioris; IO, inferior oblique; SO, superior oblique. (Modified from Demer JL, Oh SY, Poukens V. Evidence for active control of rectus extraocular muscle pulleys. *Invest Ophthalmol Vis Sci.* 2000;41:1280–1290.)

The global layer is closest to the eye and the orbital layer is closest to the extraconal fascial compartment of the orbit (**Figs. 1.19** and **1.21**).

These two portions have distinct fiber types.[14] Most orbital layer fibers are specialized for oxidative metabolism and fatigue resistance, whereas most global layer fibers are less fatigue resistant and more suited to generating force pulses.[15]

MRI, gross anatomic, and histologic observations indicate that global layer fibers extend from the annulus of Zinn to

their insertions onto the sclera, as classically recognized. By contrast, however, and supporting the evolving understanding of the pulley system, it has been shown that the orbital fibers actually insert onto the pulleys rather than to the globe (**Fig. 1.19**).[16]

Light microscopy shows the difference between the fibers of the global portion of the muscle and the orbital portion of the muscle. It demonstrates clear connections with the fascial sleeves surrounding the muscle and with

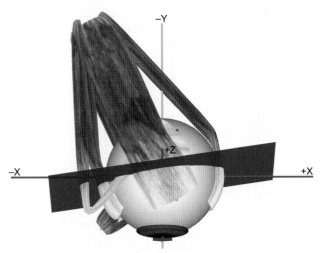

FIGURE 1.20 Drawing of a left eye as seen from above, relative to Listing's plane in blue. In motions of the eye from primary gaze, all rotational axes of eye (X, Y, Z—also called Fick's axes) lie in this fixed plane. (Courtesy of T. Kaltofen, S. Priglinger. See-kid—Computer assisted eye motility diagnostics—Listing's plane. http://www.see-kid .at/. Accessed January 2017.)

the interwoven bands of fascial collagen and elastin that connect the fascial pulleys to the orbital wall, via their slings (**Fig. 1.21**).

Although certain functional implications of this anatomy remain controversial, this revised view of extraocular muscle anatomy strongly suggests that extraocular muscle movements are more readily subject to

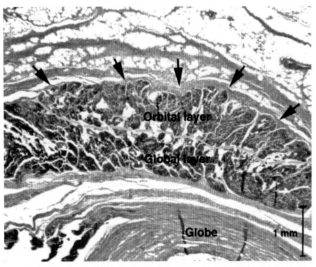

FIGURE 1.21 Photomicrograph of the lateral rectus of a 17-month-old human stained with Masson's trichrome allowing distinction between the orbital and global layers of the muscle and insertion of the orbital layer onto fine, collagenous tendons (*arrows*) contiguous with the dense collagen of the muscle pulley. Global layer fibers are brighter red than orbital layer fibers with this stain. The plane of separation between these parts of the muscle is demarcated by the green line. (From Oh SY, Poukens V, Demer JL. Quantitative analysis of the structure of the human extraocular muscle pulley system invest. *Ophthalmol Vis Sci.* 2002;43:2923–2932.)

pharmacologic, surgical, and genetic manipulations than would be predicted when it was assumed that motilities were governed almost entirely through a brain-directed system of simplistically arranged muscles, contracting in a straight line in response to impulses from cranial nerves. At the very least, this represents another reminder that believing anatomy to be a discipline that has been fully explored is simply wrong.

Neural Pathways within the Orbit

The cranial nerves entering the orbit include:
- The optic nerve (CN II)
- The oculomotor nerve (CN III)
- The trochlear nerve (CN IV)
- The ophthalmic division of the trigeminal nerve (CN V)
- Portions of the maxillary division of the trigeminal nerve (CN V)
- The abducens nerve (CN VI)

In addition to these cranial nerves, parasympathetic fibers leaving the brainstem as part of CN VII reach the orbit to provide stimulatory innervation for the lacrimal gland. Sympathetic innervation of the structures of the eye and orbit is discussed in the **CHAPTER 3: OVERVIEW OF THE EYE**.

Three principal apertures for the entrance of these nerves are provided near the orbital apex. Two of these, the optic canal and the superior orbital fissure, allow passage into the orbit from the middle cranial fossa. The third, the inferior orbital fissure, connects the orbit to the pterygopalatine fossa. The cranial nerves are discussed below relative to their portal of entry into the orbit.

Cranial Nerves Entering the Orbit via the Optic Canal

The only cranial nerve passing through the optic canal is the optic nerve (CN II). In its passage through the optic canal, CN II is accompanied by the ophthalmic artery and the postganglionic sympathetic fibers that form a plexus around it. En route to the optic canal, through the intraconal compartment of the orbit, the optic nerve runs an S-shaped course, providing slack for movement of the eye. At the optic canal, the sheath of the optic nerve makes connections with the superomedial aspect of the common tendinous ring (annulus of Zinn—**Fig. 1.12**). As mentioned, some sources consider this connection to represent a second point of origin for the superior and medial rectus muscles. After transiting the optic canal, the optic nerve enters the middle cranial fossa, passing below the anterior clinoid process of the sphenoid bone but above the cavernous sinus, to join with the contralateral optic nerve at the optic chiasm. Between the retina

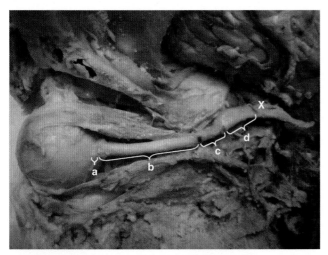

FIGURE 1.22 Dissection of the length of the optic nerve shown from above. The four segments of the nerve between the eye and optic chiasm can be identified. (a) Within the intrascleral canal; (b) within the intraconal compartment of the orbit; (c) within the optic canal; (d) within the middle cranial fossa; (X) optic chiasm. (From Selhorst JB, Chen Y. The optic nerve. *Semin Neurol.* 2009;29:29–35.)

axons from the medial half of each retina (i.e., the temporal halves of the visual field from each eye) decussate and the reorganized groups of axons that emerge from the posterior aspect of the chiasm are termed the optic tracts. Situated near the chiasm, where the optic tracts diverge toward the lateral geniculate nuclei in the thalamus, is the stalk or infundibulum of the pituitary gland (**Fig. 1.23**). The pituitary gland resides below the chiasm within the sella turcica. Expanding pituitary tumors can therefore compress the optic chiasm from below, in most cases producing a characteristic visual field loss in which the temporal half of the visual field in each eye is lost (bitemporal hemianopia). Anatomic variations occur in the relationship between the chiasm and the position of the infundibulum, in some cases, even placing the infundibular stalk anterior to the chiasm. Imaging of suspected tumors is critical in these cases, since this will change the presentation on the visual field and will likely alter the surgical approach required to safely resect the tumor.[17]

and the chiasm, the lengths of the various segments of the nerve include 1 mm within the wall of the globe, 24 to 30 mm within the orbit, 6 to 10 mm within the optic canal, and 10 to 16 mm coursing within the middle cranial fossa (**Fig. 1.22**).

The optic chiasm is bordered laterally by the two internal carotid arteries, as they emerge from the roof of the cavernous sinus (**Fig. 1.23**). Aneurysms at this location can compress the optic chiasm, producing characteristic visual field defects. At the optic chiasm, the fibers representing

◉ Cranial Nerves Entering the Orbit via the Superior Orbital Fissure

Destined to enter the orbit through the superior orbital fissure are CN III, IV, the ophthalmic division of CN V and CN VI. Just posterior to the superior orbital fissure is the cavernous sinus. All of the cranial nerves that enter the orbit through the superior orbital fissure pass through the lateral wall of, or within, the cavernous sinus to reach the orbit. The pathways of these nerves, prior to entering the cavernous sinus, are as follows.

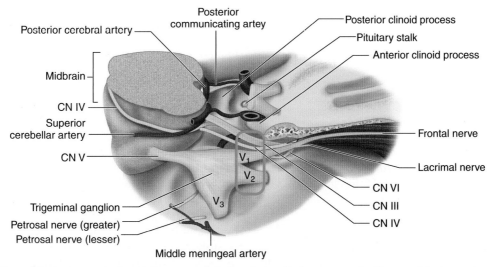

FIGURE 1.23 View of the brainstem and cranial nerves reveals the relationship between optic chiasm and the internal carotid arteries and stalk (infundibulum) of the pituitary gland. Also shown are the intracranial pathways of CN III, IV, V, and VI including the close relationship between the path of CN III and the posterior communicating artery. The green rectangle approximates the position of the cavernous sinus and the passage of CN III, IV, and V (ophthalmic, V_1 and maxillary, V_2, divisions) through the lateral wall of the sinus. CN VI passes within the sinus itself. (Modified from Mancuso AA. *Head and Neck Radiology.* Philadelphia, PA: Wolters Kluwer; 2010.)

CN III

The oculomotor nerve exits the brainstem from the ventral surface of the midbrain, between the posterior cerebral and superior cerebellar arteries. In addition to its motor fibers for movement of the orbital muscles that it serves, CN III is among the four cranial nerves (III, VII, IX, and X) that carry preganglionic parasympathetic fibers. Those traveling with CN III are destined for the eye.

Parasympathetic Component of CN III

The cell bodies of the preganglionic parasympathetic fibers conveyed by CN III originate in the Edinger–Westphal nucleus of the midbrain, at the level of the superior colliculus. As CN III exits the midbrain, these fibers are added to the superomedial surface the nerve. CN III passes forward, inferior and lateral to the posterior communicating artery that joins the circulations of the vertebrobasilar and internal carotid systems at the circle of Willis (**Fig. 1.23**). CN III then enters the superolateral wall of the cavernous sinus.

 *For a variety of reasons, normal function of CN III can be compromised. Most often, this results in a partial "third nerve palsy." In such cases, compromising the innervation to four of the six extraocular muscles renders the eye positioned inferiorly and laterally. As a way to recall this position as representing a third nerve palsy, students and residents are often told to remember that the eye points the way the patient feels— "down and out!" One of the first steps in the differential diagnosis of most probable causes of a third nerve palsy is to determine whether the pupillary fibers added to the outside of the nerve have been affected. In such cases, the ipsilateral pupil will be larger than on the contralateral side. In other cases, the pupil is "spared." Two main causes for third nerve palsies include compressive lesions (e.g., aneurysms of the posterior communicating artery) and microvascular disease (e.g., diabetes mellitus) (**Fig. 1.24**).*

CN IV

The trochlear nerve is the only cranial nerve to exit the dorsal surface of the brainstem, originating from the dorsal midbrain immediately below the inferior colliculus (**Fig. 1.23**). The nerve moves anteriorly, between the cerebral peduncle and the sharp lateral edge of the tentorium cerebelli. Its course runs parallel with, but below and lateral to, CN III, to reach the cavernous sinus (**Fig. 1.23**).

CN V (OPHTHALMIC DIVISION)

CN V emerges from the pons as a larger, superior, sensory root and a smaller, inferior, motor root. These converge

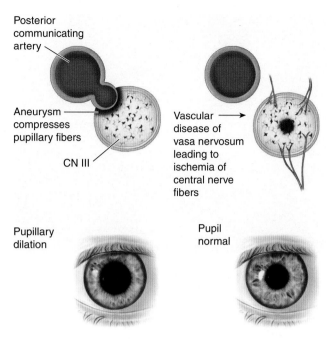

FIGURE 1.24 Because the parasympathetic fibers destined for the pupil are present on the superomedial surface of CN III, compressive lesions of the third nerve (e.g., aneurysm of the adjacent posterior communicating artery) commonly produce not only a third nerve palsy, but also involve the pupil, rendering it larger than that on the contralateral side. By contrast, because the microvascular supply of the nerve is richer near the surface than in the center, microvascular disease (e.g., diabetes mellitus) is less likely to adversely affect the pupillary fibers and will more often produce a third nerve palsy that is "pupil-sparing."

to form the trigeminal (Gasserian) ganglion (**Fig. 1.23**). From the anterior margin of the trigeminal ganglion arise the three main divisions, which give the trigeminal nerve its name. The most superior of these, the ophthalmic division (V_1), passes anteriorly and almost immediately enters the lateral wall of the cavernous sinus (**Fig. 1.25**). This branch is purely sensory, since all of the motor fibers of CN V pass into the mandibular division (V_3).

CN VI

The purely motor abducens nerve leaves the brainstem at the pontinomedullary junction, closer to the midline than the exit of CN VII. The nerve courses superiorly between the pons and the bony clivus and makes a sharp turn anteriorly, over the crest of the petrous ridge of the temporal bone. Because of its long passage between brain and bone, along the clivus and petrous ridge, it is prone to be damaged in closed-head injuries where the mass of the brain is forced downward, compressing the nerve, especially in its passage across the bony petrous ridge. Unlike CN III, IV, and the ophthalmic and maxillary divisions of CN V, which pass through the lateral wall of the cavernous sinus, CN VI passes

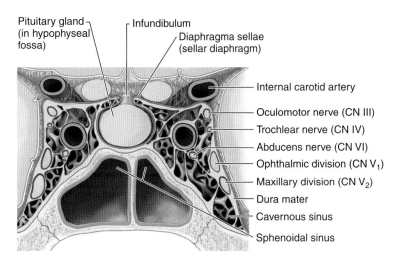

Pituitary gland (in hypophyseal fossa)

Infundibulum

Diaphragma sellae (sellar diaphragm)

Internal carotid artery

Oculomotor nerve (CN III)

Trochlear nerve (CN IV)

Abducens nerve (CN VI)

Ophthalmic division (CN V$_1$)

Maxillary division (CN V$_2$)

Dura mater

Cavernous sinus

Sphenoidal sinus

FIGURE 1.25 Coronal section through the cavernous sinus and adjacent structures, viewed from behind. Note optic nerves above the roof of the sinus, and the position of the pituitary gland and the sphenoid sinuses. Passing through the lateral wall of the cavernous sinus on each side, from superior to inferior, are CN III, CN IV, the ophthalmic division of CN V, and the maxillary division of CN V. CN VI is seen passing through the sinus in proximity to the internal carotid artery. The internal carotid artery courses anteriorly, forming a hairpin loop as it emerges from the roof of the cavernous sinus to pass lateral to the optic chiasm. (Modified from Moore KL, Argur AMR, Dalley AF. *Clinically Oriented Anatomy.* 7th ed. Philadelphia, PA: Wolters Kluwer; 2013.)

through the interior of the cavernous sinus in proximity to the internal carotid artery (**Fig. 1.25**).

Inferior Orbital Fissure

CN V (MAXILLARY DIVISION)

The maxillary division (V$_2$) emerges from the trigeminal ganglion and almost immediately enters the inferolateral wall of the cavernous sinus (**Fig. 1.23**).

Pathway of Cranial Nerves through the Cavernous Sinus to the Superior Orbital Fissure

Passing within the lateral wall of the cavernous sinus, from superior to inferior, reside CN III, CN IV, CN V (ophthalmic division) and CN V (maxillary division) (**Fig. 1.25**). As previously noted, CN VI actually passes within the sinus itself, in proximity to the internal carotid artery.

Upon emerging from the cavernous sinus, both CN III and the ophthalmic division of CN V subdivide. CN III gives rise to superior and inferior motor branches and the ophthalmic division of CN V divides into three branches—the frontal, lacrimal, and nasociliary nerves (**Fig. 1.26**).

As these nerves enter the orbit, portions of the openings through which they pass (the superior orbital fissure and optic canal) are intersected by the common tendinous ring (annulus of Zinn) that serves as the common origin for the rectus muscles. In this way, the annulus delimits a subset of nerves and nerve branches that enter the muscle cone to reach their target tissues, from others that pass into the extraconal compartment.

NERVES DESTINED FOR TARGETS WITHIN THE MUSCLE CONE

- **CN II**—Clearly, the optic nerve must enter the muscle cone to reach the posterior pole of the eye (**Fig. 1.26**).
- **CN III**—Since the orbital muscles served by CN III, like most skeletal muscles, receive their innervation from their more protected inner surfaces, both divisions of CN III enter the muscle cone to serve the inner surfaces of their target muscles. The superior division serves the superior rectus and levator palpebrae superioris and the inferior division serves the medial rectus, inferior rectus, and inferior oblique (**Fig. 1.26**). Before reaching the inferior oblique muscle, the branch of the inferior division of CN III serving this muscle gives off a communicating branch to the ciliary ganglion, conveying the preganglionic parasympathetic fibers that originate with CN III (**Fig. 1.26**). This branch is referred to as the motor root of the ciliary ganglion. The ciliary ganglion is discussed in **CHAPTER 3: OVERVIEW OF THE EYE**.
- **CN V**—Only the nasociliary branch of the ophthalmic division of the trigeminal nerve enters the muscle cone. It logically enters the muscle cone since it provides sensory fibers for the surface of the eye, via pathways beginning at the posterior surface of the globe (**Fig. 1.26**). The further course of this nerve is detailed below.
- **CN VI**—In order for the lateral rectus to receive its innervation in the conventional way, from its inner surface, the abducens nerve also enters the muscle cone (**Fig. 1.26**).

NERVES DESTINED FOR TARGETS OUTSIDE OF THE MUSCLE CONE

- **CN IV**—The superior oblique muscle is outside of the muscle cone (**Fig. 1.26**). Hence, CN IV, the

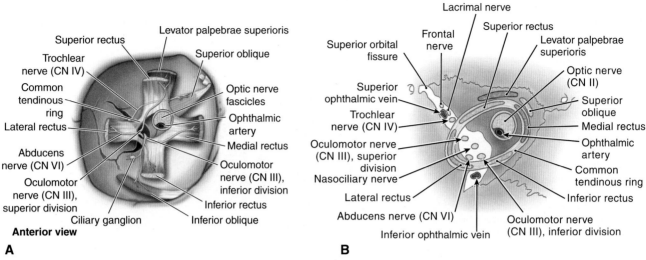

FIGURE 1.26 **A:** Anterior view of a right orbit showing the intraorbital pathway of CN III. The nerve has divided into a superior and an inferior division. The superior division innervates the levator palpebrae superioris and the superior rectus. The inferior division serves the medial rectus, inferior rectus, and the inferior oblique. The branch serving the inferior oblique conveys the preganglionic parasympathetic fibers onboard CN III to the ciliary ganglion, via a communicating branch. **B:** Sketch demonstrating the relationship between the common tendinous ring (annulus of Zinn) and both the optic canal and the superior orbital fissure, showing those structures that enter the muscle cone and those that do not. Also shown are the entry and exit points of major arteries and veins that serve the orbit. (Modified from Moore KL, Anne M. R. Agur AMR, Dalley AF. *Moore's Clinically Oriented Anatomy.* 7th ed. Philadelphia, PA: Wolters Kluwer; 2013.)

trochlear nerve, enters the superior orbital fissure but remains in the extraconal compartment of the orbit to reach this muscle. Of interest, the superior oblique muscle is an exception to the usual rule and often receives innervation from its outer surface.

- **CN V—Ophthalmic division:** Both the frontal and lacrimal branches of the ophthalmic division of the trigeminal nerve are destined to leave the orbit, providing sensory innervation to the upper lids and periorbital skin of the forehead (**Figs. 1.26** to **1.28**). Their pathways and distributions are detailed below.
- **CN V—Maxillary division:** Upon emerging from the wall of the cavernous sinus, the maxillary nerve enters the pterygopalatine fossa near it roof, via the foramen rotundum. It traverses the fossa, supporting the pterygopalatine ganglion from above. From the pterygopalatine fossa, the maxillary nerve passes anteriorly, onto the floor of the orbit, through the inferior orbital fissure. It will ultimately leave the orbit, providing sensory innervation to the lower lids, cheek, and upper lip (**Fig. 1.28**). Its further pathway and branches are detailed below.

Pathways of the Ophthalmic and Maxillary Divisions of CN V and their Branches within the Orbit

OPHTHALMIC DIVISION AND ITS BRANCHES

As noted above, the three branches of the ophthalmic division of CN V are the frontal, lacrimal, and nasociliary

nerves. All three enter the orbit via the superior orbital fissure; only one of them, the nasociliary nerve, enters the muscle cone (**Fig. 1.26**).

The Frontal Nerve

After dividing from the ophthalmic division of CN V, the frontal nerve passes anteriorly, just below the roof of the orbit. Indeed, in any dissection of the orbit from above, the frontal nerve is the first structure encountered below the periorbita. As the frontal nerve passes forward, toward the superior orbital rim, it subdivides into two branches. These include a larger supraorbital and a smaller supratrochlear nerve. This division is evident in **Fig. 1.27**. The supraorbital nerve is lateral to the supratrochlear nerve.

The supratrochlear nerve emerges from the superior orbital rim, piercing the orbital septum near the trochlea, providing sensory innervation to the skin of the forehead, laterally from the midline to the sensory field of the ipsilateral supraorbital nerve. The supratrochlear nerve also serves the medial aspect of the upper lid and superior palpebral conjunctiva (**Fig. 1.28**).

The supraorbital nerve emerges onto the forehead through the commonly palpable supraorbital notch along the superior orbital rim, in conjunction with the artery of the same name (**Figs. 1.4** and **1.6**). In some individuals, a canal is present instead of a notch and thus it may not be palpable. As the supraorbital nerve traverses the orbital rim, it provides a sensory branch to the mucosal lining of the frontal sinus. Upon emerging beyond the superior orbital rim, this nerve serves the skin and palpebral conjunctival surfaces of the upper lid and the forehead lateral to the distributional field of the supratrochlear and medial to the

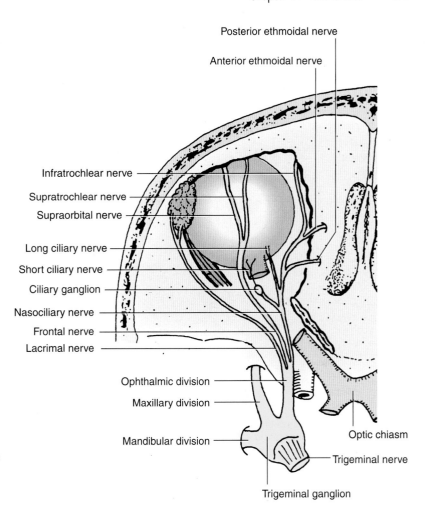

FIGURE 1.27 Sketch of dissection of left orbit, from above, shows the branches of the ophthalmic division of CN V. (Modified from Chung KW, Chung HM. *BRS Gross Anatomy*. 7th ed. Philadelphia, PA: Wolters Kluwer; 2011.)

distributions of the lacrimal nerve, the zygomaticotemporal nerve, and the auriculotemporal branch of the mandibular division of CN V (**Fig. 1.28**).

The Lacrimal Nerve

After dividing from the ophthalmic division of CN V, the lacrimal nerve passes anteriorly, in close proximity to the superior border of the lateral rectus, together with the artery of the same name (**Figs. 1.27** and **1.29**). As it passes the lacrimal gland, near the superolateral rim of the orbit, it sends a branch to the gland. This branch represents sensory fibers intrinsic to CN V and postganglionic sympathetic and parasympathetic fibers conveyed to the lacrimal nerve after it has already branched from the ophthalmic division of CN V. The sympathetic and parasympathetic pathways that convey these fibers to the lacrimal nerve are detailed in the discussion of the lacrimal gland, later in this chapter.

After passing the lacrimal gland, the lacrimal nerve pierces the orbital septum, crossing the superior orbital rim near the lateral edge of the upper lid. Continuing superiorly, it provides sensory fibers to the lateral aspect of the lids and the forehead to just above the lateral edge of the eyebrow and lateral to the field served by the supraorbital nerve (**Fig. 1.28**).

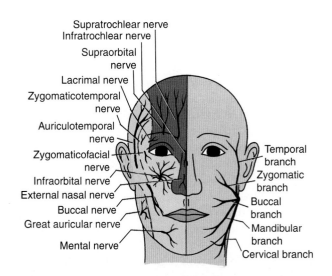

FIGURE 1.28 Distribution of nerves to the face. On right side of the face, the sensory branches derived from CN V are shown. Note that the sensory distributional fields of the ophthalmic, maxillary, and mandibular divisions of CN V are shown in different colors. The surface of the eye is served by the nasociliary branch of the ophthalmic division. On the left side of the face, the motor branches from CN VII, serving the muscles of facial expression are shown. (Modified from Snell RS. *Clinical Anatomy by Regions*. 9th ed. Philadelphia, PA: Wolters Kluwer; 2011.)

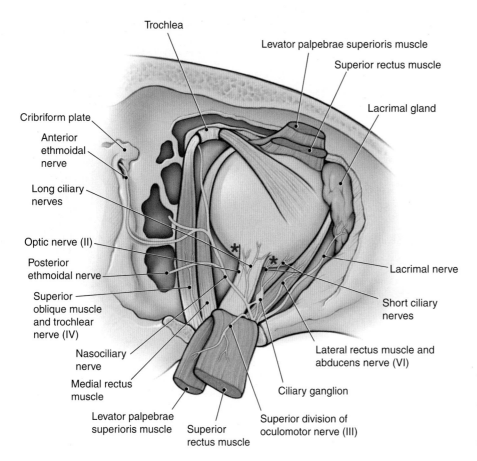

FIGURE 1.29 Sketch of dissection of right orbit from above shows distribution of branches of the nasociliary nerve, including extension of the anterior ethmoidal nerve from the anterior ethmoidal air cells to the floor of the anterior cranial fossa in the region of the cribriform plate. Also shown are the long ciliary nerves (*asterisk*). Posterior ethmoidal branch not shown. (From Detton AJ. *Grant's Dissector*. 16th ed. Philadelphia, PA: Wolters Kluwer; 2016.)

The Nasociliary Nerve

The nasociliary nerve provides sensory fibers for the cornea, bulbar conjunctiva, and uvea, but, beyond the eye, it also runs an extensive course that serves additional structures within and outside of the orbit. After dividing from the ophthalmic division of CN V, the nasociliary nerve most commonly enters the orbit between the two heads of the lateral rectus muscle, as they join the annulus of Zinn. Moving anteriorly from its point of origin near the orbital apex, the nasociliary nerve enters the muscle cone, providing two to three communicating branches to the ciliary ganglion. Their further course is discussed under the section Ciliary Ganglion in **CHAPTER 3: OVERVIEW OF THE EYE**.

Continuing anteriorly, the nasociliary nerve courses above the optic nerve, but beneath the superior rectus and superior oblique, headed toward the medial wall of the orbit. As it crosses above the optic nerve, two to three long ciliary nerves are given off (**Fig. 1.29**). It is the long ciliary nerves that enter the posterior surface of the eye to provide sensory fibers reaching the cornea, bulbar conjunctiva, and uvea. Like the communicating branches, details of this pathway are discussed under the section Ciliary Ganglion in **CHAPTER 3: OVERVIEW OF THE EYE**.

After crossing the optic nerve, the nasociliary nerve reaches the portion of the medial wall of the orbit that is formed by the lamina papyracea of the ethmoid bone. Here, the nasociliary nerve gives off a posterior ethmoidal branch, and then an anterior ethmoidal branch (**Fig. 1.29**). The posterior ethmoidal branch passes through a foramen of the same name, to provide sensory fibers to the mucosae of the posterior ethmoidal air cells and the sphenoid sinus (**Fig. 1.5**).

The anterior ethmoidal nerve enters the anterior ethmoidal foramen (**Fig. 1.5**). Like the posterior ethmoidal nerve, the anterior ethmoidal nerve provides sensation to the mucosal lining of portions of the ethmoid sinus, specifically to mucosae of the anterior and middle ethmoid air cells. Unlike the posterior ethmoidal nerve, which terminates in the ethmoid sinus, a branch of the anterior ethmoidal nerve continues beyond the ethmoid sinus. From the anterior ethmoidal air cells, this branch passes superiorly to the cribriform plate, which forms the top of the ethmoid bone and serves as the midline portion of the floor of the anterior cranial fossa, upon which rest the olfactory bulbs (**Fig. 1.29**). This extension of the anterior ethmoidal nerve runs forward along the cribriform plate and back into the bone anteriorly, where it provides internal nasal branches delivering sensory fibers to the mucosa of the upper reaches of the nasal cavity. From here, the nerve finally emerges from the junction between the inferior edge of the nasal bone and upper margin of the lateral nasal cartilage as the external nasal nerve. This terminal branch provides sensory innervation to the skin along the sides of the nose, below the nasal bones, all the way to its tip (**Fig. 1.28**).

After giving off its anterior ethmoidal branch, the nasociliary nerve continues toward the trochlea as its terminal

HUTCHINSON'S RULE

From the discussion above, it is clear that the meandering path of the nasociliary nerve reaches the ciliary ganglion and the nose, just as its name implies. From a clinical standpoint, it is important to appreciate that the cornea, the uvea, and the tip of the nose receive innervation from the same branch of the ophthalmic division of the trigeminal nerve. By adulthood, in the vast majority of individuals, the trigeminal ganglion harbors varicella (herpes zoster - chickenpox) virus that is suppressed by the immune system. If the immune system is compromised, this neurotropic virus can fan out within the branches of the trigeminal nerve, producing ipsilateral inflammatory lesions at any point receiving its innervation from the trigeminal nerve (i.e., shingles). When the nasociliary nerve is involved, it can produce skin lesions on the upper lids, forehead, and all the way to the tip of the nose (Fig. 1.30). But since this branch also serves the cornea and the uvea, any involvement of the skin of the forehead or eyelid may also involve the cornea, conjunctiva, and/or uvea. Hutchinson's rule provides fair warning that if you see a lesion on the tip of the nose, which is the most distal point in the distribution of the nasociliary nerve, it is likely that more proximal structures such as the cornea and the uvea are likely involved as well. As such, the eye must be examined especially carefully to rule out potentially blinding involvement. The principle is that since the distance from the trigeminal ganglion to the eye is shorter than the distance along the nasociliary nerve to reach the tip of the nose, a lesion at the tip of the nose portends probable, but not certain involvement of the eye. With the advent of a recently released vaccine against varicella zoster, the incidence of shingles should be reduced, especially in the elderly and immunocompromised, among whom this condition is most prevalent.

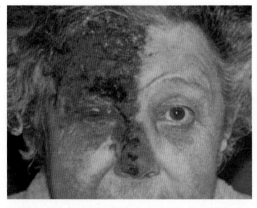

FIGURE 1.30 A patient showing pattern of encrusted herpes zoster lesions corresponding to the distributional field of the ophthalmic division of CN V and redness in adjacent areas. (Courtesy of Dr. Howard Leibowitz.)

branch, the infratrochlear nerve. The infratrochlear nerve runs anteriorly, near the superior edge of the medial rectus muscle (**Figs. 1.27** and **1.29**). As its name implies, the infratrochlear nerve emerges from the orbit, inferior to the trochlea, to provide sensory innervation to the skin of the medial edge of the upper eyelids and superior palpebral conjunctiva (**Fig. 1.28**). It also serves several other structures in the medial canthal region, including the lacrimal sac, the lacrimal punctum, and the bridge of the nose.

MAXILLARY DIVISION AND ITS BRANCHES

Branches of the maxillary division of CN V enter the orbit from the pterygopalatine fossa, via the inferior orbital fissure. The maxillary division gives rise to the zygomatic nerve, the alveolar nerves (posterior, middle, and anterior), and the infraorbital nerve.

The Zygomatic Nerve

This branch passes to the lateral wall of the orbit subdividing into zygomaticofacial and zygmaticotemporal branches that enter foramina bearing the same names in the lateral wall of the orbit (**Fig. 1.31**). Before entering its foramen, the zygomaticotemporal nerve passes a communicating branch to the lacrimal branch of the ophthalmic division of CN V. This communicating branch delivers postganglionic sympathetic and parasympathetic fibers destined for the lacrimal gland. Details of their specific pathway are discussed later in this chapter, under Lacrimal Gland.

The zygomaticotemporal nerve emerges onto the lateral surface of the skull to provide sensory innervation to a portion of skin adjacent to the field served by the lacrimal nerve (**Fig. 1.28**). The zygomaticofacial nerve emerges lower and more anteriorly to provide sensory fibers to the lateral portion of the lower lid and the skin overlying the bony prominence of the cheek (**Fig. 1.28**).

Posterior Superior Alveolar Nerve

After giving off the zygomatic nerve, the maxillary nerve gives off a posterior superior alveolar (dental) branch that extends inferiorly to provide sensory innervation to the posterior portion of the superior alveolar ridge including the upper gums and teeth (**Fig. 1.31**). This branch also serves the mucosa of the maxillary sinus.

The Infraorbital Nerve

The infraorbital branch is the direct extension of the maxillary division, after all of its other branches have been given off (**Fig. 1.31**). This branch passes into the infraorbital groove in the floor of the orbit, continuing anteriorly into the infraorbital canal to the infraorbital foramen on the cheek. While traversing the infraorbital canal, this nerve gives off the middle and anterior superior alveolar branches. These provide sensation to the mucosa of the maxillary sinus and the lateral and anterior portions of the superior

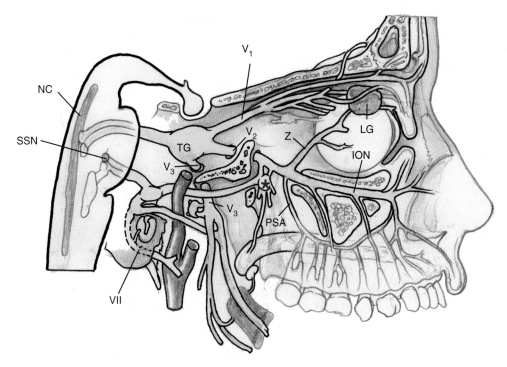

FIGURE 1.31 Sketch showing distribution of branches of the ophthalmic (V_1), maxillary (V_2), and mandibular (V_3) divisions of CN V arising from the Trigeminal ganglion (TG) in a lateral view. Also shown are branches of CN VII as they relate to the orbit. The maxillary division (V_2) emerges onto the floor of the orbit from the pterygopalatine fossa, via the inferior orbital fissure. It gives rise to a zygomatic branch (Z) with its communicating branch to the lacrimal nerve, shown ascending toward the lacrimal gland (LG). The posterior superior alveolar (PSA) branch serves the posterior teeth and gums of the upper jaw and the mucosa of the maxillary sinus before the remainder of the maxillary nerve continues anteriorly as the infraorbital nerve (ION). Preganglionic parasympathetic nerves destined for the LG originate in the superior salivatory nucleus (SSN) and join CN VII. These fibers are ultimately conveyed to the pterygopalatine ganglion (*asterisk*), which is suspended below the maxillary nerve (V_2) in the pterygopalatine fossa. The fibers synapse in the ganglion and the postganglionic fibers are then conveyed toward the LG along V_2 and its zygomatic branch. The zygomatic nerve then conveys the parasympathetic fibers for the LG to the lacrimal branch of V_1 and it is the lacrimal nerve that finally delivers these fibers to the LG. NC, Trigeminal nucleus. (From Johnson J, ed. *Bailey's Head and Neck Surgery.* 5th ed. Philadelphia, PA: Wolters Kluwer; 2013.)

alveolar ridge, including the teeth and gums (**Fig. 1.31**). Upon emerging from the infraorbital foramen, below the inferior orbital rim, this nerve provides palpebral branches that serve the skin of the lower eyelid, inferior palpebral conjunctiva, upper lip and nasal branches that serve the mucosa lining of the anterior portion of the nasal cavity (**Figs. 1.28** and **1.31**). It is a useful clinical reminder that fractures of the orbital floor can give rise to numbness of a portion of the upper gums and the area of skin served by the infraorbital nerve.

Vascular Supply

The arterial blood supply to the orbit arises from two major vessels, the ophthalmic artery and the infraorbital artery. The ophthalmic artery is the first branch of the internal carotid artery. The infraorbital artery is ultimately a branch of the external carotid artery, arising from one of its terminal branches, the maxillary artery, within the pterygopalatine fossa.

The venous return from the eye and the orbit converges on two principal vessels, the superior and inferior ophthalmic veins. As is generally the case, there is greater

variability between individuals in the distribution of their venous system than their arterial system. While the superior ophthalmic vein consistently returns to the cavernous sinus the inferior ophthalmic vein may join either the cavernous sinus or the pterygoid venous plexus in the infratemporal fossa. The pterygoid plexus of venous vessels coalesces at its posterior margin to form the maxillary vein.

Arterial Anatomy

THE OPHTHALMIC ARTERY

The ophthalmic artery arises just as the internal carotid emerges through the roof of the cavernous sinus, beneath the anterior clinoid process (**Fig. 1.25**). The artery immediately enters the orbit, passing beneath the optic nerve within the optic canal (**Fig. 1.26**). In the head, most of the postganglionic sympathetic fibers derive from the carotid plexus that surrounds the internal carotid artery. Fibers from this plexus distribute to their target tissues along the various vascular branches of the ophthalmic artery. As such, most tissues within the orbit and eyelids receive their sympathetic innervation from the plexus of

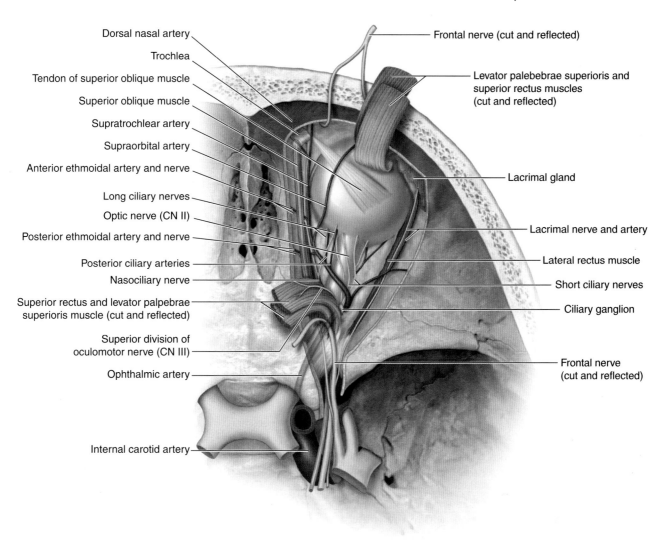

FIGURE 1.32 Idealized depiction of the branches of the ophthalmic artery. Note that the long and short posterior ciliary arteries do not arise directly from the ophthalmic artery. They arise from the medial and lateral posterior ciliary arteries that are the direct branches from the ophthalmic artery. (Modified from Tank PW. *Grant's Dissector*. 15th ed. Philadelphia, PA: Wolters Kluwer; 2012.)

fibers surrounding the vessels that provide their vascular supply. These postganglionic sympathetic fibers enter the orbit through the optic canal as a plexus surrounding the ophthalmic artery.

The branches of the ophthalmic artery are most conveniently discussed in two groups—an orbital group and an ocular group. The orbital group is discussed below and the ocular group is discussed in **CHAPTER 3: OVERVIEW OF THE EYE.**

The orbital group of branches from the ophthalmic artery includes the following (**Fig. 1.32**).

- Lacrimal artery
- Supraorbital artery
- Supratrochlear artery (i.e., frontal artery)
- Posterior ethmoidal artery
- Anterior ethmoidal artery
- Medial palpebral artery
- Dorsal nasal artery

The additional orbital branches, the superior and inferior muscular arteries, serve the extraocular muscles, but the specific branches of these vessels that serve the rectus muscles, also give rise to the anterior ciliary arteries that serve the eye itself. The anterior ciliary arteries are described in **CHAPTER 3: OVERVIEW OF THE EYE.**

ORBITAL BRANCHES OF THE OPHTHALMIC ARTERY

Lacrimal Artery

The main trunk of the ophthalmic artery emerges from beneath the optic nerve, under its lateral edge, crossing above the nerve and moving toward the medial wall of the orbit. The lacrimal artery is the main branch provided to serve the structures near the lateral wall of the orbit, with a continuation into the eyelids (**Figs. 1.32 and 1.33**).

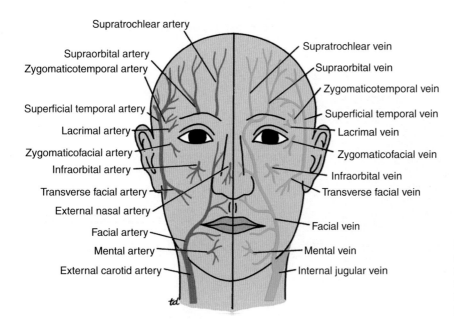

FIGURE 1.33 Distribution of major arterial and venous vessels of the face. Note that there are rich anastomoses between the vessels that serve the forehead and scalp. (Modified from Snell RS. *Clinical Anatomy by Regions.* 9th ed. Philadelphia, PA: Wolters Kluwer; 2011.)

The lacrimal artery follows the same course as the nerve of the same name, along the superior edge of the lateral rectus (**Fig. 1.32**). Along its path, it gives rise to zygomatic branches that divide and follow the course of the zygomaticotemporal and zygomaticofacial nerves. It also gives rise to a recurrent branch that passes through the posterolateral wall of the orbit, into the adjacent middle cranial fossa. Here, the recurrent branch of the lacrimal artery anastomoses with the middle meningeal artery, the branch of the maxillary artery that enters the cranium via the foramen spinosum and passes within the groove provided for it on the interior surface of the cranium.

Continuing anteriorly, the lacrimal artery supplies the lacrimal gland and pierces the orbital septum, dividing to enter both the upper and lower lids as the lateral palpebral arteries (**Fig. 1.33**). These are discussed in detail in **CHAPTER 2: THE EYELIDS AND ADNEXA.**

Supraorbital Artery

The supraorbital artery branches from the ophthalmic artery as the latter crosses above the optic nerve. The supraorbital artery passes along the medial edges of the superior rectus and levator palpebrae superioris, traveling with the supraorbital nerve. This vessel reaches the scalp of the forehead via the supraorbital notch or foramen, at the superior orbital rim. In the scalp, the vascular field of this vessel anastomoses with the field of the ipsilateral supratrochlear artery medially and the superficial temporal branch of the external carotid artery laterally (**Figs. 1.32** and **1.33**).

Supratrochlear Artery (i.e., Frontal Artery)

The supratrochlear artery passes anteriorly, medial to the supraorbital artery. Along with the dorsal nasal artery, it

is one of the terminal branches of the ophthalmic artery. The supratrochlear artery emerges onto the scalp above the orbit, accompanied by the nerve of the same name. The vascular field of this vessel, in the scalp of the forehead, anastomoses across the midline with the contralateral supratrochlear artery and laterally with the ipsilateral supraorbital artery (**Figs. 1.32** and **1.33**).

Posterior Ethmoidal Artery

The posterior ethmoidal artery enters the posterior ethmoidal foramen, accompanied by the nerve of the same name. It serves the mucosa of the posterior ethmoid air cells and continues through the ethmoid sinus to serve the mucosa of the midline nasal septum.[18]

Anterior Ethmoidal Artery

The anterior ethmoidal artery enters the anterior ethmoidal foramen, following the tortuous pathway of the anterior ethmoidal branch of the nasociliary nerve. The artery serves the mucosae of the anterior and middle ethmoid air cells. As with the nasociliary nerve, this vessel continues superiorly, within the ethmoid bone to the floor of the anterior cranial fossa, delivering vascular branches to the mucosa of the superior portion of the nasal cavity along its path. In the anterior cranial fossa, it makes small contributions to the dura mater before giving rise to a terminal branch that follows the external nasal nerve onto the bridge of the nose.

Medial Palpebral Arteries

Additional anterior branches include the superior and inferior medial palpebral arteries, which pass below the trochlea, pierce the orbital septum, and pass into the upper and lower eyelids. Each branch passes laterally within the lid, to anastomose with the lateral palpebral arteries. These vessels are discussed in greater detail in **CHAPTER 2: THE EYELIDS AND ADNEXA**.

The inferior palpebral artery anastomoses with the angular artery, at the medial canthus. The angular artery is a terminal branch of the facial artery, itself a branch of the external carotid artery. From this anastomosis in the medial canthus, a branch passes to the mucosa of the lacrimal duct. This branch continues serving the mucosa of the lacrimal drainage system inferiorly, to its entry into the inferior meatus of the nasal cavity.

Dorsal Nasal Artery

The dorsal nasal artery, along with the supratrochlear artery, are considered to be the terminal branches of the ophthalmic artery. The dorsal nasal artery emerges from the orbit, passing through the orbital septum, superior to the medial palpebral ligament. This vessel also anastomoses with the angular artery and provides branches that serve the side and bridge of the nose and the superior portion of the lacrimal sac (**Fig. 1.32**).

Superior and Inferior Muscular Arteries

The superior muscular branch of the ophthalmic artery supplies the lateral and superior rectus muscles, the superior oblique, and the levator palpebrae superioris.

The inferior muscular branch supplies the inferior oblique, the inferior rectus, and the medial rectus. The inferior rectus and inferior oblique also receive branches from the infraorbital artery, described below. As the lacrimal artery passes anteriorly, along the superior edge of the lateral rectus, it may contribute to the arterial supply of this muscle as well.

The muscular branches serving the four rectus muscles give rise to terminal branches termed the anterior ciliary arteries. The anterior ciliary arteries emerge onto the sclera from the anterior margins of the tendons of the rectus muscles. Each muscle provides two anterior ciliary arteries, except for the lateral rectus, which provides only one. The further course of these vessels is discussed in **CHAPTER 3: OVERVIEW OF THE EYE**.

The Infraorbital Artery

While the ophthalmic artery is the sole source of arterial blood to the eye, it is not the sole source of blood to the orbit. The infraorbital artery is an indirect branch of the external carotid artery, arising from the maxillary artery in the pterygopalatine fossa. It enters the orbit via the inferior orbital fissure to serve structures near the floor of the orbit including the inferior rectus, inferior oblique, and lacrimal sac. The artery continues anteriorly into the infraorbital groove and canal, giving rise to the anterior superior alveolar artery before emerging from the infraorbital foramen, with the nerve of the same name. This terminal branch serves the side of the nose, the cheek, and upper lip (**Fig. 1.33**).

Venous Anatomy

The venous blood from the eye, the orbit and portions of the eyelids, and the face returns to either the superior or inferior ophthalmic vein. The vascular fields leading to these two principal vessels freely anastomose.

As mentioned previously, there is greater individual variability in the anatomy of the human venous system than the arterial system. Recent evidence suggests that this variability is taken to an extreme in the orbit. For simplicity, it is generally accurate to say that the veins converging upon the superior ophthalmic vein drain the vascular field served by the branches of the ophthalmic artery. Those returning to the inferior ophthalmic vein, in addition to the inferior vortex veins, generally include the tissues served by the branches of the infraorbital artery.[19] But even this generality is contested.[20–24] Most available drawings of the branches contributing to the superior and inferior ophthalmic veins, such as **Fig. 1.34**, are generalized.

Detailed delineations of orbital venous anatomy were recently described, based upon dissections of 34 orbits from 17 preserved cadaveric specimens and from two non-preserved, cadaveric specimens.[25] The discussion of the venous distribution within the orbit presented below relies heavily upon this recent work including clinical imaging, rather than highly idealized classical presentations.

THE SUPERIOR OPHTHALMIC VEIN

The superior ophthalmic vein can be defined as arising at its anastomosis with the angular vein in the medial canthal region.[25] From its origin, the general course of this vein is posterolateral. It initially runs parallel to the medial border of the superior rectus. It then enters the muscle cone and continues laterally, to leave the orbit above the annulus of Zinn, via the superior orbital fissure (**Fig. 1.26**).

Along this path, the vein consistently receives the following branches:

- **Superior vortex veins.** The superior vortex veins, commonly two in number, drain into the superior ophthalmic vein. The medial of these two always drains directly into the superior ophthalmic vein. The superolateral vortex vein drains either into the lacrimal vein or directly into the superior ophthalmic vein. The pathways leading to the formation of the vortex veins, prior to their exit from the sclera, are described in detail in **CHAPTER 3: OVERVIEW OF THE EYE, CHAPTER 7: THE IRIS, CHAPTER 8: THE CILIARY BODY, AND CHAPTER 12: CHOROID AND CHOROIDAL CIRCULATION**.

- **Lacrimal vein.** The lacrimal vein drains the lacrimal gland, passing posteriorly in conjunction with the lacrimal artery and lacrimal nerve, along the superior edge of the lateral rectus. This vein receives most of the venous blood from this muscle and commonly receives most of the venous blood from the superior rectus. Before joining

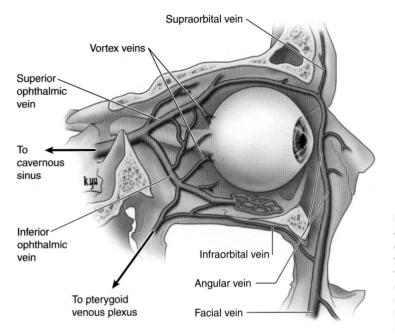

FIGURE 1.34 Sketch showing an idealized representation of the venous drainage of the orbit. In reality, the pattern of venous drainage from the orbit is quite variable. Note that recent dissections suggest that the inferior ophthalmic vein takes origin as a plexus that forms beneath the globe, continuing posteriorly from that point and with no connection to the face. (Modified from Moore KL, Agur AMR, Dalley AF. *Clinical Oriented Anatomy.* 7th ed. Philadelphia, PA: Wolters Kluwer; 2013.)

the superior ophthalmic vein, this vessel occasionally receives the superolateral vortex vein from the eye.

- **Ethmoidal veins.** Along its path posteriorly, the superior ophthalmic vein receives small branches conveying blood returning from the ethmoid sinuses.
- **Collateral veins.** Several connections, principally a medial and lateral collateral vein, join the drainage fields of the superior and inferior ophthalmic veins.
- **Muscular veins.** The superior ophthalmic vein receives numerous, variable, venous branches from the extraocular muscles, primarily the superior rectus and superior oblique, plus the levator palpebrae superioris.
- **Central retinal vein.** The classical depiction of the drainage pathway for the central retinal vein is to the superior ophthalmic vein and then to the cavernous sinus. It is included here for that reason. From the recent dissections of Cheung and McNab,[25] however, their conclusion is that when the central retinal vein could be identified definitively, it drained directly into the cavernous sinus. This result contrasts with the reports of earlier dissections such as those of Whitnall,[26] and speaks to the degree of interindividual variability that is common to the anatomy of the venous system.

THE INFERIOR OPHTHALMIC VEIN

Despite classical renditions of gross anatomy, the inferior ophthalmic vein is less reliably identified than its superior counterpart. From recent dissections, the inferior ophthalmic vein appears to take origin from a venous plexus that is present in the mid-orbit, just superior to the inner surface of the inferior rectus muscle[25] and may not make direct connections with the veins of the face (**Fig. 1.34**).

Anteriorly, this plexus receives the inferior vortex veins. This plexus also receives contributions from the inferior rectus and oblique, and variably, from the medial rectus. It is from the posterior confluence of this plexus that the inferior ophthalmic vein arises, and almost immediately receives the lateral and medial collaterals from the superior ophthalmic vein.

Consistent with classical depictions, the inferior ophthalmic vein, in most cases, reaches the cavernous sinus by passing initially through the inferior orbital fissure. In a smaller number of cases, the vein reaches the pterygoid plexus, in the infratemporal fossa (**Fig. 1.34**).

 From a clinical standpoint, the detailed anatomy of the orbital veins is less critical (except in orbital surgery) than appreciating that the orbital veins represent a connection between the veins draining a portion of the face and the cavernous sinus. This triangular area of the face, from the bridge of the nose to the lateral edges of the upper lips, is termed the "danger triangle of the face" (Fig. 1.35). Infections in this region can be conveyed to the cavernous sinus and lead to life-threatening complications including cavernous sinus thrombosis, meningitis, or brain abscess.[27]

Lymphatic Anatomy

It remains the consensus that there are few, if any, lymphatic channels in the human orbit, with the exception of those serving the lacrimal gland.

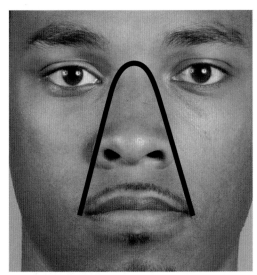

FIGURE 1.35 Curved line from the bridge of the nose to the corners of the mouth delimits the danger area of the face, which drains to the cavernous sinus.

Lacrimal Gland

The lacrimal gland is situated just posterior to the lateral aspect of the superior orbital rim, nested within the fossa provided for it along the orbital surface of the frontal bone (**Figs. 1.7** and **1.36**). The lacrimal gland produces much of the aqueous component of the tear film. It is divided into superior and inferior lobes by the aponeurosis of the levator palpebrae superioris as the aponeurosis moves into the eyelid from the orbit (**Fig. 1.36**). The larger orbital lobe resides above the aponeurosis while the smaller palpebral lobe is situated beneath the aponeurosis, making it easily visualized by pulling the upper lid superiorly and

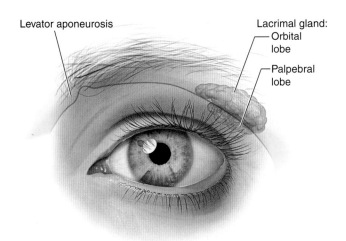

Levator aponeurosis

Lacrimal gland:
— Orbital lobe

— Palpebral lobe

FIGURE 1.36 Sketch shows position of lacrimal gland and separation of the gland into a larger orbital lobe and smaller palpebral lobe by the passage of the aponeurosis of the levator palpebrae superioris (shown in *yellow*) into the upper lid. (Modified from the Anatomical Chart Company. *Eye Anatomical Chart*. Philadelphia, PA: Wolters Kluwer; 2000.)

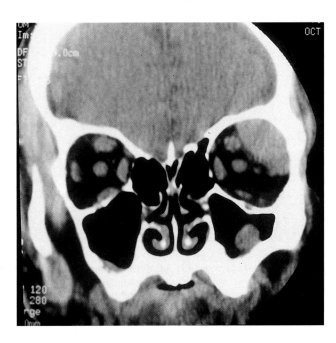

FIGURE 1.37 Note expanding tumor compressing left orbital contents. (From Penne RB, ed. *Wills Eye Institute—Oculoplastics*. 2nd ed. Philadelphia, PA: Wolters Kluwer; 2011.)

laterally. Ducts from both lobes are ultimately conveyed to the conjunctival surface in the superior fornix.

 Despite its greater accessibility, the inferior palpebral lobe of the gland is less often chosen when biopsies of the lacrimal gland are required. It is most common to make an incision through the eyelid at the lid crease (sulcus) in order to biopsy the larger superior lobe (https://vimeo.com/123406342 - Lacrimal gland biopsy on Vimeo). In this way, there is less risk of post-incisional scarring of the ducts draining the lacrimal gland onto the surface of the eye. As a practical matter as well, most tumors affecting this gland originate in the orbital lobe and hence biopsy of this lobe is more likely to render useful material. Note the enlarging lacrimal gland tumor in Figure 1.37.

HISTOLOGY OF THE LACRIMAL GLAND

The lacrimal gland is classified as a compound tubuloacinar gland. It is made up of many acini arranged into lobules that are separated by an interstitial fibrovascular matrix (**Fig. 1.38**). The secretory cells line the acini and are partially surrounded on their basal surface by a discontinuous ring of myoepithelial cells (**Fig. 1.38**). Within the interstitial tissue is a resident population of B cells, T cells, and plasma cells. The latter of these make principally secretory immunoglobulin A, dimerized by linking with a J-chain, and to which the acinar cells add a secretory piece before releasing this immunoglobulin as part of the normal tears. The central lumina of the acini converge onto myoepithelial

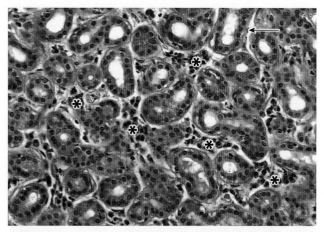

FIGURE 1.38   Light micrograph shows lacrimal gland acini lined by secretory cells and surrounded by a layer of flattened myoepithelial cells (*arrow*). The lumina of the acini converge on intralobular ducts, which anastomose to finally form the terminal ducts that drain into the cul-de-sac of the conjunctiva. Within the fibrovascular interstitium of the gland is a resident population of B cells, T cells, and plasma cells (*asterisks*). (From Mills SE, ed. *Histology for Pathologists.* 4th ed. Philadelphia, PA: Wolters Kluwer; 2012.)

cell-lined intralobular ducts. These intralobular ducts anastomose to form larger ducts that are lined by a not well-characterized third type of cell, which is capable of modifying the composition of the secretion before it ultimately drains onto the ocular surface from both lobes.

INNERVATION OF THE LACRIMAL GLAND

The lacrimal gland receives sensory, sympathetic, and parasympathetic fibers. All of these fibers are conveyed to the gland via a branch from the lacrimal nerve, itself a branch of the ophthalmic division of CN V. The sensory fibers

conveyed to the gland are intrinsic to CN V. The autonomic fibers, both sympathetic and parasympathetic, are conveyed to the lacrimal nerve, after this nerve has branched from the main trunk of the ophthalmic division of CN V.

The preganglionic parasympathetic fibers destined for the lacrimal gland originate in the lacrimal nucleus (a portion of the superior salivatory nucleus) within the pontine tegmentum. These fibers join CN VII and emerge with it from the pontinomedullary junction, traveling with CN VII into the temporal bone via the internal acoustic meatus. At the external genu of CN VII, in the middle ear cavity, these fibers leave as the greater petrosal branch of the nerve, emerging onto the floor of the middle cranial fossa, via the hiatus of the facial canal. From here, it passes anteriorly and medially toward the foramen lacerum where they leave the base of the skull and enter the pterygoid (vidian) canal (**Fig. 1.39**).

The foramen lacerum borders the carotid canal of the skull. Most of the postganglionic sympathetic fibers that reach the head arrive as a plexus around the internal carotid artery. Some of these fibers leave the internal carotid artery where the foramen lacerum and carotid canal cross. These fibers, called the deep petrosal nerve, join with the greater petrosal below the carotid canal to become the vidian nerve. The vidian nerve (i.e., nerve of the pterygoid canal) passes anteriorly within the pterygoid (vidian) canal to reach the pterygopalatine ganglion within the pterygopalatine fossa (**Fig. 1.39**). Upon reaching this parasympathetic ganglion, the preganglionic parasympathetic fibers synapse. The postganglionic sympathetic fibers arriving at the ganglion pass through without synapsing.

The postganglionic parasympathetic fibers destined for the lacrimal gland, in conjunction with some of the postganglionic sympathetic fibers that traversed the ganglion,

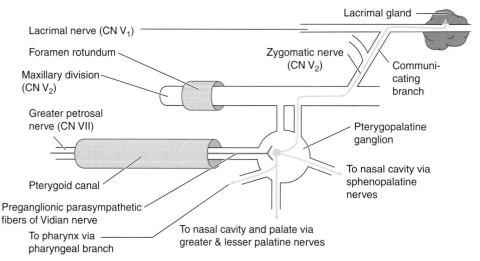

FIGURE 1.39   Preganglionic parasympathetic fibers destined for the lacrimal gland reach the pterygopalatine ganglion via the greater petrosal nerve (a branch of CN VII), which becomes part of the vidian nerve (nerve of the pterygoid canal). The parasympathetic fibers synapse in the ganglion and the postganglionic parasympathetic fibers join the maxillary division of V_2, which conveys them into the zygomatic branch of the maxillary division and then its zygomaticotemporal branch. The zygomaticotemporal branch passes them to the lacrimal nerve, a branch of the ophthalmic division of CN V, for delivery to the lacrimal gland. (Modified from Moore KL, Agur AMR, Dalley AF. *Clinical Oriented Anatomy.* 7th ed. Philadelphia, PA: Wolters Kluwer; 2013.)

leave the ganglion to join the maxillary division of CN V. The Maxillary division suspends the ganglion from above, as it passes from the middle cranial fossa via the foramen rotundum, traverses the pterygopalatine fossa, and enters the orbit via the inferior orbital fissure (**Figs. 1.31** and **1.39**). The sympathetic and parasympathetic fibers pass into the zygomatic nerve and, in turn, its zygomatico-temporal branch. Before the zygomaticotemporal nerve reaches its foramen on the lateral wall of the orbit, the autonomic fibers are given off to the lacrimal branch of the ophthalmic division of CN V via a communicating branch (**Figs. 1.31** and **1.39**). The lacrimal nerve then conveys these sympathetic and parasympathetic fibers to the lacrimal gland. The parasympathetic fibers predominate in the lacrimal gland. They stimulate production and release of the lacrimal gland's contribution to the aqueous component of the tear film, while the sympathetic fibers provide vascular tone for the vessels within the gland. An array of regulatory neurotransmitters have been identified in the lacrimal gland and their neuroregulation of the gland has recently been reviewed.[28]

Secretion of tears occurs at a basal rate but can be augmented as part of a reflex arc beginning with sensory nerves in the cornea and conjunctiva or via psychogenic stimuli (crying).[29]

BLOOD SUPPLY TO THE LACRIMAL GLAND

As noted earlier, the arterial supply to the lacrimal gland is via the lacrimal artery, a branch of the ophthalmic artery (**Fig. 1.32**). The venous return from the lacrimal gland is via the lacrimal vein, which joins the superior ophthalmic vein.

LYMPHATICS

Lymphatics within the lacrimal gland drain primarily into the preauricular (i.e., superficial parotid) nodes.

Acknowledgment

Thanks to Dr. Richard Hertle for his contributions to the Muscle Pulleys section of this chapter.

REFERENCES

1. Sevel D. The origins and insertions of the extraocular muscles: development, histologic features, and clinical significance. *Trans Am Ophthalmol Soc.* 1986;84:488–526.
2. Fink WH. Ligament of Lockwood in relation to surgery of the inferior oblique and inferior rectus muscles. *Arch Ophthal.* 1948;39(3):371–382.
3. Zide BM, Jelks GW. *Surgical Anatomy around the Orbit: The System of Zones.* Philadelphia, PA: Wolters Kluwer; 2005.
4. Mallajosyula S. *Surgical Atlas of Orbital Diseases.* New Delhi, India: Jaypee Brothers Medical Publishers; 2008.
5. Porter JD, Baker RS, Ragusa RJ, et al. Extraocular muscles: basic and clinical aspects of structure and function. *Surv Ophthalmol.* 1995;39(6):451–484.
6. Miller JM, Robins D. Extraocular muscle sideslip and orbital geometry in monkeys. *Vision Res.* 1987;27(3):381–392.
7. Kono R, Poukens V, Demer JL. Quantitative analysis of the structure of the human extraocular muscle pulley system. *Invest Ophthalmol Vis Sci.* 2002;43(9):2923–2932.
8. Demer JL. The orbital pulley system: a revolution in concepts of orbital anatomy. *Ann N Y Acad Sci.* 2002;956:17–32.
9. Demer JL, Miller JM, Poukens V, et al. Evidence for fibromuscular pulleys of the recti extraocular muscles. *Invest Ophthalmol Vis Sci.* 1995;36(6):1125–1136.
10. Demer JL, Clark RA. Magnetic resonance imaging of human extraocular muscles during static ocular counter-rolling. *J Neurophysiol.* 2005;94(5):3292–3302.
11. Clark RA, Miller JM, Demer JL. Location and stability of rectus muscle pulleys muscle paths as a function of gaze. *Invest Ophthalmol Vis Sci.* 1997;38(1):227–240.
12. Von Helmholtz H. *Handbuch der physiologischen optik.* Vol 9. Leipzig: Leopold Voss; 1867.
13. Oh SY, Poukens V, Demer JL. Quantitative analysis of rectus extraocular muscle layers in monkey and humans. *Invest Ophthalmol Vis Sci.* 2001;42(1):10–16.
14. Scott AB, Collins CC. Division of labor in human extraocular muscle. *Arch Ophthalmol.* 1973;90(4):319–322.
15. Miller JM. Functional anatomy of normal human rectus muscles. *Vision Res.* 1989;29(2):223–240.
16. Clark RA, Demer JL. Magnetic resonance imaging of the effects of horizontal rectus extraocular muscle surgery on pulley and globe positions and stability. *Invest Ophthalmol Vis Sci.* 2006;47(1):188–194.
17. Griessenauer CJ, Raborn J, Mortazavi MM, et al. Relationship between the pituitary stalk angle in prefixed, normal, and postfixed optic chiasmata: an anatomic study with microsurgical application. *Acta Neurochir.* 2014;156(1):147–151.
18. Hyrtl J. *Lehrbuch der anatomie des menschen.* Leipzig: Wilhelm Braumüller; 1875.
19. Duke-Elder S. The foundations of ophthalmology. In: *System of Ophthalmology.* Vol 7. London, UK: H. Kimpton; 1962.
20. Soemmering ST. *Abbildungen des menschlichen auges. cited by: Gurwitsch M. Über die anastomosen zwischen den gesichtsund orbitalvenen. graefes arch ophthalmol. 1883. 29:31–83.* Vol 29. Frankfurt, Germany: Warrentrapp und Wenner; 1801:31–88.
21. Bergen MP. A literature review of the vascular system in the human orbit. *Acta Morphol Neerl Scand.* 1981;19(4):273–305.
22. Bergen MP. A spatial reconstruction of the orbital vascular pattern in relation with the connective tissue system. *Acta Morphol Neerl Scand.* 1982;20(2):117–137.
23. Bergen MP. Relationships between the arteries and veins and the connective tissue system in the human orbit. *Acta Morphol Neerl Scand.* 1982;20(1):1–15.
24. Bergen MP. Some histological aspects of the structure of the connective tissue system and its relationships with the blood vessels in the human orbit. *Acta Morphol Neerl Scand.* 1982;20(4):293–308.
25. Cheung N, McNab AA. Venous anatomy of the orbit. *Invest Ophthalmol Vis Sci.* 2003;44(3):988–995.
26. Whitnall S. Anatomy of the human orbit and accessory organs of vision. New York, NY: Oxford University Press; 1932.
27. Maes U. Infections of the dangerous areas of the face: their pathology and treatment. *Ann Surg.* 1937;106(1):1–10.
28. Dartt DA. Neural regulation of lacrimal gland secretory processes: relevance in dry eye diseases. *Prog Retin Eye Res.* 2009;28(3):155–177.
29. Acosta MC, Peral A, Luna C, et al. Tear secretion induced by selective stimulation of corneal and conjunctival sensory nerve fibers. *Invest Ophthalmol Vis Sci.* 2004;45(7):2333–2336.

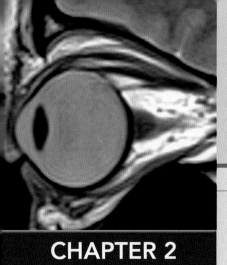

CHAPTER 2

The Eyelids and Adnexa

Overview

The primary functions of the eyelids and their adnexal structures include physical protection of the eye, protection from excessive light, and lubrication of the surface of the eye. Actions of the lids can be:

- Reflexive (rapid closure of the lid if an object approaches the eye or touches the eye or the lashes).
- Voluntary (squeezing the eyes tightly shut or winking).
- Involuntary (a routine blink).

By blinking, the lids spread newly formed tears across the eye. In this way, each blink sweeps cell debris, dust, and microbes toward the lacrimal drainage system and provides the equally important function of resurfacing the primary optical surface of the eye. Contraction of the muscles and tendons that close the eye also contributes to the pumping action of the lacrimal drainage system, to move tears through the lacrimal drainage channels, toward the inferior meatus of the nasal cavity and then to the gastrointestinal system.

Surface Landmarks

Readily identifiable surface landmarks of the eyelids (palpebrae) and adnexa include the eyebrows, the eyelashes, the palpebral margins, the superior and inferior sulci, and the medial and lateral canthi (singular: canthus) (**Fig. 2.1**). Each of these landmarks is discussed in greater detail below.

With the eyelids open, the space between the upper and lower lids, in which the surface of the eye is exposed, is termed the *interpalpebral fissure*. The fissure averages 9 mm in height in normal adults. For comparison, most soft contact lenses average 13 to 14 mm in diameter, ensuring that the upper and lower edges of the lens remain behind the upper and lower lid margins.

When the lids are closed, the eyes reflexively elevate behind them, in what is called the Bell's phenomenon.[1] As a result, it is the inferior cornea and not the central cornea that becomes exposed if the lids are open slightly during sleep (**Fig. 2.2**). The Bell's phenomenon can be viewed by holding open the upper lids while asking the subject to blink. The attempted blink will force the eyes upward.

The free edges of the eyelids, termed the *superior and inferior palpebral margins*, run an arcuate course over the eyeball. The arcuate course of the upper lid normally covers a portion of the iris above or tangential to the superior edge of the

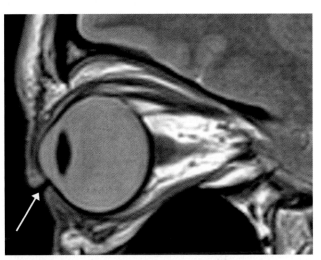

FIGURE 2.2 Sagittal, T2-weighted MRI of human eye, eyelids and orbit. Note slight opening between mostly closed lids aligns with inferior portion of the cornea and not the central cornea (*arrow*). (Courtesy of Dr. Robert Bert.)

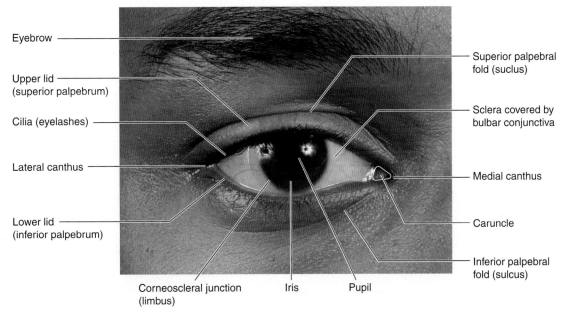

FIGURE 2.1 Principal anatomical landmarks of the eyelids and visible portion of the eye.

pupil. The lower lid runs an arcuate course that is normally tangential to the inferior limbus, where the clear cornea and white sclera are joined (**Fig. 2.1**). Another metric of normal lid height is measurement of the distance between the upper or lower lid margin and pupillary light reflex. The upper lid margin-reflex distance (MRD-1) usually measures 4 mm, and the lower lid margin-reflex distance (MRD-2) averages 5 mm.

THE EYEBROW

The eyebrow is a strip of hair-bearing skin that roughly parallels the superior orbital rim, though the arching course of eyebrows can be quite variable (**Fig. 2.1**). These hairs are generally coarser and stiffer than other hairs. The brow bulges slightly forward from the forehead owing to the presence of an underlying focal fat pad, primarily beneath the medial half of the brow. The brow is thus able to help shield the eye from dust, sweat of the forehead, and excessive light coming from above the eye. Additionally, voluntary alteration of the arc of the brow is used in facial expressions such as frowning.

THE SUPERIOR AND INFERIOR PALPEBRAL SULCI

These are the furrows or creases in the lids that occur when the eyes are open. The superior palpebral sulcus is significant enough to create a redundant fold of lid tissue. An inferior palpebral sulcus is also present in the lower eyelid, but it is much less prominent and does not produce a fold (**Figs. 2.1** and **2.3**). The magnitude of the superior palpebral sulcus differs between Oriental individuals and those of other races. In Oriental eyes, the fold commonly extends inferiorly, almost to the lash line. In other races, the edge of this fold does not normally reach the lash line at the margin of the upper lid (**Fig. 2.3**). The anatomical basis for this difference is discussed later in this chapter.

THE LATERAL AND MEDIAL CANTHI

These are the points where the upper and lower lids are joined. The architecture of the medial and lateral canthi differs. Examination of the upper lid margin reveals that it has a smooth, arcing contour that extends from the lateral to the medial canthus (**Figs. 2.3** and **2.4**). In the arcing contour of the lower lid, however, the lid margin arcs inferiorly from the lateral canthus but rises to a peak,

termed the lacrimal crest, which is just lateral to the medial canthus. From this crest, the contour of the lower lid dips inferiorly in a shorter arc, rising again to reach the medial canthus (**Fig. 2.4**). At the crest of the peak is the inferior lacrimal punctum into which the tears drain (**Fig. 2.5**). There is a superior punctum as well. Like the inferior punctum, the superior punctum has a surrounding crest of lid tissue, but its presence does not as significantly alter the contour of the upper lid margin.

Along both the upper and lower lid margins are thin strips of tears referred to as the tear menisci (**Figs. 2.4** and **2.6**). The superior tear meniscus extends along the entire upper lid margin, from the lateral canthus to the medial canthus. The inferior tear meniscus, however, terminates at the medially located crest containing the inferior lacrimal

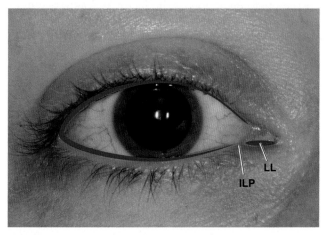

FIGURE 2.4 Figure depicts distribution of lacrimal tear meniscus along upper and lower lid margin, plus position of inferior lacrimal punctum (ILP) at inferior lacrimal crest. Note difference in arc of upper and lower lid margins. Arcing contour of upper lid is essentially continuous from the lateral to medial canthus while lower lid margin exhibits a continuous arc only as far as the inferior lacrimal crest at ILP. Medial to the ILP, the lower lid contour dips again before reaching the medial canthus. It is here that the lacrimal lake (LL) is present. (From Shields JA, Shields CL. *Eyelid, Conjunctival, and Orbital Tumors: An Atlas and Textbook*. 3rd ed. Philadelphia, PA: Wolters Kluwer; 2015.)

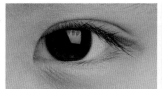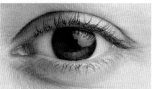

FIGURE 2.3 Oriental eye with superior palpebral sulcus nearly aligned with lid margin over medial half (**left**). Occidental eye with superior palpebral sulcus well above lid margin (**right**).

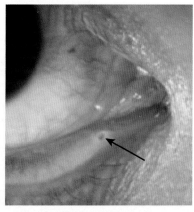

FIGURE 2.5 Clinical photograph of everted inferior lid margin showing inferior lacrimal punctum. (Courtesy of Dr. Derek Ho.)

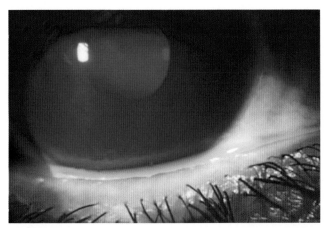

FIGURE 2.6 Clinical photograph shows fluorescent dye mixed with tears in the inferior tear meniscus. A similar but thinner strip of tears also clings to the inferior surface of the upper lid (unseen). (Courtesy of Dr. Derek Ho.)

punctum. An additional reservoir of tears resides along the inferior lid margin, between the punctum and the medial canthus. This reservoir is termed the *lacrimal lake*.

THE PALPEBRAL MARGINS

Along the superior and inferior palpebral margins, a series of parallel, linearly oriented features are identifiable (**Fig. 2.7**). From anterior to posterior these include the following:

- The lash line
- The gray line
- The Meibomian gland orifices
- The mucocutaneous junction (i.e., Marx's line)

The Lash Line

Along both the superior and inferior lid margins, two rows of cilia, or eyelashes, are present. The eyelashes protect the eye from dust and debris and most recently have been shown to assist in retarding the evaporation of the tear film that covers the surface of the eye.[2] The arrangement of these rows of eyelashes, paralleling the contour of the lids, creates the lash line. The upper eyelid exhibits

approximately 100 lashes. The lower lid exhibits only half as many, making them appear more sparsely distributed. The lashes of the upper lid are longer than those of the lower lid and curl upward. Those of the lower lid curl downward. In this way, the lashes do not interfere with the field of vision. This feature also appears to minimize entanglement of the upper and lower lashes during blinking. Under normal conditions, the life cycle of a lash is 5 to 11 months.[3] Topical administration of certain prostaglandin compounds, available by prescription, will make lashes grow faster, longer, and thicker.[4]

The lashes receive sensory innervation: those of the upper lid from the ophthalmic division of the trigeminal nerve and those of the lower lid from the maxillary division. Touching the lashes results in a reflex closure of the eyelids.

*Appreciating the contour of the lash line is important. Some lesions near the lid margin may alter the direction of individual lashes from the base to the tip (**Fig 2.8A**). However, lesions that appear to alter the continuity of the lash line, generally carry a greater suspicion of malignancy (**Fig. 2.8B**).*

The histologic structure of the eyelashes is essentially the same as other terminal hairs. They are composed of a pilosebaceous unit, including the hair bulb, the hair shaft, and associated sebaceous glands. In the case of the lashes, the sebaceous glands associated with the lash follicle are named. They are the glands of Zeis. An additional feature distinguishing the lash follicle from other terminal hair follicles is the absence of a sympathetically innervated arrector pili muscle to stand the hair erect. Hence, when you get "goose bumps" your lashes do not tingle.

With age, the eyelashes do not generally turn gray, but they can become white in certain systemic disorders such as Vogt–Koyanagi–Harada syndrome. Whitening of the lashes is termed *poliosis*. Loss of lashes due to an array of disease processes is termed *madarosis*. The lashes are not the

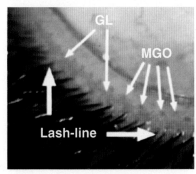

FIGURE 2.7 Clinical photograph of the inferior lid margin shows, from anterior to posterior, the lash line, the gray line (GL) and the series of Meibomian gland orifices (MGO).

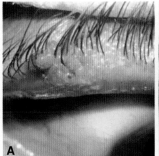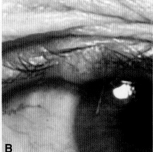

FIGURE 2.8 **A:** Papillomatous lesion at the lash line. Note that it diverts the direction of individual lashes but has not altered the contour of the lash line. **B:** By contrast, this lesion has caused diversion/interruption of the lash line, a more worrisome clinical sign.

only hairs associated with the eyelids. It is not uncommon to also find sparse, fine, vellus hairs on the skin surface of the upper lid.

 *Distichiasis is the term used to describe a rare condition in which extra rows of lashes are present (**Fig. 2.9**). These additional lashes often emerge from Meibomian gland orifices. Most cases are congenital, but acquired forms can be encountered.*

The Gray Line

The gray line is a variably visible line along the lid margin, between the lash line and the row of Meibomian gland orifices (**Fig. 2.7**). Its histologic analog remains under debate, but most sources attribute its gray color to the presence of a strip of skeletal muscle, called the muscle of

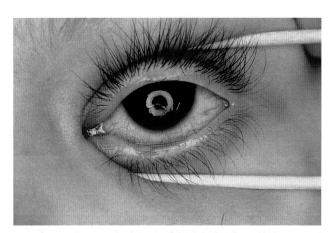

FIGURE 2.9 Note multiple rows of densely distributed lashes typical of distichiasis. (Modified from Penne RB, ed. *Wills Eye Institute— Oculoplastics.* 2nd ed. Philadelphia, PA: Wolters Kluwer; 2011.)

Riolan, just beneath the surface of the skin.[5] The gray line serves as a useful surgical landmark. An incision along the posterior edge of the gray line, followed by blunt dissection into the lid from that point, will find a natural cleavage plane between the orbicularis oculi muscle and the tarsal plate, separating the eyelid into anterior and posterior lamellae (**Fig. 2.10A**).

 *The surgical splitting of the lid margin, along the posterior edge of the gray line, is also known as a "split-lid" procedure. This is the initial step in an array of reconstructive lid surgeries (**Fig. 2.10B**).*

Meibomian Gland Orifices

Along the upper and lower lid margins, posterior to the gray line, are a series of circular openings corresponding to orifices of the ducts of the Meibomian glands (**Fig. 2.7**). These are sebaceous glands that reside within the tarsal plates. The tarsal plates are composed of dense irregular connective tissue and provide shape and some stiffness to the upper and lower eyelids. The Meibomian glands that are resident within the tarsal plates contribute most of the oily layer of the tear film and are discussed in greater detail later in this chapter.

Mucocutaneous Junction

The mucocutaneous junction of the lid margin is the area of transition between the keratinized skin of the eyelid and the mucosal lining of the conjunctiva. It begins at, or is just posterior to, the Meibomian gland orifices. Another term, *Marx's line*, is also used to describe this transition. As a practical matter, both terms are equivalent. Marx's

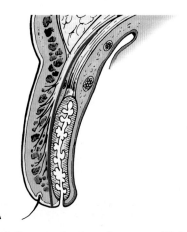
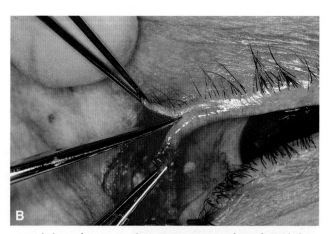

FIGURE 2.10   **A:** Cross section through upper eyelid shows natural plane of separation between anterior surface of tarsal plate and posterior surface of orbicularis oculi muscle that can be reached with an incision along the posterior edge of the gray line. (Modified from Tse DT, ed. *Color Atlas of Oculoplastic Surgery.* 2nd ed. Philadelphia, PA: Wolters Kluwer; 2011.) **B:** Clinical photograph of surgical incision along the gray line. (From Tse DT, ed. *Color Atlas of Oculoplastic Surgery.* 2nd ed. Philadelphia, PA: Wolters Kluwer; 2011.)

line was originally defined by the presence of a stippled line of vital dye staining along the lid margin in normal individuals. This line of stippled staining began at the posterior margin of the Meibomian orifices and extended posteriorly for approximately 0.1 to 0.3 mm.[6] These early findings suggested that, at the lid margin, the keratinized stratified squamous epithelium of the skin does not abruptly transition to the typical mucosal epithelium of the conjunctiva.

More recent studies of the transition area have shown that the fully keratinized epidermis of the eyelid skin gives way to an area of epithelial transition, exhibiting a stratified squamous epithelium, but one in which neither a granular cell layer (stratum granulosum) nor layers of anucleate, keratinized surface cells (stratum corneum) are present (**Fig. 2.11**). Instead, there are individual, flattened, keratinized cells that retain their nuclei. All of these features bear similarity to changes that one would expect to see in the pathologic process of parakeratosis. It is for this similarity in appearance to parakeratosis that these cells are referred to as "para-keratinized" (**Fig. 2.11**). And it is likely that these individual para-keratinized cells were those that produced the stippled line of vital dye staining identified by Marx. This region of para-keratinized cells transitions posteriorly to the normal conjunctival mucosal epithelium, which is nonkeratinized, contains goblet cells, and exhibits either a stratified cuboidal or stratified columnar epithelium. This mucosal lining of the posterior surface of the eyelids, including the epithelium and its underlying stroma, is called the palpebral portion of the conjunctiva.

Posterior to the series of lid margin landmarks discussed earlier is a recently identified, specialized region of the palpebral conjunctiva termed the *lid wiper* (**Fig. 2.12**). From these recent studies, it appears that most of the posterior surface of the normal lid does not make contact with the eye during a blink. Only a thin band of thickened,

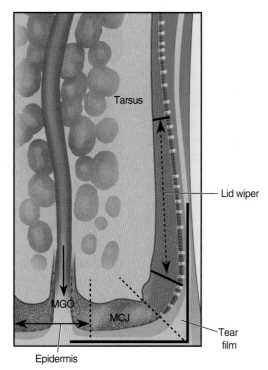

FIGURE 2.12 Lid wiper. Diagram of transition from epidermis straddling the Meibomian gland orifices (MGO), through the muco-cutaneous junction (MCJ) to the lid wiper portion of the palpebral conjunctiva.

palpebral conjunctival epithelium, contacts the eye. This strip of conjunctiva exhibits a thickened epithelium that is stratified cuboidal or columnar and includes a modest complement of goblet cells. Beyond the lid wiper region of the palpebral conjunctiva, the epithelium of the conjunctiva retains the same general architecture, but it is thinner. The lid wiper region of the palpebral conjunctiva is likely held firmly in place against the eye by tension imparted along the lid margin by the muscle of Riolan. From this recently documented anatomy, it appears that a blink should be thought of less as the broad inner surface of the lid wiping tears across the eye than as a thin windshield wiper blade, represented by the lid wiper region. The "lid wiper" skims debris and spreads a thin uniform layer of tears onto the surface of the eye. With each blink, a new smooth, optical surface is created for the eye.[7]

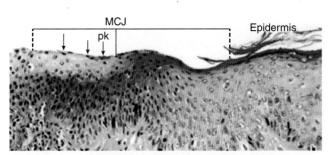

FIGURE 2.11 Light micrograph shows the mucocutaneous junction (MCJ) of the eyelid margin. Note that the non-nucleated, keratinized layers of the stratum corneum of the epidermis **(right)** give way to surface cells containing keratin (*red stain*) but with retention of their nuclei, reminiscent of parakeratosis. Posterior to this area only individual para-keratinized cells are sporadically present (*pk-arrows*). Eventually, these disappear and the typical mucosal epithelium of the conjunctiva emerges. (From Knop E, Knop N, Zhivov A, et al. The lid wiper and muco-cutaneous junction anatomy of the human eyelid margins: an in vivo confocal and histological study. *J Anat*. 2011;218(4):449–461.)

In some patients who wear silicon-hydrogel contact lenses, the edge of the contact lens can irritate the lid wiper portion of the palpebral conjunctival epithelium, as the lid wiper encounters the edge of the lens with each blink. This is called lid wiper syndrome. Affected patients may report symptoms of dry eyes because the impaired lid wiper cannot properly distribute the tear film onto the surface of the eye.[8] Both the upper and lower lids can be involved.

Gross Anatomical Organization of the Lids

The organization of the tissues within the eyelids is complex because of intricate connections with structures originating within the orbit and structures that must attach to the eye in ways that do not restrict its movement. The arrangement of these tissues is shown in **Figures 2.13** and **2.14**. In a cross section of the upper eyelid, from the anterior to the posterior surface, the following major structures are identified in the upper lid:

- Skin (epidermis and dermis)
- Orbicularis oculi muscle
- Orbital septum
- Aponeurosis of the levator palpebrae superioris
- The tarsal plate (tarsus) and its integral sebaceous glands (tarsal/Meibomian glands)
- Müller's muscle
- The palpebral conjunctiva and its associated accessory lacrimal glands of Krause and Wolfring

SKIN

As an organ, the skin is customarily divided into three layers—the epidermis, the dermis, and the hypodermis. The skin of the eyelids is very thin. The eyelid skin is also unusual in that it exhibits a highly attenuated hypodermal layer. Note the absence of a layer of adipose tissue (hypodermis) between the dermis of the lid skin and the orbicularis oculi muscle in **Figures 2.13** and **2.14**.

Epidermis

Like epidermis elsewhere, the epidermis of the lids is a keratinized, stratified squamous epithelium, including a single layer of basal cells known as the stratum germinativum, a multiple cell-layered stratum spinosum (prickle cell layer), a thin stratum granulosum (granular cell layer) and a very thin stratum corneum (keratiniazed layer) (**Fig. 2.15**). Typical rete pegs convolute the basal surface of the epidermis. Compared with most other locations on the body surface, however, the epidermis of the eyelids carries only a very thin stratum

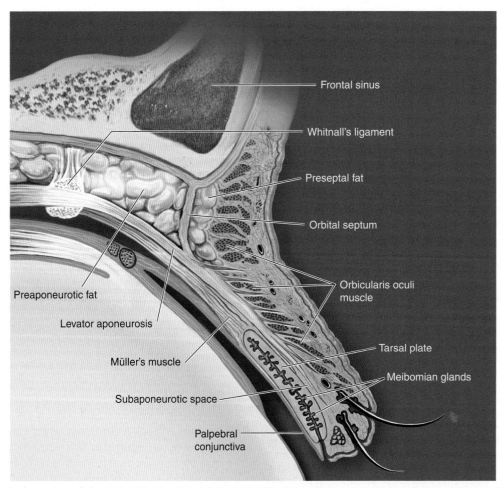

FIGURE 2.13   Cross section of the upper lid, identifying layers. (Modified from Rootman J. *Orbital Surgery.* 2nd ed. Philadelphia, PA: Wolters Kluwer; 2013.)

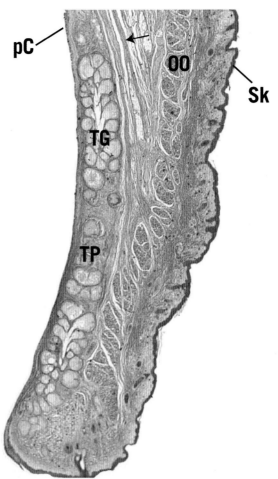

FIGURE 2.14 Photomicrograph of cross-section of the Occidental upper lid demonstrates eyelid skin (Sk), orbicularis oculi muscle (OO), tarsal plate (TP), Meibomian (tarsal) gland (TG) and palpebral conjunctiva (pC). Aponeurosis of the levator palpebrae superioris is also seen (*arrow*). Following the strands of the aponeurosis into the upper lid, it can be seen that branches insert between the fascicles of the OO muscle to reach the dermis of the lid skin anteriorly. This branching of the aponeurosis is much less prominent in the Oriental lid. (From Gartner LP, Hiatt JL. *Color Atlas and Text of Histology.* 6th ed. Philadelphia, PA : Wolters Kluwer; 2013.)

corneum of three to four layers of anucleate, fully keratinized cells. Within the epithelial layer, two other cell types are found, namely, melanocytes and Langerhan's cells. Melanocytes are distributed among the basal cells, producing the pigment that the keratinocytes carry with them as they differentiate and keratinize. The Langerhan's cells serve an immune surveillance role and are capable of antigen recognition and processing.

> *With age, loss of elastic tone in the connective tissue of the lid can result in sagging of the skin of the eyelids. This is referred to as dermatochalasis. In some cases, this redundancy can begin to interfere with vision by creating a "pseudo-ptosis" that may require surgical repair (**Fig. 2.16**).*

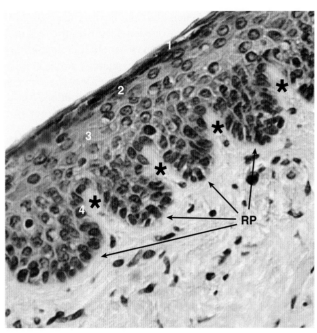

FIGURE 2.15 Photomicrograph of eyelid skin showing stratum corneum (*1*), stratum granulosum (*2*), stratum spinosum (*3*), and stratum germinativum (*4*). Rete pegs (RPs) are evident. The underlying dermis is divided into papillary dermis between adjacent rete pegs (*asterisks*) and reticular dermis below the RP.

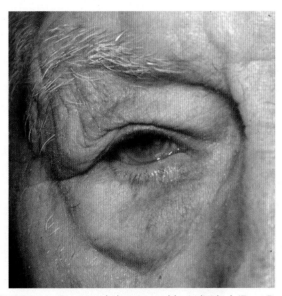

FIGURE 2.16 Dermatochalasis in an older individual. (From Penne RB, ed. *Wills Eye Institute—Oculoplastics.* 2nd ed. Philadelphia, PA: Wolters Kluwer; 2011.)

Dermis

The dermis of the skin is similar to the dermis elsewhere and is divided into two principal layers: the papillary and reticular dermis. The papillary dermis is the portion of the dermis between adjacent rete pegs of the epidermis (**Fig. 2.15**). The reticular dermis is the continuous layer of dermis below the rete pegs and above the underlying orbicularis oculi muscle (**Fig. 2.15**). The reticular dermis forms a loose areolar matrix that can be distended substantially if there is hemorrhage or edema. Within the reticular dermis are the usual skin appendages including the follicles of vellus hairs and their sebaceous glands, sweat glands, blood vessels, lymphatic channels, and sensory nerve fibers. Innervation, blood supply, and lymphatic drainage of the skin of the eyelids are described later in this chapter.

In the clinic, it is easy to forget anatomical structures that are usually seen only by microscopy of sectioned tissue, such as eccrine sweat glands in the skin. In some patients, however, ductal elements of the eccrine sweat glands, within the dermis of the eyelids, undergo benign hyperplastic changes. As they enlarge, they focally elevate the overlying skin revealing their presence and location. When they occur, their first appearance is usually after puberty. These focal, elevated lesions, called syringomas, are usually bilateral, but are rarely treated, except for cosmesis (Fig. 2.17).

ORBICULARIS OCULI MUSCLE

The orbicularis oculi muscle is responsible for closing the eyelids and is innervated by the temporal and zygomatic branches of the facial nerve (CN VII). The orientation of the muscle fibers of the orbicularis oculi muscle is parallel to the orbital rim and the lid margins around their entire circumference. The orbicularis oculi muscle extends beyond the orbital rim, onto the forehead and the cheek. This is called the orbital portion of the muscle. The portion of the muscle that is actually within the eyelid is termed the *palpebral portion* (Fig. 2.18). The palpebral portion is divided into an upper pre-septal portion and lower pre-tarsal portion, designating the lid structures that they overlie (Fig. 2.18). Additional anatomical subdivisions of the pretarsal portion that are not visible from the anterior view include Horner's muscle (pars lacrimalis) and the muscle of Riolan (pars ciliaris). All of these will be described in more detail.

The orbicularis oculi muscle is composed of skeletal muscle fibers, which when seen in cross section, are packaged

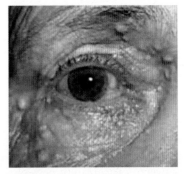

FIGURE 2.17   Multiple syringomas of the peri-orbital skin. (From Syringoma - Treatment, Removal, Pictures, Causes, Surgery, Prevention. Cancer Wall website. http://cancerwall.com/syringoma-treatment-removal-pictures-causes-surgery-prevention/. 2013. Accessed March 21, 2017.)

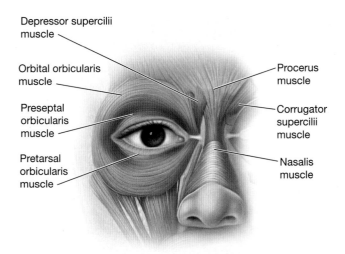

FIGURE 2.18   Sketch shows relationship between parts of the orbicularis oculi (OO) muscle and procerus, nasalis, corrugator supercilii, and depressor supercilii muscles. Visible are the orbital portion of the OO, and the palpebral segment represented by the preseptal and pretarsal portions of the muscle. (From Thorne CH, Gurtner GC, Chung K, et al, eds. *Grabb and Smith's Plastic Surgery.* 7th ed. Philadelphia, PA: Wolters Kluwer; 2013.)

into parallel fascicles separated by septae of fibrovascular connective tissue (Fig. 2.14). In all but Oriental lids, these fibrovascular septae allow for passage of strands of the aponeurosis of the levator palpebrae superioris anteriorly, making connections into the dermis (Figs. 2.13 and 2.14). These anterior extensions of the levator aponeurosis into the dermis contribute to the difference in appearance of the sulci in Oriental lids versus those of other races.

Orbital Portion

The orbital portion of the muscle does not participate in closure of the eyelids as part of the normal blink. It contracts only as part of forced closure in the presence of very bright light, or the approach of an object toward the eye. It is the thickest portion of the muscle, overlying the orbital rim, and extending onto the forehead and cheek (Fig. 2.18). This portion of the muscle blends with the frontalis muscle and corrugator (depressor) superciliaris muscle superiorly.

The corrugator (depressor) superciliaris muscle pulls the eyebrows medially, toward the bridge of the nose. Together with the procerus, which pulls the midline skin of the forehead inferiorly, they extend the tissue of the superior orbital rim anteriorly and medially, furrowing the brow and creating a ridge extending forward above the eye, to shield it from excessive light from above (Fig. 2.19). The frontalis, originating in the scalp above the orbit, pulls the periorbital skin above the orbit superiorly, raising the eyebrow and wrinkling the forehead while widening the interpalpebral fissure.

Examination of the fibers that form the orbital portion of the orbicularis oculi muscle reveals that they circumscribe a continuous arch around the lateral orbital rim as shown

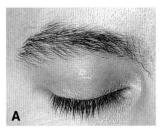 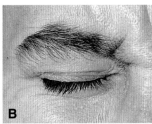

FIGURE 2.19 **A:** During a blink, or when the lid is gently closed, only the palpebral (preseptal and pretarsal) portions of the orbicularis oculi muscle contract. **B:** When tight closure is required, the orbital portion of the muscle is recruited. Simultaneous contractions of the procerus and corrugator supercilii muscles draw the brow medially and inferiorly, producing furrows. (Modified from Moore KL, Agur AMR, Dalley AF. *Clinically Oriented Anatomy.* 7th ed. Philadelphia, PA: Wolters Kluwer; 2013.)

in **Figure 2.18**. As such, the fibers of the orbicularis oculi can be thought of as originating from and inserting onto the medial orbital rim, including the maxillary process of the frontal bone above and the frontal process of the maxillary bone below. These attachments are shared with the anterior head of the medial palpebral (canthal) ligament.

Palpebral Portion

The palpebral portion of the orbicularis oculi muscle resides within the mobile portion of the eyelid. It functions as a single unit but is anatomically divided into preseptal and pretarsal portions, named for the tissues that these portions of the muscle overlie. Both of these portions contract with each blink (**Fig. 2.18**). The fibers of the palpebral portion of the orbicularis oculi in the upper and lower lids are arranged as half ellipses that are attached to the lateral and medial canthal (palpebral) ligaments. In the lateral canthal region, the hemi-ellipses of the upper and lower palpebral portions of the orbicularis oculi are described as interweaving to form what is termed the *lateral horizontal raphe*, which overlies the lateral canthal (palpebral) ligament.[9] From recently reported studies, including numerous dissections, however, the actual existence of the classically described raphe, in all lids, regardless of race, has been challenged.[10,11]

The anatomy of the medial canthal region is far more complex than that of the lateral canthal region. This is due to the presence of multiple insertions of various structures, relations with the several parts of the orbicularis oculi, and their relationships with the structures of the lacrimal drainage system. Bands of fibers, referred to as *crura*, extend medially and laterally from the tarsal plates to stabilize them in the upper and lower lids. In the medial canthal region, these bands of fibers fuse to join the medial canthal (palpebral) ligament. This ligament splits to insert as three heads (**Fig. 2.20**). The anterior head inserts onto the maxilla, anterior to the anterior lacrimal crest. This

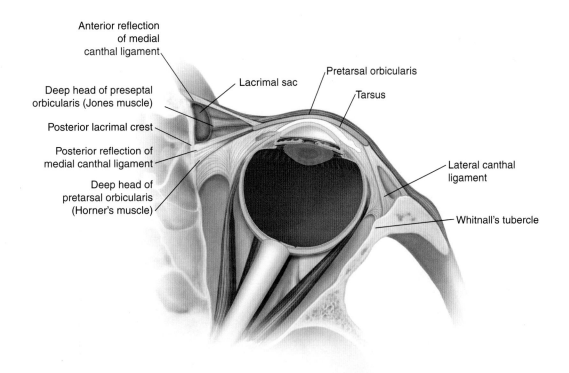

FIGURE 2.20 Horizontal section of right eye, lids and orbit viewed from above shows complex anatomical relationships between anterior and posterior reflections of the medial canthal (palpebral) ligament, orbicularis oculi muscle, and the lacrimal sac. Lateral canthal (palpebral) ligament also shown in relation to Whitnall's tubercle. Notice that both the medial and lateral canthal ligaments attach to and stabilize the edges of tarsus. (From Thorne CH, Gurtner GC, Chung K, et al, eds. *Grabb and Smith's Plastic Surgery.* 7th ed. Philadelphia, PA: Wolters Kluwer; 2013.)

positions the anterior head anterior to the lacrimal sac (**Fig. 2.20**). The posterior head inserts onto the posterior lacrimal crest, posterior to the lacrimal sac (**Fig. 2.20**). The third, superior head of the medial (canthal) palpebral ligament draws together fibers from the anterior and posterior heads and inserts onto the frontal bone above the lacrimal sac, where it is joined by the deep head of the preseptal portion of the orbicularis, a muscle segment sometimes referred to as *Jones' muscle* (**Fig. 2.20**).

Insertion of the lateral crura, together with fibers from the pretarsal portions of the orbicularis oculi muscle in the upper and lower lids, occurs at the lateral orbital (Whitnall's) tubercle, which is along the lateral orbital wall, but posterior to the orbital rim (**Fig. 2.20**). Note that the path of the medial (canthal) palpebral ligament is readily visible beneath the skin in the medial canthus, while the path of the lateral (canthal) palpebral ligament, attaching to the deeper Whitnall's tubercle, is not (**Fig. 2.18**). This more posterior position of the attachment of the lateral (canthal) palpebral ligament is believed to assist in holding the lid margins close to the surface of the eye.

Horner's Muscle: The pretarsal portion of the orbicularis oculi muscle, like the medial (canthal) palpebral ligament, inserts medially as two heads, one superficial and one deep. The superficial head merges with the anterior head of the medial (canthal) palpebral ligament to insert anterior to the lacrimal sac. The deeper heads from the upper and lower lids fuse medially to insert onto the posterior lacrimal crest, posterior to the posterior head of the medial (canthal) palpebral ligament as what is termed *Horner's muscle*. As a result, the anterior head of the medial (canthal) palpebral ligament and the superficial head of the pretarsal portion of the orbicularis insert anterior to the lacrimal sac. The posterior head of the medial (canthal) palpebral ligament, and Horner's muscle, which runs posterior to the ligament, both insert posterior to the lacrimal sac (**Fig. 2.20**).

Muscle of Riolan: The pretarsal portion of the orbicularis oculi muscle extends along the lid margin in a plane just anterior to the follicles of the eyelashes. At the lid margins, an additional, thin band of striated muscle is found posterior to the follicles of the eyelashes. This strip of muscle contracts with the palpebral portion of the orbicularis oculi. Its exact function remains under debate, but it most likely plays a role in ensuring that the lid margin, or at least the lid wiper portion of the palpebral conjunctiva, is held firmly against the surface of the eye. As noted earlier, its presence along the lid margin is generally considered to be the histologic counterpart for the grossly observable gray line.[12]

ORBITAL SEPTUM

Posterior to the plane of the orbicularis oculi muscle is the orbital septum. The orbital septum is an extension of the periorbita from the orbital rim into the lids (**Fig. 2.22**).

The line of origin for the septum, around the orbital rim, is termed the *arcus marginalis*. The septum forms the important anterior wall of the extraconal fascial compartment of the orbit. It simultaneously defines the posterior limit of a fascial compartment in the eyelids, which is termed the *preseptal space*. Infections occurring in the extraconal compartment of the orbit are prevented from unimpeded access to the lids by the orbital septum. Such infections are referred to as *orbital cellulitis*. Infections occurring anterior to the orbital septum are similarly prevented from disseminating readily into the orbit. Such infections are referred to as *preseptal cellulitis*, and these are generally less severe. Most anatomical structures passing from the extraconal compartment of the orbit onto the face must pierce this orbital septum to leave the orbit anteriorly. Exceptions include those structures passing through foramina or notches to leave the orbit, including the supraorbital and infraorbital arteries and nerves (see the section on the blood supply of the lids later in this chapter).

 *With increasing age, the elastic resiliency of the orbital septum can decrease, resulting in prolapse of the orbital fat (**Fig. 2.21**). Prolapse appears to be more common in men and occurs most often in the lateral canthal region but may appear in other locations as shown in Fig. 2.21.[13] In most cases, there are no complications. Repair is done only for cosmetic purposes.*

APONEUROSIS OF THE LEVATOR PALPEBRAE SUPERIORIS MUSCLE

The aponeurosis of the levator palpebrae superioris muscle is the medial and lateral expansion of the levator muscle's tendon, near the orbital rim (**Fig. 2.22**). This expansion allows the tendon to span across the breadth of the lid, inserting across the anterior surface of the tarsal plate. The broad insertion of the aponeurosis ensures that elevation of the lid margin occurs in a uniform manner. As discussed

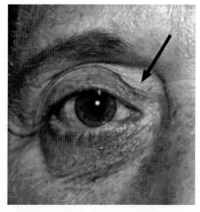

FIGURE 2.21   Mild superior medial prolapse of orbital septum (*arrow*). (Courtesy of Dr. Howard Leibowitz.)

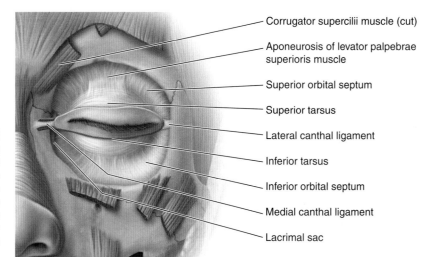

Corrugator supercilii muscle (cut)

Aponeurosis of levator palpebrae
superioris muscle

Superior orbital septum

Superior tarsus

Lateral canthal ligament

Inferior tarsus

Inferior orbital septum

Medial canthal ligament

Lacrimal sac

FIGURE 2.22 Sketch shows the superior orbital septum and inferior orbital septum extending into the lids from the orbital rim, separating the extraconal compartment of the orbit from the preseptal space of the eyelids. Also visible superiorly is the aponeurosis of the levator palpebrae superioris muscle as it broadens to attach to the superior tarsus. (Modified from Moore KL, Agur AMR, Dalley AF. *Clinically Oriented Anatomy.* 7th ed. Philadelphia, PA: Wolters Kluwer; 2013.)

in **CHAPTER 1: THE ORBITS**, the lateral edge of the aponeurosis indents all but the most lateral portion of the lacrimal gland as it passes from the orbit into the lids. In doing so, it divides the gland into two lobes, a superior orbital lobe and an inferior palpebral lobe. The latter is visible beneath the upper lid when everted. Providing support for the aponeurosis, across its breadth, just posterior to the orbital rim, is Whitnall's ligament, which is also discussed in detail in **CHAPTER 1: THE ORBITS**.

THE ORIENTAL EYELID AND THE EYELIDS OF OTHER RACES

The principal factors accounting for the difference in the superior sulcus and fold of the Oriental eyelid, compared with the sulcus of other races, are the anatomical relationships between the aponeurosis of the levator palpebrae

superioris muscle, the orbital septum, and orbicularis oculi muscle (**Fig. 2.23**). In the eyelid of Oriental individuals, the aponeurosis typically fuses with the orbital septum at a point below the superior border of the tarsus. As such, the orbital septum extends further into the eyelid. This allows for the extraconal fat pad to extend anteriorly and inferiorly within the lid. As a consequence, the typical interweaving of the aponeurosis through the pretarsal portion of the orbicularis oculi muscle and into the dermis of the eyelid skin is not present.

In the eyelids of other races, the aponeurosis fuses with the orbital septum above the superior border of the tarsus and its terminal fibers extend into and through the muscle fascicles of the orbicularis oculi muscle to insert into the dermis of the skin. This extension of the aponeurosis creates the superior palpebral sulcus typical of the eyelid appearance in these races.

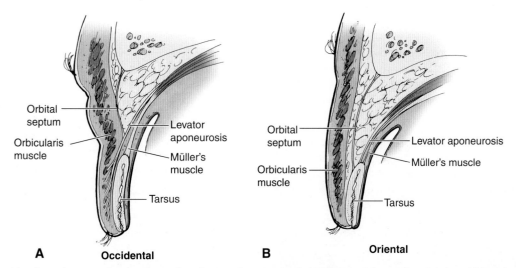

Orbital septum

Orbicularis muscle

Levator aponeurosis

Müller's muscle

Tarsus

A   **Occidental**

Orbital septum

Orbicularis muscle

Levator aponeurosis

Müller's muscle

Tarsus

B   **Oriental**

FIGURE 2.23 Sketches of cross sections of Occidental **(A)** and Oriental **(B)** eyelids. Note that in the Occidental lid, the orbital septum connects to the levator aponeurosis at a point above the tarsus. In the Oriental lid, the orbital septum extends much further into the lid, connecting directly to the tarsus. This allows the fat of the extraconal compartment of the orbit to extend into the space between the orbital septum and levator aponeurosis, all the way to the superior margin of the tarsus. (Modified from Tse DT, ed. *Color Atlas of Oculoplastic Surgery.* 2nd ed. Philadelphia, PA: Wolters Kluwer; 2011.)

THE TARSAL PLATES OR TARSI AND THE MEIBOMIAN GLANDS

The tarsal plates, or tarsi (singular: tarsus), are thick bands of dense irregular connective tissue that span most of the breadth of the upper and lower lids and provide form and additional stiffness to the structure of the lids (**Figs. 2.13** and **2.14**). The superior tarsus extends from the lid margin, approximately 9 mm into the lid. As a practical clinical matter, applying pressure to the midpoint of the upper lid, along the superior edge of this tarsal plate, allows it to be used as a pivot point to evert the upper lid for inspection of the palpebral conjunctiva.

The smaller inferior tarsus extends into the lower lid only 4 to 5 mm. The tarsal plates are stabilized by the crura that extend laterally and medially to the lateral and medial (canthal) palpebral ligaments. Within the tarsal plates are the elongated sebaceous glands called the *Meibomian glands* (**Fig. 2.14**). The upper lid usually contains approximately 30 of these glands and the lower lid contains fewer, approximately 25. The ducts of these glands exit at the lid margin, and their sebum product contributes to the oily layer of the tear film (**Fig. 2.7**).

 Using available clinical techniques, it is possible to readily image the Meibomian glands within the tarsal plates in situ and monitor changes in these glands with age and in certain diseases. In Figure 2.24, the upper lid has been everted. As such, the superior edge of the tarsal plate is at the bottom of the picture, and the lid margin, with its lashes, is at the top. With this method, it is easy to appreciate the lobules of the glands, clustered around their main ducts, all of which lead to orifices at the lid margin.[14]

MÜLLER'S MUSCLE

Unlike the levator palpebrae superioris and the orbicularis oculi muscle, Müller's muscle (i.e., the tarsal muscle) is a smooth muscle, innervated by postganglionic sympathetic nerve fibers. Within the upper lid, this muscle originates from the interior surface of the aponeurosis of the levator

palpebrae superioris muscle and inserts onto the superior edge of the tarsal plate (**Fig. 2.13**).[15] Müller's muscle assists in raising the upper lid and lowering the lower lid and in the sustained effort of holding the lids open. Interruption of the sympathetic innervation of this muscle (as in Horner's syndrome) results in a drooping of the upper lid and slight elevation of the inferior lid margin. The term used to describe an upper lid that is too low, or a lower lid that is too high, is *ptosis*.

THE RETRACTORS OF THE LOWER LID

In the absence of a skeletal muscle entering the lower lid to pull it down, there is also no aponeurosis in the lower lid. There is, however, a fascial analog that extends into the lower lid that is termed the *capsulopalpebral fascia*. In the lower lid, Müller's muscle takes origin in the capsulopalpebral fascia and from fascial extensions of the inferior extraocular muscles that form the ligament of Lockwood. From here, Müller's muscle extends into the inferior lid to reach the inferior edge of the inferior tarsal plate (**Fig. 2.25**). The Müller's muscle in the lower lid is part of a system of structures that are collectively referred to as the "lid retractors." Despite the absence of a levator palpebrae superioris analog in the lower lid, during inferior gaze, the margin of the lower lid retracts inferiorly. This appears to occur because of fascial connections between the sheath of the inferior rectus, the ligament of Lockwood, and the inferior edge of the tarsal plate. Contraction of the inferior rectus and the inferior "tarsal" muscle (Müller's muscle) pulls the tarsal plate inferiorly and, with it, the lower lid.

THE PALPEBRAL CONJUNCTIVA

The structure of the palpebral conjunctiva, beyond the lid wiper region that was described earlier, is presented in detail in **CHAPTER 5: THE CONJUNCTIVA AND THE LIMBUS**.

◉ The Glands of the Eyelids

Both unicellular and multicellular glands are found within the eyelids. The eccrine sweat glands of the eyelid skin have been mentioned earlier. The unicellular glands, termed *goblet cells*, which are distributed within the conjunctival epithelium, and the crypts of Henle in the palpebral conjunctiva are discussed in **CHAPTER 5: THE CONJUNCTIVA AND THE LIMBUS**. The remaining multicellular glands within the eyelids include the following:

- Meibomian glands
- Glands of Zeis
- Glands of Moll
- Glands of Krause
- Glands of Wolfring

An overview of the distribution of these various glands is summarized in **Figure 2.26**.

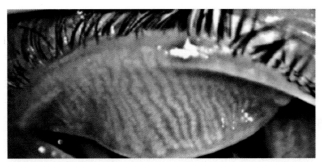

FIGURE 2.24 Clinical image of everted superior lid optimized to reveal outlines of Meibomian glands within the tarsal plate. (Courtesy of Genoptic Healthcare, South Africa.)

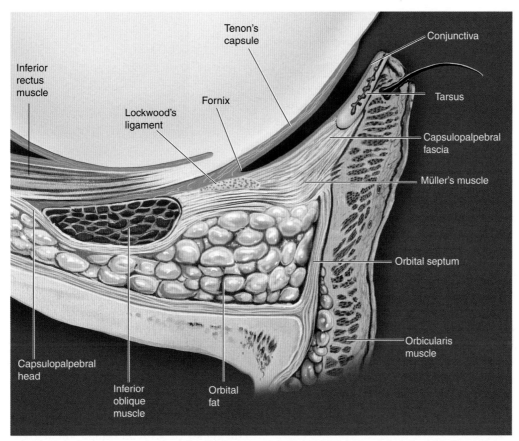

FIGURE 2.25 Sketch shows sagittal cross section through lower eyelid. The inferior rectus muscle is seen in longitudinal section and the inferior oblique muscle in cross section. The inferior Müller's (tarsal) muscle is seen taking origin from the fascia that forms the ligament of Lockwood. The inferior Müller's (tarsal) muscle then extends into the inferior lid to reach the inferior edge of the tarsal plate, together with the capsulopapebral fascia. (Updated from Rootman J. *Orbital Surgery.* 2nd ed. Philadelphia, PA: Wolters Kluwer; 2013.)

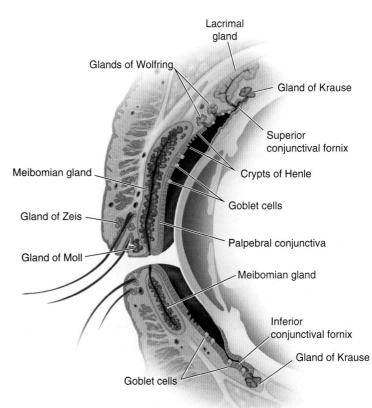

FIGURE 2.26 Artist's rendering of the relative positions and locations of the various unicellular and multicellular glands associated with the eyelids and palpebral conjunctiva.

THE MEIBOMIAN GLANDS

Meibomian glands are composed of modified sebaceous cells arranged into acini (**Fig. 2.27**). Individual cells have a small central nucleus and a cytoplasm that appears foamy because their lipid content is removed during tissue processing, leaving only the delicate intracellular matrix visible. The acini of the gland are arranged to form clusters termed *lobules*, which secrete their sebum product into lobular ductules. Ductules from each lobule lead to a single central duct, running the long axis of the gland (**Fig. 2.24**). This duct releases the product of the gland through its orifice, onto the lid margin (**Fig. 2.7**). As noted earlier, this sebum product represents most of the oily layer of the normal tear film.[16]

Although the Meibomian glands receive both sympathetic and parasympathetic fibers, it appears that regulation is not as simple as the usual "push–pull" between these two divisions of the autonomic nervous system. Immunohistochemical studies have demonstrated the existence of estrogen and androgen receptors in the glandular cells but not the cells of the ducts.[17,18] It appears that the androgen receptors support secretion and that the estrogen receptors inhibit secretion. Vasoactive intestinal peptide (VIP) positive nerves have also been identified in human Meibomian glands.[19]

The normal secretion of the Meibomian glands is clear and oily. In some conditions, however, the composition of this secretion can change, rendering it viscous and opaque. In such cases, manual expression of the contents of the gland produces a ribbon of material with a consistency more like toothpaste. Figure 2.28 shows ribbons of this expressed material clinging to the corneal surface.

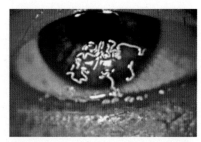

FIGURE 2.28 Expression of altered Meibomian gland secretions seen as ribbons on the corneal surface in Meibomian gland disease. (Courtesy of Dr. Howard Leibowitz.)

GLANDS OF ZEIS

Like virtually all hair follicles, the follicles of the eyelashes have sebaceous glands associated with them. In the case of the eyelashes, these sebaceous glands have gained a name. They are called the *glands of Zeis*. The cells within the glands of Zeis are virtually identical to those of the Meibomian glands. These cells are clustered into several lobules that convey their sebaceous product, via a duct, to the hair shaft of each eyelash. This oily secretion lubricates the eyelash as it grows and advances through the shaft of the follicle, toward the lid margin.

GLANDS OF MOLL

The glands of Moll are simple tubular glands that also terminate within the shafts of the eyelashes or into the duct of the follicle-associated sebaceous glands of Zeis (**Fig. 2.29**). Initially the tubules, with their relatively wide lumina, are wound into a spiral. These glands are more widely distributed in the lower than the upper lid and are less numerous than the lashes themselves, suggesting that their product is not essential to the normal maintenance of the eyelash. These glands appear similar to sweat glands; they are lined by a single row of columnar cells with their nuclei displaced toward their basal surface. Surrounding this ring of secretory cells is a variable layer of flattened myoepithelial cells, which do not appear to continue into the walls of the draining ducts. Unlike sweat glands, the glands of Moll secrete their product through the process of apocrine rather than eccrine secretion. The function of the watery product of these glands remains uncertain.

GLANDS OF KRAUSE

The glands of Krause are termed *accessory lacrimal glands*. They are found in the deep stroma and subconjunctival connective tissue of the conjunctival fornices, where the palpebral conjunctiva reflects onto the surface of the anterior third of the sclera as the bulbar conjunctiva (**Fig. 2.26**). The majority of these glands are found in the superior fornix. Current estimates are that approximately 40 such glands are found along the superior fornix and fewer than 10 are found distributed along the inferior fornix. Their histologic organization is very similar to that of the main

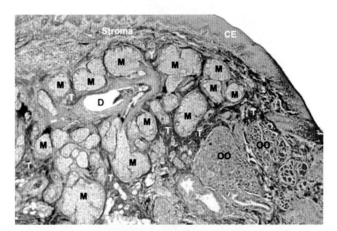

FIGURE 2.27 Photomicrograph of lid margin showing tarsal plate (*T-dark blue*) within which reside acini of a Meibomian gland (*M*) and their connections via lobular ducts to the main duct of the gland (*D*). CE, conjunctival epithelium; OO, orbicularis oculi muscle. (Courtesy of Mission for Vision and Dr. Ben Glasgow [www.missionforvision.org].)

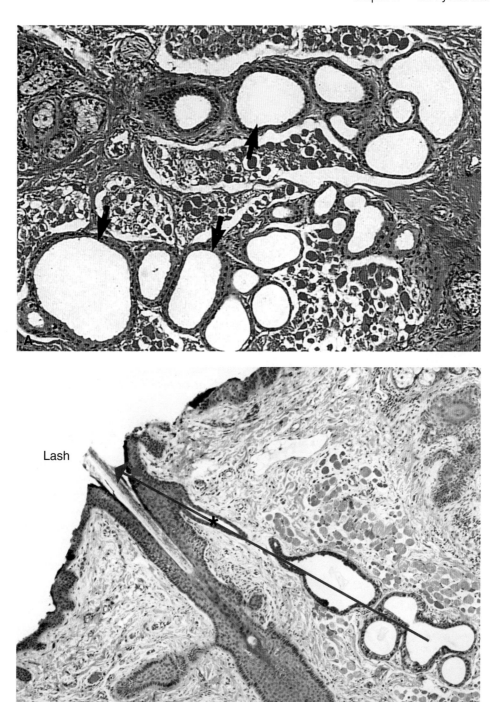

FIGURE 2.29   A: Photomicrograph of glands of Moll showing cross sections through the coils of this gland (*arrows*) that are similar to sweat glands and are lined with simple columnar epithelium surrounded by a discontinuous layer of flattened myoepithelial cells. **B:** Photomicrograph shows relationship between lash follicle and associated gland of Moll extending its duct (*asterisk*) to the shaft surrounding the eyelash (*tip of pink arrow*). (Modified from Mills SE, ed. *Histology of Pathologists.* 4th ed. Philadelphia, PA: Wolters Kluwer; 2012.)

lacrimal gland, which is discussed in **Chapter 1: The Orbits**. These glands receive both sympathetic and parasympathetic nerve fibers that work in opposition to regulate secretion. VIP positive nerves have also been found, but their function remains uncertain.[19] These glands contribute to the aqueous layer of the tear film by secreting their watery product onto the surface of the conjunctiva.

GLANDS OF WOLFRING

The glands of Wolfring are also categorized as *accessory lacrimal glands.* They differ from the glands of Krause only in their location. In the upper lids, they are located anterior to the insertion of Müller's muscle along the superior edge of the tarsal plate (**Fig. 2.26**). In the lower lid, they are distributed along the inferior edge of the tarsal plate. The glands of Wolfring are fewer in number than the glands of Krause, numbering less than 10 in the upper and 5 in the lower lid. For many years, it was assumed that the accessory lacrimal glands made only a minor and functionally insignificant contribution to the tear film. More recent data suggest that these glands can sustain a basal tear film in the absence of the main lacrimal gland. Logically, because of their greater numbers, it appears that glands of Krause are the more critical of the two. As evidence from one study, resection of glands of Wolfring, occurring during eyelid ptosis repair procedures (Fasanella-Servat), gave rise to dry eye signs and symptoms in only 6 of 144 patients after this procedure.[20]

◉ Vascular Supply

ARTERIES

The eyelids are richly vascularized. As a result, bleeding from a lid laceration can be profuse, but this rich vascular supply also assists in minimizing scarring compared with other areas of the skin. All of the tissues of the eyelids, including the palpebral conjunctiva and its associated glands, receive their arterial supply from vascular arcades, formed by the anastomosis of the medial and lateral palpebral arteries. The lateral palpebral arteries of the upper and lower lid

arise from the lacrimal artery, with a small contribution from the frontal branch of the superficial temporal artery. (**Fig. 2.30**). The medial palpebral arteries arise as direct branches of the ophthalmic artery and pierce the orbital septum above and below the trochlea to reach the medial aspect of the upper and lower lids. The orbital pathways of the lateral and medial palpebral arteries in the orbit are described in greater detail in **CHAPTER 1: THE ORBITS**.

In the upper lids, the medial and lateral palpebral arteries branch and anastomose to form two vascular arcades: the peripheral tarsal arcade and the marginal tarsal arcade. In the lower lid, there may be either one or two arcades (**Fig. 2.30**). When only a single arcade is present, its distribution within the lower lid and inferior palpebral conjunctiva is most analogous to the marginal arcade of the upper lid. These arcades anastomose with several vessels near the orbital rim, including the superficial temporal artery, the transverse facial artery and the infraorbital artery. The medial palpebral arteries also make important anastomoses with the angular artery, a terminal branch of the facial artery arising from the external carotid artery (**Fig. 2.30**).

The Peripheral Tarsal Arcade

The peripheral tarsal arcade traverses the lid, superior to the tarsal plate, in a tissue plane that is posterior to the aponeurosis of the levator palpebrae superioris and anterior to Müller's muscle (**Fig. 2.31**). Branches from this arcade

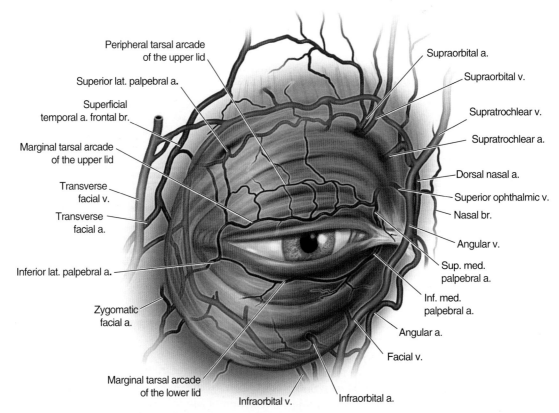

FIGURE 2.30 Arterial (*red*) and venous (*blue*) vessels of the eyelids. Note that, in this case, two arcades (peripheral and marginal) are present in the upper lid and only a single marginal arcade is present in the lower lid.

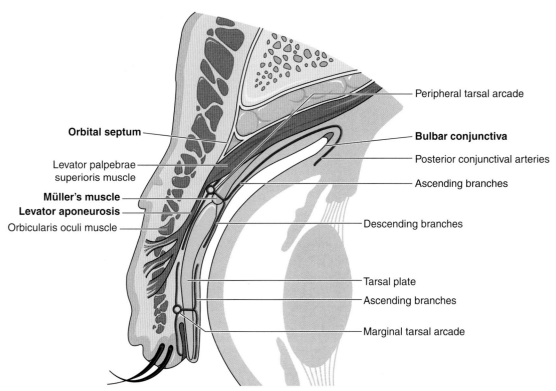

FIGURE 2.31 Sketch shows tissue planes through which the vascular arcades of the lids pass. Note an ascending branch that passes above the superior conjunctival fornix to enter the bulbar conjunctiva as the posterior conjunctival artery.

serve the superior aspect of the lid and additional branches pierce Müller's muscle to provide ascending and descending branches within the palpebral conjunctiva.

The ascending branches supply the superior palpebral conjunctiva. They then pass over and above the superior fornix to descend into the bulbar conjunctiva as the posterior conjunctival arteries (**Fig. 2.31**). The posterior conjunctival arteries serve the bulbar conjunctiva, except for a 2 to 3 mm ring around the limbus. This perilimbal area of the conjunctiva is served by superficial branches of the anterior ciliary arteries that contribute to a perilimbal marginal plexus from which the *anterior conjunctival arteries* arise. These are described in greater detail in **CHAPTER 3: OVERVIEW OF THE EYE** and **CHAPTER 5: THE CONJUNCTIVA AND THE LIMBUS**. The descending branches anastomose with ascending branches that reach the palpebral conjunctiva from the marginal tarsal arcade described below.

The Marginal Tarsal Arcade

The marginal tarsal arcade traverses the lid just above the lid margin in a tissue plane between the anterior surface of the tarsus and the posterior surface of the palpebral part of the orbicularis oculi muscle (**Fig. 2.31**). It sends branches to anastomose with descending branches from the peripheral tarsal arcade and, like the peripheral arcade, it sends branches posteriorly to reach the palpebral conjunctiva. Upon reaching the palpebral conjunctiva, ascending and descending branches arise. The ascending branches anastomose with the descending branches of the peripheral

tarsal arcade and the descending branches extend to the lid margin. Again, when only a single arcade is present in the lower lid, its vascular distribution mimics the pattern of the marginal tarsal arcade in the upper lid.

VEINS

As is generally the case in the venous system as a whole, the arrangement of the venous system within the lids is less consistent between individuals than the distribution of the arteries. The veins of the eyelids appear to form plexi in front of and behind the tarsal plate and near the superior and inferior fornices of the conjunctiva. The venous drainage of the lids, via superior and inferior papebral veins, reaches several larger veins, including the superficial temporal, supraorbital, supratrochlear, and infratrochlear veins (**Fig. 2.30**). These venous plexi also reach the anastomosis of the angular and superior ophthalmic vein.

Innervation

The skin of the eyelids and the mucosal surface of the palpebral conjunctiva receive sensory fibers from the trigeminal nerve (CN V). But what is most important clinically is appreciation of the fact that the upper lid, like the surface of the eye, lies within the sensory distributional field of the ophthalmic division of the trigeminal nerve, while the lower lid lies within the sensory distributional field of the maxillary division of the trigeminal nerve.

The central portion of the upper lid is served by branches from the supraorbital and supratrochlear nerves (**Fig. 2.32**). The lateral edge of the upper lid is served by the lacrimal nerve and medial edge of the upper lid is served by the supratrochlear and infratrochlear nerves (**Fig. 2.32**). The lower lid is served over most of its surface by branches from the infraorbital nerve, with a minor contribution from the zygomaticofacial nerve at the lateral canthal margin (**Fig. 2.32**).

INNERVATION OF THE LEVATOR PALPEBRAE SUPERIORIS

Innervation of the levator palpebrae superioris is from the superior motor division of the oculomotor nerve (CN III). Details of this motor pathway are presented in **CHAPTER 1: THE ORBITS**, as is the path of the sympathetic fibers that innervate Müller's muscle.

INNERVATION OF THE ORBICULARIS OCULI MUSCLE

Innervation of the orbicularis oculi muscle is from the facial nerve (CN VII), via its temporal and zygomatic branches, both of which enter the muscle from its temporal side

(**Fig. 2.32**). However, the innervation of the orbicularis oculi muscle is unique.

Unlike the muscles of facial expression below the eye, the orbicularis oculi muscle and the frontalis muscle exhibit bilateral cortical representation. This means that the facial motor nucleus on each side receives innervation from both sides of the cortex (**Fig. 2.33**). For the remainder of the facial muscles below the level of the eyes, innervation to the facial motor nucleus of CN VII is received solely from the contralateral side. Thus, if there is a supranuclear lesion ("X" in **Figure 2.33**) affecting the cortical fibers on the left side (which innervates the right side of the face and the frontalis and orbicularis oculi muscles on both sides) the patient can still wrinkle their forehead and partially close their eyelid on both sides, but they cannot elevate the corner of their mouth to smile on the right side. This "sparing" of the orbicularis oculi and frontalis muscles in supranuclear lesions (i.e., upper motor neuron lesions) of the seventh nerve pathway is not because peripheral nerve branches of the temporal and zygomatic branches of the two facial nerves cross the midline to innervate both sets of muscles.

By contrast, if a lesion occurs at a point below the facial motor nucleus of CN VII (i.e., lower motor neuron lesions, "Z" in **Figure 2.33**), where the inputs from the right and

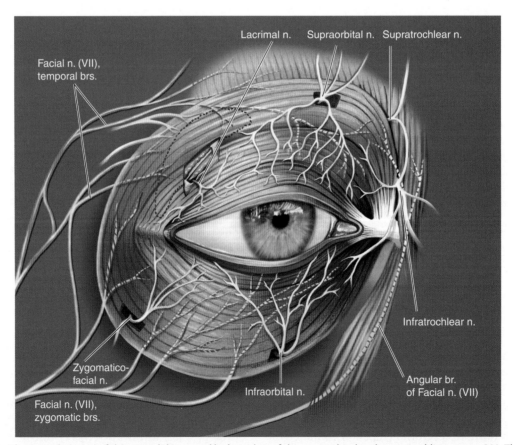

FIGURE 2.32   The central portion of the upper lid is served by branches of the supraorbital and supratrochlear nerves (V₁). The lateral edge of the upper lid is served by the lacrimal nerve (V₁) and the medial edge is served by the supratrochlear and infratrochlear nerves (V₁). The inferior lid is served primarily by branches from the infraorbital nerve (V₂). Motor innervation of the orbicularis oculi muscle from branches of the facial nerve (CN VII) are also shown. (Modified from Rootman J. *Orbital Surgery*. 2nd ed. Philadelphia, PA: Wolters Kluwer; 2013.)

left cortex have been joined together into the right or left facial nerves, sparing of the orbicularis oculi and frontalis muscles will not occur. The resulting difficulty with lid closure will leave the surface of the cornea very vulnerable and can result in dryness, corneal ulceration, and blindness.

 Fortunately, in most cases of lower motor neuron disease, partial or complete recovery occurs within months. In such cases, interim palliative measures such as use of artificial tear supplements may be sufficient to protect the cornea. In severe cases, or those that do not recover sufficiently, a surgical partial closure of the interpalpebral fissure of the lid (i.e., tarsorrhaphy) may be required, in order to protect the cornea from damaging dryness (Fig. 2.34).

Lymphatic Drainage

Lymphatics from the lateral two-thirds of the upper lid and the lateral one-third of the lower lid drain to the preauricular (superficial parotid) and occasionally to retroauricular and deep parotid lymph nodes. Drainage from the medial one-third of the upper lid and medial two-thirds of the lower lid drain to the submandibular nodes and eventually the anterior cervical nodes (**Fig. 2.35**).

The Lacrimal Drainage System

The lacrimal puncta at the medial end of the upper and lower lid margins (**Figs. 2.5** and **2.36**) are the openings into small canals (i.e., canaliculi) that drain tears, cell debris, dust, and microbes from the ocular surface, to the inferior meatus of the nasal cavity and ultimately to the gastrointestinal system. The superior canaliculus initially travels upward for 2 to 3 mm and then turns medially, running an inferomedial course that is approximately 8 mm in length. The transition from the vertical to the inferomedial part of the canaliculus is referred to as its *ampulla*. The inferior canaliculus runs initially downward for 2 to 3 mm before turning superomedially at its ampulla to reach the lacrimal sac. In most cases, the superior and inferior canaliculi join to form a common canaliculus, which then enters the lateral wall of the lacrimal sac at a point approximately 2 to 3 mm below the superior limit of the sac (**Fig. 2.36**). In a minority of cases, the upper and lower canaliculi do not form a common canaliculus, but enter the wall of the lacrimal sac separately. By following movement of a tracer with imaging methods, it has been shown that the superior and inferior lacrimal canaliculi share equally in the volume of tears they convey.[21]

The lacrimal canaliculi are approximately 0.5 mm in diameter and are lined by a nonkeratinized, stratified squamous epithelium, surrounded by elastic connective tissue.

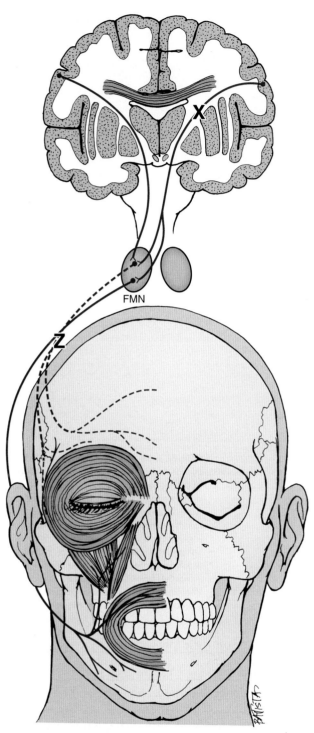

FIGURE 2.33 Cranial nerve VII (CN VII) innervation of the orbicularis oculi (OO) muscle. Sketch depicts bilateral cortical input to right facial motor nucleus (FMN), serving the right OO muscle via the temporal and zygomatic branches of CN VII (*dashed red lines*). Bilateral cortical representation of this muscle is projected to the FMN. The same is not true for muscles of facial expression served by lower branches of CN VII in the face (*solid red line*), which receive input from only the contralateral motor cortex. If a lesion occurs at *X*, the patient will have continued function of their orbicularis oculi and frontalis muscle on the right side but will lose function of muscles below the eyes. If a lesion occurs below the facial motor nucleus (*Z*), normal function of all facial muscles on the right side will be compromised. (From Oatis CA. *Kinesiology.* 3rd ed. Philadelphia, PA: Wolters Kluwer; 2016.)

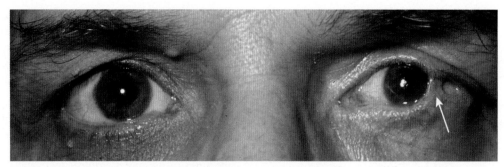

FIGURE 2.34 Tarsorrhaphy of left eyelids narrows interpalpebral fissure (*arrow*) to reduce tear loss from evaporation. (Courtesy of Dr. Howard Leibowitz.)

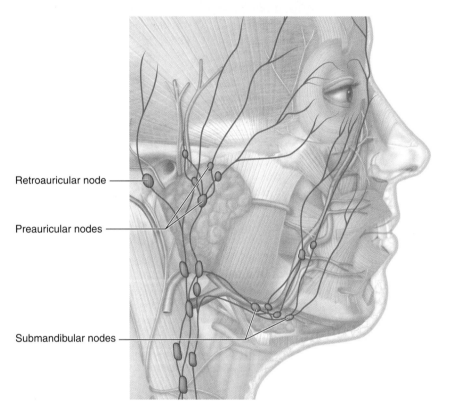

Retroauricular node

Preauricular nodes

Submandibular nodes

FIGURE 2.35 Lymphatic drainage from the eyelids and conjunctiva. The lateral two-thirds of the upper lid and the lateral one-third of the lower lid commonly drain to preauricular (superficial parotid) nodes. Occasional drainage to retroauricular nodes or deep parotid nodes is also found. The medial third of the upper lids and the medial two-thirds of the lower lid drain primarily to the submandibular nodes. (Modified from Tank PW, Gest TR. *Lippincott Williams & Wilkins Atlas of Anatomy*. 1st ed. Philadelphia, PA: Wolters Kluwer; 2008.)

Because of its thin wall and elasticity, the canaliculus can be dilated with graduated diameter probes to nearly three times its normal width, when blockages occur. The lacrimal sac, situated within the lacrimal fossa, is enveloped by fascia derived from the periorbita. This fascia extends from the posterior to the anterior lacrimal crest.

From the lacrimal sac, the nasolacrimal drainage system continues inferiorly as nasolacrimal duct. A rich vascular plexus surrounds the inferior portions of the nasolacrimal system in the canal and is continuous with a similar plexus within the mucosa of the inferior turbinate process. This plexus is termed the *cavernous body*. The opening of the nasolacrimal duct is in the lateral wall of the nasal cavity, beneath the inferior turbinate process. From this opening, tears drain onto the floor of the nasal cavity (i.e., roof of the hard palate). The floor of the nasal cavity is sloped inferiorly from anterior to posterior, thus draining tears over

the soft palate onto the tongue and then to the esophagus via the oropharynx. As a result, patients can taste certain eyedrops after they are administered.

As a reminder that the lacrimal sac and nasolacrimal duct make connections to the nasal cavity, these structures are lined by a modified form of respiratory epithelium and exhibit stratified columnar cells, microvilli, tufts of kinociliae, and a complement of goblet cells.[22]

Several "valves" have been described along the pathway of the lacrimal drainage system. Most are merely folds in the mucosa of the lacrimal sac and duct or strictures created by angulations in the anatomical position of the sac and duct. The two most constant are the valves of Rosenmuller and Hasner. The valve of Rosenmuller is simply a stricture created at the angled entry of the common canaliculus into the wall of the lacrimal sac. Incompetence of this valve can result in a reflux of air escaping the puncta when the individual

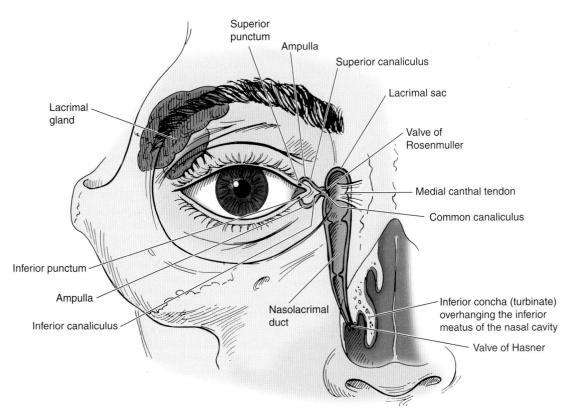

FIGURE 2.36 Major structures of the lacrimal drainage pathway are shown. (Modified from Tse DT, ed. *Color Atlas of Oculoplastic Surgery.* 2nd ed. Philadelphia, PA: Wolters Kluwer; 2011.)

In some infants, the nasolacrimal duct, at its most inferior point, fails to fully canalize at the time of birth. In cases where opening of the valve of Hasner remains incomplete, the stagnant fluid in the nasolacrimal fluid may become infected, leading to inflammation and swelling of the lacrimal sac and overlying tissues (i.e., dacryocystits). Management is usually conservative, allowing the system to open on its own. This usually occurs within 6 months of birth. Opening the duct by probing the lacrimal system can be accomplished, if required.

blows their nose or sneezes. The most constantly present valve in the lacrimal drainage system is at the inferior end of the nasolacrimal duct and is termed the *valve of Hasner.*

The position of the lacrimal drainage pathway can be revealed using imaging. Indeed, following instillation of topical contrast agents, these same methods can be used clinically to identify blockages in the system (**Fig. 2.37**).

The anatomically complex part of the lacrimal drainage system is the way in which the relationship between the canaliculi, lacrimal sac, and the muscles and ligaments that close the lids, assist in the movement of tears through the system. There are numerous theories attempting to explain how this occurs.[23–28] Recall that the pretarsal portion of the orbicularis oculi muscle splits into a superficial and

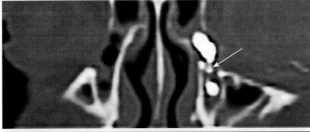
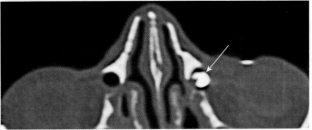

FIGURE 2.37 Upper figure shows a coronal section of the right and left lacrimal drainage system (**Orbits at top—right and left**), with the nasal cavity shown in the midline. Note contrast material in the lacrimal drainage system on left side of the image uniformly fills the lacrimal system and accumulates in the inferior meatus of the nasal cavity. On the right side of the photo, contrast material has accumulated within and distended the lacrimal sac (*just above arrow*) owing to partial obstruction of the nasolacrimal duct (*arrow*). Lower image shows axial (transverse) view in which the unobstructed side has drained its contrast material and the duct is shown as black, whereas contrast material remains in the duct on the partially obstructed side (*arrow*). (Modified from Hasso AN, ed. *Diagnostic Imaging of the Head and Neck.* Philadelphia, PA: Wolters Kluwer, 2011.)

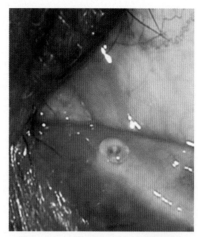

FIGURE 2.38 Note the presence of a lacrimal plug in the inferior punctum. (From Treatment of Dry Eye. Eye Plastics® website. https://www.eyeplastics.com/dry-eye-treatment-punctal-plugs-silicone-plugs-collangen-plugs.html. 2017. Accessed March 21, 2017.)

deep head. The superficial head merges with the anterior head of the medial (canthal) palpebral ligament to insert anterior to the lacrimal sac (**Fig. 2.20**). The deeper heads from the upper and lower lids fuse medially to form Horner's muscle, which inserts onto the posterior lacrimal crest (**Fig. 2.20**). En route to their insertions, the superficial and deep heads encircle the canaliculi. Both of these portions of the pretarsal orbicularis oculi muscle contract with the blink, squeezing the lacrimal sac between them. Most theories concur that this contraction initially creates a positive pressure in the sac that moves its aliquot of tears from the previous blink into the nasal cavity, leaving behind a negative pressure in the lacrimal sac that then draws tears in, via the puncta and canaliculi, as the orbicularis relaxes. Some theories also suggest that these contractions shorten the canaliculi, assisting in the movement of tears toward the lacrimal sac. But there is no consensus on the mechanics of the process overall.[29]

In cases of dry eye, symptomatic relief can sometimes be obtained by blocking the lacrimal drainage system, thus ensuring that the reduced volume of tears is lost only by evaporation and not by drainage. Commercially available punctal plugs can be inserted into one or both puncta in order to block access to the canaliculi. They can usually be removed if problems develop (Fig. 2.38).

REFERENCES

1. Francis IC, Loughhead JA. Bell's phenomenon. A study of 508 patients. *Aust J Opthalmol.* 1984;12(1):15–21.
2. Amador GJ, Mao W, DeMercurio P, et al. Eyelashes divert airflow to protect the eye. *J R Soc Interface.* 2015;12(105). doi:10.1098/rsif.2014.1294.
3. Elder MJ. Anatomy and physiology of eyelash follicles: Relevance to lash ablation procedures. *Ophthal Plast Reconstr Surg.* 1997;13(1):21–25.
4. Johnstone MA, Albert DM. Prostaglandin-induced hair growth. *Surv Ophthalmol.* 2002;47:S185–S202.
5. Wulc AE, Dryden RM, Khatchaturian T. Where is the gray line? *Arch Ophthalmol.* 1987;105(8):1092–1098.
6. Marx E. Über vitale färbungen am auge und an den lidern [in German]. *Graefes Arch Clin Exp Ophthalmol.* 1924;114(3):465–482.
7. Knop E, Knop N, Zhivov A, et al. The lid wiper and muco-cutaneous junction anatomy of the human eyelid margins: an in vivo confocal and histological study. *J Anat.* 2011;218(4):449–461.
8. Korb DR, Herman JP, Greiner JV, et al. Lid wiper epitheliopathy and dry eye symptoms. *Eye Contact Lens.* 2005;31(1):2–8.
9. Bron AJ, Tripathi RC, Tripathi BJ. *Wolff's Anatomy of the Eye and Orbit.* 8th ed. London: Chapman and Hall Medical; 1997:46.
10. Goold L, Kakizaki H, Malhotra R, et al. Absence of lateral palpebral raphe in Caucasians. *Clin Ophthalmol.* 2009;3:391–393.
11. Kakizaki H, Zako M, Nakano T, et al. No raphe identified in the orbicularis oculi muscle. *Okajimas Folia Anat Jpn.* 2004;81(5):93–96.
12. Lipham WJ, Tawfik HA, Dutton JJ. A histologic analysis and three-dimensional reconstruction of the muscle of Riolan. *Ophthal Plast Reconstr Surg.* 2002;18(2):93–98.
13. Viana GA, Osaki MH, Filho VT, et al. Prolapsed orbital fat: 15 consecutive cases. *Scand J Plast Reconstr Surg Hand Surg.* 2009;43(6):330–334.
14. Finis D, Ackermann P, Pischel N, et al. Evaluation of meibomian gland dysfunction and local distribution of meibomian gland atrophy by non-contact infrared meibography. *Curr Eye Res.* 2014;40(10):982–989.
15. Beard C. Muller's superior tarsal muscle: anatomy, physiology, and clinical significance. *Ann Plast Surg.* 1985;14(4):324–333.
16. Jester JV, Nicolaides N, Smith RE. Meibomian gland studies: histologic and ultrastructural investigations. *Invest Ophthalmol Vis Sci.* 1981;20(4):537–547.
17. Esmaeli B, Harvey JT, Hewlett B. Immunohistochemical evidence for estrogen receptors in meibomian glands. *Ophthalmology.* 2000;107(1):180–184.
18. Auw-Haedrich C, Feltgen N. Estrogen receptor expression in meibomian glands and its correlation with age and dry-eye parameters. *Graefes Arch Clin Exp Ophthalmol.* 2003;241(9):705–709.
19. Seifert P, Spitznas M. Vasoactive intestinal polypeptide (VIP) innervation of the human eyelid glands. *Exp Eye Res.* 1999;68(6):685–692.
20. Pang NK, Newsom RW, Oestreicher JH, et al. Fasanella—Servat procedure: indications, efficacy, and complications. *Can J Ophthalmol.* 2008;43(1):84–88.
21. Daubert J, Nik N, Chandeyssoun PA, et al. Tear flow analysis through the upper and lower systems. *Ophthal Plast Reconstr Surg.* 1990;6(3):193–196.
22. Paulsen F, Thale A, Kohla G, et al. Functional anatomy of human lacrimal duct epithelium. *Anat Embryol (Berl).* 1998;198(1):1–12.
23. Becker BB. Tricompartment model of the lacrimal pump mechanism. *Ophthalmology.* 1992;99(7):1139–1145.
24. Jones LT, Wobig JL. The Wendell L. Hughes lecture. Newer concepts of tear duct and eyelid anatomy and treatment. *Trans Sect Ophthalmol Am Acad Ophthalmol Otolaryngol.* 1977;83(4, pt 1):603–616.
25. Rosengren B. On lacrimal drainage. *Ophthalmologica.* 1972;164(6):409–421.
26. Jones LT. An anatomical approach to problems of the eyelids and lacrimal apparatus. *Arch Ophthalmol.* 1961;66(1):111–124.
27. Doane MG. Blinking and the mechanics of the lacrimal drainage system. *Ophthalmology.* 1981;88(8):844–851.
28. Thale A, Paulsen F, Rochels R, et al. Functional anatomy of the human efferent tear ducts: a new theory of tear outflow mechanism. *Graefes Arch Clin Exp Ophthalmol.* 1998;236(9):674–678.
29. Tanenbaum M, Mccord C Jr. Lacrimal drainage system. In: *Duane's ophthalmology on CD ROM.* Philadelphia, PA: Lippincott Williams & Wilkins; 2006.

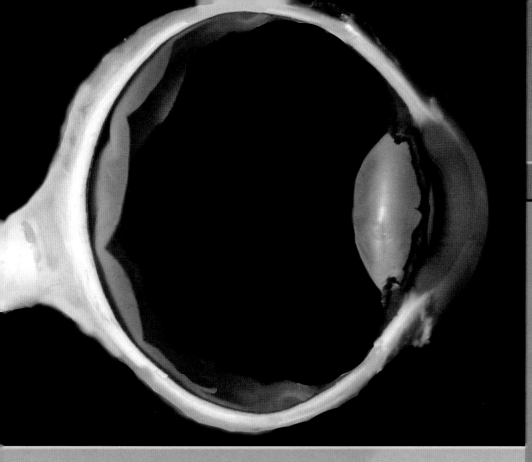

OVERVIEW OF
THE EYE

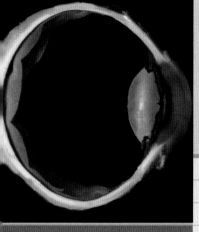

Overview of the Eye

CHAPTER 3

Overview

The eye is the organ of sight. Through a remarkable system that includes living tissues that are optically clear and remain viable without a blood supply, this organ focuses light onto photosensitive cells that can convert the absorption of photons into neural messages that, when processed by the visual pathways, provide us with a dynamic visual representation of our environment. To do so, it must provide a means of addressing all of the optical requirements of imaging, including control of the distance between the optical elements and the focal plane, minimizing optical aberrations, control of brightness and contrast, depth of focus and depth of field, and continual maintenance of the critical surface of this optical system. And it must be capable of readjusting and optimizing these parameters over a broad range of illumination levels and, ideally, at any distance. At the same time, it must provide a means of keeping all of the parts of this complex biologic system alive and healthy. This includes meeting each tissue's unique metabolic demands, replenishing certain cell populations, selectively removing or suppressing foreign antigens, warding off infection, minimizing the deleterious effects of ultraviolet and infrared light, while maintaining a relatively constant intraocular pressure and repairing tissues when injured.

Shape and Dimensions of the Eye

The eye is never a perfect sphere because the clear cornea invariably has a steeper radius of curvature than the sclera, with which it forms the external wall of the eye. The apex of the cornea is termed the anterior pole of the eye. The posterior pole of the eye is the point where a line drawn perpendicular to the corneal apex intersects the posterior surface of the sclera along the horizontal equator of the eye (**Fig. 3.1**).

Human eyes are consistently asymmetric around their horizontal equator due to the fact that the optic nerve is not at the posterior pole of the eye. Instead, the optic nerve is displaced to the nasal side of the posterior pole by approximately 3 mm and is also offset vertically, with its center lying 1 mm inferior to the horizontal equator of the eye. As a result, the circumferential distances along the horizontal equator, from the nasal and temporal sides of the optic nerve, to the center of the cornea, are unequal. The temporal dimension is invariably longer (**Fig. 3.1**). Generally, the larger the eye becomes (i.e., the more myopic), the more disparate these two dimensions become.

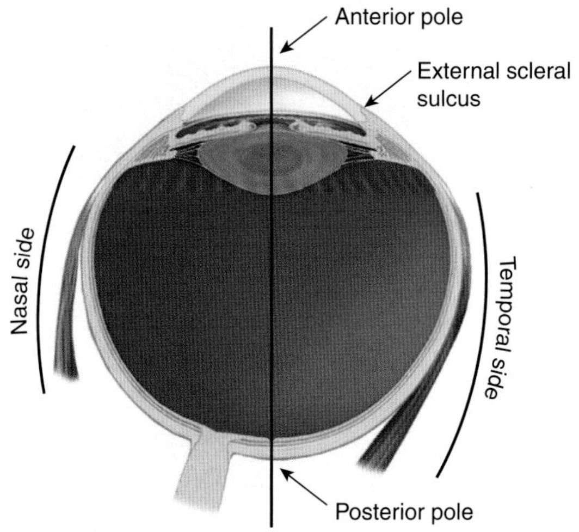

FIGURE 3.1 Sketch of a right eye sectioned at its horizontal equator showing positions of anterior and posterior poles and change in contour at external scleral sulcus. Note that the circumferential distance from the anterior pole to the optic nerve (in yellow) is greater on the temporal than the nasal side. (From Thorne CH, Gurtner GC, Chung K, et al, eds. *Grabb and Smith's Plastic Surgery*. 7th ed. Philadelphia, PA: Wolters Kluwer; 2013.)

The vertical equatorial diameter of the eye averages 23.2 mm. The horizontal equatorial diameter is slightly greater, averaging 24 mm. There is evidence that adult male eyes are slightly larger than those of adult females.[1] But these dimensions are all less variable than the anteroposterior diameter of the eye.

The average anteroposterior (i.e., axial) length of the adult human eye is 24.2 mm. Most eyes range from 22 to 27 mm.[1] Because axial length is more often the major determinant of refractive errors than is corneal curvature, eyes with shorter axial lengths are more likely to be hyperopic and those with longer axial lengths are more likely to by myopic. Highly hyperopic eyes may be as short as 20 mm and highly myopic eyes as long as 29 mm.[1]

A rough but useful clinical guide is that for every 1 mm of change in axial length, longer or shorter than the average of 24 mm, one can expect a shift in myopic or hyperopic refractive error of approximately 3 D.

Clinical measurement of the anteroposterior (i.e., axial) length of the eye can be readily obtained using commercially available ultrasonography instruments (Figs. 3.2 and 3.3). Axial length measurements (ideally, meaning measurement of the visual axis) are routinely taken before cataract surgery because anteroposterior length of the eye is one of the key parameters in algorithms that calculate the power of the intraocular lens to be used to replace the cataractous lens of the eye, once it has been removed. Figure 3.2 shows a typical scan of an eye with an axial length of 24.31 mm. Figure 3.3 shows the anatomic structures corresponding to the amplitude spikes shown in Figure 3.2. (Courtesy of Accutome, Co.)

◉ External Landmarks

The external landmarks of the anterior half of the eye are few. Among these landmarks is the line of demarcation between the clear cornea and white sclera, termed the limbus. Also visible is the iris. At its center is the variable aperture of the visual system, the pupil, which is slightly displaced to the nasal side, as evident in the enucleated left eye shown in **Figure 3.4**. Also visible in this specimen are the cut stumps of three of the four rectus muscles.

Viewed from the posterior surface, several anatomic landmarks are evident on the surface of the enucleated eye. The most obvious of these is the transected end of the optic nerve and its surrounding meningeal coverings. Upon reaching the eye, the dura mater surrounding the optic nerve blends with the sclera (**Fig. 3.5A** and **B**).

Visible in **Figure 3.5A** are the exits of the four vortex veins, one in each quadrant of the posterior segment of the eye. Temporal to the optic nerve, where a patch of blood is seen on the specimen, is the insertion of the inferior oblique (IO) muscle (**Fig. 3.5A**). On the sketch in **Figure 3.5B**, one can see all of these same landmarks, plus the locations of the extraocular muscles.

Medial to the optic nerve, running along the horizontal equator of the eye in **Figure 3.5A**, one can see the medial long posterior ciliary artery (LPCA). Unseen is the accompanying long ciliary nerve. The temporal LPCA and its accompanying long ciliary nerve are obscured in the specimen by the insertion of the IO and the surrounding patch of blood. Moving anteriorly from its entrance into the sclera, the neurovascular bundle composed of the LPCA and the long ciliary nerve gradually disappears into the thickness of the sclera. This disappearance is mirrored on the inside of the eye by the appearance of this bundle, at or near the intersection of the horizontal and vertical equators of the eye. Inside of the eye, the path of the

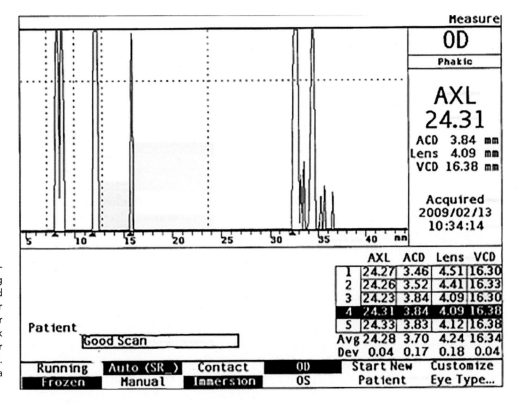

FIGURE 3.2 Print-out of clinical ultrasound scan identifying major structures of the eye and calculating antero-posterior length. Large double peak at far left represents cornea. Tall peak at far right represents posterior scleral surface (see Figure 3.3). (Courtesy of Accutome: A Halma Company.)

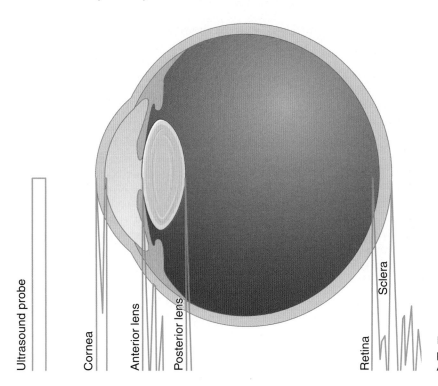

Ultrasound probe

Cornea

Anterior lens

Posterior lens

Retina

Sclera

FIGURE 3.3 Anatomical correspondence of peaks shown in Figure 3.2. (Courtesy of Accutome: A Halma Company.)

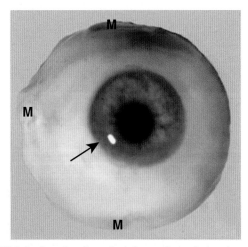

FIGURE 3.4 Anterior view of a left eye shows limbus (*arrow*) and cut stumps of superior, medial, and inferior rectus muscles (*M*). Note that the pupil is displaced slightly to the nasal side of the iris.

LPCAs provides a useful clinical landmark representing the horizontal equator of the eye.

Finally, best seen in **Figure 3.5B** are the numerous short posterior ciliary arteries that pierce the sclera very near the optic nerve. The remaining small vessels seen on the surface of the enucleated eye in **Figure 3.5A** are contained within the thin, vascularized layer of connective tissue overlying the sclera that is appropriately called the episclera. Finally, unseen but superficial to the episclera is the transparent, fascial covering of the eye, called Tenon's capsule (or the fascia bulbi). The fascia bulbi envelops the eye, beginning beneath the bulbar conjunctiva at

the limbus and blending with the dura mater of the optic nerve in the posterior pole.

Axes, Angles, and Sections of the Eye

Several axes related to the eye have been defined, largely in order to compensate for the fact that the eye is asymmetric in shape. This asymmetry accounts for why a line connecting the apical center of the cornea, with the point of maximal diameter on the posterior scleral wall (the geometrical axis of the eye), does not correspond with the line connecting the fovea of the retina with the object of regard in visual space.[2] Compensating for this offset is often critical in procedures that seek to alter one or more of the refractive elements of the eye (i.e., refractive surgery or placement of intraocular lenses), or procedures that involve assessing or changing the relative positions of the two eyes with respect to each other (e.g., strabismus surgery or measurement of interpupillary distance).[2–4]

Some of these axes are based upon anatomically definable points on and within the eye, such as the point of reflection of a small light directed at the center of the cornea, and the observable center of the pupil. Others are based upon theoretically calculated points, including the positions of nodal points and the entrance pupil of the light path within the eye. The entrance pupil of the eye is the virtual image of the anatomic pupil as viewed clinically through the aqueous humor in the anterior chamber and the cornea. It is larger than the actual size of the physical pupil.

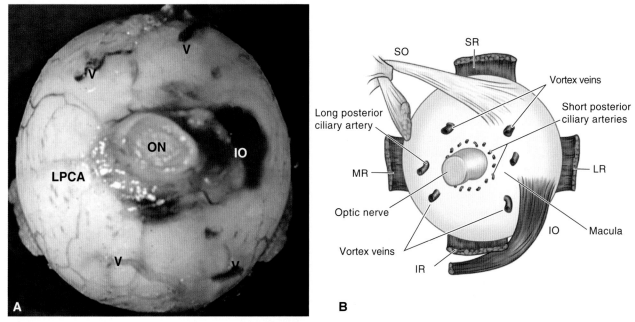

FIGURE 3.5 A: Posterior view of a right eye shows transected optic nerve (ON) and its surrounding meningeal coverings. Locations of four vortex veins (V), one in each quadrant, are seen, along with the insertion of inferior oblique (IO) muscle. The gradual disappearance of the medial long posterior ciliary artery (LPCA), as it passes anteriorly along the horizontal equator, is also seen. **B:** Sketch of the posterior view of a right eye shows landmarks visible in **(A)**, plus ring of short posterior ciliary arteries surrounding the ON. Insertions of the four, rectus muscles and two obliques are also seen. IR, inferior rectus; LR, lateral rectus; MR, medial rectus; SO, superior oblique; SR, superior rectus. (Modified from Chern KC, Saidel MA, eds. *Ophthalmology Review Manual.* 2nd ed. Philadelphia, PA: Wolters Kluwer; 2011.)

AXES OF THE EYE

The principal defined axes of the eye are illustrated in **Figure 3.6**. Each of these are discussed in the following sections.

The Visual Axis

The visual axis is the light path extending from the object of visual attention, through nodal points (N and N′) to the fovea of the retina.

The Optical Axis

The optical axis is a line perpendicular to the corneal apex that passes through the nodal points and the centers of curvature of the refracting elements of the eye. Because the fovea is temporally displaced within the retina, it does not fall along this axis. The optical axis assumes that all the optical elements of the eye and pupil are centered relative to each other and in most eyes these elements are slightly

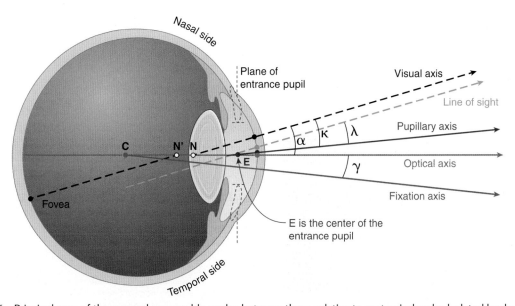

FIGURE 3.6   Principal axes of the eye and measurable angles between them, relative to anatomical and calculated landmarks such as the nodal points (N, N′), the entrance pupil (E) and the center of rotation of the eye (C). (Modified from: Thorne CH, Gurtner GC, Chung K, et al, eds. *Grabb and Smith's Plastic Surgery.* 7th ed. Philadelphia, PA: Wolters Kluwer; 2013.)

displaced. However, its location can be approximated and it serves as a useful reference axis for other axes. The term geometrical axis approximates the optical axis.

Pupillary Axis

The pupillary axis is defined by a line perpendicular to the apex of the cornea that passes through the center of the pupil (actually through the entrance pupil) of the eye. If the optical elements and the pupil in an eye were centered relative to each other, the pupillary axis and the optical axis would be coincident.

Line of Sight

The line of sight is defined as a line passing from the center of the pupil (actually the entrance pupil) to the object of visual attention. As a practical matter, the line of sight is determined by having the patient look directly and monocularly at a penlight presented directly in front of the eye, at a distance of approximately three feet, and noting the position of the point of reflection of that light from the corneal surface (i.e., Purkinje image I).

In normal adults, this light reflex is displaced approximately 0.5 mm to the nasal side of the observed center of the pupil (see left eye in **Fig. 3.7**). This same displacement in infant eyes is greater, averaging nearly 1 mm. As a result of this displacement, the pupillary axis and the line of sight (visual axis) are not anatomically the same.

Comparisons can be made between the corneal reflexes of the patient's two eyes as well (Fig. 3.7). Note that in the left eye, the light reflex is displaced just slightly to the nasal side of the center of the pupil, whereas in the right eye, the light reflex is coincident with the temporal edge of the pupil. This is called the Hirschberg test and is used in estimating the magnitude of a strabismus.

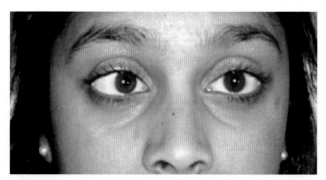

FIGURE 3.7 Comparison of corneal light reflexes in normal left eye and strabismic right eye. (Courtesy of Dr. Joseph Bonnano and the Indiana University School of Optometry, Bloomington, IN.)

As mentioned earlier, the offsets between these defined axes can be critical in an array of diverse clinical procedures, from centering the alignment of the laser system used in refractive surgery, to calculating the power of intraocular lenses, or assessment of the angle of deviation in cases of strabismus. As such, not only are these various axes important but the various angles subtended between them are important as well.

ANGLES BETWEEN AXES

The relationships between certain pairs of these various axes are defined by their angles of separation. By convention they are named using Greek letters and are summarized in **Table 3.1**. All of the principal defined angles (**Fig. 3.6**). are discussed in the following sections.

Angle Alpha (α)

The angular separation between the optical axis and visual axis.

Angle Kappa (κ)

The angular separation between the pupillary axis and the visual axis (as defined above). As a practical matter, these lines may be considered to be clinical approximations of the angle between the optical axis and the visual axis of the eye.[5]

Angle Lambda (λ)

The angle lambda is the angle formed between the pupillary axis and the line of sight. For most clinical purposes, the difference between the line of sight and the visual axis is considered to be negligible as they are very close to each other at the cornea and the center of the entrance pupil. Thus the difference between the angle kappa and angle lambda is also considered by many to be negligible.

Angle Gamma (γ)

This less broadly used term refers to the angle between the optical axis defined as above and the fixation axis. The fixation axis is defined as a line connecting the object of visual attention with the center of rotation of the eye,

TABLE 3.1 Angles Formed between Various Ocular Axes

	Visual Axis	Line of Sight	Fixation Axis
Pupillary axis	κ	λ	
Optical axis	α		γ

Adapted from Measurement of Eye Position and Motion. Oculomotor Functions and Neurology CD-ROM website for the Indiana University School of Optometry. http://www.opt.indiana.edu/v665/CD /CD_Version/CH4/CH4.HTM. 2004. Accessed March 21, 2017.

which is approximately 13 to 13.5 mm behind the surface of the cornea, in the center of the vitreous cavity (**Fig. 3.6**).

PLANE AND AXES RELATED TO MOTION

Because the eye is capable of motion in any direction, there are also axes that define its movements. In motions originating from the primary position of gaze, it is assumed that the center of rotation of the eye does not move up or down, laterally or temporally, or in or out. Instead, it theoretically remains within a fixed plane, orthogonal to the line of sight. This is called Listing's plane.[6] The axes of possible rotation in the X, Y, and Z directions are defined as Fick's axes and all three converge at the center of rotation of the eye (**Fig. 3.8**).

◉ Definition of Planes and Sections of the Eye

As in general anatomy, planes and sections are defined from the position of the eye when the individual is in anatomical position. For the eye, one must first stipulate that the head is in anatomical position. With the head in anatomical position, the eye is directed toward a distant object that is neither higher nor lower than the eye itself and no convergence of the two eyes has been induced. This is also referred to as the "primary position of gaze" and appears to be an actively maintained position rather than simply the neutral position to which the eye comes to rest when all extraocular muscles are fully relaxed and exert only tonic tension.[7]

CORONAL

Coronal sections are any sections made parallel to the coronal plane. The coronal plane is a vertical plane

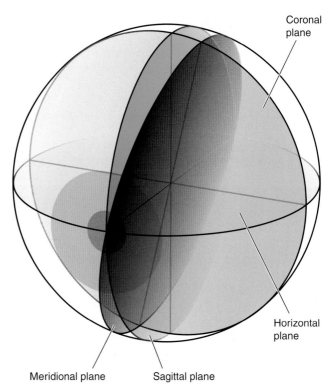

FIGURE 3.9 Coronal, horizontal, and sagittal planes of the eye. Note that an infinite number of meridional or radial planes are possible, rotating around the center of the cornea and defined most often using clock hours. As such, the midsagittal (median) and horizontal planes are special cases of meridional planes.

perpendicular to the floor, and perpendicular to the sagittal plane (**Fig. 3.9**). The coronal plane divides anterior from posterior in anatomical position and all coronal sections are parallel to this plane (**Fig. 3.10**). Whether in histology or in clinical imaging methods (e.g., MRI) most of what are labeled as coronal sections are often somewhat oblique to this ideal vertical plane. Nonetheless, the term coronal section is commonly used in most such cases. If the vertical tilt, forward or backward, is extreme, the term oblique section may be chosen.

MERIDIONAL

Because the eye is essentially a sphere, one can make anteroposterior sections along, or parallel to, any meridian for 360° from the center of the cornea.

The term radial section, as applied to the eye, is synonymous with meridional section. Meridional sections made along, or parallel to the horizontal equator of the eye (i.e., the 3- to 9-o'clock meridian at the limbus), are a defined subset referred to as transverse, axial, or horizontal sections, the terms used to describe such sections for nonspherical structures such as the head or the body as shown in **Figure 3.11**. These are parallel to the horizontal plane which separates superior from inferior (**Fig. 3.9**). Horizontal or transverse meridional sections are the most

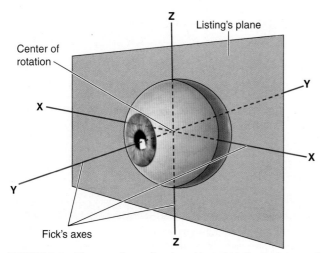

FIGURE 3.8 Diagram shows fixed position of Listing's plane and Fick's axes of rotation.

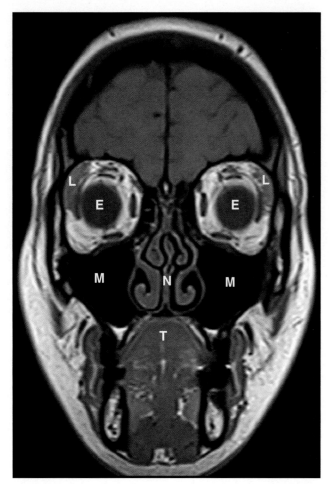

FIGURE 3.10 Coronal section of the head (T1-weighted MRI). Representative landmarks include the eyes (*E*), lacrimal glands (*L*), nasal cavity (*N*), maxillary sinuses (*M*), and tongue (*T*). (Courtesy of Dr. Robert Bert.)

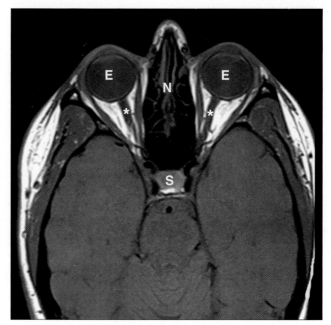

FIGURE 3.11 Horizontal (axial, transverse) section of the head at the level of the optic nerves (T1-weighted MRI). Representative landmarks include the eyes (*E*), optic nerves (*asterisks*), nasal cavity (*N*), and sella turcica (*S*). (Courtesy of Dr. Robert Bert.)

common sections of the eye that are examined in histology and pathology laboratories for the reasons outlined below in the description of how the eye is opened for pathologic examination.

SAGITTAL

Sagittal sections are any sections made parallel to the sagittal plane. The sagittal plane is a vertical plane that is perpendicular to the floor and perpendicular to the coronal plane as well (**Fig. 3.12**). Because the eye is essentially a sphere, sagittal sections of the eye, unlike the head, are a defined subset of meridional sections, and represent anteroposterior sections that transect, or are parallel to the 12- to 6-o'clock meridian at the limbus. The midsagittal plane of the eye divides temporal from nasal. Note that because of the asymmetry of the eye and the temporal displacement of the fovea, the anatomic nasal and temporal hemispheres defined by the midsagittal plane of the eye do not correspond to the nasal and temporal fields of

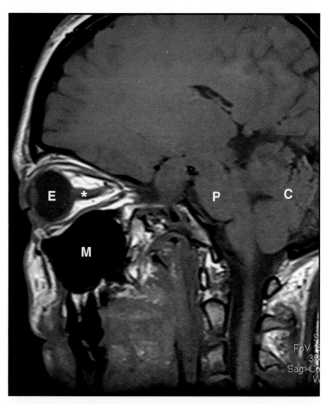

FIGURE 3.12 Sagittal section of the head (T1-weighted MRI). Representative landmarks include the eye (*E*), optic nerve (*asterisk*), maxillary sinus, (*M*), pons (*P*), and cerebellum (*C*). (Courtesy of Dr. Robert Bert.)

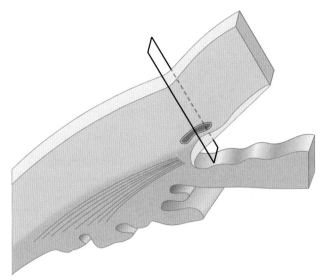

FIGURE 3.13 Frontal section, perpendicular to the surface of the eye and tangential to the corneoscleral junction at the limbus.

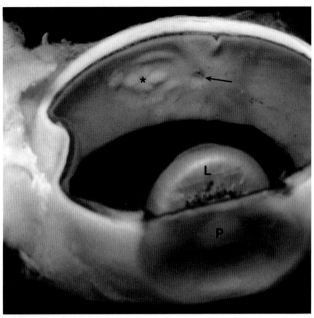

FIGURE 3.14 Pupil-optic nerve section of an eye with calottes removed. Pupil (*P*), lens (*L*), optic nerve head (*arrow*) and fovea (*asterisk*).

vision, since fields of vision are defined as they relate to the position of the fovea.

FRONTAL

The term frontal section is used primarily in examination of the aqueous outflow structures and structures near the limbus. It is a plane perpendicular to the surface of the eye and tangential to the peripheral edge of the cornea at the limbus (**Fig. 3.13**).[8]

SECTIONING THE EYE FOR PATHOLOGIC AND SUBSEQUENT HISTOLOGIC EXAMINATION

In order to appreciate all of the anatomic and pathologic features of an enucleated eye, in a way that also lends to subsequent histologic processing, the enucleated eye is customarily opened in the pathology laboratory using two transverse cuts that are made above and below the horizontal equator of the eye (**Fig. 3.14**). In this way, there is representation of all of the anatomic features of the eye within this ring. Note that if similar parallel cuts were made vertically, one would likely lose either the fovea of the retina or the optic nerve head, both important anatomic features to be examined when histologic sections are made. The parallel cuts are made above and below the optic nerve, in a posterior to anterior direction, seeking to reach the anterior surface of the eye near the limbus. Completing the cuts near the limbus reduces the risk of cutting into or dislodging the crystalline lens. In this way, the eye is rendered into three pieces, a central ring called the PO (pupil-optic nerve) section shown in **Figure 3.14** and two cup-shaped pieces from the top and bottom of the eye that are called calottes. It is the processing and sectioning of the PO section that renders the classical

section through the whole eye that includes the pupil, optic nerve, and fovea.

Layers of the Eye

The wall of the eye is arranged into three layers (**Fig. 3.15**). They are:

- The fibrous tunic or the corneoscleral layer
- The vascular tunic or the uvea
- The neural tunic or retina

THE FIBROUS TUNIC

The fibrous tunic is composed of the clear cornea anteriorly and the opaque, white sclera posteriorly. The junction between the cornea and the sclera is termed the limbus and the limbus is the point of origin for the tissues overlying the anterior sclera, including the bulbar conjunctiva, Tenon's capsule, and the episclera. The latter two of these, Tenon's capsule and the episclera, extend posteriorly and envelop the entire sclera to the point of departure of the optic nerve.

THE VASCULAR TUNIC

The vascular tunic is more commonly referred to as the uvea. The term uvea is derived from the Latin word, *uva*, for grape. If the corneoscleral coat of the eye is removed, the outside of the remaining structures of the eye will appear purplish brown due to the pigment and numerous blood vessels of the uveal layer. Without the support of the corneoscleral coat, what remains of the eye will droop

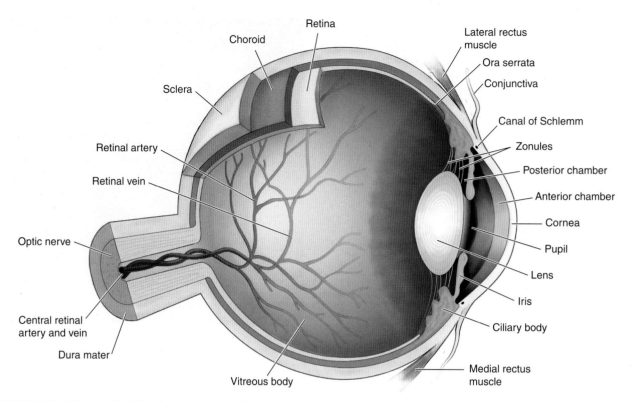

FIGURE 3.15 Diagram identifies the major tissues of the eye and their anatomical positions. (From Hinkle JL, Cheever KH, eds. *Brunner & Suddarth's Textbook of Medical-Surgical Nursing.* 13th ed. Philadelphia, PA: Wolters Kluwer; 2013.)

into a vertically oval structure when held up by the optic nerve, making it look truly reminiscent of a dark red or purple grape hanging from its stem.

Clinically, the uvea is divided into the anterior uvea and the posterior uvea. The anterior uvea is composed of the iris and the ciliary body. The iris serves as the variable optical diaphragm in the visual system, controlling the entry of light through the central pupil. The ciliary body rings the interior of the eye, posterolateral to the iris and surrounding the crystalline lens. From the ciliary body, a set of anchoring fibrils, called the zonules, suspend the crystalline lens in place behind the pupil. The posterior uvea is composed of the choroid, an intensely vascularized layer that provides metabolic support for the outer half of the retina. The anterior and posterior uvea meet at the ora serrata, which is the visible line of separation between the retina and the posterior edge of the ciliary body.

 Inflammation of the uveal tissues, called uveitis, is commonly named for its anatomic location. Anterior uveitis involves the iris and/ or ciliary body and posterior uveitis involves principally the choroid. When inflammation affects the area near the junction of the anterior and posterior uvea, the term intermediate uveitis is applied. Finally, if the entire uvea is involved, a diagnostic term panuveitis is used.

THE NEURAL TUNIC

The innermost layer of the eye, termed the neural tunic, is composed of the retina. The retina is most commonly subdivided into the neural (sensory) retina and the retinal pigment epithelium. The neural retina is composed of the photosensitive tissue that converts photons of light into chemical/electrical messages and the additional neurons and glial cells that begin the analysis of these inputs and transmit them to higher centers. Between the photoreceptor cells and the underlying choroid is a single layer of pigmented epithelial cells that assist in nourishing the outer retina—the retinal pigment epithelium of the retina.

In the clinical entity termed a retinal detachment, the detachment actually occurs between the neural (sensory) retina and retinal pigmented epithelium, not between the entirety of the retina and the underlying choroid.

The ultimate output of the retina is action potentials that are transmitted along the optic nerve to higher centers via the direct extension of the axons of its 1.2 million ganglion cells that coalesce to form the optic nerve.

The principal clinical landmarks of the retina include the optic disc, the central retinal artery and vein, and the

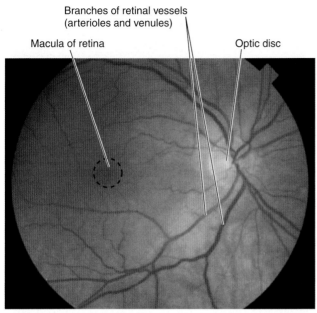

Branches of retinal vessels
(arterioles and venules)

Macula of retina

Optic disc

FIGURE 3.16   Fundus photo of posterior pole, identifying principal landmarks. (From Moore KL, Agur AMR, Dalley AF. *Clinically Oriented Anatomy.* 7th ed. Philadelphia, PA: Wolters Kluwer; 2013.)

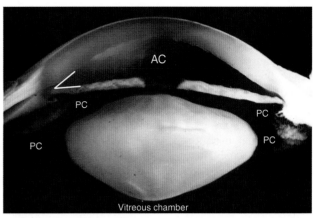

AC

PC

PC

PC

PC

PC

Vitreous chamber

FIGURE 3.17   Macrophotograph of the anterior segment of the eye shows anterior chamber (AC), posterior chamber (PC) surrounding the crystalline lens, and the vitreous chamber posterior to the lens. Converging white lines along the posterior corneal surface and the anterior iris surface designate the AC angle of the eye. (Courtesy of Mission for Vision and Dr. Ben Glasgow [www.missionforvision.org].)

slightly darker area temporal to the optic disc known as the macula (**Fig. 3.16**). At the center of the macula resides a shallow depression containing the fovea centralis, the only portion of the retina capable of 20/20 (6/6) vision.

Chambers of the Eye

The arrangement of the uveal tissues and the position of the lens divide the interior space of the eye into three compartments (**Fig. 3.17**). They are:

- The anterior chamber
- The posterior chamber
- The vitreous chamber

THE ANTERIOR CHAMBER

The anterior chamber is delimited anteriorly by the interior surface of the cornea and posteriorly by the anterior surface of the iris, its pupil, and the portion of the anterior surface of the crystalline lens upon which the pupil rests. Laterally, the anterior chamber is bounded by the angle subtended between the iris plane and the arcing dome of the cornea. This juncture is referred to as the anterior chamber angle, or simply the angle of the eye (**Fig. 3.17**). In this location reside the trabecular meshwork and the canal of Schlemm, through which most of the fluid filling the anterior chamber is drained into the bloodstream via channels weaving through the sclera to the episcleral veins.

In the average adult emmetropic eye (an eye with no refractive error), the anterior chamber subtends a volume of approximately 250 to 350 μL.[9] The anterior chamber is

filled with aqueous humor, a clear nutritive fluid that meets the metabolic needs of the avascular tissues bordering the anterior chamber, including the cornea, the lens, and the trabecular meshwork. Aqueous humor is produced by the ciliary body and secreted into the posterior chamber. Aqueous humor enters the anterior chamber solely through the pupil. In the anterior chamber, the aqueous humor circulates in a convection current driven by the temperature difference between the warm iris and the cornea, which is cooler due to its exposure to air. Aqueous humor rises along the anterior surface of the iris and falls along the inner surface of the cornea, ultimately draining from the eye via two principal pathways, both of which begin in the angle of the eye and are discussed in detail in **CHAPTER 9: ANATOMY OF THE AQUEOUS OUTFLOW PATHWAYS.**

 Because the normal aqueous humor is a clear fluid, without particulates, it is impossible to appreciate the convection current that circulates the aqueous humor in the normal eye. But in an inflamed eye, white blood cells invade the aqueous humor. Examining a moderately inflamed eye, with cells in the anterior chamber, one can confirm that all of the cells in the aqueous humor near the iris are rising and all of the cells in the aqueous humor just posterior to the inner surface of the cornea are falling.

THE POSTERIOR CHAMBER

The posterior chamber of the eye is the donut-shaped space that surrounds the crystalline lens. It is delimited anteriorly by the posterior surface of the iris and the inner surface of the ciliary body. Its posterior limit is the anterior hyaloid membrane, which also forms the anterior limit of the vitreous chamber. Extending across the posterior chamber, around its entire circumference, are the bands of zonular fibers that attach the crystalline lens to the ciliary body. The posterior chamber subtends a volume of approximately 50 µL.

Aqueous humor is secreted into the posterior chamber by the ciliary body at a rate of about 2 to 3 µL per minute.[1] As noted above, aqueous humor then enters the anterior chamber through the pupil, since it cannot traverse the intact iris. The combined volumes of the anterior and posterior chambers are approximately 350 to 400 µL. Assuming an equal rate of aqueous secretion and drainage, in order to keep intraocular pressure stable, this means that all of the aqueous humor in these chambers is replaced every 90 to 120 minutes.

 Because the iris rests against the anterior surface of the lens, a slight pressure head must develop in the posterior chamber in order to force an aliquot of aqueous humor through the pupil and into the anterior chamber. In some individuals, particularly when the pupil is at the mid-dilated position, the relative amount of resistance that aliquots of aqueous humor must overcome, in order to enter the anterior chamber at the pupillary margin, is increased. This phenomenon is termed "relative pupillary block." If relative pupillary block becomes great enough, the new aqueous being secreted accumulates in the posterior chamber, unable to pass into the anterior chamber. As fluid accumulates, pressure increases, forcing the iris forward. As the iris moves forward, the peripheral iris can obstruct the flow of aqueous humor present in the anterior chamber from draining from the eye through the trabecular meshwork (arrow in optical coherence tomogram shown in **Fig. 3.18**). *Together, these contributing factors can acutely elevate pressure significantly, causing hazy vision, eye pain, nausea, and even vomiting in an acute attack of angle-closure glaucoma.*

THE VITREOUS CHAMBER

The vitreous chamber is the largest of the spaces within the eye, with a volume of approximately 5.5 mL in emmetropic eyes.[9]

The vitreous chamber contains the vitreous body, which is a gel that is 99% water by weight. This gel contains a sparse collagenous support matrix and is enveloped by a condensation of the structural proteins that compose the additional 1% of this tissue. The envelope surrounding the entire circumference of the vitreous gel is termed the hyaloid membrane or vitreous face.

Anteriorly, the hyaloid membrane establishes the posterior limit of the posterior chamber, but does not represent a

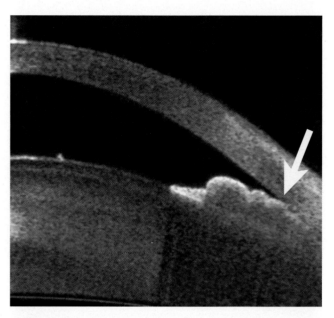

FIGURE 3.18 Optical coherence tomogram of anterior chamber angle. Note that the iris is nearly touching the posterior surface of the cornea (arrow) and obstructing the flow of aqueous humor to the drainage pathways in the anterior chamber angle. (Courtesy of Dr. Douglas Rhee. In: Rhee DJ, ed. *Color Atlas and Synopsis of Clinical Ophthalmology—Wills Eye Institute—Glaucoma.* 2nd ed. Philadelphia, PA: Wolters Kluwer; 2012.)

diffusion barrier between the vitreous and aqueous compartments. Water, ions, and even cells (including leaked red blood cells or even tumor cells from the posterior segment of the eye) can leave the vitreous to enter the circulating aqueous humor and be carried into the anterior chamber.

The hyaloid membrane surrounds and contains the more liquid, central vitreous humor and connects the vitreous body to tissues that surround it. With increasing age, the vitreous gel becomes more liquid. The firmest attachment of the vitreous body to the wall of the eye is called the vitreous base. It is a 360° band of attachment spanning across the most anterior portion of the retina and the most posterior portion of the ciliary body (**Fig. 3.19**).

Overview of the Ocular Vasculature

The source of arterial blood for the eye is the ophthalmic artery, which is the first branch of the internal carotid artery. It arises just as the internal carotid artery emerges from the roof of the cavernous sinus, beneath the anterior clinoid process of the sphenoid bone, in the middle cranial fossa. The ophthalmic artery enters the orbit through the optic canal, beneath the optic nerve.

The branches of the ophthalmic artery are most conveniently discussed in two groups—an orbital group and an ocular group. The orbital group is discussed in **CHAPTER 1: THE ORBITS**. The ocular group is discussed below.

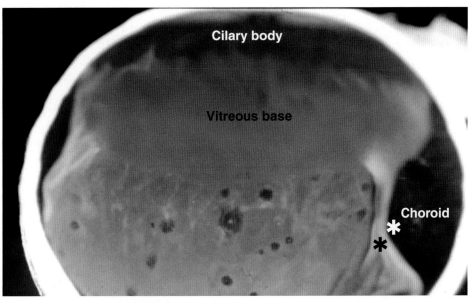

FIGURE 3.19   This macrophotograph shows the interior of a calotte from an eye of a patient who died from leukemia. Recall that a calotte removes the top or bottom of the eye wall, and thus neither the lens nor and iris is present. The anterior segment of the eye is at the top. Numerous white-centered hemorrhages, typical of leukemia, are seen within the retina. At one edge of the specimen, the sensory retina has been artifactually detached (*black asterisk*) revealing the underlying retinal pigment epithelium and choroid (*white asterisk*). Hemorrhage into the vitreous required removal of the vitreous in vivo but the heme has infiltrated the ring of remaining vitreous at the vitreous base, rendering it orange in color and readily identifying its location. The vitreous base straddles the underlying ora serrata, that divides the ciliary body at top from the retina below.

THE OCULAR GROUP

Arterial Supply of the Eye

The branches of the ophthalmic artery that serve the eye are depicted in simplified form **Figure 3.20** and include the:

- **Central retinal artery: 1**
- **Posterior ciliary arteries: 2 to 3**

The posterior ciliary arteries give rise to:

- ○ **10 to 20 Short posterior ciliary arteries**
- ○ **Two long posterior ciliary arteries**
- **Anterior Ciliary Arteries – 7** (derived from branches of the ophthalmic artery serving the four rectus muscles).

The following discussion is intended as an introductory overview. Greater detail regarding the microvascular supply to each specific ocular tissue is provided in the chapters on those respective tissues.

The Central Retinal Artery (CRA)

The CRA arises from the ophthalmic artery while the ophthalmic artery is still inferior to the optic nerve at the orbital apex. Based upon dissections, 50% to 90% of CRAs arise as a separate and distinct branch. In the remainder, the CRA arises from a common trunk that also gives rise to the medial posterior ciliary artery.[10,11] In approximately 58% of the cases, where the CRA arises as a separate branch, the CRA is the first branch of the ophthalmic artery. In the remaining 42%, it is the medial posterior ciliary that arises first, followed by the CRA.[11] The CRA runs beneath the optic nerve to a point 5.3 to 15.2 mm

(average 7 to 8 mm) behind the eye where it pierces the meningeal coverings inferiorly (70%) or inferomedially (21%) to take its position within the center of the optic nerve.[10–12] During embryogenesis, the CRA gains access to the inferiorly directed cleft in the optic stalk that is termed the fetal fissure. It is closure of this cleft that envelops the CRA and its companion central retinal vein (CRV) within the optic nerve (for more details, **SEE CHAPTER 16: EMBRYOLOGY OF THE EYE AND ORBIT**).

The CRA emerges from the optic nerve head slightly nasal to its center as a vessel that is approximately 100 μm in diameter. The vessel usually divides into branches for each retinal quadrant that travel arcuate courses and are termed arcades (**Fig. 3.16**).

The 100 μm diameter of the CRA can be used as a clinically valuable scale to estimate the size of lesions and other anomalies of the retina that are microns in size in the posterior pole of the eye. By comparison, the normal horizontal diameter of the optic nerve head (optic disc) is 1.5 mm and the "disc diameter" is a clinically useful unit

The ratio of the diameters of the CRA and CRV is routinely recorded during a comprehensive eye examination. The expected ratio between the diameter of the CRA and CRV is commonly 2/3. As arteriolar sclerosis of the CRA ensues, with increasing age, the arteriolar diameter increases and this ratio approaches 1/1.

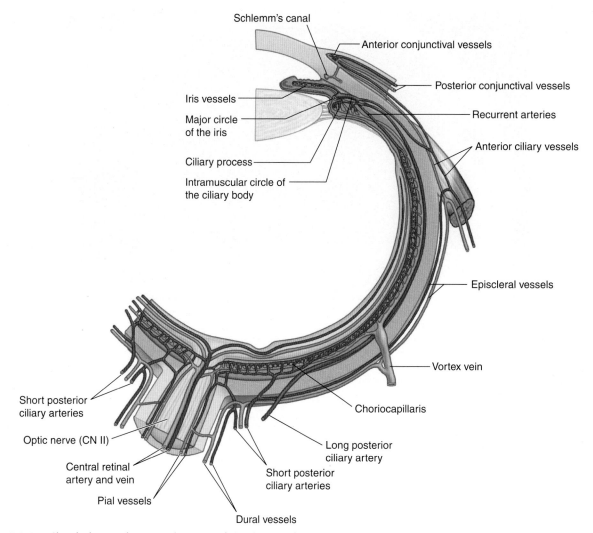

FIGURE 3.20   Sketch depicts the general pattern of distribution of the blood supply to the eye, including the central retinal artery, the short and long posterior ciliary arteries and the anterior ciliary arteries. Blood from the retina leaves the eye via the central retinal vein and the remainder of the blood within the eye exits principally via the vortex veins. (Modified from Moore KL, Agur AMR, Dalley AF. *Clinically Oriented Anatomy.* 7th ed. Philadelphia, PA: Wolters Kluwer; 2013.)

of measure for estimating both size and distances between objects that are on a mm scale in the posterior pole of the eye.

The Branches of the Posterior Ciliary Arteries

The Short Posterior Ciliary Arteries: Confusion in nomenclature often arises in discussing the short and long posterior ciliary arteries, because both sets of vessels represent branches from vessels called the posterior ciliary arteries. The posterior ciliary arteries are the direct branches from the ophthalmic artery. The long and short posterior ciliary arteries are branches of these vessels. Over 80% of humans have either two or three posterior ciliary arteries serving each eye. These run forward, parallel to the medial and lateral sides of the optic nerve. Rarely a third posterior ciliary artery may also run above optic nerve[13] (**Fig. 3.21**).

Numerous short posterior ciliary arteries arise from the two to three posterior ciliary artery trunks, arriving at the posterior scleral surface as three groups of vessels. A small group of 10 to 20 short posterior ciliary arteries pierce the sclera in a partial ring around the insertion of the optic nerve. These have been termed paraoptic short posterior ciliary arteries (**Fig. 3.21**). Two additional clusters of short posterior ciliary arteries, termed distal short posterior ciliary arteries, pierce the sclera along the horizontal equator of the eye. One group pierces the sclera nasal to the paraoptic ring and another group pierces the sclera temporal to the paraoptic ring, in the vicinity of the macula and near the tendinous insertion of the IO muscle (**Fig. 3.21**).[13]

The paraoptic short posterior ciliary arteries make contributions to the vascular supply of the optic nerve head, the peripapillary choroid and anastomose with vessels of the pia mater, surrounding the optic nerve (**Fig. 3.21**).

The distal short posterior ciliary arteries ramify inside the sclera to become the principal blood supply for the choroid, at least as far anteriorly as the vertical equator of the eye. The remainder of the choroid, anterior to this

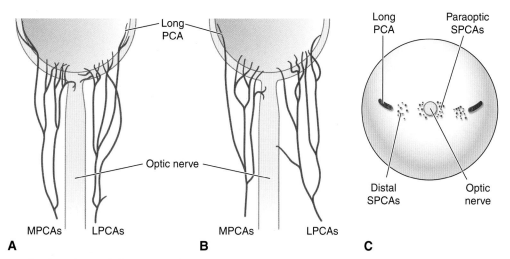

FIGURE 3.21 **A** and **B** show the Medial (MPCA) and Lateral posterior ciliary arteries (LPCA) of two right eyes from above, and variations in branching and distribution of the long and short posterior ciliary arteries that arise from them. **C:** Shows a posterior view of an eye, noting the positions of entry of the two Long posterior ciliary arteries (Long PCA) and the three groups of short posterior ciliary arteries (SPCA). Paraopitc SPCAs surround optic nerve, with two clusters of distal SPCAs between the optic nerve and the entry of the Long PCAs. (Redrawn from Hayreh SS. Posterior ciliary artery circulation in health and disease: the Weisenfeld Lecture. *Invest Ophthalmol Vis Sci.* 2004;45(3):749–757.)

point, is commonly served by recurrent arterial vessels, moving posteriorly from the ciliary body (**Fig. 3.20**).

A summary of the blood vessels contributing to the vascular supply of each of the uveal tissues is provided in **Table 3.2**. Greater detail on the microvascular anatomy of the optic nerve head and choroid is provided in the respective chapters on these tissues.

The Long Posterior Ciliary Arteries: Two LPCAs arise, one from each of the posterior ciliary artery trunks. They enter the eye along the horizontal equator of the eye, outside of the ring of vessels created by the paraoptic and distal short posterior ciliary arteries. One enters nasal to the optic nerve and the other temporal. These two vessels traverse the thickness of the sclera at a very oblique angle in conjunction with the long ciliary nerves (**Figs. 3.5A, B** and **3.20**).

Reaching the interior of the sclera near the crossing point of the horizontal and vertical equators of the eye, the LPCAs run anteriorly within the suprachoroidal space and its anterior continuation as the supraciliary space (**Fig. 3.20**). These vessels bifurcate and ramify further to become the major contributors to the formation of the major circle of the iris.[14] In some individuals, branches of the LPCAs pass directly into the iris to become radial iris arterioles, bypassing the major circle of the iris completely. Notwithstanding these few direct branches, it is from the major circle of the iris that most of the blood supply for the iris arises.

Finally, the temporal LPCA commonly provides a recurrent branch that contributes to the blood supply of a wedge of choroid extending anteriorly from the point at which the vessel completely emerges from its long course through the thickness of the sclera.[15]

The remainder of the anterior choroid is served by recurrent vessels that run posteriorly from the major circle of the iris, with additional vessels that come directly from both the anterior ciliary arteries and the LPCAs before either joins the major circle of the iris or the intramuscular circle. Whether this system of vessels serving the anterior choroid anastomoses with the posterior choroid served by the short posterior ciliary arteries remains heavily contested.[16]

The Anterior Ciliary Arteries

The anterior ciliary arteries arise from the vascular supply of the four rectus muscles. The rectus muscles are served by the muscular branches of the ophthalmic artery. The anterior ciliary arteries extend forward, onto the sclera, anterior to the tendinous insertions of the rectus muscles. Each rectus muscle usually gives rise to two anterior ciliary arteries, except for the lateral rectus, which provides only one (**Fig. 3.22**). Posterior to the limbus, the main trunks of these seven vessels pass through scleral emissaria, to reach the ciliary body (**Fig. 3.23**). These branches make only minor contributions to the major circle of the iris but make anastomotic connections with the LPCAs in all quadrants (**Fig. 3.24A**). The penetrating branches of the anterior ciliary arteries contribute only minimally to the major circle of the iris, and these are primarily limited to the most superior and inferior portions of the circle. These arteries do contribute significantly to another discontinuous vascular circle that runs circumferentially within the ciliary muscle and is called the intramuscular circle (**Fig. 3.24A**).

Like the branches of the LPCAs, branches of the anterior ciliary arteries may also enter the iris directly. Despite these small, direct branches to the iris from the long posterior and anterior ciliary arteries, most of the blood supply to the iris is derived from the major circle of the iris (**Table 3.2**).

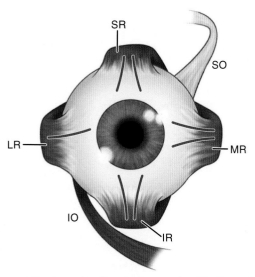

FIGURE 3.22 Curved red lines indicate paths of the 7 anterior ciliary arteries from rectus muscle insertions to their points of entry into the sclera. SR, superior rectus; SO, superior oblique; MR, medial rectus; IR, inferior rectus; IO, inferior oblique; LR, lateral rectus. (Modified from Chern KC, Saidel MA. *Ophthalmology Review Manual*. 2nd ed. Philadelphia, PA: Wolters Kluwer; 2011.)

Additional branches of the anterior ciliary arteries do not pierce the sclera. Instead, they remain more superficial, contributing the anterior conjunctival arteries that serve the perilimbal conjunctiva, and both the superficial and

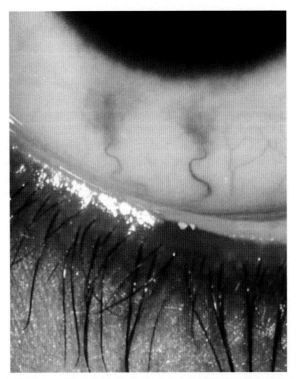

FIGURE 3.23 Clinical photograph shows anterior view of the inferior limbal region and lower lid margin, including lashes. Two S-shaped anterior ciliary arteries are seen entering the sclera near the limbus. Surrounding the points of entry are diffuse episcleral deposits of bluish uveal pigment that has emigrated from the uvea via the scleral emissarial canals through which these penetrating branches of the anterior ciliary arteries enter the eye.

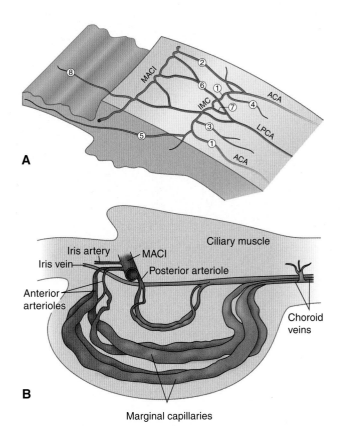

FIGURE 3.24 Diagram of ciliary body vasculature. **A:** Branches of anterior ciliary arteries (ACA) and the long posterior ciliary arteries (LPCA). ACA branches: (*1*) Branches forming the intramuscular circle (IMC); (*2*) branch to of the major arterial circle of the iris (MACI), especially contributing to the superior and inferior portions of the circle; (*3*) branch to outer and posterior ciliary muscle; (*4*) recurrent artery to peripheral choroid; (*5*) branch to iris. LPCA branches; (*6*) primary branches supplying the major arterial circle of the iris (MACI); (*7*) branch to the intramuscular circle; (*8*) radial iris artery. **B:** MACI and its principal branches to each ciliary process and venous drainage to the choroid.

deep episcleral vessels. Connections also exist between this episcleral circle and the major circle of the iris in the ciliary body. Indeed there is angiographic evidence that several of these branches flow from the major circle of the iris toward the episcleral circle rather than the reverse. This suggests that flow through these connections between the major circle of the iris and the episcleral circle, serving the perilimbal conjunctiva and episclera, may be bidirectional and can change depending on the relative pressure dynamics of the two circles to which they are connected.[17] The episclera overlying the posterior sclera receives its vascular supply primarily from the posterior ciliary arteries and their branches. (**Fig 3.20**).

Venous Drainage of the Eye

The venous blood leaves the eye via four pathways.
- The central retinal vein
- The vortex veins
- The anterior ciliary veins
- The episcleral veins

TABLE 3.2   Summary of Arterial Blood Supplies for Uveal Tissues

Tissue	Primary Supply	Additional Supply
Iris	Major circle of the iris	Direct branches from anterior ciliary arteries and long posterior ciliary arteries
Ciliary muscle (anterior) Ciliary muscle (posterior) Ciliary processes	Major circle of the iris Intramuscular circle Major circle of the iris	
Anterior choroid	Recurrent arteries from major circle of the iris and directly from anterior ciliary arteries	Recurrent branch only on temporal side from long posterior ciliary artery
Posterior choroid	Distal short posterior ciliary arteries	

THE CENTRAL RETINAL VEIN

The venous return from the capillary beds of the retina converges onto a set of venules that roughly parallel the course of the CRA and its branches. These venules, from the quadrants of the retina, ultimately anastomose to form a single CRV at the optic nerve head (**Fig. 3.16**). The diameter of the normal CRV is approximately 150 μm.

 Venous pressure within the CRV is often nearly the same as intraocular pressure. In at least 50% of eyes, the CRV can be seen to pulse and this is generally considered a normal finding.[18] By contrast, pulsation of the CRA is invariably pathologic and usually indicates a very elevated intraocular pressure, a decreased vascular perfusion pressure,[19] or an increase in systemic pulse pressure, most commonly due to an aortic valve insufficiency.[20]

The CRV leaves from the inferior surface of the optic nerve at the point where the CRA enters. In classical descriptions, the CRV joins the superior ophthalmic vein, which leaves the orbit via the superior orbital fissure to enter the cavernous sinus. More recent dissections of 34 orbits suggest that the CRV may, in some cases, join the cavernous sinus directly.[21]

THE VORTEX VEINS

Almost all of the venous blood from the iris and ciliary body drains posteriorly to join the choroidal venous system. Some of the anterior portion of the ciliary muscle may drain via anterior ciliary veins, which parallel the path of the penetrating branches of the anterior ciliary arteries. Except for the limited drainage to the anterior ciliary veins, the majority of venous blood leaving the anterior uveal tissues, plus the venous blood from the choroid, converge onto the several vortex vein ampullae. The convergence of these vessels toward the ampullae occurs in a somewhat vorticeal pattern that gives these vessels their name (**Fig. 3.25**). An average of seven vortex veins are found in each eye. These commonly coalesce, with an average of four vortex veins exiting posterior to the coronal equator of the eye, through emissaria in each quadrant (**Fig. 3.5A and B**). The superior and inferior vortex veins most commonly join their respective superior or inferior ophthalmic veins.

THE ANTERIOR CILIARY VEINS

The anterior ciliary veins parallel the course of the anterior ciliary arteries and drain the venous blood from the anterior portion of the ciliary muscle. These veins return to the muscular veins of the rectus muscles and from there to the superior and inferior ophthalmic veins (**Fig. 3.20**).

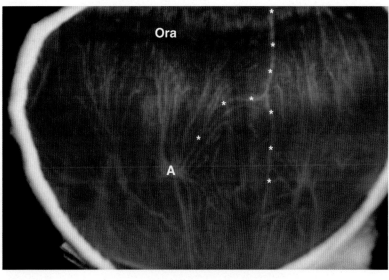

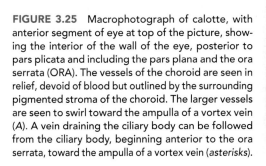

FIGURE 3.25 Macrophotograph of calotte, with anterior segment of eye at top of the picture, showing the interior of the wall of the eye, posterior to pars plicata and including the pars plana and the ora serrata (ORA). The vessels of the choroid are seen in relief, devoid of blood but outlined by the surrounding pigmented stroma of the choroid. The larger vessels are seen to swirl toward the ampulla of a vortex vein (*A*). A vein draining the ciliary body can be followed from the ciliary body, beginning anterior to the ora serrata, toward the ampulla of a vortex vein (*asterisks*).

THE EPISCLERAL VEINS

From angiographic studies, the episcleral veins initially form by receiving small venules from the perilimbal conjunctiva and anterior episclera, draining a perilimbal venous circle.[22] These vessels proceed posteriorly and are joined by venous vessels emerging from the sclera that do not drain the uvea. These vessels instead drain deep episcleral and perilimbal plexi. Importantly, some of these receive the aqueous humor from Schlemm's canal. Finally, the episcleral veins return their blood and aqueous humor to the venous drainage of the extraocular muscles and from there to the inferior and superior ophthalmic veins.

 It is important to appreciate that most of the aqueous humor leaving the eye from the anterior chamber traverses the sclera through a complex system of intrascleral channels to enter the venous circulation of the episclera. If pressure in the venous system leaving the eye and orbit is elevated for any reason, the pressure in the eye will rise until it exceeds that of the episcleral venous pressure. Only then can aqueous outflow resume. Until the pressure is reduced, the risk of permanent vision loss remains high.

 Innervation

The eye receives sensory fibers and autonomic fibers, both sympathetic and parasympathetic. The pathways taken by these fibers, from their origin to their entry into the ciliary ganglion, are presented in **CHAPTER 1: THE ORBITS**. Their pathways into, through, and beyond the ciliary ganglion, to reach their target tissues within the eye, are detailed below.

SENSORY INNERVATION

Sensory innervation reaches the eye on both the long and short ciliary nerves, which arise from the nasociliary branch of the ophthalmic division of CN V. The relationship between the long and short ciliary nerves and the ciliary ganglion, including the passage of these fibers to their target tissues, is detailed below under Ciliary Ganglion.

PARASYMPATHETIC INNVERATION

Parasympathetic fibers destined for the eye travel to the orbit as a bundle added to the superotemporal surface of CN III as it emerges from the midbrain. The pathway of these fibers, from their origin in the brainstem to their entry into the ciliary ganglion, is discussed in **CHAPTER 1: THE ORBITS**.

The preganglionic parasympathetic fibers serving the eye are conveyed to the ciliary ganglion as a branch from the nerve to the inferior oblique muscle, which is a branch of the inferior division of CN III. The further path of these fibers to the eye is detailed below, under Ciliary Ganglion.

SYMPATHETIC INNERVATION

The preganglionic sympathetic fibers destined for the eye originate in the intermediolateral column of the spinal cord, between levels C8–T2, in a region collectively termed the ciliospinal center of Budge (**Fig. 3.26**). From here, these preganglionic fibers pass superiorly, in the paravertebral sympathetic chain, in close proximity to the apex of the lung, up to the superior cervical ganglion.

 Tumors near the apex of the lung (e.g., Pancoast's tumor) may invade and interrupt the continuity of the cervical sympathetic pathways. Any interruption of the sympathetic pathways to the head and neck may result in Horner's syndrome, which is characterized by ipsilateral partial ptosis, miosis, and anhydrosis. The partial ptosis results from loss of sympathetic tone to Müller's muscle in the lids, the miosis results from loss of sympathetic innervation to the pupillary dilator muscle, and the anhydrosis results from loss of sympathetic innervation to the sweat glands of the face. Because sympathetic fibers also provide a sustaining neurotrophic effect on melanophores in the iris, there may be atrophic changes in the anterior border layer of the iris, leading to a change in iris color (heterochromia). This latter feature is more common in congenital forms of Horner's syndrome but Horner's syndrome is not the sole cause of heterochromia.

Upon reaching the superior cervical ganglion, the preganglionic sympathetic fibers synapse and the postganglionic fibers leave as a plexus wrapped around the internal carotid artery as it enters the carotid canal at the base of skull. When the internal carotid artery emerges from the roof of the cavernous sinus, beneath the anterior clinoid process of the sphenoid bone, it gives off its first branch, the ophthalmic artery.

The vasomotor sympathetic fibers destined for the eye leave the plexus of the internal carotid artery to form a smaller plexus surrounding the ophthalmic artery and pass with the artery through the optic canal, beneath the optic nerve. Upon emerging into the orbit, some of the postganglionic sympathetic fibers form a communicating branch to the ciliary ganglion. Since the ciliary ganglion is primarily a parasympathetic system ganglion, these postganglionic sympathetic fibers do not synapse before continuing to their target vessels in the uvea along the short ciliary nerves.

The postganglionic fibers destined for the pupil leave the plexus surrounding the internal carotid artery at the point where the artery and the ophthalmic division of the trigeminal nerve come into close proximity, as both emerge from the wall of the cavernous sinus near its anterolateral margin. At this location, postganglionic sympathetic fibers are conveyed from the internal carotid plexus to the nasociliary branch of the ophthalmic division of the trigeminal nerve and then into the long ciliary nerves, which convey them to the eye and ultimately to the anterior myoepithelium of the iris. Unlike the sphincter muscle of the pupil, which is smooth muscle, it is the "myo" component of these myoepithelial cells that constitutes the dilator muscle of the pupil. The pathway of the sympathetic fibers in relation to the ciliary ganglion is detailed in the Ciliary Ganglion section.

CILIARY GANGLION

It is at the ciliary ganglion that most of the sensory, sympathetic, and parasympathetic pathways to and form the eye converge. The ciliary ganglion resides within the orbit, most often positioned between the optic nerve and the lateral rectus within the muscle cone. In dissection, the easiest way to find this pinhead-sized ganglion is to find the branch of the oculomotor nerve that is headed to the inferior oblique muscle and then follow its connection to

the ganglion. The ciliary ganglion is functionally associated with the parasympathetic division of the autonomic nervous system. It is one of four principal parasympathetic ganglia in the head and neck, together with the otic, pterygopalatine, and submandibular ganglia.

The ciliary ganglion is not merely a synaptic station for the preganglionic parasympathetic fibers destined for the eye. Because of its central location behind the eye, both sensory and postganglionic sympathetic fibers that are conveyed to and from the eye also pass through the ganglion, but without synapsing.

The ciliary ganglion receives three connections (**Fig. 3.27**). These are:

- **The motor root**—arises from the oculomotor nerve's (CN III) branch to the inferior oblique.
- **The sensory root**—arises from the nasociliary branch of the ophthalmic division of the trigeminal nerve (CN V)
- **The sympathetic root**—arises from the sympathetic plexus surrounding the internal carotid artery and that of the internal carotid's first branch, the ophthalmic artery.

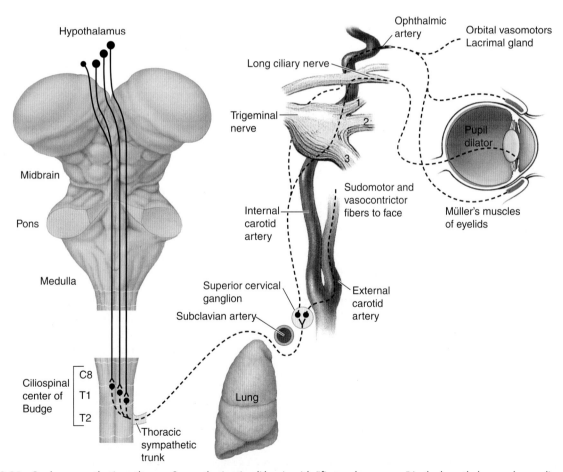

FIGURE 3.26 Ocular sympathetic pathways. Sympathetic stimuli begin with "first-order neurons" in the hypothalamus, descending through the brainstem to reach the intermediolateral column of the spinal cord at levels C8–T2. This region is termed the ciliospinal center of Budge. The second-order neuron follows the sympathetic chain to the superior cervical ganglion where these "preganglionic" sympathetic fibers synapse. Third-order neurons (postganglionic fibers) leave the ganglion as a plexus surrounding the internal carotid artery and are distributed to the orbit via the ophthalmic artery and ophthalmic division of the trigeminal nerve. (Modified from the Anatomical Chart Company. *Eye Anatomical Chart*. Philadelphia, PA: Wolters Kluwer; 2000.)

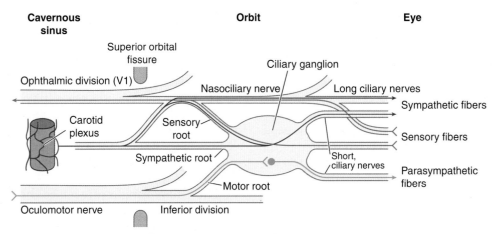

FIGURE 3.27   Relationship between sensory fibers (*blue*), sympathetic fibers (*red*) and parasympathetic (secretomotor) fibers (*green*) entering and leaving the ciliary ganglion and pathways to the eye.

The outputs of the ciliary ganglion are the short ciliary nerves. These nerves convey the sensory fibers from the intraocular tissues, plus the sclera and the anterior surface of the eye. They also convey the postganglionic parasympathetic fibers to the ciliary muscle for accommodation and to the pupillary sphincter for pupillary constriction (miosis). Far greater numbers of fibers serve the ciliary muscle than serve the pupillary sphincter.

Finally, the short ciliary nerves also convey the postganglionic sympathetic fibers that provide vascular tone to the intraocular vasculature. As noted earlier, the postganglionic sympathetic fibers conveyed to the long ciliary nerves from the carotid plexus innervate the myo component of the anterior myoepithelium of the iris. And it is these cells that constitute the dilator muscle of the iris.

Lymphatic Drainage

Traditionally, the shortest section of any text on anatomy of the eye would be the section on the lymphatic supply to the tissues inside of the eye. It has been an accepted fact that there are lymphatic channels in the conjunctiva, and these are detailed in **CHAPTER 5: THE CONJUNCTIVA AND THE LIMBUS**. It has been equally accepted that there are no lymphatic channels anywhere inside of the eye. This contention is supported by years of clinical experience that intraocular malignancies will metastasize via the bloodstream but spread to regional lymph nodes is rare. This is in contrast to the behavior of conjunctival malignancies in which metastasis to regional lymph nodes is regularly encountered. As a routine practice, clinicians were taught to palpate regional lymph nodes in the workup of a potential conjunctival malignancy but not when the malignancy was within the eye (e.g., choroidal melanoma).

While the immunology of the conjunctiva is more like other mucosae, in having what is often termed a "classical" lymphatic system that drains to regional lymph nodes, the immunology within the eye is quite unique, whether there are anatomically identifiable lymphatics or not. The details of what make the immune system of the eye so unique will not be described in detail here. Numerous comprehensive textbooks on this subject are available.[23]

Briefly, when foreign antigens are presented within the eye, they are met with long-term tolerance rather than an aggressive inflammatory response as would occur in the skin. And this is not because the immune system is unaware of the presence of the antigen. Indeed the eye not only tolerates the antigen, it simultaneously suppresses potential systemic responses to antigen harbored within the eye that could be mounted through the mechanisms of delayed hypersensitivity. It appears that this is of benefit to an organ where the consequence of an aggressive response might be more devastating to its function than to tolerate the continued presence of the antigen. While this seems a logical means of preserving sight, the downside is that this failure to respond often extends to a tolerance of intraocular tumors.

In the last few years, however, some investigators have proposed that the ciliary body and choroid have lymphatic vessels. Much of the data is based upon positive immunohistochemical staining, with antibodies believed to bind to unique markers for lymphatic lineage. There is increasing evidence that, with inflammation, the cornea can draw both blood vessels and lymphatic channels toward the central cornea from the limbal region where both normally exist.[24,25] There is also some evidence that when the integrity of the sclera is compromised, lymphatics may be drawn through the sclera and into the eye, but neither of these conditions presumes the presence of lymphatic channels inside the eye under physiologic conditions.[26,27]

Because a conclusion that there are lymphatics within the eye would so completely change long-held views on not only the anatomy but the physiology and immunology of the eye, and conventions of clinical practice, a consensus group was recently convened to review the literature on this subject. The reader is urged to read this consensus document.[28] The conclusion of this consensus panel was that "The evidence for a 'classical' lymphatic system in the inner portions of the eye under physiological conditions remains controversial." From a purely anatomic perspective, one of the difficulties in accepting the presence of classical lymphatic channels within the eye comes from the fact that identification of lymphatic capillaries in routine histologic sections of human intraocular tissues has not been possible, even for well-trained and experienced observers.[29] By contrast, identification of lymphatic channels in the conjunctival stroma is quite simple, as the reader will discover in **CHAPTER 5: THE CONJUNCTIVA AND THE LIMBUS.** This yet to be resolved controversy also serves as a useful reminder that the notion of there being nothing left to be discovered in anatomy is simply wrong.

◉ Acknowledgment

Thanks to Dr. Natalie Hutchings for her contributions to the Visual Axes sections of this chapter.

REFERENCES

1. Bron AJ. *Wolff's Anatomy of the Eye and Orbit.* 8th ed. London, UK: Chapman & Hall Medical; 1997.
2. Lauinger N. The two axes of the human eye and inversion of the retinal layers: the basis for the interpretation of the retina as a phase grating optical, cellular 3D chip. *J Biol Phys.* 1993;19(4):243–257.
3. Agarwal A, Kumar D, Jacob S. Angle kappa may play important role in success of multifocal IOLs. Ocular Surgery News, U S Edition. http://www.healio.com/ophthalmology/cataract-surgery/news/print/ocular-surgery-news/%7B9a3596d2-2129-488c-adee-8f2d763a2027%7D/angle-kappa-may-play-important-role-in-success-of-multifocal-iols. May 10, 2010. Accessed January 19, 2017.
4. Clark T. Measure visual, not pupillary, axis for accurate progressive addition lenses placement. Optometry Times. http://optometrytimes.modernmedicine.com/optometrytimes/news/modernmedicine/modern-medicine-feature-articles/measure-visual-not-pupillary-axi?page=full. November 1, 2011. Accessed January 19, 2017.
5. Moshirfar M, Hoggan RN, Muthappan V. Angle kappa and its importance in refractive surgery. *Oman J Ophthalmol.* 2013;6(3):151–158.
6. Wong AM. Listing's law: clinical significance and implications for neural control. *Surv Ophthalmol.* 2004;49(6):563–575.
7. Jampel RS, Shi DX. The primary position of the eyes, the resetting saccade, and the transverse visual head plane head movements around the cervical joints. *Invest Ophthalmol Vis Sci.* 1992;33(8):2501–2510.
8. Lu Z, Overby DR, Scott PA, et al. The mechanism of increasing outflow facility by rho-kinase inhibition with Y-27632 in bovine eyes. *Exp Eye Res.* 2008;86(2):271–281.
9. Xu HM, Zhou YX, Shi MG. Exploration of three-dimensional biometric measurement of emmetropic adult eye-ball by using magnetic resonance imaging technology [in Chinese]. *Zhonghua Yan Ke Za Zhi.* 2008;44(11):1007–1010.
10. Kocabiyik N, Yalcin B, Ozan H. The morphometric analysis of the central retinal artery. *Ophthalmic Physiol Opt.* 2005;25(4):375–378.
11. Erdogmus S, Govsa F. Topography of the posterior arteries supplying the eye and relations to the optic nerve. *Acta Ophthalmol Scand.* 2006;84(5):642–649.
12. Tsutsumi S, Rhoton AL Jr. Microsurgical anatomy of the central retinal artery. *Neurosurgery.* 2006;59(4):870–878; discussion 878, 879.
13. Hayreh SS. Posterior ciliary artery circulation in health and disease: The Weisenfeld Lecture. *Invest Ophthalmol Vis Sci.* 2004;45(3):749–757.
14. Funk R, Rohen J. Scanning electron microscopic study on the vasculature of the human anterior eye segment, especially with respect to the ciliary processes. *Exp Eye Res.* 1990;51(6):651–661.
15. Hayreh SS. The long posterior ciliary arteries. An experimental study. *Albrecht Von Graefes Arch Klin Exp Ophthalmol.* 1974;192:197–213.
16. Hayreh SS. Segmental nature of the choroidal vasculature. *Br J Ophthalmol.* 1975;59(11):631–648.
17. Meyer PA, Watson PG. Low dose fluorescein angiography of the conjunctiva and episclera. *Br J Ophthalmol.* 1987;71(1):2–10.
18. Legler U, Jonas JB. Assessment of the spontaneous pulsations of the central retinal vein in daily ophthalmic practice. *Clin Experiment Ophthalmol.* 2007;35(9):870–871.
19. Brown GC, Magargal L. The ocular ischemic syndrome. *Int Ophthalmol.* 1988;11(4):239–251.
20. Babu AN, Kymes SM, Fryer SMC. Eponyms and the diagnosis of aortic regurgitation: what says the evidence? *Ann Intern Med.* 2003;138(9):736–742.
21. Cheung N, McNab AA. Venous anatomy of the orbit. *Invest Ophthalmol Vis Sci.* 2003;44(3):988–995.
22. Meyer PA. Patterns of blood flow in episcleral vessels studied by low-dose fluorescein videoangiography. *Eye.* 1988;2(5):533–546.
23. Dartt DA, Dana R, D'Amore P. *Immunology, Inflammation and Diseases of the Eye.* Oxford, UK: Academic Press; 2011.
24. Cursiefen C, Schlotzer-Schrehardt U, Kuchle M, et al. Lymphatic vessels in vascularized human corneas: immunohistochemical investigation using LYVE-1 and podoplanin. *Invest Ophthalmol Visual Sci.* 2002;43(7):2127–2135.
25. Cursiefen C, Chen L, Borges LP, et al. VEGF-A stimulates lymphangiogenesis and hemangiogenesis in inflammatory neovascularization via macrophage recruitment. *J Clin Invest.* 2004;113(7):1040–1050.
26. Heindl LM, Hofmann TN, Knorr HL, et al. Intraocular lymphangiogenesis in malignant melanomas of the ciliary body with extraocular extension. *Invest Ophthalmol Vis Sci.* 2009;50(5):1988–1995.
27. Wessel JM, Hofmann-Rummelt C, Kruse FE, et al. Invasion of lymphatic vessels into the eye after open globe Injuries: intraocular lymphatic vessels after open globe injuries. *Invest Ophthalmol Vis Sci.* 2012;53(7):3717–3725.
28. Schroedl F, Kaser-Eichberger A, Schlereth SL, et al. Consensus statement on the immunohistochemical detection of ocular lymphatic vessels: consensus ocular lymphatics. *Invest Ophthalmol Vis Sci.* 2014;55(10):6440–6442.
29. Sleeman JP, Krishnan J, Kirkin V, et al. Markers for the lymphatic endothelium: in search of the holy grail? *Microsc Res Tech.* 2001;55(2):61–69.

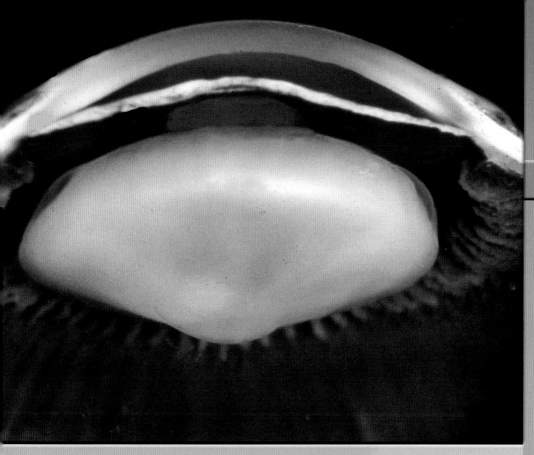

ANTERIOR SEGMENT
OF THE EYE

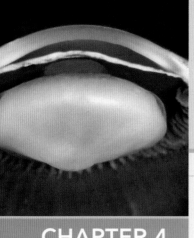

The Cornea

CHAPTER 4

Overview

The cornea is the dominant optical element in the visual system, providing approximately 75% to 80% of the refractive power of the human eye. The cornea is continuous with the conjunctiva, Tenon's capsule, the episclera, and sclera at its peripheral edge. This transition area is termed the *limbus*. Together, the cornea and sclera serve as a fibrous exoskeleton for the globe, providing support and attachment for the more delicate intraocular tissues. The cornea and sclera also serve an important role in protecting the intraocular contents. The corneal surface, together with the conjunctival surface and the tear film, present physical, chemical, and immunologic barriers to infection. The corneal surface and tear film also serve as the smooth optical surface of the eye that is resurfaced with each blink.

Macroscopic and Clinical Anatomy of the Cornea

CORNEAL DIMENSIONS

To serve its role as a refractive element, the cornea is optically clear. Neither blood vessels nor lymphatic vessels are found within the normal central cornea. As an optical element of the eye, taking measurements of the cornea's various anatomic dimensions are a common part of clinical practice, whether as preparation for refractive surgery, cataract surgery or contact lens fitting.[1]

Corneal Diameter

The cornea is nearly its adult size at birth. The horizontal diameter of the newborn cornea measures approximately 10 mm, reaching an average of about 11.7 mm by 2 years of age.[2] Viewed from its anterior aspect, the cornea appears wider than it is high; its vertical diameter measures an average of 10.6 mm. This disparity in horizontal versus vertical dimensions results from the way the cornea and sclera overlap at the limbus. A disparity in vertical versus horizontal dimensions is not observed when the cornea is viewed from its posterior surface. In a posterior view, both dimensions measure an average of 11.7 mm (**Fig. 4.1**).

 *Departures from the normal range of corneal diameters are rare and can occur either as isolated developmental anomalies or as a part of several genetic syndromes. Corneas with horizontal diameters from 7 to 10 mm are termed microcornea (**Fig. 4.2**), while those with horizontal diameters of 12 mm or more in the neonate, or 13 mm or more in the adult, are termed megalocornea.*

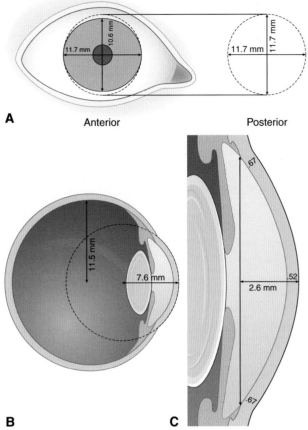

A   Anterior   Posterior

B   **C**

FIGURE 4.1   A: Viewed from its anterior surface, the cornea appears wider than it is high due to the manner of overlap of the cornea and sclera at the limbus. Viewed from its posterior surface, the cornea appears round. **B:** The average radius of curvature of the cornea and radius of curvature of the scleral shell. **C:** The corneal height is shown, measured from a transverse line connecting the peripheral edges of the posterior corneal surface. Also, the comparative thicknesses of the central and peripheral cornea are shown (0.52 and 0.67 mm). (Modified from Hogan MJ, Alvarado JA, Weddell JE. *Histology of the Human Eye.* Philadelphia, PA: WB Saunders; 1971:61.)

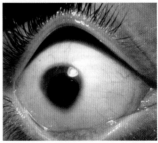

FIGURE 4.2   Note the unusually small size of this cornea and its inverted teardrop shape. This is termed microcornea. (Courtesy of Dr. William Charles Caccamise, Sr, and EyeRounds.org at the University of Iowa, Iowa City, IA.)

Corneal Thickness

Reports on the average thickness of the central cornea vary between approximately 520 and 550 μm. At the limbus, the corneal thickness averages 670 μm.[3] Of importance, the corneas of African-Americans are generally thinner than those of all other races. And thinner corneas are a known risk factor for glaucoma.[4-6] Presenting data on corneal thickness merely as numbers understates the remarkable durability of this tissue. Instead, consider the last time you watched someone rub their eyes hard, really dug those knuckles in and rubbed hard. Now consider the fact that the tissue they were rubbing so hard is only half of 1 mm thick and it did not rupture.

> *Central corneal thickness is most readily measured using one of several types of pachometers (i.e., pachymeters). Measuring corneal thickness has become increasingly important in clinical practice. As a general rule, patients should not undergo refractive surgery if the amount of tissue that must be removed in order to render an optimal refractive power could structurally and functionally destabilize the cornea, rendering a poor visual result. Measuring corneal thickness has also become an important adjunct to the measurement of intraocular pressure. Thinner corneas are more readily flattened by applanation-type tonometers, such as the commonly used Goldmann type. A thinner than average cornea, which flattens too readily under the pressure of the tonometer tip, will underestimate intraocular pressure. Conversely, a thicker than average cornea will flatten less readily, rendering an overestimate of intraocular pressure.*

Radius of Curvature and Index of Refraction

The average radius of curvature of the adult human cornea at its center is 7.6 to 7.7 mm (**Fig. 4.1**). The corneal curvature is usually flatter in men and the corneas of Orientals are usually steeper than the corneas of Occidental individuals. The cornea is actually aspheric, becoming progressively flatter in curvature toward the periphery. **Figure 4.3** shows a clinically obtained topographic map of the curvatures across a normal cornea. Note the progression from steeper curvatures (red) to flatter curvatures (blue) toward the periphery (i.e., lower dioptric power).

The index of refraction of the tear film/cornea overall is 1.376.[7] By most calculations, the anterior surface of the cornea provides an average of +49.00 D of power and the posterior surface −6.00 D, producing an average total power of +43.00 D.[8] Most refractive errors are axial, meaning they result from a longer or shorter eye, rather than from a more or less steeply curved cornea in eyes of similar lengths.[9]

> *Because the cornea is aspheric, most corneal contact lenses have both a central radius of curvature on their inside surface (i.e., base curve) and at least one flatter radius of curvature in their periphery (**Fig. 4.4**).*

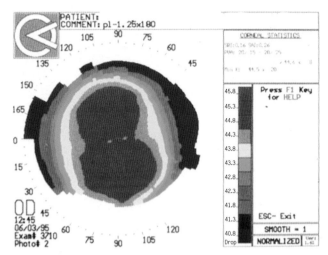

FIGURE 4.3 A topographical map showing the asphericity of a normal cornea, with its central area of steeper curvature (*red*) and a transition to the less steeply curved periphery (*blue*). (Courtesy of Dr. Timothy McMahon, University of Illinois, Chicago, IL.)

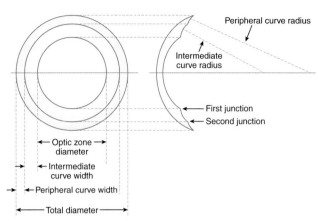

FIGURE 4.4 These figures show a posterior and cross-sectional view of a typical corneal contact lens. Note that the central portion of the posterior surface of the lens (the optical zone) has a steeper radius of curvature (the base curve) than the peripheral portion of the lens (the peripheral curve) in order to accommodate the asphericity of the normal cornea. Contact lenses commonly have several, progressively flatter, peripheral curves.

The majority of adult corneas exhibit different curvatures vertically and horizontally and the principal meridians of these two curvatures are commonly 90° apart. The difference between these measurements defines the amount of corneal astigmatism and, if the principal meridians are 90° apart, the astigmatism is considered to be "regular." Because most corneas exhibit a steeper curvature vertically than horizontally, this pattern is referred to as "with the rule" astigmatism. The converse is called "against the rule" astigmatism. When the principal meridians are not 90° apart, the astigmatism is considered to be irregular.

CORNEAL STRUCTURE

The cornea is subdivided into five layers (**Fig. 4.5**).
1. The corneal epithelium
2. Bowman's layer
3. The corneal stroma
4. Descemet's membrane
5. The corneal endothelium

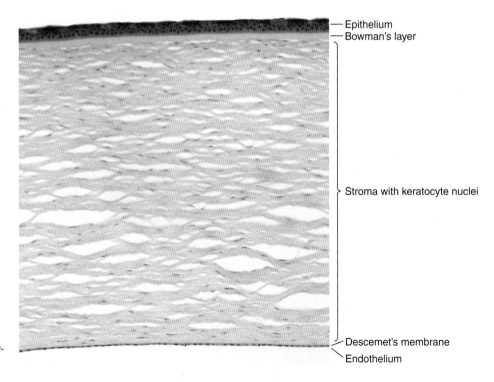

FIGURE 4.5 Light micrograph showing the layers of the cornea.

The Corneal Epithelium

The corneal epithelium is usually five to seven cell layers thick, representing a nonkeratinized, stratified squamous epithelium with an overall thickness of approximately 50 µm. These five to seven layers are composed of a single layer of columnar basal cells, two to three layers of "wing" cells, and two to three layers of nonkeratinized, squamous cells at the surface (**Fig. 4.6**).[10,11] Corneal epithelial thickness appears to remain constant throughout life in the central cornea, whereas the paracentral and peripheral epithelium thins with age, especially near the medial and temporal limbus.[12]

The Basal Layer and the Epithelial Basement Membrane: The basal layer, which produces the corneal epithelial basement membrane, consists of a single layer of columnar cells. It is only this single layer of cells that normally undergoes mitotic division and it appears that both daughter cells of this division leave the basal layer and differentiate together (**Fig. 4.7**). The mitotic rate in the basal layer is lower than would be predicted based upon the projected number of cells needed to sustain the average turnover rate for the epithelium as a whole, which is 7 to 10 days. This is because the principal source of stem cells for the epithelium is found at the limbus (SEE CHAPTER 5: THE CONJUNCTIVA AND THE LIMBUS). These stem cells migrate centripetally within the basal layer and are termed *transient amplifying cells*.[13] This migration toward the center of the cornea is not radial but occurs in a vorticeal pattern.[14]

Certain metabolic conditions and medications (e.g., Fabry's disease and amiodarone) can add non-melanin, pigmented deposits to corneal epithelial cells and in such cases vorticeal patterns are observed in the corneal epithelium as these pigments are carried toward the central corneal during normal cell migration[14] (Fig. 4.8).

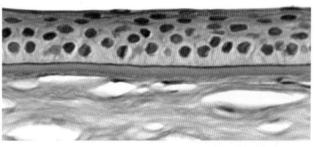

FIGURE 4.6   The five to seven layers of the corneal epithelium are shown, resting on a thin, basement membrane (*thin dark pink line*), which separates the basal layer of the epithelium from the homogeneous, acellular, Bowman's layer and underlying corneal stromal lamellae with keratocyte nuclei.

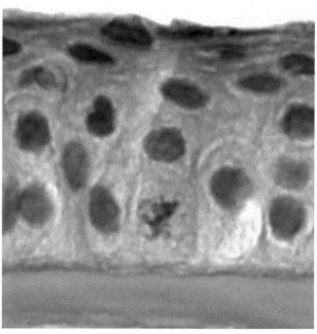

FIGURE 4.7   A basal cell undergoing mitotic division is shown.

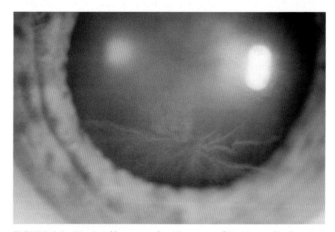

FIGURE 4.8   Vorticeal keratopathy. (Courtesy of Dr. Howard Leibowitz.)

Scattered among the basal epithelial cells, another cell type is occasionally found in the periphery. Particularly in heavily pigmented individuals it is not uncommon for melanocytes to migrate into the corneal epithelium from the limbus, producing a band of light, superficial pigmentation of the epithelium that is usually difficult to see with the naked eye.[15]

Another critical cell type found within the epithelium of the peripheral cornea is the Langerhan's cell. Langerhan's cells populate the epithelia of the skin, conjunctiva, and the peripheral cornea, where they function in antigen recognition and processing.[16] In infants, Langerhan's cells are regularly found across the entire corneal epithelial surface.[17] But in the normal adult, they are present only in the corneal periphery, where their density is approximately 15 to 20 per mm^2, which is less than 10% of the Langerhan's cell density in the conjunctiva.[18] The absence of Langerhan's cells in the central corneal epithelium limits the types of immune responses that the central cornea can mount under normal circumstances, in order to minimize central scarring that could be worse than the damage caused by the initial insult.[19]

A number of agents, from herpes virus to extended wear contact lenses, can induce Langerhan's cells to migrate into the central cornea in adults. This unfavorably changes the spectrum of immune responses the cornea can then mount, increasing the risk of scarring.[20–22]

The basal layer of the corneal epithelium produces the basal lamina (basement membrane) (**Fig. 4.9**). The basal layer of the epithelium is attached to and through the basement membrane (lamina lucida and lamina densa of the basal lamina) by adhesion complexes. Adhesion complexes are formed by actin-based focal adhesions and intermediate filament-based hemidesmosomes, linked to anchoring fibrils of type VII collagen. These fibrils traverse the type IV collagen found in the basement membrane, to reach anchoring plaques tied into the type I collagen of the corneal stroma (**Fig. 4.10**).[23] The interaction of the hemidesmosomes and focal adhesions of the basal cells, with the matrix proteins of the basement membrane including fibronectin, are mediated by integrin heterodimers.[24]

Bullous pemphigoid antigen is among the components of hemidesmosomes in the cornea. Aberrant autoantibodies to this antigen likely underlie the epithelial blisters (bullae) that affect the cornea in this disease.[25]

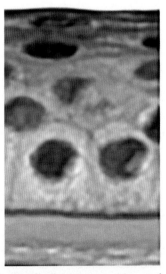

FIGURE 4.9 Two basal cells are seen, resting on their basal lamina. Note clear color difference between the more darkly stained basal lamina and more lightly stained, homogeneous, Bowman's layer in this periodic acid Schiff (PAS) stained section.

In general, the epithelium of the central cornea is less adherent to its basement membrane than the peripheral cornea because the latter forms a tighter adhesion complex with the basal lamina and underlying stroma.[26]

Above the single layer of columnar basal cells are two to three layers of "wing" cells that are named for the wing-like appearance of their dramatically extended lateral cell processes (**Fig. 4.11**). These cells are the intermediate stage in corneal epithelial differentiation, analogous to the stratum spinosum, or prickle cell layer in keratinized epithelia. Wing cells are attached to each other by numerous desmosomes and gap junctions (**Fig. 4.12**). As wing cells move to the surface, they flatten into squamous cells, which develop tight junctions. These tight junctions represent the intercellular permeability barrier of the corneal epithelium.

Figure 4.12 shows the overall pattern of distribution of the various intercellular junctions in the corneal epithelium. These include tight junctions between apical epithelial cells plus desmosomes and gap junctions between cells of all of the cell layers. Hemidesmosomes are confined to the basal surface of the basal epithelial layer.

The integrity of the corneal epithelial tight junctions is compromised temporarily by certain preservatives used in various eye drops, such as benzalkonium chloride. This temporarily increases corneal epithelial permeability.[27]

The Corneal Surface and the Tear Film: In addition to tight junctions, the fully differentiated squamous cells on the corneal surface develop microplicae. Microplicae on the corneal surface serve to increase the surface area available for oxygen/carbon dioxide exchange, an essential factor in corneal metabolism since the avascular cornea depends upon oxygen uptake from the tear film rather than the bloodstream (**Fig. 4.13**). Microplicae also assist in maintaining the tear film adherent to the surface of the cornea. Adherence of the tear film is critical since the tear film provides the requisite smooth optical surface for the eye that is constantly resurfaced with each blink. Even modest surface irregularities of the cornea and tear film are more likely to compromise vision than numerous focal opacities within the stroma.

The Tear Film: Estimates of normal tear film thickness vary with the methods used to obtain the measurement. The most recently developed methods indicate that the tear film of the normal eye is approximately 3 μm in thickness.[28–32]

In addition to its biologic protective functions as lubricant and antimicrobial agent, the tear film also serves as the critical first optical surface of the eye, the point in the light path where the index of refraction changes from the 1.0 of air to the 1.336 of the tear film and then the

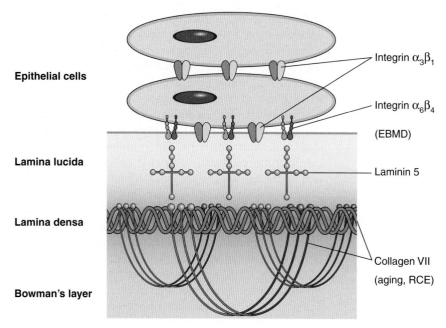

Epithelial cells

Integrin $\alpha_3\beta_1$

Integrin $\alpha_6\beta_4$

(EBMD)

Lamina lucida

Laminin 5

Lamina densa

Collagen VII

(aging, RCE)

Bowman's layer

FIGURE 4.10 Integrin $\alpha_3\beta_1$ is located inter-cellularly or at the cell–matrix junction and forms focal adhesions. Integrin $\alpha_6\beta_4$ is only located at the cell–matrix junction and forms adhesions with hemidesmosomes. Laminin 5 and collagen VII are essential components of, respectively, the lamina lucida and the lamina densa of the basement membrane (BM). The BM is anchored to the underlying Bowman's layer by collagen VII fibrils. Diseases associated with abnormalities in each type of adhesion molecule are listed as: epithelial basement membrane dystrophy (EBMD), recurrent corneal erosion (RCE). (Modified from Chen YT, Huang CW, Huang FC, et al. The cleavage plane of corneal epithelial adhesion complex in traumatic recurrent corneal erosion. *Mol Vis.* 2006;12:196–204.)

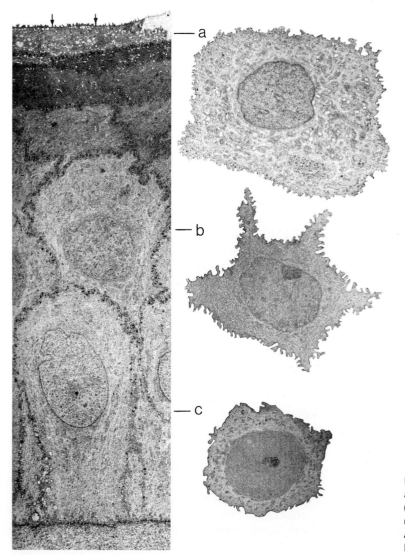

a

b

c

FIGURE 4.11 Ultrastructure of the corneal epithelium and individual appearance of surface squamous cells (*a*), wing cells (*b*), and basal cells (*c*). Arrows indicate microplicae on the corneal surface. (From Hogan MJ, Alvarado JA, Weddell JE. *Histology of the Human Eye.* Philadelphia, PA: WB Saunders; 1971:67.)

FIGURE 4.12 Distribution of intercellular junctions in the corneal epithelium. *Yellow lines* correspond to tight junctions joining the entire circumference of surface squamous cells. *Blue dots* correspond to gap junctions and green ovals correspond to desmosomes. *Orange ovals* along the basal surface of the epithelium correspond to hemidesmosomes attaching the basal layer of the epithelium to and through the basement membrane and Bowman's layer.

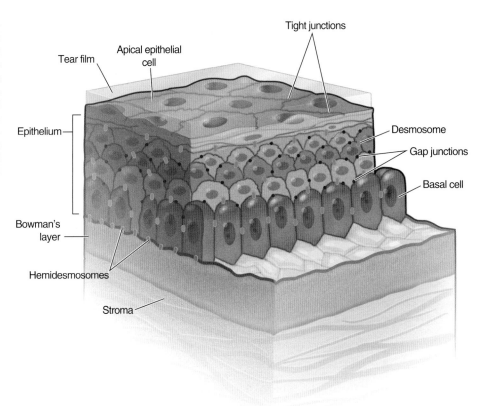

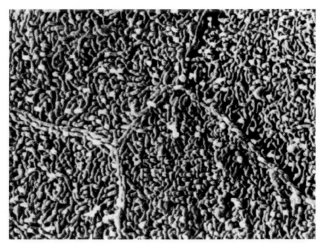

FIGURE 4.13 Scanning electron micrograph of the corneal surface showing complex pattern of surface microplicae and borders between surface cells. (From Smolek MK, Klyce SD. Cornea. In: Tasman WS, Jaeger EA, eds. *Duane's Clinical Ophthalmology on CD-ROM*. Philadelphia, PA: Lippincott Williams and Wilkins; 2006.)

1.3376 of the cornea itself. With each blink, a new, smooth, optical surface for the eye is created. Classically this film is described as having three components.

The innermost layer of the tear film is mucoid and derived primarily from the goblet cells of the conjunctiva.

The middle aqueous layer is derived from the main lacrimal gland and accessory lacrimal glands of Krause and Wolfring within the eyelids. Finally, an oily layer is present that partitions principally to the surface. This layer is derived from the sebaceous glands of the eyelids, termed the Meibomian glands and the glands of Zeis. The latter are associated with the follicles of the eyelashes.

More recently available research methods show a more complex relationship between the layers of the tear film themselves and between the microplicae of the epithelium and the mucoid layer of the tear film. The layers of the tear film do not form discrete layers. Instead, they form a colloidal matrix, the surface of which exhibits aggregates of lipid held together by hydrophobic forces (i.e., a coacervate) and beneath which are aqueous components including both soluble and gel-forming mucins. These interact with a base layer of epithelial membrane-bound mucins.[33,34] The corneal epithelial cells at the surface produce a glycocalyx that includes several transmembranous mucins, including MUC1, MUC4, and MUC16. These mucins interact with the submembranous actin matrix of the surface cells at their cytoplasmic end and with highly glycosylated and hydrophilic glycoproteins in their extracellular domains. By doing so, these transmembranous mucins play a major role in tear film adherence to the vertically-oriented surface of the cornea (**Fig. 4.14**).[35]

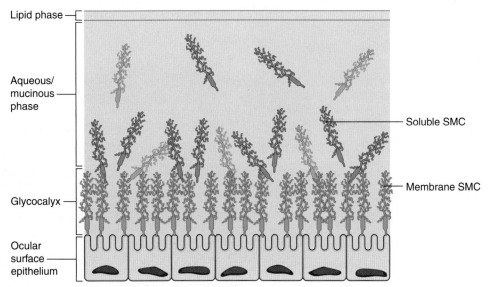

Lipid phase

Aqueous/ mucinous phase

Soluble SMC

Glycocalyx

Membrane SMC

Ocular surface epithelium

FIGURE 4.14 This schematic shows a model of the structure of the tear film, including membrane-bound surface sialomucins (SMC) that form a part of the epithelial glycocalyx and soluble SMC distributed within the aqueous/mucinous phase, beneath the lipid phase of the tear film. (From Carraway KL, Price-Schiavi SA, Komatsu M, et al. Multiple facets of sialomucin complex/MUC4, a membrane mucin and ERBB2 ligand in tumors and tissues. *Front Biosci.* 2000;5:D95–D107.)

Corneal Innervation: The sensory nerve endings in the corneal epithelium are mediated through the nasociliary branch of the ophthalmic division of the fifth cranial nerve, and conveyed to the eye via the long ciliary nerves.[36]

Pattern of Innervation: Most of the nerves serving the cornea enter from the nasal and temporal limbus (**Fig. 4.15**).[37] As they move radially, through the corneal stroma, they lose their myelin sheaths. This makes these nerves difficult to see clinically, except in certain abnormal conditions in which their prominence increases (e.g., keratoconus). The nerve branches penetrate Bowman's layer, and then take a 90° turn to travel within the basement membrane of the corneal epithelium as a subbasal plexus. Thin, sensory fibers then turn toward the surface, between basal cells, to provide nerve endings near the corneal surface (**Fig. 4.16**).[37,38]

The density of corneal nerve endings is greater centrally than peripherally, consistent with the greater sensitivity known to exist in the central cornea. Although the corneal surface is exquisitely sensitive, these nerve endings provide less precise localization of the source of pain than is found on the skin.

Neurotropic viruses such as herpes simplex can travel within the branches of the fifth cranial nerve, giving rise to inflammatory lesions along nerve endings. In these cases, the branching pattern of the affected nerves becomes evident, creating a dendriform lesion on the cornea that stains with fluorescein dye (Fig. 4.17).

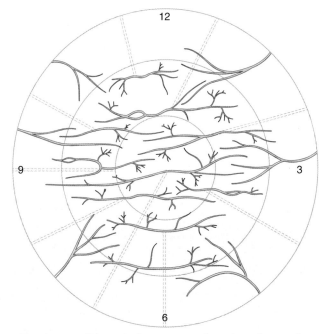

FIGURE 4.15 Schematic demonstrates the points of entry of corneal sensory nerves at the corneal limbus and their general pattern of distribution. (Modified from Muller LJ, Vrensen G, Pels L, et al. Architecture of human corneal nerves. *Invest Ophthalmol Vis Sci.* 1997;38:985–994.)

Bowman's Layer

Bowman's layer is not the basement membrane of the corneal epithelium. These two structures are readily identified as separate in sections stained with periodic acid–Schiff (PAS), a stain commonly used to identify

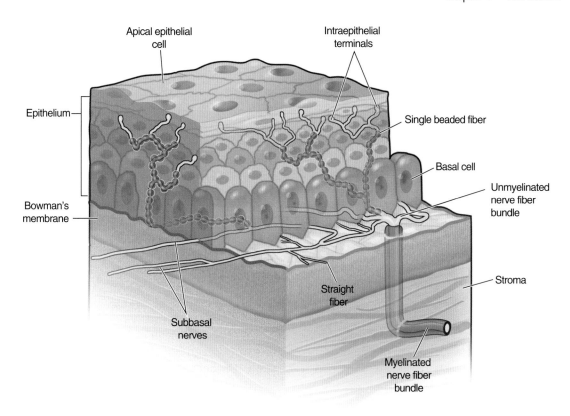

FIGURE 4.16 Three-dimensional drawing of the penetration and distribution of stromal nerve bundles into the subbasal plexus of the corneal epithelium. The unmyelinated nerve fiber bundles (*yellow*) arising from myelinated nerves that traverse Bowman's layer sometimes divide, with bifurcations at almost right angles. These consist of several straight and single-beaded (*green*) fibers. Single-beaded fibers bifurcate obliquely and turn upward between the basal cells to reach the wing cells and extend to intraepithelial terminals near the surface. (Modified from Muller LJ, Vrensen G, Pels L, et al. Architecture of human corneal nerves. *Invest Ophthalmol Vis Sci.* 1997;38:985–994.)

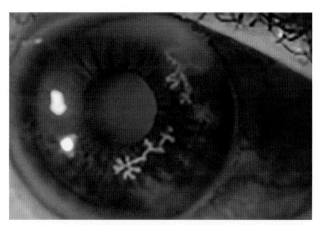

FIGURE 4.17 Dendriform lesion of corneal epithelium stained with fluorescein dye. (Courtesy of Dr. Howard Leibowitz.)

basement membranes. Note in **Figure 4.18** that the basement membrane of the corneal epithelium stains a deep magenta, while the thicker, more homogeneous Bowman's layer beneath it does not. Bowman's layer represents a remarkably resilient, acellular condensation of collagen types I and III, but with a smaller fiber diameter than those found in the stroma. Unlike the epithelial basement membrane above it, and the corneal stroma below it, Bowman's layer does not extend all the way to the corneoscleral junction; it stops approximately 1 mm short of the corneoscleral junction. In vivo estimates of Bowman's layer thickness vary from 11 to 17 μm and there is evidence that Bowman's layer thins by about one-third between the ages of 20 and 80.[10,43]

The anatomic integrity of the corneal epithelium is dependent upon an intact sensory innervation (i.e., neurotrophic effect). Prolonged loss of sensory innervation can lead to the development of corneal epithelial defects, ulcers, and perforation (neurotrophic keratitis).[39–42]

Penetrating corneal injuries (incisional or traumatic) that are deep enough to involve Bowman's layer cannot fully repair to optical clarity. Such defects produced in Bowman's layer result in scarring and opacification of varying degrees.[44]

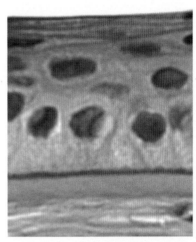

FIGURE 4.18 Bowman's layer is seen as a homogeneous layer between the thinner, darker basal lamina of the corneal epithelium and the anterior lamellae of the corneal stroma.

The importance of Bowman's layer to the maintenance of normal corneal function remains uncertain since some species exhibit no discernable Bowman's layer and yet their corneas remain optically clear and structurally stable. Additionally, photorefractive keratectomy, a form of refractive surgery, completely ablates Bowman's layer without destabilizing the cornea.

The Corneal Stroma

The stroma represents 90% of the total corneal thickness. It is the ultimate example of a dense, regular connective tissue and is composed of very regularly ordered layers of type I/V heterotypic collagen fibrils, microfibrillar structures of type VI collagen, FACIT collagens (XII and XIV) and other non-fibrillar collagens. Proteoglycans (principally decorin, lumican, and smaller amounts of osteoglycin and keratocan) are present and they anchor the hydroscopic glycosaminoglycans. These proteoglycans appear to regulate fibrillar diameter and their anatomic spacing, both of which are critical for transparency.[45]

Interspersed within this matrix, and responsible for its maintenance and repair, are resident connective tissue cells termed keratocytes.[46] Keratocytes appear fusiform and send thin processes to each other. Together they produce an integrated cell matrix throughout the breadth and depth of the cornea, communicating by way of gap junctions.[47] The number of keratocytes in the corneal stroma decreases with age. In addition to keratocytes, the normal stroma contains a small resident population of patrolling phagocytes including histiocytes and occasional polymorphonuclear leukocytes. To move through the stroma these cells become very flattened and thus are easily mistaken for keratocytes at the light microscopic level.

Each layer of the stroma is called a lamella. Lamellae can be surgically separated, permitting partial thickness replacement of diseased cornea in a lamellar keratectomy, without postoperative scarring centrally. The collagen fibrils within adjacent lamellae have been traditionally assumed to be oriented 90° apart from their next adjacent layers. This arrangement is similar to that seen in the construction of plywood, in which the grain of the wood is turned 90° in each adjoining leaflet of the plywood's thickness, thus producing more strength than a single board of the same total thickness. More recent assessments indicate that the angles between adjacent lamellae are less stringent but vary within a range of about 20° of the horizontal and vertical axes.[48] At the limbus, these lamellae interdigitate with a circumferentially oriented ring of collagen sometimes referred to as the "ligamentum circulare corneae," which appears to stabilize the structure of the eye at the zone of dramatic change in the outside contour of the eye, as the more steeply curved peripheral cornea transitions to the less steeply curved sclera at what is termed the external scleral sulcus (SEE CHAPTER 6: THE SCLERA, EPISCLERA, AND TENON'S CAPSULE).[48,49]

Within each lamella, all of the collagen fibrils are parallel to one another, separated by a constant distance determined by the relative hydration of their surrounding layer of proteoglycans and glycosaminoglycans. This regular arrangement is widely regarded as essential to the maintenance of corneal transparency (**Fig. 4.19**).[50] When the stromal collagen fibers are optimally spaced, the scattering of light that each produces is out of phase with the scattering originating from its surrounding fibers. This destructive interference of stromal collagen light scattering increases transparency. If the spacing between adjacent collagen fibrils is irregularly increased, as when excess fluid enters the stroma in corneal edema, the light scattering of adjacent fibrils no longer creates destructive interference, resulting in loss of corneal transparency.[51]

To think of the corneal stroma as a uniform matrix is inaccurate. Increasing evidence suggests that various stromal components are distributed asymmetrically, concentrating preferentially either in the anterior or posterior lamellae. Keratocytes are more abundant in the anterior third of the stroma than in deeper layers. So too, plasma-derived proteins such as albumin, which diffuse into the corneal stroma from normally leaky blood vessels in the perilimbal conjunctiva, tend to concentrate in the anterior third of the corneal stroma (**Fig. 4.20**).[52] Even the proteoglycans of the corneal stroma are asymmetrically distributed. In the anterior stroma, the ratio of keratan sulfate to dermatan sulfate is 1.59/1, whereas in the posterior stroma, this same ratio is 2.23/1.[53]

Recent evidence suggests that the posteriormost lamellae of the stroma, adjacent to Descemet's membrane, may be particularly durable and it appears that it is from this same posterior stromal region that collagen extends into the cores of the beams of the trabecular meshwork, beyond the periphery of the cornea.[54]

Normal stromal collagen arrangement

Abnormal stromal collagen arrangement

Destructive interference

Constructive interference

FIGURE 4.19 **Top:** Arrangement of collagen fibrils within adjacent stromal lamellae. Intervening between lamellae are the flattened cell profiles of keratocytes with their nuclei shown in green. **Middle:** Cross-sectional organization of collagen fibril spacing in the normal, clear cornea at left and cross-sectional organization of collagen fibril spacing in edematous, hazy corneal stroma at right. **Lower:** Waveform showing destructive interference that reduces light scattering and improves transparency **(left)**. Waveform in which scattering from adjacent collagen fibrils becomes additive, creating constructive interference and leading to reduced transparency **(right)**. (Modified from Hogan MJ, Alvarado JA, Weddell JE. *Histology of the Human Eye.* Philadelphia, PA: WB Saunders; 1971:92.)

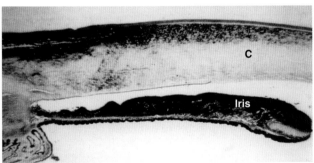

FIGURE 4.20 Light micrograph shows immunohistochemical localization of albumin within the normal cornea (*C*). Note that the majority of the albumin is restricted to the anterior third of the stroma. The source of this albumin is the perilimbal vasculature. (From Gong H, Ye W, Johnson M, et al. The nonuniform distribution of albumin in human and bovine cornea. *Exp Eye Res.* 1997;65:747–756.)

Descemet's Membrane

Unlike Bowman's layer, which is not a true basement membrane, Descemet's membrane is the basement membrane of the corneal endothelium. Together with the posteriormost stromal lamellae, they constitute the most resilient of all of the corneal layers. The peripheral edge of Descemet's membrane is visible clinically by gonioscopy and is termed Schwalbe's line (**SEE CHAPTER 9:**

ANATOMY OF THE AQUEOUS OUTFLOW PATHWAYS). This membrane thickens slowly but continuously throughout life. The prenatal and postnatal portions of Descemet's membrane can be distinguished ultrastructurally. The prenatal portion exhibits a peculiar "banding" evident by electron microscopy, which is not found in the more posterior portions of Descemet's membrane that develop postnatally (**Fig. 4.21**). Age-related thickening of Descemet's membrane is usually uniform except in the far periphery where focal, nodular thickenings are produced that are termed Hassal–Henle bodies.

 Nodular excrescences that appear histologically similar to Hassal–Henle bodies can occur as a pathologic finding in the central portion of Descemet's membrane where they are called guttata and are seen readily with a slit-lamp. Figure 4.22 shows irregular droplet-like guttata of Descemet's membrane. Guttata are a characteristic finding of a condition known as Fuchs' dystrophy, in which progressive corneal endothelial cell degeneration leads to corneal edema and vision loss.

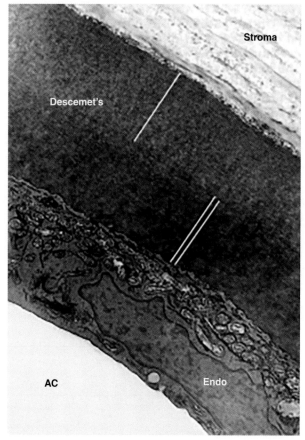

FIGURE 4.21 Electron micrograph shows the prenatal (*single line*) and postnatal portions (*double line*) of Descemet's membrane, between the corneal stroma and corneal endothelium (*Endo*). AC, anterior chamber. (From Leibowitz HM, Waring GO, eds. *Corneal Disorders: Clinical Diagnosis and Management*. 2nd ed. Philadelphia, PA: WB Saunders; 1998.)

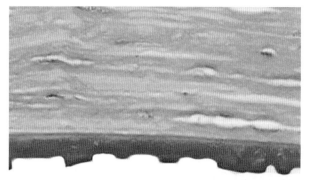

FIGURE 4.22 Light micrograph shows numerous drop-like deposits (guttata) on the posterior surface of Descemet's membrane in Fuchs' dystrophy.

The Corneal Endothelium

The corneal endothelium is a simple, cuboidal epithelium that lines the posterior corneal surface (**Fig. 4.21**). The density of the endothelial cell population is less in the central than in the paracentral and peripheral regions of the cornea.[55]

The membranes of the corneal endothelial cell contain Na-K, ATPase pumps that continually pump fluid from the corneal stroma to maintain the hydrophilic glycosaminoglycans

of the corneal stroma in a less than fully hydrated state (i.e., a state of deturgescence). The tight junctions between adjacent endothelial cells are discontinuous and permit a flux of aqueous humor from the anterior chamber into the corneal stroma.[56] If not removed by the Na-K pumps and other channels and ion ports, this fluid would more fully hydrate the stromal glycosaminoglycans, irregularly separating the stromal collagen fibrils and swelling the cornea, rendering it opaque (**Fig. 4.19**).

In the child and young adult, the average diameter of corneal endothelial cells is approximately 20 µm. These cells are approximately 4 to 6 µm thick in young and middle-aged adults.[57] At the corneal periphery, the monolayer of corneal endothelial cells becomes continuous with the single layer of endothelial cells that wraps the beams of the trabecular meshwork.

The corneal endothelium has a very limited capacity for mitotic division.[58] While there is increasing evidence that there is a resident stem cell population in the transition area between the corneal endothelium and the trabecular meshwork, the low mitotic rate is unable to maintain corneal endothelial cell numbers.[59] As a result, there is an age-related decrease in endothelial cell numbers.[60,61]

In order to provide the requisite coverage of the entire posterior corneal surface with fewer cells, each cell spreads to cover a larger surface area and thus, in cross section, these cells appear thinner with age, looking more squamous than cuboidal (**Fig. 4.23**).

Using specular microscopy, endothelial cells can be viewed en face and cell size, shape, and numbers can be assessed noninvasively in the clinical setting. Young, healthy endothelial cells look fairly uniform in size and shape (**Fig. 4.24A**). Loss of corneal endothelial cells, with increasing age, leads to variability of cell shape (pleomorphism) and variability in cell size (polymegathism) (**Fig. 4.24B**). Endothelial cell counts in infancy range from 3,500 to 4,000 cells per mm[2]. In normal adult corneas, cell density is approximately 3,000 to 3,500 cells per mm[2]. If cell density falls below 500 to 700 cells per mm[2], it is increasingly difficult to maintain optical clarity.[62–64]

ARLT'S TRIANGLE
*Although its anatomic borders are imaginary, there is an area of the posterior corneal surface that has particular clinical importance as an anatomic location. This area of the posterior corneal surface is termed Arlt's triangle, which has its apex at the center of the cornea and its curved base along the inferior limbus (**Fig. 4.25**). Within the limits of Arlt's triangle is the most common area for circulating pigment or inflammatory cells in the aqueous humor to sediment out onto the endothelial surface. Identifying distributions of endothelial deposits that are within and outside of Arlt's triangle can be useful in differential diagnosis, especially in the distribution of inflammatory cells on the corneal endothelium (keratic precipitates) in various forms of anterior uveitis.*

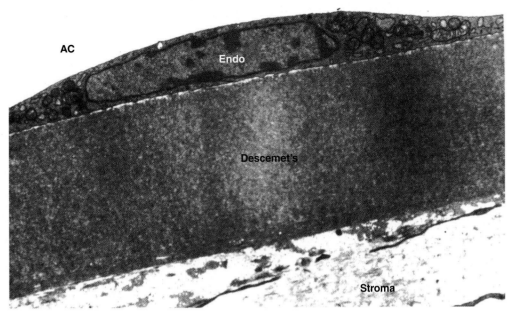

FIGURE 4.23 Electron micrograph of posterior corneal layers of an elderly normal cornea shows thickened Descemet's membrane and flattened corneal endothelial cell (*Endo*). AC, anterior chamber. (From Leibowitz HM, Waring GO, eds. *Corneal Disorders: Clinical Diagnosis and Management.* 2nd ed. Philadelphia, PA: WB Saunders; 1998.)

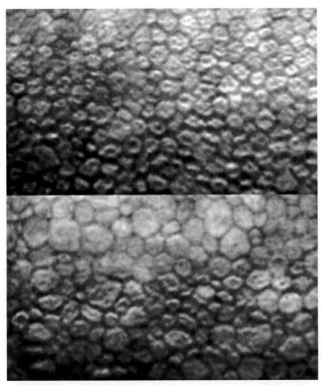

FIGURE 4.24 **Top:** En face specular microscopic image of young corneal endothelial mosaic, showing relative uniformity of cell size and shape. **Bottom:** Specular micrograph of elderly normal cornea shows generally larger cells (polymegathism) and greater heterogeneity in shape (pleomorphism). (Courtesy of Setsuo Oak, Konan Corp.)

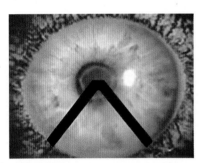

FIGURE 4.25 Arlt's triangle.

REFERENCES

1. Rio-Cristobal A, Martin R. Corneal assessment technologies: current status. *Surv Ophthalmol.* 2014;59(6):599–614.
2. Rufer F, Schroder A, Erb C. White-to-white corneal diameter: Normal values in healthy humans obtained with the orbscan II topography system. *Cornea.* 2005;24(3):259–261.
3. Doughty MJ, Zaman ML. Human corneal thickness and its impact on intraocular pressure measures: a review and meta-analysis approach. *Surv Ophthalmol.* 2000;44(5):367–408.
4. Brandt JD, Beiser JA, Kass MA, et al. Central corneal thickness in the ocular hypertension treatment study (OHTS). *Ophthalmology.* 2001;108(10):1779–1788.
5. La Rosa FA, Gross RL, Orengo-Nania S. Central corneal thickness of Caucasians and African Americans in glaucomatous and nonglaucomatous populations. *Arch Ophthalmol.* 2001;119(1): 23–27.
6. Aghaian E, Choe JE, Lin S, et al. Central corneal thickness of Caucasians, Chinese, Hispanics, Filipinos, African Americans, and Japanese in a glaucoma clinic. *Ophthalmology.* 2004;111(12):2211–2219.

7. Trinkaus-Randall V, Edelhauser HF, Leibowitz H, et al. *Corneal Structure and Function. Corneal Disorders; Clinical Diagnosis and Management*. 2nd ed. Philadelphia, PA: WB Saunders; 1998:21–27.

8. Ruben M. *Contact Lens Practice*. Baltimore, MD: Williams and Wilkins; 1975.

9. Sorsby A. Biology of the eye as an optical system. *Clin Ophthalmol*. 1995;1:1–17.

10. Tao A, Wang J, Chen Q, et al. Topographic thickness of bowman's layer determined by ultra-high resolution spectral domain-optical coherence tomography. *Invest Ophthalmol Vis Sci*. 2011;52(6):3901–3907.

11. Reinstein DZ, Silverman RH, Rondeau MJ, et al. Epithelial and corneal thickness measurements by high-frequency ultrasound digital signal processing. *Ophthalmology*. 1994;101(1):140–146.

12. Yang Y, Hong J, Deng SX, et al. Age-related changes in human corneal epithelial thickness measured with anterior segment optical coherence tomography. *Invest Ophthalmol Vis Sci*. 2014;55(8):5032–5038.

13. Thoft RA, Friend J. The X, Y, Z hypothesis of corneal epithelial maintenance. *Invest Ophthalmol Vis Sci*. 1983;24(10):1442–1443.

14. Bron AJ. Vortex patterns of the corneal epithelium. *Trans Ophthalmol Soc U K*. 1973;93(0):455–472.

15. Cowan T. Striate melanokeratosis in negroes. *Trans Am Ophthalmol Soc*. 1963;61:61–74.

16. Dana MR. Corneal antigen-presenting cells: diversity, plasticity, and disguise: the Cogan lecture. *Invest Ophthalmol Vis Sci*. 2004;45(3):721–727.

17. Chandler JW, Cummings M, Gillette TE. Presence of Langerhans cells in the central corneas of normal human infants. *Invest Ophthalmol Vis Sci*. 1985;26(1):113–116.

18. Rodrigues MM, Rowden G, Hackett J, et al. Langerhans cells in the normal conjunctiva and peripheral cornea of selected species. *Invest Ophthalmol Vis Sci*. 1981;21(5):759–765.

19. Hori J, Joyce NC, Streilein JW. Immune privilege and immunogenicity reside among different layers of the mouse cornea. *Invest Ophthalmol Vis Sci*. 2000;41(10):3032–3042.

20. Miller JK, Laycock KA, Nash MM, et al. Corneal Langerhans cell dynamics after herpes simplex virus reactivation. *Invest Ophthalmol Vis Sci*. 1993;34(7):2282–2290.

21. Hazlett LD, McClellan SM, Hume EB, et al. Extended wear contact lens usage induces Langerhans cell migration into cornea. *Exp Eye Res*. 1999;69(5):575–577.

22. Cursiefen C, Schlotzer-Schrehardt U, Kuchle M, et al. Lymphatic vessels in vascularized human corneas: immunohistochemical investigation using LYVE-1 and podoplanin. *Invest Ophthalmol Visual Sci*. 2002;43(7):2127–2135.

23. Chen YT, Huang CW, Huang FC, et al. The cleavage plane of corneal epithelial adhesion complex in traumatic recurrent corneal erosion. *Mol Vis*. 2006;12:196–204.

24. Stepp MA. Corneal integrins and their functions. *Exp Eye Res*. 2006;83(1):3–15.

25. Anhalt GJ, Jampel HD, Patel HP, et al. Bullous pemphigoid autoantibodies are markers of corneal epithelial hemidesmosomes. *Invest Ophthalmol Vis Sci*. 1987;28(5):903–907.

26. Gipson I. Anatomy of the conjunctiva, cornea, and limbus. In: *The Cornea*. 3rd ed. Boston, MA: Little, Brown and Company; 1994:3–24.

27. Ramselaar JA, Boot JP, van Haeringen NJ, et al. Corneal epithelial permeability after instillation of ophthalmic solutions containing local anaesthetics and preservatives. *Curr Eye Res*. 1988;7(9):947–950.

28. King-Smith PE, Fink BA, Fogt N. Three interferometric methods for measuring the thickness of layers of the tear film. *Optom Vis Sci*. 1999;76(1):19–32.

29. King-Smith PE, Fink BA, Fogt N, et al. The thickness of the human precorneal tear film: evidence from reflection spectra. *Invest Ophthalmol Vis Sci*. 2000;41(11):3348–3359.

30. King-Smith PE, Fink BA, Nichols JJ, et al. Interferometric imaging of the full thickness of the precorneal tear film. *J Opt Soc Am A Opt Image Sci Vis*. 2006;23(9):2097–2104.

31. Huang D, Swanson EA, Lin CP, et al. Optical coherence tomography. *Science*. 1991;254(5035):1178–1181.

32. Azartash K, Kwan J, Paugh JR, et al. Pre-corneal tear film thickness in humans measured with a novel technique. *Mol Vis*. 2011;17:756–767.

33. Bron A, Tiffany J, Gouveia S, et al. Functional aspects of the tear film lipid layer. *Exp Eye Res*. 2004;78(3):347–360.

34. Prydal JI, Artal P, Woon H, et al. Study of human precorneal tear film thickness and structure using laser interferometry. *Invest Ophthalmol Vis Sci*. 1992;33(6):2006–2011.

35. Carraway KL, Price-Schiavi SA, Komatsu M, et al. Multiple facets of sialomucin complex/MUC4, a membrane mucin and erbb2 ligand, in tumors and tissues (Y2K update). *Front Biosci*. 2000;5:D95–D107.

36. Marfurt CF, Cox J, Deek S, et al. Anatomy of the human corneal innervation. *Exp Eye Res*. 2010;90(4):478–492.

37. Muller LJ, Vrensen GF, Pels L, et al. Architecture of human corneal nerves. *Invest Ophthalmol Vis Sci*. 1997;38(5):985–994.

38. He J, Bazan NG, Bazan HE. Mapping the entire human corneal nerve architecture. *Exp Eye Res*. 2010;91(4):513–523.

39. Sigelman S, Friedenwald JS. Mitotic and wound-healing activities of the corneal epithelium; effect of sensory denervation. *AMA Arch Ophthalmol*. 1954;52(1):46–57.

40. Simone S. De ricerche sul contenuto in acqua totale ed in azoto totale della cornea di coniglio in condizioni di cheratite neuroparalitica sperimentale. *Arch Ottalmol*. 1958;62:151.

41. Alper MG. The anesthetic eye: an investigation of changes in the anterior ocular segment of the monkey caused by interrupting the trigeminal nerve at various levels along its course. *Trans Am Ophthalmol Soc*. 1975;73:323–365.

42. Mackie IA. Role of the corneal nerves in destructive disease of the cornea. *Trans Ophthalmol Soc U K*. 1978;98(3):343–347.

43. Germundsson J, Karanis G, Fagerholm P, et al. Age-related thinning of bowman's layer in the human cornea in vivo. *Invest Ophthalmol Vis Sci*. 2013;54(9):6143–6149.

44. Wilson SE, Hong JW. Bowman's layer structure and function: critical or dispensable to corneal function? A hypothesis. *Cornea*. 2000;19(4):417–420.

45. Hassell JR, Birk DE. The molecular basis of corneal transparency. *Exp Eye Res*. 2010;91(3):326–335.

46. West-Mays JA, Dwivedi DJ. The keratocyte: corneal stromal cell with variable repair phenotypes. *Int J Biochem Cell Biol*. 2006;38(10):1625–1631.

47. Watsky MA, Rae JL. Initial characterization of whole-cell currents from freshly dissociated corneal keratocytes. *Curr Eye Res*. 1992;11(2):127–134.

48. Ruberti J, Roy AS, Roberts C. Corneal structure and function. Corneal biomechanics and biomaterials (supplementary material).

49. Meek KM, Boote C. The organization of collagen in the corneal stroma. *Exp Eye Res*. 2004;78(3):503–512.

50. Maurice D. The physical basis of corneal transparency. *XVII Council Ophthalmol*. 1954:465–469.

51. Maurice DM. The structure and transparency of the cornea. *J Physiol*. 1957;136(2):263–286.

52. Maurice DM, Watson PG. The distribution and movement of serum albumin in the cornea. *Exp Eye Res*. 1965;4(4):355–363.

53. Smolin G, Thoft RA. *The Cornea: Scientific Foundations and Clinical Practice*. Boston, MA: Little, Brown and Company; 1994.

54. Dua HS, Faraj LA, Branch MJ, et al. The collagen matrix of the human trabecular meshwork is an extension of the novel pre-descemet's layer (dua's layer). *Br J Ophthalmol*. 2014;98(5):691–697.

55. Amann J, Holley GP, Lee SB, et al. Increased endothelial cell density in the paracentral and peripheral regions of the human cornea. *Am J Ophthalmol*. 2003;135(5):584–590.

56. Noske W, Fromm M, Levarlet B, et al. Tight junctions of the human corneal endothelium: morphological and electrophysiological features. *Ger J Ophthalmol*. 1994;3(4–5):253–257.

57. Hiles DA, Biglan AW, Fetherolf EC. Central corneal endothelial cell counts in children. *J Am Intraocul Implant Soc.* 1979;5(4):292–300.

58. Laing RA, Sandstrom MM, Berrospi AR, et al. Changes in the corneal endothelium as a function of age. *Exp Eye Res.* 1976;22(6):587–594.

59. Yu WY, Sheridan C, Grierson I, et al. Progenitors for the corneal endothelium and trabecular meshwork: a potential source for personalized stem cell therapy in corneal endothelial diseases and glaucoma. *J Biomed Biotechnol.* 2011;2011:412743.

60. McGowan SL, Edelhauser HF, Pfister RR, et al. Stem cell markers in the human posterior limbus and corneal endothelium of unwounded and wounded corneas. *Mol Vis.* 2007;13:1984–2000.

61. Braunger BM, Ademoglu B, Koschade SE, et al. Identification of adult stem cells in schwalbe's line region of the primate eye. *Invest Ophthalmol Vis Sci.* 2014;55(11):7499–7507.

62. Ayala G, Dıaz M, Martınez-Costa L. Granulometric moments and corneal endothelium status. *Pattern Recognit.* 2001;34(6): 1219–1227.

63. Gutierrez J, Ayala G. Set descriptors for visual evaluation of human corneal endothelia. *Comput Vis Image Underst.* 2001;84(2):249–263.

64. Sanchis-Gimeno JA, Lleo-Perez A, Alonso L, et al. Corneal endothelial cell density decreases with age in emmetropic eyes. *Histol Histopathol.* 2005;20(2):423–427.

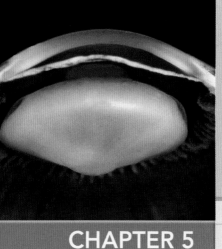

The Conjunctiva and the Limbus

CHAPTER 5

Overview

The conjunctiva is a semitransparent mucosa that serves an array of functions. The conjunctiva contributes to lubrication of the ocular surface, reducing friction of the mucosal surfaces and allowing for pain-free eye movements and lid closure. It also provides both physical and chemical antimicrobial barriers and is an integral part of the body's mucosa-associated lymphoid tissue system.[1] In addition, the limbal conjunctival epithelium provides the stem cell population for corneal epithelial renewal.

Macroscopic and Clinical Anatomy of the Conjunctiva

The conjunctiva is continuous with the cornea at the limbus and with the skin at the mucocutaneous junction of the lid margins (**Fig. 5.1**). Extending from the limbus 360°, this mucosa overlies the anterior third of the sclera and then reflects onto the inner surface of the eyelids. The portion of the conjunctiva overlying the sclera is termed the bulbar conjunctiva. The portion of the conjunctiva lining the inside surfaces of the upper and lower lids is termed the palpebral conjunctiva. Superiorly, inferiorly, and laterally, the reflection of the conjunctiva from the sclera onto the inner surface of the eyelids forms a blind pouch termed either the fornix or the cul-de-sac. Remarkably, the reflection of the conjunctiva from the surface of the eye onto the inside of the eyelids does not restrict movement of the eye.

 *Certain inflammatory conditions (ocular cicatricial pemphigoid) can lead to scarring and contraction (cicatrization) of the conjunctiva. Note vertical ridge of abnormal conjunctival tissue connecting the inferior lid margin and the edge of the cornea (arrows) in (**Fig. 5.2**). The resulting "foreshortening" of the fornix (symblepharon) can produce restrictions of eye movements and interfere with blinking.*

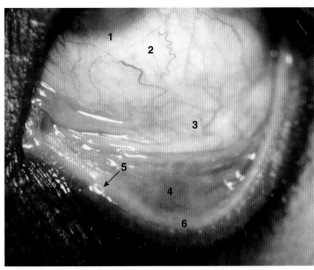

FIGURE 5.1 Clinical photograph of conjunctiva with lower eyelid pulled inferiorly. (*1*) Limbus; (*2*) bulbar conjunctiva; (*3*) fornix; (*4*) palpebral conjunctiva; (*5*) lacrimal punctum; (*6*) mucocutaneous junction of lid margin. (Courtesy of Mission for Vision and Dr. Ben Glasgow [www.missionforvision.org].)

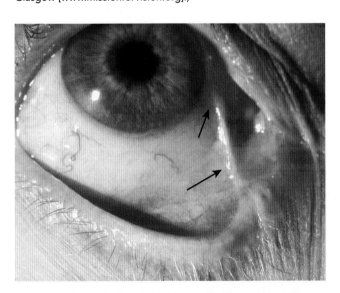

FIGURE 5.2 Band of scarring (cicatrization—*black arrows*), connecting lid margin and perilimbal conjunctiva (symblepharon) in ocular cicatricial pemphigoid. (Courtesy of Dr. Howard Leibowitz.)

THE PLICA SEMILUNARIS AND THE CARUNCLE

Near the medial canthus, the bulbar conjunctiva forms a half-moon-shaped fold called the plica semilunaris (**Fig. 5.3**). The plica is the vestigial remnant of the nictitating membrane or "third eyelid" found in other species. The plica partially unfolds on lateral gaze.

The caruncle is a yellowish nodule of tissue, medial to the plica semilunaris, occupying the interpalpebral space in the medial canthus (**Fig. 5.3**). Its true function remains uncertain. It is covered by a nonkeratinized stratified squamous epithelium, with an underlying stroma that differs from the rest of the conjunctival stroma in that it

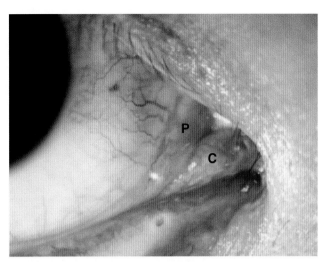

FIGURE 5.3 Clinical photograph shows medial canthus including plica semilunaris (*P*) and caruncle (*C*). Along the everted inferior lid margin, the inferior punctal opening of the lacrimal drainage system is also evident. (Courtesy of Dr. Derek Ho.)

contains pilosebaceous units with cilia, accessory lacrimal gland tissue, and numerous sebaceous glands as well. The sebaceous glands can undergo benign hypertrophy with age, producing a concerning increase in size of the caruncle termed an oncocytoma. The caruncle is well vascularized, with its blood supply arising solely from the superior palpebral vessels. Similarly, its sensory nerve supply arises from the infratrochlear nerve, which enters the nasal side of the upper eyelid below the trochlea (**SEE CHAPTER 2: THE EYELIDS AND ADNEXA**). The infratrochlear nerve is a branch of the ophthalmic division of the trigeminal nerve (CN V). Lymphatic drainage of the caruncle is initially to the submandibular lymph nodes.

Histology

CONJUNCTIVAL EPITHELIUM

The conjunctival epithelium is invariably stratified but varies in its cellular morphology in different locations (**Fig. 5.4**). At the fornix, and over most of the palpebral conjunctiva, the epithelium is categorized as stratified columnar. On the bulbar conjunctiva, the surface cells are more often cuboidal and finally, near the lid margins, the surface cells become progressively more squamous in their appearance.[2,3] The transition from conjunctival mucosal epithelium to the keratinized skin of the eyelid is termed the mucocutaneous junction. Details of this transition, and of the recently identified "lid wiper" region of the palpebral conjunctiva, near the lid margin, are presented in **CHAPTER 2: THE EYELIDS AND ADNEXA**.

The epithelial cells of the conjunctival surface exhibit microvilli. These microvilli vary in height by location, with forniceal epithelial cells having taller microvilli than elsewhere (**Fig. 5.5**).[4] Microvilli increase the surface area

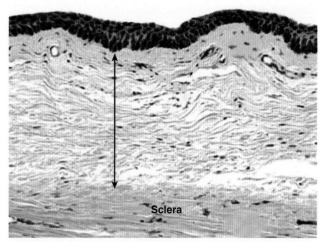

FIGURE 5.4   Light micrograph of bulbar conjunctiva within the interpalpebral fissure. Notice the paucity of goblet cells and the loose stroma between overlying conjunctival epithelium and underlying sclera (*double-headed arrow*). The stroma of the palpebral conjunctiva is not as thick or as loose. (Modified from Gartner LP, Hiatt JL. *Color Atlas and Text of Histology.* 6th ed. Philadelphia, PA: Wolters Kluwer; 2013.)

for secretion and absorption at the conjunctival surface and serve to assist in holding the mucin layer of the tear film to the vertically-oriented surface of the conjunctiva (**Fig. 5.5**). The surface cells of the conjunctiva are joined at their apicolateral surfaces by a junctional complex consisting of a zonula occludens (tight junction) and zonula adherens. The zonula adherens holds each epithelial cell

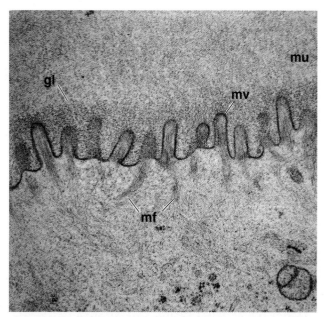

FIGURE 5.5   Electron micrograph of conjunctival surface demonstrates microvilli (mv) and their content of cytoplasmic microfibrils, (mf). On the epithelial surface, the glycocalyx (gl) is evident, along with its continuity with the surface layer of mucins (mu). (From Nichols BA. Conjunctiva. *Microsc Res Tech.* 1996;33:296–319.)

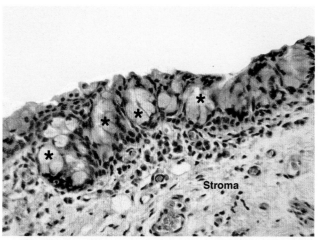

FIGURE 5.6   Light micrograph shows numerous goblet cell-lined crypts within the conjunctival epithelium (*asterisks*).

to its neighbors, around its entire circumference, while the zonula occludens seals the intercellular clefts between the surface cells. In doing so, they form the intercellular permeability barrier of the epithelium.[5] The actual junctional proteins of the zonula occludens between conjunctival epithelial cells include claudins 1, 4, and 7. Those joining epithelial cells to goblet cells include claudin 10 as well.[6]

Crypts of Henle and Stieda

The issue of whether there are truly crypts in the surface of the palpebral conjunctiva, and what their functions might be, has been controversial since the original claims made by Henle and Stieda in 1886 and 1887, respectively. More recently, in an attempt to resolve this question using more modern methods, Kessing[7] completed detailed gross and histologic assessments of 78 human conjunctival whole mounts. The conclusion was that goblet-cell-lined structures, similar to those described by both Henle and Stieda, were present (**Fig. 5.6**). In additional studies, crypt-like surface folds have been shown to result from parallel, linear, subepithelial accumulations of lymphoid aggregates in the underlying stroma. This arrangement creates a surface groove that is proposed to be a part of the conjunctiva-associated lymphoid tissue system.[8] The true function of these structures remains uncertain, but it is suspected that these grooves, crypts, and troughs trap bacteria and antigenic material, allowing it to be neutralized by the various defense mechanisms of the conjunctiva.[9]

Additional Cell Types within the Epithelial Layer

Goblet Cells: Interspersed within the conjunctival epithelium are goblet cells, unicellular glands common to various mucosae, especially in the gastrointestinal and respiratory systems. These glands produce most of the mucous layer of the tear film. The mucus is secreted from these cells in the manner utilized by apocrine glands. That is, all or most of the secretory granules of

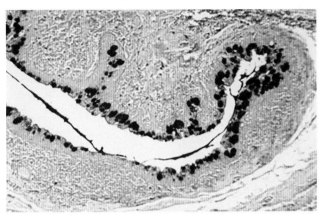

FIGURE 5.7 Light micrograph of conjunctival fornix showing numerous periodic acid–Schiff positive goblet cells within the conjunctival epithelium.

It was long assumed that goblet cells received no autonomic innervation. This assumption has recently been disproven. Human conjunctival goblet cells do receive both parasympathetic and sympathetic nerve terminals and have receptors for several neurotransmitters. As elsewhere, these two divisions of the autonomic nervous system work in opposition to regulate goblet cell secretion.[11] Parasympathetic neruotransmitters, acetylcholine and vaso-intestinal peptide, as well as purinergic nucleotides, are stimulatory.

While goblet cells are the principal source of mucins for the ocular surface, it is important to appreciate that non-goblet cells of the conjunctival epithelium are also capable of producing neutral mucin, sialomucin, and sulfomucin in limited amounts.[12]

the cells are discharged at once, following stimulation.[10] The distribution of goblet cells within the conjunctiva is nonuniform. The lowest concentration of goblet cells is found near the limbus (**Figs. 5.4** and **5.8**) and the highest concentration of goblet cells is found in the forniceal conjunctiva (**Figs. 5.7** and **5.8**). From the fornices, the concentration of goblet cells diminishes toward both the limbus and the lid margin. Overlain on this distributional pattern, the normal conjunctiva usually exhibits greater numbers of goblet cells nasally than temporally (**Fig. 5.8**). Compare the paucity of goblet cells seen in the conjunctival epithelium near the limbus (**Fig. 5.4**) with the abundance of goblet cells at the fornix (**Fig. 5.7**).

 *The two figures (**Fig. 5.9A and B**) show epithelial inclusion cysts produced by injuries to the surface of the conjunctiva. Note that the content of the cyst near the limbus is clear, whereas the content of the cyst near the fornix is opaque. Near the fornix, where there is a greater concentration of goblet cells within the epithelium, there are also greater numbers of goblet cells within the wall of the cyst that was derived from the overlying epithelium. This has resulted in the addition of opaque mucus to the contents of that cyst. Near the limbus, fewer goblet cells are present and so there are fewer of them to become incorporated into the walls of such cysts, rendering the contents more clear.*

Langerhan's Cells: The conjunctival epithelium also contains Langerhan's cells, which function as immune system sentinels and are capable of antigen recognition and processing. The density of Langerhan's cells in the human conjunctiva is approximately 250 to 300 per mm^2, roughly half the density found in the skin. By contrast, in the peripheral third of the corneal epithelium, their density is only 15 to 20 per mm^2. In the central cornea of the normal adult eye, no Langerhan's cells are found (**Fig. 5.10**).[13]

Dendritic Melanocytes: In some individuals, the conjunctival epithelium may include a complement of dendritic melanocytes. These are especially common in more heavily pigmented races and can produce a densely pigmented ring at the limbus (**Fig. 5.11**) or diffusely scattered patches of pigmentation, primarily on the bulbar conjunctiva (i.e., racial melanosis). It is not uncommon for such areas to further darken during puberty, in some cases creating the impression that they are newly acquired. It is assumed that this darkly pigmented limbal ring serves to protect the constantly dividing limbal stem cell population from damaging UV radiation in populations indigenous to sunny climates.

FIGURE 5.8 Pattern of goblet cell distribution within the conjunctival epithelium. The perilimbal conjunctiva has the lowest density of goblet cells. Generally, the goblet cell density increases from the limbus or lid margin, toward the fornices, and the goblet cell density is generally greater nasally than temporally.

- Meibomian gland orifices
- Superior palpebral conjunctiva
- Superior fornix
- Superior punctum
- Limbus
- Caruncle
- Inferior punctum
- Bulbar conjunctiva
- Inferior fornix
- Inferior palpebral conjunctiva

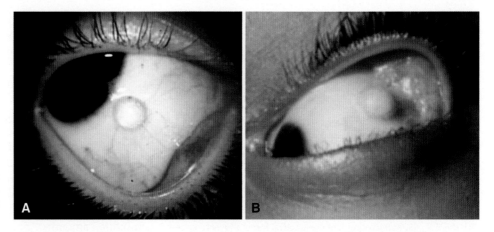

FIGURE 5.9 Epithelial inclusion cysts of the bulbar conjunctiva. **A:** clear cyst near limbus; **B:** opaque cyst near fornix.

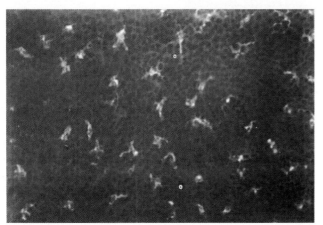

FIGURE 5.10 En face view of conjunctival epithelium shows the distribution of Langerhan's cells (white dendriform cells). (From Rodrigues MM, Rowden G, Hackett J, et al. Langerhan's cells in the normal conjunctiva and peripheral cornea of selected species. *Invest Ophthalmol Vis Sci.* 1981;21:759–765.)

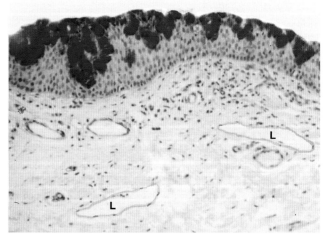

FIGURE 5.11 Clinical photograph shows perilimbal distribution of melanin pigment. (Courtesy of Jon Miles Research.)

CONJUNCTIVAL STROMA *(SUBSTANTIA PROPRIA)*

The conjunctival stroma is a fibrovascular matrix. The stroma of the bulbar conjunctiva forms a looser matrix than that of the palpebral conjunctiva and is less firmly attached to underlying tissues of the episclera. Within the stroma are the nerves, blood vessels, and lymphatic vessels that serve this tissue (**Fig. 5.12**).

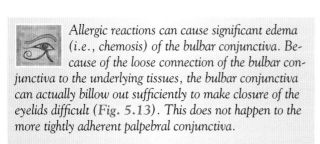

Allergic reactions can cause significant edema (i.e., chemosis) of the bulbar conjunctiva. Because of the loose connection of the bulbar conjunctiva to the underlying tissues, the bulbar conjunctiva can actually billow out sufficiently to make closure of the eyelids difficult (Fig. 5.13). This does not happen to the more tightly adherent palpebral conjunctiva.

FIGURE 5.12 Light micrograph shows conjunctival epithelium including numerous goblet cells and underlying conjunctival stroma, including blood vessels and lymphatic channels (*L*).

The stroma of the palpebral conjunctiva contains diffusely distributed lymphoid cells including lymphocytes and plasma cells, which secrete predominantly immunoglobulin A and are a normal finding. There are also concentrated lymphoid

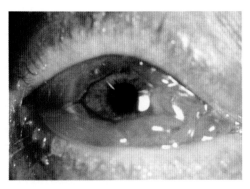

FIGURE 5.13 Billowing chemosis of the bulbar conjunctiva. (Courtesy of Dr. Howard Leibowitz.)

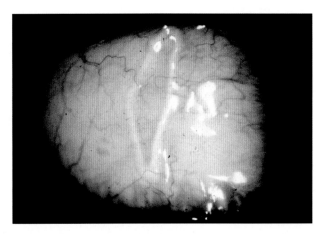

FIGURE 5.15 Lympangiectasis. (Courtesy of Dr. Rodney Gutner.)

aggregates that are more prevalent in the superior than the inferior palpebral stroma and occasionally manifest organized lymphoid follicles. The presence of quiescent, raised follicles in the palpebral conjunctiva is not an uncommon finding in normal, asymptomatic children. In the normal conjunctiva, these follicles are usually devoid of germinal centers (**Fig. 5.14**).

Some investigators believe that there is a functional association between these lymphoid aggregates and conjunctival crypts.[8] M cells have been demonstrated in the conjunctival epithelium overlying such lymphoid aggregates in guinea pig and rabbit conjunctiva.[14,15] M cells transport antigens from the lumen or surface of mucosae to underlying cellular components of the immune system, thereby initiating an immune response or tolerance. Whether the human conjunctival epithelium has true M cells, facilitating transepithelial transport of antigens, bacteria, and lectins, to the underlying lymphoid aggregates, as occurs in the gut appears probable but remains uncertain at this time.

The vascular elements of the conjunctival stroma in the normal eye are surrounded by large numbers of mast cells, with typical granules containing vasoactive compounds such as histamine. The density of mast cells in the normal human conjunctiva has been estimated to be as high as 6,000 per mm^3.[16] Antigen-induced release of these granules, mediated by immunoglobulin E, gives rise to the signs and symptoms of allergic conjunctivitis.

Lymphatics

Unlike most of the cornea, the conjunctiva is served directly by lymphatics. Because these small channels are clear, they are difficult to appreciate in vivo. They are readily identified in histologic sections by their thin walls (**Fig. 5.12**).

Recent in vivo studies that involved following the drainage of injected vital dyes have demonstrated a complex system of lymphatic vascular elements, including a convergence of lymphatic channels to a circular perilimbal vessel termed the lymphatic circle of Teichmann.[17]

> *In the presence of chronic irritation, lymphatic channels can become dilated and congested.*
> *In these cases, they increase in diameter sufficiently to be seen clinically and this is termed lymphangiectasis (**Fig. 5.15**).*

The lymphatic channels of the conjunctiva drain to regional lymph nodes. Lymphatics from the lateral two-thirds of the upper lid and the lateral one-third of the lower lid drain to the preauricular (i.e., superficial parotid) and occasionally to retroauricular and deep parotid lymph nodes. Drainage from the medial one-third of the upper lid and medial two-thirds of the lower lid drain to the submandibular nodes and eventually the anterior cervical nodes. It is these areas that should be palpated to reveal enlarged lymph nodes in the workup of certain clinical presentations of red eyes or tumors of the eyelids and conjunctiva (**Fig. 5.16**).

Innervation

The superior palpebral conjunctiva and the bulbar conjunctiva are provided with sensory innervation by branches of the ophthalmic division of the trigeminal nerve, including the nasociliary, lacrimal, and frontal

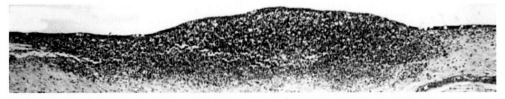

FIGURE 5.14 Light micrograph shows aggregates of lymphoid cells (conjunctiva-associated lymphoid tissue) within the superficial conjunctival stroma, beneath the conjunctival epithelium. (From Knop N, Knop E. Conjunctiva-associated lymphoid tissue in the human eye. *Invest Ophthalmol Vis Sci.* 2000;41:1270–1279, Figure 6C.)

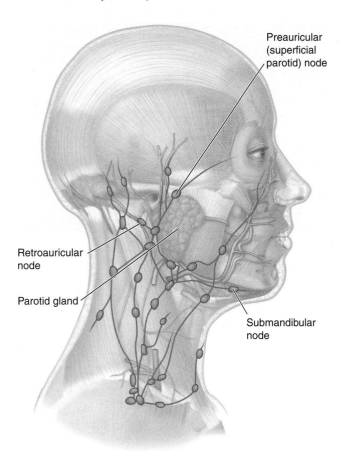

Preauricular
(superficial
parotid) node

Retroauricular
node

Parotid gland

Submandibular
node

FIGURE 5.16 Diagram showing the general pattern of lymphatic drainage from the face. The lateral two-thirds of the upper lid and the lateral one-third of the lower lid drain to the preauricular (i.e., superficial parotid) and occasionally to retroauricular lymph nodes. Drainage from the medial one-third of the upper lid and medial two-thirds of the lower lid drain to the submandibular nodes. (Modified from Tank PW, Gest TR. *Lippincott Williams & Wilkins Atlas of Anatomy.* 1st ed. Philadelphia, PA: Wolters Kluwer; 2008.)

nerves. The inferior palpebral conjunctiva is served by branches of the maxillary division of the trigeminal nerve, via its infraorbital branch. Based upon studies done in cynomolgus monkeys, the conjunctiva receives postganglionic parasympathetic fibers from the pterygopalatine ganglion. Sympathetic fibers are derived from the carotid plexus, via the vascular branches of the ophthalmic artery. These autonomic fibers primarily serve the vasculature. Unlike sensory fibers, their distribution to the epithelium appears to be very limited.[18]

Vascular Supply

The vascular supply of the conjunctiva arises from multiple sources. The superior palpebral conjunctiva is served by branches entering the eyelid from the orbit, including the supraorbital artery centrally, the supratrochlear artery medially, and the lacrimal artery laterally. The inferior palpebral conjunctiva is served principally by the infraorbital artery. The vascular supply for the bulbar conjunctiva, except for the 2 to 3 mm surrounding the limbus, is derived from the

vascular arcades within the eyelids. Branches from these arcades loop around the conjunctival fornices and proceed into the bulbar conjunctiva as the posterior conjunctival arteries (**Fig. 5.17**).

The vascular supply for the 2 to 3 mm of bulbar conjunctiva at the limbus arises from the anterior ciliary arteries that are derived from the blood supply of the rectus muscles. Two anterior ciliary arteries arise from each rectus muscle, except for the lateral rectus, which provides only one. The main trunks of the anterior ciliary arteries pierce the perilimbal sclera to contribute to the major circle of the iris and hence, to the vascular supply of the anterior uvea (**Fig. 5.18**). But additional branches are given off from the anterior ciliary arteries before they pierce the sclera. These branches that ultimately give rise to the anterior conjunctival arteries, remain superficial and serve the superficial marginal plexus at the limbal region (**Fig. 5.19**). The capillaries in the limbal region are fenestrated and therefore leak macromolecules into the conjunctival stroma.[19–21] These macromolecules also enter the corneal stroma and diffuse to its center along a concentration gradient (see Fig. 4.20).[22]

 The blood supply for the 2 to 3 mm of perilimbal conjunctiva is linked primarily to the anterior ciliary artery circulation, whereas the remainder of the bulbar conjunctiva is served by the posterior conjunctival arteries that derive from the vasculature of the eyelids. Inflammation of the anterior uvea causes dilation and vascular congestion in the entire anterior ciliary artery vascular network, often giving rise to a telltale pattern of redness in which the perilimbal conjunctiva is intensely red compared with the remainder of the bulbar conjunctiva. This pattern is referred to as "ciliary injection" and is an indication that the focus of the inflammation is more likely intraocular rather than conjunctival in origin. Note the arc of intense redness along the superior limbus (Fig. 5.20).

Conjunctiva-Associated Glands

Two sets of accessory lacrimal glands are present at specific locations in and beneath the stroma of the palpebral and forniceal conjunctiva. Each of these several glands conveys its exocrine contribution to the tear film via ducts that reach the conjunctival surface. These two sets of glands are termed the glands of Krause and the glands of Wolfring. The glands of Wolfring are found within the palpebral conjunctiva at the superior edge of the tarsus and the glands of Krause are found in the forniceal conjunctiva. They are described in detail in **CHAPTER 2: THE EYELIDS AND ADNEXA**.

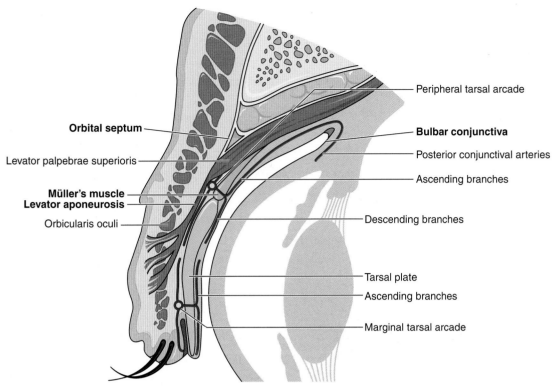

FIGURE 5.17   Arterial supply of the conjunctiva. Most of the bulbar conjunctiva, except near the limbus, is served by the posterior conjunctival arteries. These arteries arise from the vascular arcades of the eyelids and loop around the fornices to reach the bulbar conjunctiva. (Modified from LifeArt. Philadelphia, PA: Wolters Kluwer; 2017.)

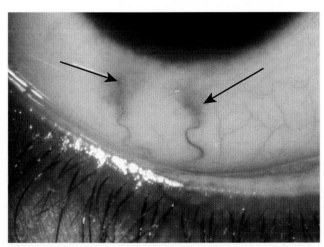

FIGURE 5.18   Clinical photograph of inferior bulbar conjunctiva, sclera, and lid margin shows entry of two anterior ciliary arteries and surrounding fine distribution of *gray-blue* uveal pigment in the surrounding episclera (*black arrows*).

Macroscopic and Clinical Anatomy of the Limbus

Defined in its simplest clinical terms, the limbus is the junction between the clear cornea and white sclera. This is not a specific point but a transitional area approximately 1 to 2 mm in width. This grossly visible transition zone does not have a clear analog in histologic sections. As such, somewhat awkward definitions of the limbus have emerged. Classically these are referred to as the "histologist's limbus" and the "pathologist's limbus." The differences between them are shown in **Figure 5.21**.

The histologist's limbus attempts to outline the edge of where the regularity of corneal stromal lamellae can still be distinguished from the more random arrangement observed in the opaque sclera. Despite being called the histologist's limbus, this transition is actually more readily seen in macrophotographs of sectioned whole eyes than in histologic sections. Note that the outline of this transition has a contour remarkably similar to the beveled edge of a lens (**Fig. 5.22**).

By contrast, the pathologist's limbus delimits more strictly defined boundaries. The anterior boundary is an imaginary line drawn from the peripheral edge of Bowman's layer of the cornea to the peripheral edge of Descemet's membrane. The edge of Descemet's membrane is also known as Schwalbe's line (**Fig. 5.21**). The posterior margin of the pathologist's limbus is a line drawn perpendicular to the surface of the eye and transecting the sclera spur. This much broader zone of transition places the trabecular meshwork and the primary aqueous outflow pathway within the limbus (**Fig. 5.21**). Despite this, given the complexity of the trabecular meshwork and aqueous outflow pathways, these are discussed in a separate chapter. (**SEE CHAPTER 9: ANATOMY OF THE AQUEOUS OUTFLOW PATHWAYS**).

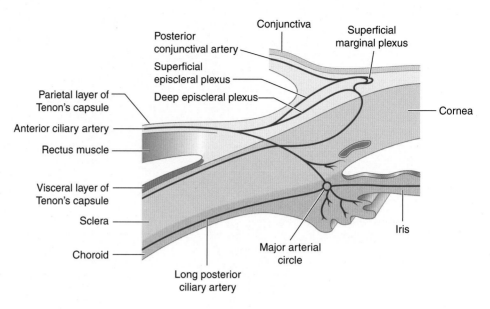

FIGURE 5.19 This simplified sketch demonstrates the distribution pattern of the anterior ciliary arteries. These vessels originate from the blood supply to the rectus muscles. Passing anteriorly from their origin, they pierce the sclera to join the major circle of the iris, while superficial branches serve the perilimbal conjunctiva. Peripheral to the superficial marginal plexus, the remainder of the bulbar conjunctiva is served by the posterior conjunctival arteries, arising as shown in **Figure 5.17**.

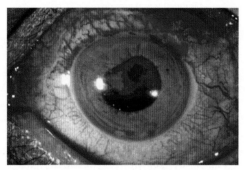

FIGURE 5.20 Acute anterior uveitis showing perli-limbal "ciliary injection" from 10 o'clock to 2 o'clock.

THE SURGICAL LIMBUS

Viewed externally, through an operating microscope, the limbus appears as a blue-gray ring that is an important and consistent anatomic landmark (**Fig. 5.23A**). This landmark is broader superiorly and inferiorly than it is medially and temporally. As one dissects away the outer layers of the limbus, moving progressively deeper, this blue-gray structure gradually gains better definition, revealing where clear cornea begins anteriorly. This important landmark corresponds to the anterior limit of the trabecular meshwork at the peripheral edge of Descemet's membrane of the cornea (i.e., Schwalbe's line) (white arrow in **Fig. 5.23B**). Equally important, where the blue-gray transitional zone gives way to white sclera at its posterior margin corresponds to the posterior limit of Schlemm's canal at the scleral spur (black arrow in **Fig. 5.23B**). Numerous glaucoma surgeries rely on a thorough understanding of these anatomic relationships and the ability to identify the positions of internal structures, such as Schwalbe's line, Schlemm's canal, and the scleral spur with certainty, before entry into the anterior chamber is made.

HISTOLOGY OF THE LIMBUS

The limbus is actually a complex area of transition from the cornea to the several tissue layers with which the cornea is joined at its periphery. Beginning at the surface, the tissues that overlie the sclera include the limbal conjunctival epithelium, which harbors the stem cells for corneal epithelial renewal (**Fig. 5.24**).

 The limbal stem cell population is the most mitotically active portion of the conjunctival epithelium. With this high mitotic rate and constant exposure to damaging UV rays, it is not surprising that conjunctival epithelial malignancies (e.g., conjunctival intraepithelial neoplasia and squamous cell carcinoma) occur most frequently at the limbus (Fig. 5.25).

Beneath the limbal epithelium, in sequential order, are the conjunctival stroma, Tenon's capsule, and the episclera, including its superficial and deep layers of vessels (**Fig. 5.24**). Tenon's capsule can be difficult to discern from the deep conjunctival stroma in histologic sections, but is more readily appreciated as a definable layer during dissection. These layers are described in greater detail in **CHAPTER 6: THE SCLERA, EPISCLERA, AND TENON'S CAPSULE.** Also present at the limbus are anatomically distinct vascularized ridges referred to as the palisades of Vogt.

PALISADES OF VOGT

The palisades of Vogt are a series of radially oriented and bifurcating fibrovascular channels between ridges of thickened conjunctival epithelium. They reside closer to the clear cornea than the peripheral vascular loops of the

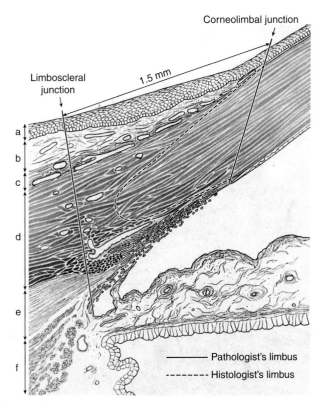

Corneolimbal junction

Limboscleral junction

1.5 mm

a
b
c
d
e
f

—— Pathologist's limbus
------ Histologist's limbus

FIGURE 5.21 Drawing of a meridional section of the limbal region. The "histologist's limbus" corresponds to the dashed line and represents the approximate location where the regular arrangement of collagen lamellae in the cornea gives way to the more irregular pattern of organization that characterizes the sclera. This feature is more readily appreciated in macrophotographs (e.g., **Fig. 5.22**) than in histologic sections. Alternatively, the limbus can be defined by the limits of the "pathologist's limbus." The pathologist's limbus corresponds to an area approximately 1.5 mm long on the anterior surface of the eye and a narrower region on the internal side of the cornea and sclera. Its defined limits lie between two lines transecting the corneoscleral coat of the eye. The anterior limit is a line connecting the peripheral terminus of Bowman's layer of the cornea with the peripheral edge of Descemet's membrane, also known as Schwalbe's line. The posterior limit is defined by a line perpendicular to the ocular surface that transects the root of the scleral spur and the posterior limit of Schlemm's canal. The identifiable layers of the wall of the eye, just posterior to the limbus include: (*a*) the conjunctival epithelium, (*b*) the conjunctival stroma, (*c*) Tenon's capsule and the episclera, (*d*) the sclera, (*e*) the longitudinal bundle of the ciliary muscle, and (*f*) the radial and circular bundles of the ciliary muscle. (From Hogan MJ, Alvarado JA, Weddell JE. *Histology of the Human Eye.* Philadelphia, PA: WB Saunders; 1971:113.)

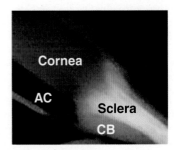

Cornea

AC

Sclera

CB

FIGURE 5.22 Macrophotograph of meridional section of limbus showing the transition between the corneal stroma and surrounding sclera. Note that the contour of the transition, from clear cornea to opaque sclera corresponds to the histologist's limbus depicted in **Figure 5.21**. AC, anterior chamber; CB, ciliary body.

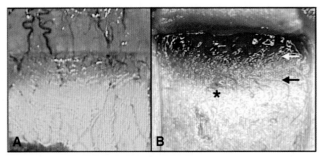

A   B

FIGURE 5.23 Surgical limbus in human eye viewed under conjunctiva (**A**) and under a split-thickness scleral flap (**B**). **A:** shows bluish area corresponding to the surgical limbus. **B:** White arrow indicates the anterior margin of the surgical limbus corresponding to the most anterior border of the trabecular meshwork and the peripheral edge of Descemet's membrane (Schwalbe's line). Black arrow (**B**) indicates the posterior margin of the surgical limbus corresponding to the scleral spur. Schlemm's canal lies just anterior to the scleral spur. Asterisk is situated just below a glistening drop of aqueous escaping from an external collector channel leading to episcleral vessels from Schlemm's canal. (Courtesy of Drs. John Morrison and Kelly Ma.)

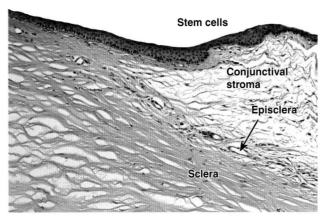

Stem cells

Conjunctival stroma

Episclera

Sclera

FIGURE 5.24 Light micrograph of the limbus shows focal thickenings of the conjunctival epithelium where the corneal stem cell population is found. Also shown are the conjunctival stroma, episcleral vessels, and sclera.

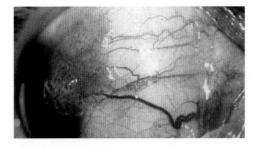

FIGURE 5.25 Limbal squamous cell carcinoma.

conjunctival marginal plexus. These linear projections average 0.36 mm in length and 0.04 mm in width and are most obvious at the superior and inferior limbal margins. The palisades are more readily seen in more heavily pigmented individuals in whom the palisades are commonly outlined with pigment (**Fig. 5.26**).[23]

The palisades are covered by an attenuated conjunctival epithelium that overlies a fibrovascular core conveying

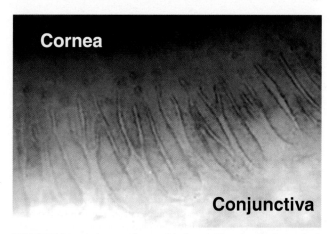

FIGURE 5.26 High magnification black and white clinical photograph of the limbus shows the outlines of the palisades of Vogt at the inferior limbus. (From Patel DV, Sherwin T, McGhee CNJ. Laser scanning in vivo confocal microscopy of the normal human corneoscleral limbus. *Invest Ophthalmol Vis Sci.* 2006;47:2823–2827.)

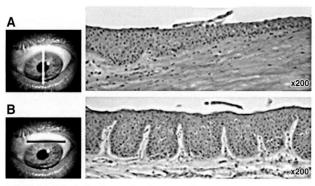

FIGURE 5.27 Histology of palisades of Vogt. **A:** A radial section through the limbus shows the region of the palisades of Vogt and the limbal stem cell population. **B:** A frontal section tangential to the limbus in the same region shows the alternating pattern of epithelial thickening and thinning that outline fibrovascular connective tissue channels containing arterial, venous, and lymphatic vessels. (From Chen Z, de Paiva CS, Luo L, et al. Characterization of putative stem cell phenotype in human limbal epithelia. *Stem Cells.* 2004;22:355–366.)

arterial, venous, and lymphatic vessels. Between adjacent palisades, the conjunctival epithelium regains its normal thickness. This alternate thickening and thinning gives a cross-sectional appearance that is reminiscent of the rete pegs exhibited by the epidermis of the skin (**Fig. 5.27**). Clearly, the palisades and the corneal stem cell population reside within the same area. The question of whether the epithelium of the palisades is a unique subset of limbal epithelium that corresponds to the entirety of the limbal stem cell population for the cornea remains uncertain.[24]

By angiography, the vessels of the palisades have been shown to be leaky, but less so than the terminal vascular arcades of the conjunctiva mentioned earlier.[25] This increase in permeability facilitates leakage of metabolites that diffuse into the anterior corneal stroma.

Acknowledgments

Thanks to Drs. John Morrison and Kelly Ma for their contributions to the Limbus section of this chapter.

REFERENCES

1. Chandler J, Axelrod A. *Conjunctiva-associated Lymphoid Tissue: A Probable Component of the Mucosa-associated Lymphoid System. Immunologic Diseases of the Mucous Membranes.* New York, NY: Masson and Cie; 1980:63–70.
2. Steuhl KP. Ultrastructure of the conjunctival epithelium. *Dev Ophthalmol.* 1989;19:1–104.
3. Weingeist T. Fine structure and function of ocular tissues: the conjunctiva. *Int Ophthalmol Clin.* 1973;13(3):85–91.
4. Nichols BA. Conjunctiva. *Microsc Res Tech.* 1996;33(4):296–319.
5. Huang AJ, Tseng SC, Kenyon KR. Paracellular permeability of corneal and conjunctival epithelia. *Invest Ophthalmol Vis Sci.* 1989;30(4):684–689.
6. Yoshida Y, Ban Y, Kinoshita S. Tight junction transmembrane protein claudin subtype expression and distribution in human corneal and conjunctival epithelium. *Invest Ophthalmol Vis Sci.* 2009;50(5):2103–2108.
7. Kessing SV. Mucous gland system of the conjunctiva. A quantitative normal anatomical study. *Acta Ophthalmol (Copenh).* 1968:Suppl 95:1+.
8. Knop N, Knop E. Conjunctiva-associated lymphoid tissue in the human eye. *Invest Ophthalmol Vis Sci.* 2000;41(6):1270–1279.
9. Greiner JV, Henriquez AS, Covington HI, et al. Goblet cells of the human conjunctiva. *Arch Ophthalmol.* 1981;99(12):2190-2197.
10. Specian RD, Oliver MG. Functional biology of intestinal goblet cells. *Am J Physiol.* 1991;260(2, pt 1):C183–C193.
11. Diebold Y, Rios JD, Hodges RR, et al. Presence of nerves and their receptors in mouse and human conjunctival goblet cells. *Invest Ophthalmol Vis Sci.* 2001;42(10):2270–2282.
12. Greiner JV, Weidman TA, Korb DR, et al. Histochemical analysis of secretory vesicles in nongoblet conjunctival epithelial cells. *Acta Ophthalmol (Copenh).* 1985;63(1):89–92.
13. Rodrigues MM, Rowden G, Hackett J, et al. Langerhans cells in the normal conjunctiva and peripheral cornea of selected species. *Invest Ophthalmol Vis Sci.* 1981;21(5):759–765.
14. Latkovic S. Ultrastructure of M cells in the conjunctival epithelium of the guinea pig. *Curr Eye Res.* 1989;8(8):751–755.
15. Liu H, Meagher CK, Moore CP, et al. M cells in the follicle-associated epithelium of the rabbit conjunctiva preferentially bind and translocate latex beads. *Invest Ophthalmol Vis Sci.* 2005;46(11):4217–4223.
16. Allansmith MR, Kajiyama G, Abelson MB, et al. Plasma cell content of main and accessory lacrimal glands and conjunctiva. *Am J Ophthalmol.* 1976;82(6):819–826.
17. Singh D. Conjunctival lymphatic system. *J Cataract Refract Surg.* 2003;29(4):632–633.
18. Ruskell G. Innervation of the anterior segment of the eye. In: *Basic Aspects of Glaucoma Research.* Stuttgart, Germany: FK Schattauer Verlag; 1982:49.
19. Scarpelli P, Pellegrini M, Brancato R. L'ultrastruttura dei capillari della congiuntiva umana. *Ann Ottalmol Clin Ocul.* 1966;92:977–993.
20. Tamura T. Ultrastructure of human conjunctival capillaries [in Japanese]. *Nippon Ganka Gakkai Zasshi.* 1967;71(6):625–637.
21. Raviola G. Conjunctival and episcleral blood vessels are permeable to blood-borne horseradish peroxidase. *Invest Ophthalmol Vis Sci.* 1983;24(6):725–736.
22. Allansmith M, de Ramus A, Maurice D. The dynamics of IgG in the cornea. *Invest Ophthalmol Vis Sci.* 1979;18(9):947–955.
23. Patel DV, Sherwin T, McGhee CN. Laser scanning in vivo confocal microscopy of the normal human corneoscleral limbus. *Invest Ophthalmol Vis Sci.* 2006;47(7):2823–2827.
24. Chen Z, de Paiva CS, Luo L, et al. Characterization of putative stem cell phenotype in human limbal epithelia. *Stem Cells.* 2004;22(3):355–366.
25. Goldberg MF, Bron AJ. Limbal palisades of vogt. *Trans Am Ophthalmol Soc.* 1982;80:155–171.

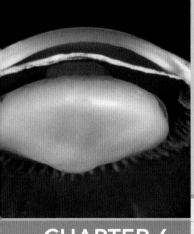

The Sclera, Episclera, and Tenon's Capsule

Overview

The sclera is a viscoelastic tissue, providing a distensible and opaque exoskeleton for the eye. Together with the intraocular pressure that provides internal support, it gives the eye its shape. It is to the inside of the sclera that all of the intraocular contents are directly or indirectly anchored. And it is to the outside of the sclera that the six extraocular muscles that move the eye are attached via tendons and fascial connections. A loosely attached fibrovascular connective tissue, termed the episclera, envelops the sclera. The episclera is in turn surrounded by a layer of fascia termed the fascia bulbi or Tenon's capsule.

The tendons of the extraocular muscles pierce Tenon's capsule and the episclera to attach directly to the sclera. The four rectus muscles insert near the limbus. From farthest to closest, it is easiest to remember the positions of each muscle insertion, relative to the limbus, with the acronym SLIM. The superior rectus inserts approximately 7.7 mm from the limbus, the lateral rectus–6.9, the inferior rectus–6.5, and the medial rectus–5.5. A line connecting these four muscle insertions circumscribes an asymmetric ring around the limbus referred to as the spiral of Tillaux (Fig. 6.1).

The tendon of the superior oblique, approaching the eye from the trochlea, near the superior medial rim of the orbit, passes between the superior rectus and the surface of the sclera to insert just posterior to the equator of the eye. The course of the inferior oblique, from its origin near the inferomedial orbital rim, passes beneath the inferior rectus, reaching the posterior wall of the sclera, lateral to the optic nerve. As such, the inferior oblique is closer to the orbital floor than the inferior rectus where their paths cross. Greater detail on the extraocular muscles is provided in **CHAPTER 1: THE ORBITS**.

The sclera itself is avascular, and meets its modest metabolic needs by receiving nutrients diffusing through its inner surface from the vasculatures of the choroid and ciliary body and through its outer surface from the vessels of the episclera. Although avascular itself, the sclera provides

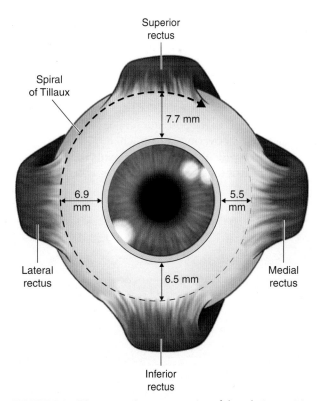

FIGURE 6.1 Diagrammatic representation of the relative positions of the rectus muscles. Farthest to closest they are the superior, lateral, inferior, and medial (SLIM), and the imaginary ring connecting them, termed the spiral of Tillaux. (Modified from Chern KC, Saidel MA, eds. *Ophthalmology Review Manual.* 2nd ed. Philadelphia, PA: Wolters Kluwer; 2012.)

conduits, known as emissaria, for the entry and exit of all of the vessels and nerves that enter or leave the eye. Unfortunately, these emissaria can also serve as conduits for extraocular extension of intraocular tumors (**Fig. 6.2**).

The sclera also provides a stable ring of insertion for the peripheral cornea and support for the optic nerve as the nerve leaves the eye via the intrascleral canal. Surrounding the optic nerve, the sclera also provides an attachment for the meningeal coverings around the optic nerve, which bring cerebrospinal fluid to the posterior surface of the globe. The details of this relationship are provided in **CHAPTER 15: THE OPTIC NERVE AND THE VISUAL PATHWAYS**. Finally, the sclera forms a part of the alternate pathway for aqueous humor outflow known as the uveoscleral outflow pathway.

◉ Macroscopic and Clinical Anatomy of the Sclera

The sclera covers the posterior 80% of the eye and its diameter, measured at the vertical equator of the eye, is approximately 22 mm. Note that the average anteroposterior diameter of the eye is greater than this, due to the more steeply curved cornea, which completes the corneoscleral tunic of the eye. The transition area over which this change in curvature occurs is referred to as the external scleral sulcus (**Fig. 6.3**). In this area, a circumcorneal annulus of collagen fibrils is present.[1] This ring assists in maintaining corneal curvature, by analogy with the architectural tension rings designed to support the base of a masonry dome.[2]

Beyond the ring of support that the sclera provides for the cornea, it also provides a ring of support in the posterior segment of the eye for the exit of the optic nerve. As the optic nerve leaves the eye, it is provided with meningeal coverings and it is to the posterior surface of the sclera that these meningeal coverings are attached. The intrascleral canal, through which the optic nerve exits the eye, is not cylindrical but cone-shaped. Its conical shape accommodates

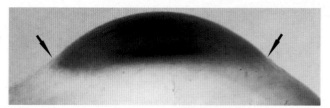

FIGURE 6.3 Macroscopic photograph of the anterior segment of the eye, with the cornea at the top, showing the inflection in the contour of the eye at the transition from the sclera to the more steeply curved cornea at the external scleral sulcus on each side (*arrows*).

the doubling of the optic nerve diameter when each axon takes on a myelin sheath within the intrascleral canal. As such, the canal widens from a diameter of 1.5 mm at the optic nerve head to a diameter of 3.0 mm along the 1 mm of the length of the canal. Details of the microanatomy of the relationship between the optic nerve and the intrascleral canal are found in **CHAPTER 15: THE OPTIC NERVE AND THE VISUAL PATHWAYS**.

Just as there is an external scleral sulcus, there is also an internal scleral sulcus (**Fig. 6.4**). Careful examination of the anterior chamber angle and the aqueous outflow pathways reveals that the trabecular meshwork and Schlemm's canal reside within a sulcus along the inner surface of the sclera. This sulcus is delimited anteriorly by the transition between the trabecular meshwork and the cornea. Posteriorly, the sulcus is delimited by a projecting lip of sclera termed the scleral spur. This cleft on the internal side of the sclera is the internal scleral sulcus. The posterior surface of the scleral spur plays an important role in anchoring the longitudinal

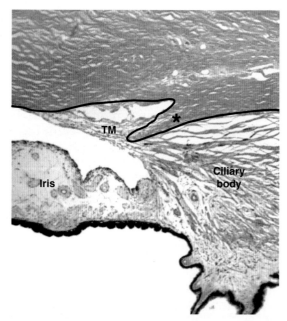

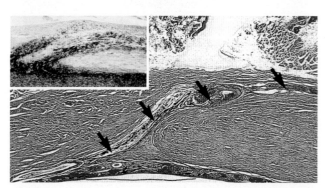

FIGURE 6.2 Histologic section demonstrates emissary canal through the thickness of the sclera and the blood vessel within it (*arrows*). Inset: An eye with choroidal melanoma in which the tumor has exploited an emissary canal to spread outside of the eye. (Main Figure: From Mills SE, ed. *Histology for Pathologists*. 4th ed. Philadelphia, PA: Wolters Kluwer; 2012.)

FIGURE 6.4 Light micrograph of the anterior segment of the eye showing the root of the iris and the ciliary body. The *black line* traces the inner surface of the sclera, demonstrating the internal scleral sulcus, which contains the canal of Schlemm and the trabecular meshwork (TM). The tongue of sclera forming the posterior limit of the internal scleral sulcus is termed the scleral spur (*asterisk*).

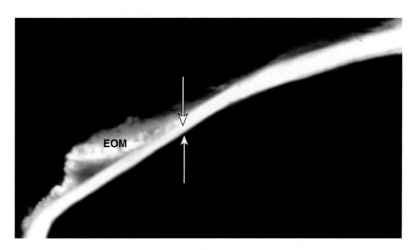

FIGURE 6.5 Macroscopic section through the thickness of the sclera, near the point of insertion of an extraocular muscle (EOM), shows how thin the sclera becomes just posterior to the muscle insertion and how the sclera thickens in both directions from this point.

bundle of the ciliary muscle. Contraction of this group of smooth muscle fibers pulls the spur posteriorly. In doing so, it alters the architecture of the trabecular meshwork, which is attached to the anterior surface of the spur. In this way, contraction of the ciliary muscle increases aqueous outflow and reduces intraocular pressure. The scleral spur is described in greater detail in **CHAPTER 9: ANATOMY OF THE AQUEOUS OUTFLOW PATHWAYS**.

The sclera varies in thickness by location and with age. The thickness of the adult sclera at the limbus is 0.7 to 0.8 mm. The thickness of the cornea at the limbus is most often quoted as 0.67 mm. The sclera is thickest surrounding the exit of the optic nerve (1.0 mm) and thinnest (0.3 mm) just posterior to the insertions of the rectus muscles (**Fig. 6.5**).

 When the eye ruptures from severe blunt trauma, the site of the rupture(s) is most commonly at the insertions of the rectus muscles, where the sclera is thinnest (Fig. 6.6).

Anterior to the rectus muscle insertions, the thickness of the sclera averages 0.6 mm and the thickness of the sclera at the equator[3] averages 0.5 mm. Although the sclera thickens as the eye grows to maturity, in old age the sclera is found to be thinner, denser, and less hydrated, with focal areas of age-related, dystrophic calcification.[4] More recent studies have extended these early findings to document that the matrix of the sclera stiffens with age as well.[5,6]

 By the age of 80, it is common to see vertically oval, gray-brown deposits in the sclera just anterior to the insertions of the medial and lateral rectus muscles. These slightly calcified deposits, presumably resulting from wear and tear at the muscle insertions, are termed (senile) hyaline plaques. Careful examination reveals that these areas are thinner than the surrounding sclera and their coloration is due, in part, to the color imparted by the dusty gray calcium deposition and, in part, due to the thinning of the sclera, which reveals the coloration of the underlying uveal pigment (Fig. 6.7).

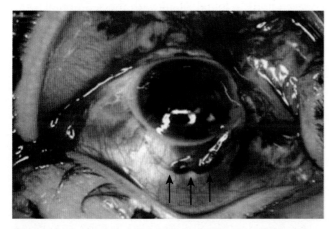

FIGURE 6.6 Rupture of the globe following blunt trauma. Note linear opening through the sclera coincident with the insertion of the inferior rectus muscle (*arrows*). (From Kertes PJ, Johnson M, eds. *Evidence-Based Eye Care.* 2nd ed. Philadelphia, PA: Wolters Kluwer; 2013.)

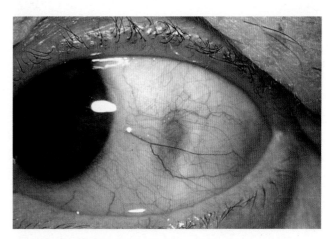

FIGURE 6.7 Clinical photograph demonstrates gray vertically oval hyaline plaque anterior to the insertion of the lateral rectus in an older individual. (© www.doc-stock.com. CMSP/F1online.)

Despite the thinness of the corneoscleral tunic, it is remarkably durable. The static rupturing pressure of the enucleated human eye has been shown to vary from 0.16 to 0.56 MPa. The average in one set of studies was 0.36 ± 0.20 MPa, which converts to approximately 23 to 81 psi or 1190 to 4189 mm Hg.[6] As an indication of how well engineered the corneoscleral coat is, recall that the pressure in a normally inflated automobile tire is about 32 to 36 psi (1,650 to 1,860 mm Hg). The eye can withstand a static pressure of nearly twice that amount but normal intraocular pressure is only about 15 mm Hg. And even in an acute attack of angle-closure glaucoma, the pressure rarely exceeds 80 mm Hg.

In addition to its durability, however, the arrangement of collagen fibers in the sclera provides a remarkable degree of viscoelasticity. If the pressure in the eye is raised rapidly, as by injecting a volume of fluid into the eye, this leads to stretching of the scleral fibers that is not initially proportional to the increase in pressure inside the eye. If this pressure elevation persists, these fibers will slowly become stretched. In the mature eye, with a sclera of normal thickness, this effect becomes asymptotic and as the fibers are stretched more and more, their rigidity increases.[7]

 In very young eyes, the sclera is thin and more distensible than in the normal adult eye. If intraocular pressure becomes elevated, as in congenital glaucoma, distention of the sclera occurs and the eye enlarges, sometimes dramatically as in the left eye of the patient shown in Figure 6.8. This condition is called buphthalmos. Scleral thinning can also occur in other conditions such as high myopia. These cases result in bulging of the posterior sclera and choroid termed a staphyloma. New methods to stabilize and strengthen such weakened scleras in high myopia are under development and include chemical cross-linking of scleral collagen.[8]

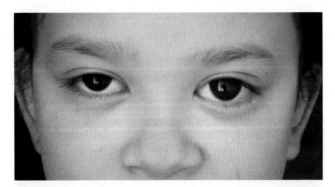

FIGURE 6.8   Buphthalmos of the left eye. (Courtesy of Dr. Beth Edmunds.)

Histology of the Sclera

The sclera has two layers, the scleral stroma and a thin layer of pigmented connective tissue on its inner surface known as the lamina fusca.

THE SCLERAL STROMA

The scleral stoma is composed of dense, irregular connective tissue that is not inert. Its extracellular matrix is under regular, albeit slow, turnover. Scleral fibroblasts produce and degrade its stroma, using conventional and regulated enzyme systems such as metalloproteinases and their inhibitors.[9] There is some evidence that when the sclera is put under strain, as when intraocular pressure is acutely increased, these fibroblasts can convert into myofibroblasts, which express α-smooth muscle actin. These cells appear to contribute to the viscoelasticity of the sclera under these conditions.[10] An excellent review of scleral stromal matrix turnover, and its alteration in progressive myopia, is available elsewhere.[11]

The fibroblasts of the sclera in several primate species have been shown to communicate through gap junctions.[12] More recently, gap junctions have also been reported to join fibroblasts of the human sclera as well.[13]

 The limited metabolic activity of the sclera allows it to be among the few tissues that can be frozen or even lightly fixed in ethanol and stored for later use in the emergency surgical repair of scleral defects, if fresh tissue is unavailable.[14]

The extracellular matrix of the scleral stroma is composed principally of collagens, surrounded by proteoglycans and glycosaminoglycans. Unlike the cornea, where collagen fibrils of uniform diameter are packed into regularly ordered lamellae, a much less ordered structure is found within the sclera. Scleral lamellae commonly branch and interweave within the outer layers of the stroma. But in the deeper stroma an even more random and denser arrangement of collagen fibrils is found, along with the addition of some elastic fibers.[15]

The collagen fibers of the scleral stroma are of nonuniform diameter, varying from 25 to 300 nm, and their packing is irregular as well (**Fig. 6.9**).[15,16] It appears that this less ordered arrangement of the stromal lamellae, combined with the irregular spacing of collagen fibers of nonuniform diameters, is likely the greatest contributor to the fact that the sclera is opaque.[15,17]

Approximately 50% of the dry weight of the sclera is composed of collagens, more than 90% of which are type I fibers.[18] Additional collagen types that have been identified in human sclera include collagen types III, IV, V, VI, VIII, XII, and XIII.[7,18,19–21]

As elsewhere, the size and arrangement of collagen fibrils in the sclera is governed by the proteoglycans and the degree of hydration of the glycosaminoglycans with which they are associated. Certain core proteins of proteoglycans found in the sclera, including decorin and

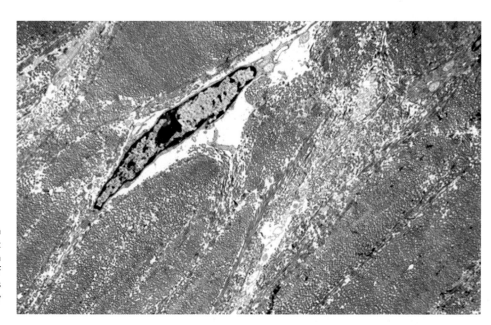

FIGURE 6.9 Transmission electron micrograph shows scleral fibroblast and surrounding matrix of collagen demonstrating variable pattern of collagen arrangement that contributes to opacity of the sclera. (Courtesy of Dr. Haiyan Gong.)

biglycan, belong to a group called "small leucine-rich proteoglycans" (SLRPs), which are known to bind matrix components, especially type I collagen. These SLRPs are known to influence matrix formation and organization.[22] In addition, aggrecan, a proteoglycan commonly found in cartilage, is present.[23]

> As noted, the proteoglycan aggrecan is found in the sclera and in cartilage. It has been hypothesized that this link to cartilage may contribute to the development of scleritis in rheumatoid arthritis, an autoimmune disease that destroys the cartilage in synovial joints and can destroy the sclera as well.[24]

The glycosaminoglycans associated with scleral proteoglycans are principally dermatan sulfate and chondroitin sulfate, with smaller amounts of heparan sulfate and the non-sulfated hyaluronan.[25] The latter of these, hyaluronan, increases in amount during limbal scleral wound healing, but gradually disappears after remodeling of the healed wound has been completed.

Other structural proteins found in the sclera include elastic fibers, which are composed of an elastin core, surrounded by microfibrils that are composed principally of fibrillin.[26]

> Thinning and distention of the sclera, resulting in high myopia, can occur in Marfan syndrome, a condition resulting from a mutation in the gene for fibrillin.[27]

THE LAMINA FUSCA

The lamina fusca, also described as the suprachoroidea in the posterior segment, and the supraciliaris anteriorly, is a loose, thin, fibrocellular layer that has a large complement of intensely pigmented, fusiform melanocytes. It is within the lamina fusca that elastic fibers are most prevalent in the sclera (**Fig. 6.10**).[26] It is also within this tissue that the potential space identified as the suprachoroidal space resides. This "space" normally subtends a zero volume, but under pathologic conditions can expand significantly as described in **CHAPTER 12: CHOROID AND CHOROIDAL CIRCULATION**. Within this same space is the principal route taken by aqueous humor leaving the eye via the uveoscleral outflow pathway. This pathway is described in detail in **CHAPTER 9: ANATOMY OF THE AQUEOUS OUTFLOW PATHWAYS**.[28]

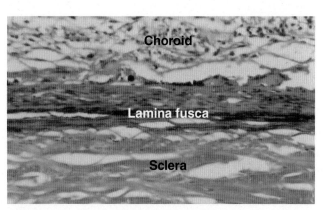

FIGURE 6.10 Light micrograph of junction between inner surface of sclera and deepest layers of the choroid demonstrates the irregular pigmented layer on the inner surface of the sclera that is termed the lamina fusca. These are stromal melanocytes of neural crest origin, not an epithelium.

INNERVATION OF THE SCLERA

Although the sclera is essentially avascular, it is well innervated with sensory fibers. The short ciliary nerves supply sensory fibers to the posterior sclera as they pierce the sclera in a ring surrounding the optic nerve. The two long ciliary nerves pierce the sclera outside of this ring, in parallel with the long posterior ciliary arteries. The two long ciliary nerves run anteriorly, along the horizontal equator of the eye, taking a tangential course through the thickness of the sclera to reach the tissues of the anterior segment.[29] Though not well described, it appears that the long ciliary nerves also send small fibers that provide sensory innervation to the remainder of the sclera. In about 12% of normal individuals, a branch of the long ciliary nerves may reach the surface of the sclera, forming a visible nodule 3 to 5 mm beyond the limbus, which is often surrounded by a cuff of extruded, bluish-gray uveal pigment. These anatomic variants are termed nerve loops of Axenfeld (**Fig. 6.11**).[30]

As further evidence of the rich sensory innervation of the sclera, it is important to recognize that inflammation of the sclera (scleritis) is commonly associated with debilitating pain. The pain is often severe enough to wake the patient from sleep and radiate through the orbit and the head. This pain is often worsened by movement of the eye as the extraocular muscles pull on the inflamed scleral tissue.

Macroscopic and Clinical Anatomy of Tenon's Capsule and the Episclera

TENON'S CAPSULE

Tenon's capsule, also referred to as the fascia bulbi is found between the deepest portions of the conjunctival stroma and the underlying episclera (**Fig. 6.12**). It is better appreciated as a gross anatomic plane in dissection than it is in histologic sections. Its anterior margin begins as a pericorneal ring of insertion into the sclera approximately 1.5 mm posterior to the corneoscleral junction.[31] From this anterior insertion, the capsule continues posteriorly, overlying the episclera to merge with the meningeal coverings of the optic nerve. Clearly, for the tendons of the extraocular muscles to move the eye precisely, they must attach directly to the sclera, thus requiring them to pierce Tenon's capsule. At these locations, Tenon's capsule is interrupted, blending with the perimysial coverings of the inner and outer bellies of the muscles to envelop the muscle insertions. The anatomic connections of Tenon's capsule are more extensive and are discussed in **CHAPTER 1: THE ORBITS**. The anterior portion of Tenon's capsule is thicker than the posterior portion and is composed of a dense irregular collagen matrix containing both elastic tissue and a small complement of smooth muscle fibers.[32,33] The capsule is separated from the sclera by the thin, loose episclera.

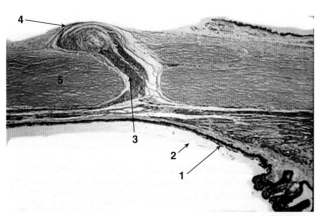

FIGURE 6.11 Histologic section showing loop of long ciliary nerve extending to the subconjunctival surface of the sclera where it would be visible clinically as a slightly raised slate blue/black focal nodule beneath the conjunctiva, on the anterior scleral surface. (*1*) the ciliary body; (*2*) anterior limit of the vitreous base; (*3*) long ciliary nerve passing through the sclera; (*4*) Axenfeld's loop; (*5*) sclera. (Courtesy of Mission for Vision and Dr. Ben Glasgow [www.missionforvision.org].)

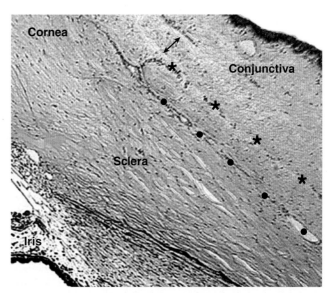

FIGURE 6.12 Histologic section of the limbal region shows the conjunctival surface at upper right and the iris root at lower left. Beneath the conjunctival epithelium, the conjunctival stroma is seen (Conjunctiva). A slightly denser layer of tissue (Tenon's capsule—*double arrowhead*) separates the conjunctival stroma from the superficial (*asterisk*) and deep (*filled circle*) layers of episcleral vessels.

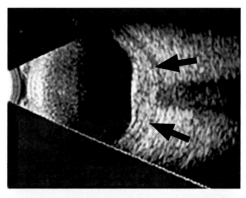

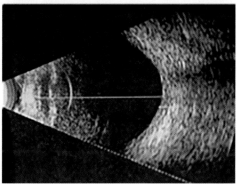

FIGURE 6.13 B-scan ultrasound images showing the anterior segment of the eye at the left and the posterior segment of the eye at the right. In the upper figure a space is evident (*arrows*) separating the sclera from Tenon's capsule in a case of posterior scleritis. Following resolution, in the lower figure, this space between Tenon's capsule and the sclera can no longer be resolved. (From Shukla D, Agrawal D, Dhawan A, et al. Posterior scleritis presenting with simultaneous branch retinal artery occlusion and exudative retinal detachment. *Eye.* 2009;23:1475–1477.)

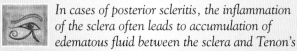 *In cases of posterior scleritis, the inflammation of the sclera often leads to accumulation of edematous fluid between the sclera and Tenon's capsule. Although one normally cannot discern these layers as being separate using clinical imaging methods, the edematous cleft between Tenon's capsule and the sclera can be discerned using B-scan ultrasound imaging of the posterior wall of the eye (arrows). This cleft disappears once the scleritis has resolved (**Fig. 6.13**).*[34]

THE EPISCLERA

The episclera is a fibrovascular layer that separates Tenon's capsule from the underlying sclera (**Fig. 6.12**). It is thickest anteriorly and thins progressively, posterior to the rectus muscle insertions. Its anatomic and clinical importance lies mostly in its vascular connections. The sources of the blood supply for the episclera are discussed in **CHAPTER 3: OVERVIEW OF THE EYE**.

Two layers of vessels reside within the episclera, a superficial capillary plexus that lies just beneath Tenon's capsule and a deeper plexus that resides on the surface of the sclera (**Fig. 6.12**). As a practical result, the vessels of the conjunctiva and the superficial episcleral plexus will move with manipulation of conjunctival surface. Those of the deepest layer will not. The vessels of the conjunctival stroma, superficial to Tenon's capsule, become dilated and congested in conjunctivitis. The superficial layer of episcleral vessels is involved in a condition termed episcleritis (**Fig. 6.12**).

But there is also an inflammatory condition known as scleritis, which is somewhat confusingly accompanied by redness, despite the fact that the sclera is essentially avascular. This begs the question, "What are the vessels that become dilated and engorged in scleritis?" It is the deeper layer of episcleral vessels that become dilated and congested in scleritis (**Fig. 6.12**). Due to their closer proximity to the surface of the sclera, the deep episcleral vessels do not move with manipulation of the conjunctiva.

The vessels of the episclera are also important beyond merely providing the vascular supply for the superficial sclera. The veins of the episclera also receive all of the aqueous humor draining from the eye via Schlemm's canal. The details of the pathway, from Schlemm's canal to the episcleral veins, are described in **CHAPTER 9: ANATOMY OF THE AQUEOUS OUTFLOW PATHWAYS**.

 Because aqueous humor drains from the eye down a passive pressure gradient, from the anterior chamber to the episcleral veins, any condition that raises episcleral venous pressure (e.g., carotid-cavernous sinus fistula) will give rise to an elevation of intraocular pressure. In order to leave the eye, aqueous humor must reach a pressure greater than episcleral venous pressure.

REFERENCES

1. Newton RH, Meek KM. Circumcorneal annulus of collagen fibrils in the human limbus. *Invest Ophthalmol Vis Sci.* 1998;39(7):1125–1134.
2. Varma MN, Jangid RS, Achwal VG. Tension ring in masonry domes. In: *Structural Analysis of Historical Constructions.* New Delhi; 2006:1–8.
3. Hogan MJ, Alvarado JA, Weddell JE. *Histology of the Human Eye: An Atlas and Textbook.* Philadelphia, PA: Saunders; 1971.
4. Friedenwald JS. Contribution to the theory and practice of tonometry. *Am J Ophthalmol.* 1937;20(10):985–1024.
5. Coudrillier B, Pijanka J, Jefferys J, et al. Collagen structure and mechanical properties of the human sclera: analysis for the effects of age. *J Biomech Eng.* 2015;137(4):041006.
6. Pallikaris IG, Kymionis GD, Ginis HS, et al. Ocular rigidity in living human eyes. *Invest Ophthalmol Vis Sci.* 2005;46(2):409–414.
7. Watson PG, Young RD. Scleral structure, organisation and disease. A review. *Exp Eye Res.* 2004;78(3):609–623.

8. Wollensak G, Spoerl E. Collagen crosslinking of human and porcine sclera. *J Cataract Refract Surg.* 2004;30(3):689–695.

9. Di Girolamo N, Lloyd A, McCluskey P, et al. Increased expression of matrix metalloproteinases in vivo in scleritis tissue and in vitro in cultured human scleral fibroblasts. *Am J Pathol.* 1997;150(2):653–666.

10. Phillips JR, McBrien NA. Pressure-induced changes in axial eye length of chick and tree shrew: significance of myofibroblasts in the sclera. *Invest Ophthalmol Vis Sci.* 2004;45(3):758–763.

11. Harper AR, Summers JA. The dynamic sclera: extracellular matrix remodeling in normal ocular growth and myopia development. *Exp Eye Res.* 2015;133:100–111.

12. Raviola G, Sagaties MJ, Miller C. Intercellular junctions between fibroblasts in connective tissues of the eye of macaque monkeys. *Invest Ophthalmol Vis Sci.* 1987;28:834–841.

13. McNeilly CM, Banes AJ, Benjamin M, et al. Tendon cells in vivo form a three dimensional network of cell processes linked by gap junctions. *J Anat.* 1996;189(pt 3):593–600.

14. Kuhn F, Pieramici DJ. *Ocular Trauma: Principles and Practice.* New York, NY: Thieme; 2011.

15. Komai Y, Ushiki T. The three-dimensional organization of collagen fibrils in the human cornea and sclera. *Invest Ophthalmol Vis Sci.* 1991;32(8):2244–2258.

16. Spitznas M. The fine structure of human scleral collagen. *Am J Ophthalmol.* 1971;71(1 pt 1):68.

17. Marshall GE, Konstas AG, Lee WR. Collagens in ocular tissues. *Br J Ophthalmol.* 1993;77(8):515–524.

18. Keeley FW, Morin JD, Vesely S. Characterization of collagen from normal human sclera. *Exp Eye Res.* 1984;39(5):533–542.

19. Rada J, Johnson J. Sclera. In: Krachmer J, Mannis M, Holland E, eds. *Cornea.* St Louis, MO: Mosby; 2004.

20. Sandberg-Lall M, Hägg PO, Wahlström I, et al. Type XIII collagen is widely expressed in the adult and developing human eye and accentuated in the ciliary muscle, the optic nerve and the neural retina. *Exp Eye Res.* 2000;70(4):401–410.

21. Wessel H, Anderson S, Fite D, et al. Type XII collagen contributes to diversities in human corneal and limbal extracellular matrices. *Invest Ophthalmol Vis Sci.* 1997;38(11):2408–2422.

22. Rada JA, Cornuet PK, Hassell JR. Regulation of corneal collagen fibrillogenesis in vitro by corneal proteoglycan (lumican and decorin) core proteins. *Exp Eye Res.* 1993;56(6):635–648.

23. Rada JA, Achen VR, Perry CA, et al. Proteoglycans in the human sclera. Evidence for the presence of aggrecan. *Invest Ophthalmol Vis Sci.* 1997;38:1740–1751.

24. Sainz de la Maza M, Foster CS, Jabbur NS. Scleritis associated with rheumatoid arthritis and with other systemic immune-mediated diseases. *Ophthalmology.* 1994;101(7):1281–1288.

25. Trier K, Olsen EB, Ammitzbøll T. Regional glycosaminoglycans composition of the human sclera. *Acta Ophthalmol.* 1990;68(3):304–306.

26. Marshall GE. Human scleral elastic system: an immunoelectron microscopic study. *Br J Ophthalmol.* 1995;79(1):57–64.

27. Maumenee IH. The eye in the Marfan syndrome. *Trans Am Ophthalmol Soc.* 1981;79:684–733.

28. Wood RL, Koseki T, Kelly DE. Uveoscleral permeability to intracamerally infused ferritin in eyes of rabbits and monkeys. *Cell Tissue Res.* 1992;270(3):559–567.

29. Foster CS, de la Maza MS. *The Sclera.* Berlin, Germany: Springer Science & Business Media; 2013.

30. Stevenson TC. Intrascleral nerve loops: a clinical study of frequency and treatment. *Am J Ophthalmol.* 1963;55(5):935–939.

31. Kakizaki H, Takahashi Y, Nakano T, et al. Anatomy of tenons capsule. *Clin Exp Ophthalmol.* 2012;40(6):611–616.

32. Doxanas MT, Anderson RL. *Clinical Orbital Anatomy.* Baltimore, MD: Williams & Wilkins; 1984.

33. Whitnall SE. *Anatomy of the Human Orbit and Accessory Organs of Vision (reprint).* New York, NY: Krieger Publishing Company; 1979.

34. Shukla D, Agrawal D, Dhawan A, et al. Posterior scleritis presenting with simultaneous branch retinal artery occlusion and exudative retinal detachment. *Eye.* 2009;23(6):1475–1477.

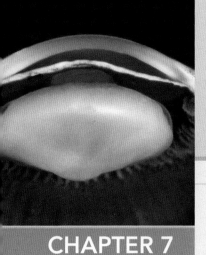

The Iris

CHAPTER 7

Overview

The iris serves as an optical diaphragm, limiting the passage of light into the eye except through its variable aperture called the pupil. The size of the pupil varies in response to ambient illumination levels and the state of accommodation. As illumination levels increase, or the object of visual attention is tracked closer to the eye, the pupil becomes smaller. With age, it is common to witness a progressive reduction in pupil size, although the reason for this remains unclear.[1] The edge of the pupil rests on the anterior surface of the crystalline lens, at virtually all pupil sizes. In doing so, the iris forms an important one-way valve, allowing passage of aqueous humor from the posterior to the anterior chamber while preventing reversal of this flow.

Macroscopic and Clinical Anatomy of the Iris

The iris varies substantially in color and surface texture among individuals, but the principal landmarks of the iris surface are constant. A corrugated border, termed the pupillary ruff or frill, lines the edge of the pupil (**Fig. 7.1A** and **B**). The pupillary ruff is created by the posterior pigmented epithelial layers of the iris, which come forward through the pupillary aperture and are visible anteriorly at the pupil's edge (**Fig. 7.1B**). The scalloped appearance of the pupillary ruff results from the convergence of a series of radially oriented furrows on the posterior surface of the iris (contraction folds of Schwalbe) (**Fig. 7.1C**). The pupil itself is most often displaced toward the nasal side of the iris.

Midway between the pupil and the peripheral iris is an irregularly branched, circularly oriented surface feature termed the collarette (**Fig. 7.1A** and **D**). The portion of the iris closer to the pupil than the collarette is termed the pupillary part and the portion peripheral to the collarette is termed the ciliary part of the iris. Near the collarette, irregularly shaped apertures in the anterior border layer are commonly seen. These apertures into the underlying stroma are called the crypts of Fuchs (**Fig. 7.1D**).

The collarette is the adult vestige of the ring of attachment of the embryonic pupillary membrane to the surface of the iris. In early development, the pupillary membrane vaults over the pupillary aperture but it is later resorbed entirely in most cases. Finding minimal remnants of the pupillary membrane is not uncommon (**Fig. 7.2A**). These most often appear as wispy, cobweb-like strands connecting

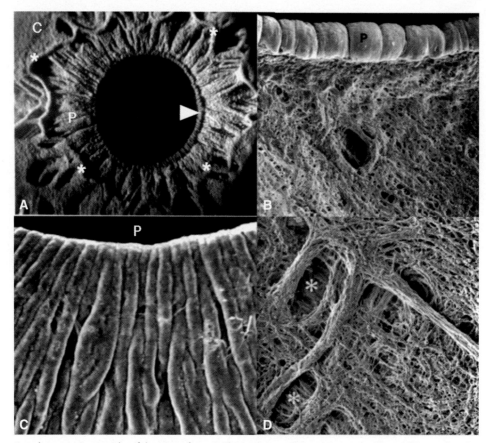

FIGURE 7.1 Scanning electron micrographs of the iris surface. **A:** Shows the pupillary aperture, pupillary ruff (*arrowhead*), and collarette (*asterisks*) separating the pupillary (P) from the ciliary (C) portion of the iris. **B:** Higher magnification of the pupillary margin showing the corrugation of the pupillary ruff (P) and texture of iris surface. **C:** Shows the pupillary margin (P) from the posterior surface of the iris demonstrating the linear contraction folds of the posterior epithelia of the iris that are termed the contraction furrows of Schwalbe. **D:** Shows higher magnification of the branching surface processes of the collarette region and clefts in the anterior iris surface termed crypts of Fuchs (*asterisks*). (Modified from Freddo T. Ultrastructure of the iris. *Micros Res Tech*. 1996;33(Special Issue, The Anterior Segment of the Eye, Freddo T, ed.):369–389.)

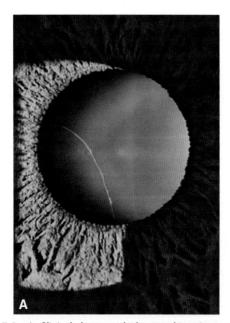

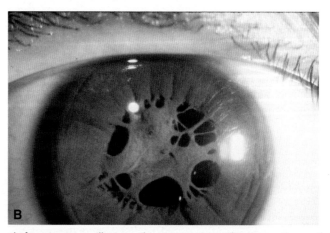

FIGURE 7.2   A: Clinical photograph shows a thin, wispy strand of persistent pupillary membrane tissue extending across the pupil. Although not visible in this image, it is important to appreciate that these strands do not attach to the pupillary margin but to the collarette. (Courtesy of Dr. Derek Ho.) **B:** Clinical photograph shows rare, visually significant, persistent pupillary membrane extending across the pupil and attached to the collarette. In this case, the collarette is folded over the pupillary margin, obscuring it from view. (Courtesy of Dr. Howard Leibowitz.)

from one place on the collarette to another, or from the collarette to the surface of the lens. Alternatively, they may appear as threads with one end attached to the collarette and the other end wafting in the aqueous humor circulation of the anterior chamber. Despite their name, these minor remnants are invariably anchored to the iris surface at the collarette, not the pupil and they are of no clinical significance. More rarely, these remnants can be large enough to be of visual consequence. In such cases, removal by laser or incisional surgery is required (**Fig. 7.2B**).

VARIANTS IN THE GROSS ANATOMY OF THE IRIS THAT ARE OF CLINICAL CONSEQUENCE

There are clinically important variations in the anatomic relationship between the contour of the iris and contour of the posterior surface of the cornea. The angle subtended between these two structures defines the anterior chamber angle of the eye. Flatter corneal curvatures, most commonly found in hyperopic eyes, usually produce a narrower anterior chamber angle, while those of highly myopic eyes tend to create a wider, more open anterior chamber angle (**Fig. 7.3**). Narrower angles put the eye at greater risk of occluding aqueous outflow and acutely elevating intraocular pressure when the pupil is dilated and the iris tissue is compressed toward the anterior chamber angle. For this reason, an estimation of the angle depth by various methods is a customary prelude to instilling drops to dilate the pupil.

Another anatomic variant of clinical importance in the relationship between the iris and the angle tissues is "plateau iris configuration." In these eyes, the ciliary body is anteriorly displaced such that the ciliary processes are rotated forward, toward the anterior chamber. The ciliary

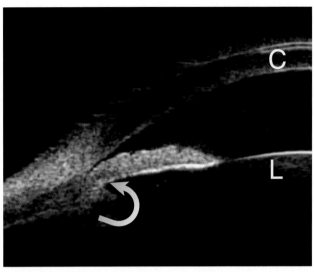

FIGURE 7.4 Ultrasound biomicroscopy image of plateau iris configuration shows arrow indicating how anterior rotation of the ciliary body has brought the root of the iris forward and rotated the iris surface toward the outflow pathways. C, cornea; L, lens. (Courtesy of the Echography Department at Bascom Palmer Eye Institute, Miami, FL.)

processes push the iris root forward such that it closely parallels the arching course of perilimbal corneosclera for a short distance. When viewed in an ultrasound biomicroscopic or optical coherence tomography image, this gives the iris the overall appearance of a plateau (**Fig. 7.4**).

The anatomic configuration of the iris can also be altered by changes in the crystalline lens. The crystalline lens of the eye continues to grow throughout life. As it increases in thickness with age, it pushes the central portion of the iris forward, making the overall contour of the iris convex, in some cases narrowing the anterior chamber angle approach as well.

MORPHOLOGY OF THE IRIS IN MIOSIS VS MYDRIASIS

Several features distinguish the morphology of the iris with a constricted pupil (miosis, **Fig. 7.5A**) from that with a dilated pupil (mydriasis, **Fig. 7.5B**).

As the pupil dilates, iris thickness increases. But this thickening of the iris is nonuniform. The pupillary portion of the iris does not appreciably thicken. At the collarette, the junction between the pupillary and ciliary portions of the iris, mydriasis results in the formation of a fold and sulcus to accommodate the thickening of the iris stroma. The most peripheral portion of the iris, where it joins the ciliary body, is termed the iris root. Like the pupillary portion of the iris, the iris root does not thicken appreciably in mydriasis, at least in Occidental eyes (**Fig. 7.5B**). The minimal thickening of the iris root presumably minimizes interference with aqueous humor outflow through the trabecular meshwork when the pupil is maximally dilated pharmacologically, or in low light conditions. The iris of the Oriental eye is general thicker than that in the

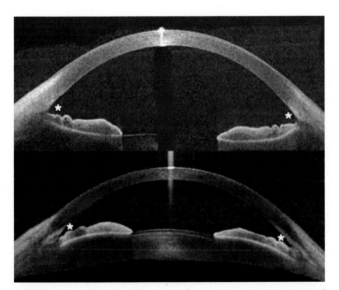

FIGURE 7.3 These clinical images show anterior segment optical coherence tomograms of eyes with relatively open (**top**) and relatively closed (**bottom**) anterior chamber angles (*asterisks*). (Courtesy of the Tomey Corporation.)

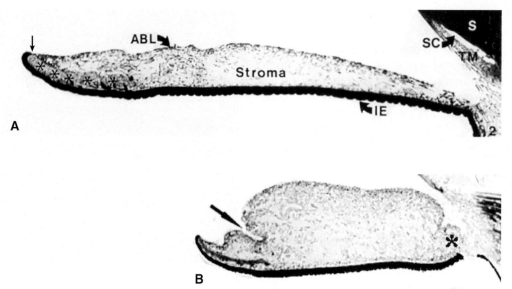

FIGURE 7.5   A: Light microscopy of normal iris in miosis. ABL, anterior border layer; IE, iris epithelium; small arrow, pupillary ruff; asterisks, pupillary sphincter muscle; SC, Schlemm's canal; TM, trabecular meshwork; S, sclera. **B:** Light microscopy of normal iris in mydriasis shows prominent fold at collarette (*arrow*) and minimal thickening of iris root (*asterisk*). (From Freddo T. Ultrastructure of the iris. *Micros Res Tech.* 1996;33(Special Issue, The Anterior Segment of the Eye, Freddo T, ed.):369–389.)

Occidental eye and this thickening appears to involve the iris root. This likely contributes to the greater incidence of closed-angle glaucoma in eastern Asia, compared with Europe and North America.

Because the root of the iris is peripheral to the limbus, direct visualization of a small iris root tear can be a challenge unless special examination methods such as gonioscopy are employed. But such tears may be revealed indirectly by the fact that the tear releases radial tension on the iris, causing the pupillary margin to flatten parallel to the tear, creating a "D-shaped" pupil. A larger and more obvious "D" shaped pupil is shown (Fig. 7.6).

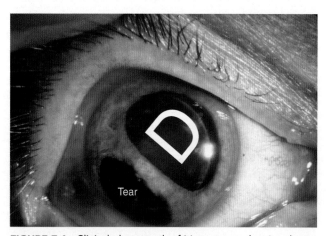

FIGURE 7.6   Clinical photograph of iris root tear showing the resulting "D" shape of the pupil. (Courtesy of Dr. Howard Leibowitz.)

As evident in **Figure 7.5A** and **B**, the iris root is overall the thinnest part of the iris, whether in mydriasis or miosis, and is the most prone to tearing following blunt trauma.

Histology

Layering of the iris is somewhat imprecise but four layers are generally recognized (**Fig. 7.7**).
1. The anterior border layer
2. The stroma and sphincter muscle
3. The anterior myoepithelium (of which the dilator muscle is a part)
4. The posterior pigmented epithelium

THE ANTERIOR BORDER LAYER

The anterior border layer has this awkward name to emphasize the fact that the anterior surface of the iris is not covered by an epithelium. Instead, the anterior surface of the iris is merely a condensation of the same cell types found in the underlying stroma—fibroblasts and melanocytes—in a collagenous matrix (**Figs. 7.7** and **7.8**). Thus, aqueous humor in the anterior chamber freely permeates the iris surface and enters the underlying stroma. The cells of the anterior border layer are interconnected by gap junctions for communication and intermediate junctions to provide focal points of intercellular adhesion.[2]

Iris Coloration

The iris varies substantially in color among individuals. The variations in iris coloration, excluding albinos, are principally due to the amount and subtypes of melanin

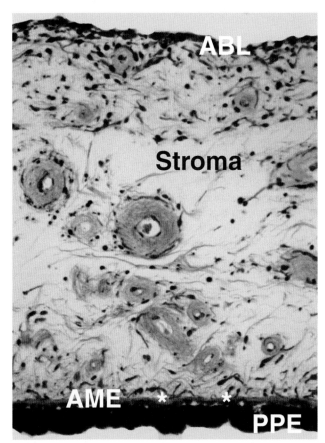

FIGURE 7.7 Light micrograph showing the layers of the iris. Both layers of the iris epithelium are pigmented and are difficult to distinguish from one another at the light microscopic level. The layer closest to the stroma includes the dilator muscle of the iris (*) and is termed the anterior myoepithelium (AME). Facing the posterior chamber of the eye is the single layer of cells termed the posterior pigmented epithelium (PPE). ABL, anterior border layer.

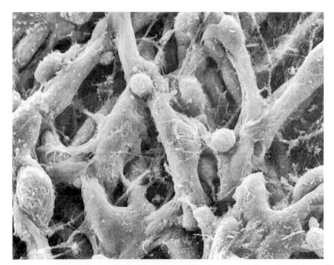

FIGURE 7.8 High magnification scanning electron micrograph of the anterior border layer shows its open matrix composed of thin, flat cell processes of surface fibroblasts covering cylindrical cellular processes of surface melanocytes. These are interspersed in a filamentous collagen matrix. Ovoid structures represent nuclear regions of these cells. Small, round structures represent wandering phagocytes.

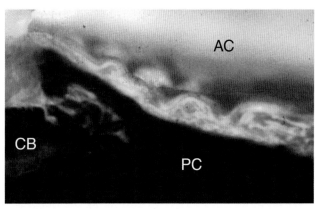

FIGURE 7.9 Macrophotograph of cross section through brown iris showing white coloration of stroma underlying brown anterior border layer. CB, ciliary body; AC, anterior chamber; PC, posterior chamber.

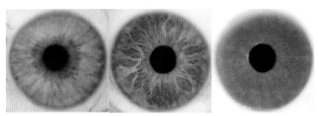

FIGURE 7.10 Variations in color and texture of the anterior surface of the iris. (Courtesy of Jon Miles Research.)

pigment found in the anterior border layer. Note that even a brown iris is nearly devoid of pigmentation beneath its anterior surface (**Fig. 7.9**).

The array of colors of the human iris is not due to different pigments but to variations in the distribution and amounts of two subtypes of a single pigment—melanin. These two melanin subtypes are eumelanin and pheomelanin (**Fig. 7.10**).[3] Eumelanin gives black and brown coloration, while pheomelanin gives reddish brown tones such as in red hair and the skin of the lips. Albinotic irides are essentially devoid of melanin pigment, despite having stromal melanocytes with mature melanosomes.[4] They appear pink due to the blood circulating within the iris and the background of the chorioretinal red reflex.

Although it may seem counterintuitive, a deep blue iris has the least melanin pigment of any other non-albinotic iris color, including paler blues and gray-blues. A deep blue iris has dense eumelanin pigment within the two layers of epithelia that line the posterior iris surface but only a modest complement of melanocytes, containing little melanin of either subtype, on the anterior surface of the iris, or in the underlying stroma.[3]

The blue color arises from stromal absorption of the long wavelengths of light, and reflection of the shorter blue wavelengths. The less melanin pigment that is present in the anterior border layer, the deeper blue the iris appears, much in the way the sky becomes deeper blue as a thin layer of clouds moves away. And as with the addition of thin clouds to a deep blue sky, as pigment is added to the surface of a deep blue iris, the deep blue color becomes a paler blue, moving toward a gray-blue.[5]

Iris colors between gray-blue and dark brown (i.e., gray, hazel, green) result from increasing amounts and differing ratios of the two melanin subtypes being added to the anterior border layer. Green irides exhibit eumelanin in their posterior epithelial layers, just as in a blue iris, but they also have moderate amounts of pheomelanic pigment in their anterior border layer melanocytes and the melanocytes within their stroma.[3] A dark brown iris has not only the two pigmented epithelial layers on its posterior surface, but a discontinuous layer of heavily pigmented melanocytes on its anterior surface as well. In brown irides, the melanosomes of the posterior epithelia contain eumelanin, as do blue and green irides, but the anterior border layer melanocytes, and the complement of stromal melanocytes, exhibit a mixture of both eumelanin and pheomelanin.[3]

As further evidence that the pigment in the anterior border layers is the principal contributor to iris coloration, there is a recently developed cosmetic surgical technique in which a laser is used to photoablate pigment from the anterior surface of the iris. The goal is to permanently change the color of the iris. As seen in the partially treated iris in **Figure 7.11**, removal of some of the anterior border layer has resulted in a lightning of iris color from brown to green.

> *In some conditions, the iris undergoes atrophy. As pigment is lost from the anterior border layer, during this process, a brown iris will change toward green, then hazel and finally gray-blue, just as depicted in Figure 7.11, following laser removal of pigment from the anterior border layer. Somewhat less intuitively, for the reasons noted earlier, a pale blue iris will lose whatever amount of gray it has and will become deeper blue as it atrophies.*

Anatomic Variants of the Anterior Border Layer

Several pigmented and nonpigmented spots are found as congenital, anatomic variants on the normal iris surface. Some of these can also be diagnostic cues to underlying congenital disorders. These anatomic variants have gathered an array of names.

Brushfield Spots/Kunkmann-Wolffian Bodies: Brushfield spots appear as a ring of small, white, slightly elevated nodules concentric with the pupil in the ciliary portion of the iris and they are most common in individuals with Down syndrome (Trisomy 21). They can also be found, however, in individuals with light colored irides, but with no known genetic anomaly. In these cases, they are referred to as Kunkmann-Wolffian bodies (**Fig. 7.12**).[6] Histologically, these "bodies" correspond to small focal nodules of anterior border layer hyperplasia surrounded by a thin ring of hypoplasia.

Iris Mammillations: Iris mammillations (**Fig. 7.13**)[7] are most commonly a unilateral finding. Their large numbers and dark coloration commonly result in the two irides appearing different in color (heterochromia). The mammillations appear as numerous focal pigmented elevations with the same color as the surrounding iris surface. A system of ridge-like linear elevations may interconnect adjacent mammillations. When associated with pigmentary changes in the conjunctiva, this finding is sometimes associated with congenital ocular melanocytosis, but is generally considered to be simply an anatomic variant.

Iris Nevi: Nevi, like those found in other tissues, are pigmented, congenital hamartomas that do not distort

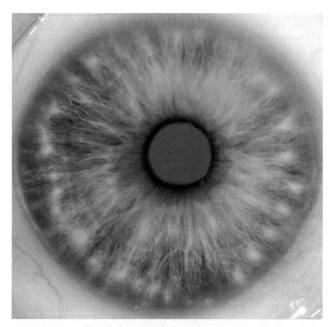

FIGURE 7.12 Clinical photograph demonstrating ring of yellow-white spots in iris periphery. (Courtesy of Jon Miles Research.)

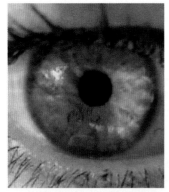

FIGURE 7.11 Clinical photograph shows human iris following partial laser ablation of the 9 o'clock–5 o'clock portion of the anterior border layer, rendering an originally blown iris, green. (Courtesy of the Stroma Medical Corporation and Jon Miles Research.)

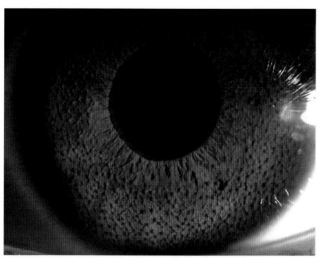

FIGURE 7.13 Clinical photograph demonstrating iris mammillations. (From Kiratli H. Head and neck: iris hamartomas. *Atlas Genet Cytogenet Oncol Haematol.* 2010;14(1):83–86. http://atlasgenetics oncology.org/Tumors/IrisHamartomaID5100.html. Accessed April 21, 2016.)

the surface anatomy of the surrounding iris. They often give the appearance of brown moss growing on the surface of the iris. These may occur as multiple focal nevi (**Fig. 7.14A**) or cover an entire iris sector (**Fig. 7.14B**). In the latter case, the inferomedial sector is most commonly affected.

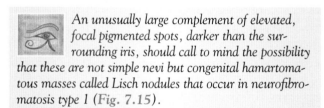

> *An unusually large complement of elevated, focal pigmented spots, darker than the surrounding iris, should call to mind the possibility that these are not simple nevi but congenital hamartomatous masses called Lisch nodules that occur in neurofibromatosis type 1 (Fig. 7.15).*

STROMA AND SPHINCTER MUSCLE

The stroma of the iris is continuous with the stroma of the ciliary body at the iris root (**Fig. 7.5**). The ample open spaces of the stroma are permeated with aqueous humor and contain a reservoir of plasma-derived proteins. This reservoir is not the result of leakage from iris blood vessels. It is, instead, sustained by proteins leaked from the permeable vessels of the ciliary body, which diffuse from the ciliary body stroma into the iris stroma, via their bridge of continuity at the iris root.[8] This small amount of plasma-derived protein, less than 1% of that found in blood plasma, ultimately enters the aqueous humor.

The structure of the iris stroma is a fine, veil-like matrix of types I and III collagen that are surrounded by

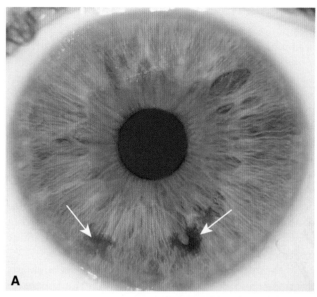

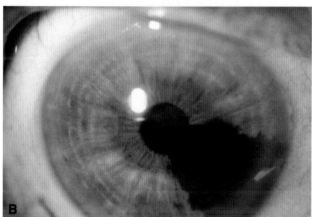

FIGURE 7.14 **A:** Clinical photograph shows two small iris nevi of the iris surface (*arrows*). (Courtesy of Jon Miles Research.) **B:** Clinical photograph shows congenital sectorial iris nevus. (Courtesy of Dr. Howard Leibowitz.)

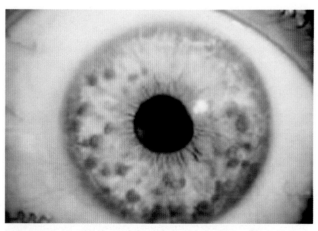

FIGURE 7.15 Lisch nodules of the iris in Neurofibromatosis, type I. (From Diab M, Staheli LT. *Practice of Pediatric Orthopedics.* 3rd ed. Philadelphia, PA: Wolters Kluwer; 2015.)

type VI (**Fig. 7.16**). Within the stroma, fibroblasts and melanocytes are also found.[9,10] The sparse complement of fibroblasts and melanocytes distributes principally surrounding the iris nerves and blood vessels that run toward and away from the pupil in this layer. Like the fibroblasts and melanocytes of the anterior border layer, the cells of the stroma are joined by gap junctions for communication and intermediate junctions that provide focal, intercellular adhesion.[2]

In addition to the fibroblasts and melanocytes, the iris stroma contains an important complement of macrophages, mast cells, and an integrated matrix of immune-system dendritic cells. These dendritic cells exhibit major histocompatibility complex (MHC) class II receptors that play a central role in regulating antigen-specific immune responses.[11]

Within the pupillary portion of the iris is a circularly oriented band of smooth muscle called the sphincter pupillae muscle (**Fig. 7.17**). Contraction of the sphincter pupillae muscle makes the pupil smaller in diameter (miosis). Innervation of this muscle is principally from parasympathetic fibers leaving the midbrain as a group of preganglionic fibers layered onto the outer surface of cranial nerve III, the oculomotor nerve. These preganglionic fibers synapse in the ciliary ganglion. After synapsing, the postganglionic fibers join the short ciliary nerves, which

pierce the posterior sclera around the optic nerve head and run forward in the suprachoroidal and supraciliary spaces to reach the iris sphincter muscle.

*Note in **Figure 7.17** that the sphincter muscle is surrounded by stroma on both its anterior and posterior surfaces, except at the pupillary margin. Recall that the pupil normally rests on the surface of the lens. In certain intraocular inflammatory diseases, the edge of the pupil, which is formed by the posterior epithelial layers of the iris, can become fused to the lens surface by the inflammatory response, producing what is termed a posterior synechia. Because the sphincter muscle is not directly attached to the posterior epithelial layers of the iris over its entire length, it remains free to contract, even when the edge of the pupil cannot move. As such, when checking pupillary responses in an inflamed eye, it is important not to mistake the continued contraction of the pupillary portion of the stroma for actual movement of the pupil itself.*

In microscopic sections of the pupillary portion of the iris, near the sphincter muscle, are rounded pigmented cells called clump cells of Koganei. As seen by electron microscopy, these cells have pigment granules sequestered in "clumps." These cells vary in size to a maximum of about 100 μm and have been divided into two groups (**Fig. 7.18**).[12] Those classified as type 1 cells (because they are more abundant) appear to function principally as macrophages, scavenging pigment released from damaged or dead cells of uveal tissues. The number of such cells increases with age. Type II cells have more homogeneously distributed melanosomes and have features of smooth muscle cells as well. Their function remains uncertain.

![iris micrograph labeled ABL and IE]

FIGURE 7.16 Scanning electron micrograph of cross section through the iris. ABL, anterior border layer; *asterisk*, iris blood vessel lumen surrounded by cylindrical processes of stromal melanocytes embedded in a fine collagenous matrix. Note the fine granular appearance given to the two layers of iris epithelia (IE) by their high content of melanosomes. (From Freddo T. Ultrastructure of the iris. *Micros Res Tech.* 1996;33(Special Issue, The Anterior Segment of the Eye, Freddo T, ed.):369–389.)

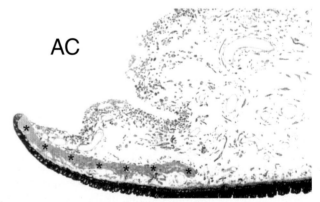

FIGURE 7.17 Light micrograph of pupillary portion of the iris showing the pupillary sphincter muscle (*asterisks*) and demonstrating that the posterior surface of the muscle is attached to the posterior epithelial layers of the iris only at the pupillary margin. AC, anterior chamber.

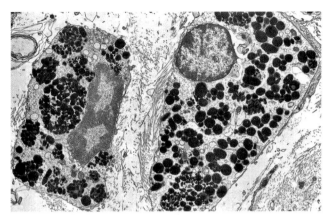

FIGURE 7.18 Transmission electron micrograph of type I clump cells of Koganei near the pupil of the iris, showing "clumps" of pigment within the cytoplasm of the cell. (From Freddo T. Ultrastructure of the iris. *Micros Res Tech*. 1996;33(Special Issue, The Anterior Segment of the Eye, Freddo T, ed.):369–389.)

Iris Vasculature

The iris is well vascularized. It is served by numerous radial iris arterioles (**Fig. 7.19**). Most of these originate from the major circle of the iris. Despite its name, the major circle of the iris is neither a complete circle nor is it normally found in the iris. The major circle of the iris normally

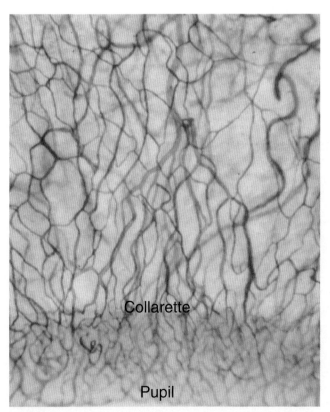

FIGURE 7.19 Whole mount preparation of iris showing stromal vascular pattern flowing toward pupil. (From Raviola G, Freddo T. A simple staining method for blood vessels in flat preparations of ocular tissues. *Invest Ophthalmol Vis Sci*. 1950;19:1518–1521.)

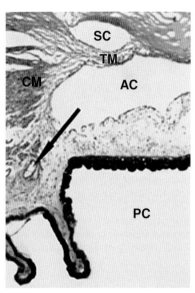

FIGURE 7.20 Light micrograph of iris root and anterior chamber angle region showing position of major circle of the iris (*arrow*) within the ciliary body. CM, ciliary muscle; AC, anterior chamber; TM, trabecular meshwork; SC, Schlemm's canal; PC, posterior chamber.

resides in the ciliary body stroma, adjacent to the iris root (**Fig. 7.20**). Although most of the radial vessels of the iris originate from the major circle of the iris, a small number represent direct branches from anterior ciliary arteries and long posterior ciliary arteries.

Angiographic evidence indicates that the radial arterioles arise mostly in pairs, running in the superficial stroma, beneath the anterior border layer of the ciliary portion of the iris, as far as the collarette. A variably well-developed minor circle of the iris, covered by fibroblasts and melanocytes of the anterior border layer, corresponds to the surface feature termed the collarette. This irregular, superficial vascular ring was the point of origin for the vessels serving the embryonic pupillary membrane prior to its resorption during development of the iris. In the pupillary portion of the iris, the arterioles ramify into a capillary plexus that drains through veins running in the deeper stroma, ultimately joining the anterior uveal venous system that leads to the vortex veins.[13]

The blood vessels of the iris meet the histologic criteria for arterioles, capillaries, and venules. These vessels are lined by a continuous endothelium, which produces a basement membrane containing collagen types I and IV, but not III.[9,10] Type VI collagen has been associated with the outer aspect of these basement membranes. The tunica media of the arterioles exhibits pericytes within splits in the basement membrane and few true smooth muscle cells are found.[14] These vessels lack an elastic lamina.

Iris blood vessels exhibit an unusual tunica adventitia, often giving them the appearance of a tube within a tube (**Fig. 7.21**). This morphology resembles a flexible, metal-encased electrical wire (i.e., coaxial cable) designed to

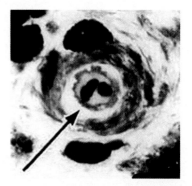

FIGURE 7.21 Light micrograph of stromal iris blood vessel shows "tube within a tube" organization of the tunica adventitia seen within the wall of many iris vessels (*arrow*). (From Freddo T, Raviola G. The homogeneous structure of blood vessels in the vascular tree of *Macaca mulatta*. *Invest Ophthalmol Vis Sci*. 1983;22:279–291.)

acuity. For this and other reasons, in the normal eye, the amount of plasma-derived protein permitted to reach the aqueous humor is only about 1% of that found in plasma.

In freeze-fracture replicas, the zonulae occludentes of iris vessels are seen as a continuous system of branching and anastomosing strands of intramembranous junctional proteins (**Fig. 7.22B**). This system of tight junctional strands seals the interendothelial clefts between iris vascular endothelial cells (**Fig. 7.23**).[16]

protect the wire from severe flexing that could weaken and sever it. This similar structure in iris vessels may function to minimize the possibility of iris vessel "kinking" and closing during the corrugations of the iris vessels that attend dilation of the pupil.[15]

The capillaries of the iris are of the continuous (nonfenestrated) type.[14] Their endothelial cells are joined by gap junctions and continuous tight junctions (zonulae occludentes), the latter of which prevent macromolecules in the bloodstream of the iris vessels from entering the iris stroma (**Fig. 7.22A**). Recall that the aqueous humor freely permeates the iris stroma due to the lack of an epithelium on the anterior surface of the iris. Therefore, leakage of plasma proteins into the iris stroma would be leakage of plasma proteins directly into the aqueous humor. Such large molecules, if present in significant amounts in aqueous humor, would scatter light in the anterior chamber, degrading visual

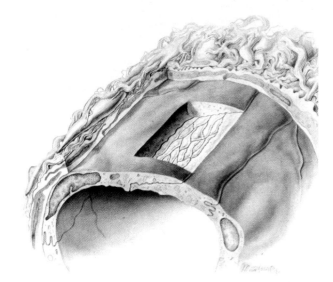

FIGURE 7.23 Sketch showing the structure of the tunica intima and tunica media of an iris blood vessel, including a cutout of overlap between adjacent vascular endothelial cells revealing the position of the branching and anastomosing pattern of tight junctional strands shown in Figure 7.22B. (From Freddo T, Raviola G. Freeze-fracture analysis of the interendothelial junctions in blood vessels of the iris in *Macaca mulatta*. *Invest Ophthalmol Vis Sci*. 1983;23:154–167.)

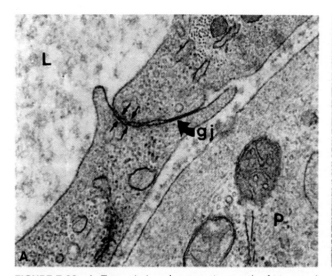

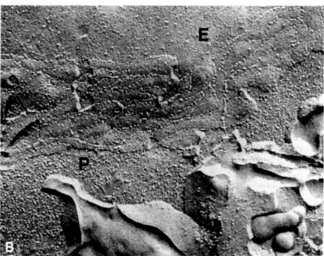

FIGURE 7.22 **A:** Transmission electron micrograph of iris vessel wall showing points of membrane attachment of tight junction (*arrows*) and gap junction (gj) between adjacent endothelial cells. L, lumen; P, pericyte in tunica media of vessel wall. **B:** Freeze-fracture electron micrograph shows continuous branching and anastomosing strands of tight junctional proteins joining adjacent iris vascular endothelial cells. P, P-face of cellular plasma membrane; E, E-face of cellular plasma membrane. (From Freddo T, Raviola G. Freeze-fracture analysis of the interendothelial junctions in blood vessels of the iris in *Macaca mulatta*. *Invest Ophthalmol Vis Sci*. 1982;23:154–167.)

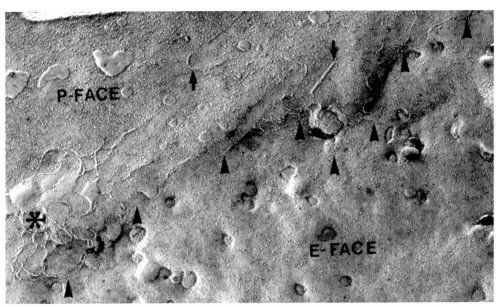

FIGURE 7.24 Freeze-fracture electron micrograph of disrupted tight junction in iris blood vessel of inflamed iris (anterior uveitis), leading to abnormal leakage of plasma proteins into the aqueous humor. A small portion of the junction remains relatively intact (*asterisk*) but most of the junction shows only isolated junctional particles (*arrowheads*) and disrupted junctional strands (*arrows*). (From Freddo TF, Sacks-Wilner R. Interendothelial junctions of the iris vasculature in anterior uveitis. *Invest Ophthalmol Vis Sci.* 1989;30:1104–1111.)

 Disruption of iris blood vessel tight junctional strands has been shown to occur in intraocular inflammatory diseases. Note in Figure 7.24 that one portion of the junction remains well preserved (asterisk), but the continuity of the remaining tight junction has been interrupted and only fragments of the tight junctional strands remain (arrows). This results in increased amounts of protein in the aqueous humor. This extra protein scatters the light of the slit-lamp and is described clinically as a "flare."[17]

Nerves within the Iris

Both unmyelinated and myelinated nerve fibers are present in the iris stroma (**Fig. 7.25**). Types of innervation known to be present in the human iris include sympathetic, parasympathetic, and substance P immune-reactive sensory nerve fibers, derived from cranial nerve V. The postganglionic parasympathetic fibers innervate the pupillary sphincter muscle as described earlier. The postganglionic sympathetic fibers provide vascular tone and innervate the myoepithelial cells that are one of the two layers of epithelium on the posterior surface of the iris. It is the "myo" portion of these cells that constitutes the dilator muscle of the iris. Iris stromal melanocytes have been shown to receive both sympathetic and parasympathetic inputs and are networked through a system of gap junctions.[2,18] The sympathetic input provides an important trophic effect that sustains iris pigmentation.

Substance P immune-reactive neurons, originating from the ophthalmic division of cranial nerve V, have also been

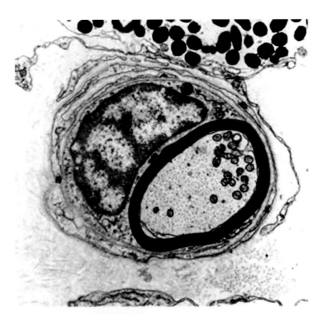

FIGURE 7.25 Transmission electron micrograph of myelinated nerve fiber in iris stroma. (From Freddo T. Ultrastructure of the iris. *Micros Res Tech.* 1996;33(Special Issue, The Anterior Segment of the Eye, Freddo T, ed.):369–389.)

Interruption of sympathetic inputs to the eye, as in congenital Horner's syndrome or Horner's syndrome acquired in childhood, commonly leads to atrophic changes in the color of the ipsilateral iris, following the sequence of color changes noted earlier. Less dramatic color changes may attend long-standing, acquired Horner's syndrome in adults.[19]

identified in the human iris. Release of substance P can stimulate contraction of the pupillary sphincter. More recent studies suggest that cholecystokinin (CCK) may be more important than substance P in contraction of the human iris sphincter.[20]

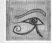 *Release of substance P or CCK into the iris, during intraocular inflammatory disease or following trauma, likely explains the miosis that commonly occurs in these conditions.[21]*

THE IRIS EPITHELIA

Two layers of pigment-containing epithelial cells line the posterior surface of the iris. These two layers do not represent a compound epithelium. Instead, they represent two simple epithelia that come to be apposed at their apical surfaces by the invagination of the embryonic optic cup during development (**SEE CHAPTER 16: EMBRYOLOGY OF THE EYE AND ORBIT**) (**Fig. 7.26**). These two layers are continuous with each other at the pupillary margin, which is the adult vestige of the rim of the embryonic optic cup. They are termed the anterior myoepithelium and the posterior pigmented epithelium of the iris.

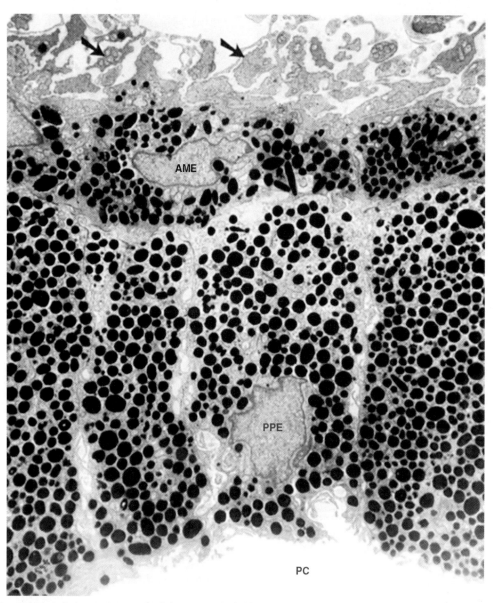

FIGURE 7.26   Transmission electron micrograph of the two epithelial layers on the posterior surface of the iris. The anterior myoepithelial (AME) layer, closest to the iris stroma, demonstrates smooth muscle-like basal processes (*arrow*) that constitute the dilator muscle of the iris and an apical portion of the cell with numerous melanosomes. The posterior pigmented epithelial (PPE) cells have no smooth muscle cell-like processes. The adjoined surfaces of these two layers are their apical surfaces. The basal surface of the AME with its smooth muscle-like processes, faces the iris stroma and the basal surface of the PPE faces the posterior chamber (PC). (From Freddo T. Intercellular junctions of the iris epithelia in *Macaca mulatta. Invest Ophthalmol Vis Sci.* 1984;25:1094–1104.)

The Anterior Myoepithelium

The anterior myoepithelium is a single layer of pigmented myoepithelial cells, the basal portions of which have been modified to function like smooth muscle (**Fig. 7.26**).[22] The basement membrane of this epithelial layer covers the smooth muscle-like basal processes of these cells and faces the iris stroma. It contains type IV collagen.

It is important to realize that, unlike the iris sphincter, the iris dilator muscle is not a separate layer of smooth muscle. The iris dilator is composed entirely of the basal, smooth muscle-like component of the anterior myoepithelial cell layer. The smooth muscle-like component of the anterior myoepithelium is stimulated by postganglionic sympathetic nerve fibers. The postganglionic fibers destined for the pupil leave the sympathetic nerve plexus surrounding the internal carotid artery, at the point where the artery and the ophthalmic division of the trigeminal nerve come into close proximity. This point of proximity occurs as both the internal carotid artery and the ophthalmic division of the trigeminal nerve emerge from the wall of the cavernous sinus, near its anterolateral margin. At this location, postganglionic sympathetic fibers are conveyed from the internal carotid plexus to the nasociliary branch of the ophthalmic division of the trigeminal nerve. They then partition into the long ciliary nerves, which convey them to the eye and ultimately to the anterior myoepithelium of the iris. The basal, smooth muscle-cell-like processes of the anterior myoepithelium cells are joined by gap junctions. These junctions coordinate dilator muscle contraction.

The apical, pigmented epithelial portions of the anterior myoepithelial cells are also joined by gap junctions and by desmosomes as well. These same two types of junctions are also found joining the apposing apical surfaces of the anterior myoepithelium and posterior pigmented epithelium.[22]

Realizing that the pupillary sphincter (S) is true smooth muscle and the dilator muscle is the "myo" component of a myoepithelium is important clinically. In diabetic eyes, excess glycogen can accumulate in both layers of the iris epithelium. When this glycogen is dissolved away during histologic processing, it gives the anterior myoepithelium and the posterior pigmented epithelium a moth-eaten appearance that is termed "lacy vacuolization" (Fig. 7.27). Because the dilator pupillae muscle is actually the "myo" component of the anterior myoepithelial layer and not a separate layer of smooth muscle cells like the pupillary sphincter, this excessive deposition of glycogen compromises myoepithelial cell function but spares the true smooth muscle cells of the pupillary sphincter. This compromise in myoepithelial cell function contributes to the commonly encountered difficulty in dilating the pupils of diabetic patients.[23]

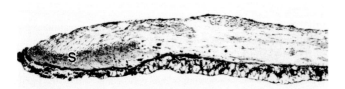

FIGURE 7.27 Light micrograph of iris from an eye with long-standing diabetes mellitus shows "moth-eaten" appearance, known as lacy vacuolization of iris epithelium. In vivo, these spaces are filled with abnormal deposits of glycogen. Both epithelial layers are involved, including the anterior myoepithelium, of which the dilator muscle is an integral part. Note that the true smooth muscle tissue of the pupillary sphincter (*S*) remains unaffected.

The Posterior Pigmented Epithelium

The posterior pigmented epithelium of the iris is a single layer of pigmented cells. The basal lamina of the posterior pigmented epithelium fronts the posterior chamber of the eye. The shape of the posterior pigmented epithelial cells varies from cuboidal to columnar depending upon the state of pupillary contraction. Studies in monkey eyes, using a protein tracer that can be visualized by electron microscopy, have shown that soluble proteins in the iris stroma can freely diffuse through the intercellular spaces between adjacent anterior myoepithelial cells and into the intercellular spaces between the apical surfaces of the two epithelial layers. But this protein is prevented from reaching the posterior chamber by zonulae occludentes joining the lateral surfaces of the posterior pigmented epithelial cells near their apical surface (**Fig. 7.28**). These tight junctions are part of an apicolateral junctional complex that also includes a zonula adherens, which provides a band of intercellular adhesion that parallels the encircling band of the tight junctions around each cell. In addition to this junctional complex, the posterior pigmented epithelial cells are also joined to one another by numerous gap junctions for intercellular communication and desmosomes for focal adhesion. These focal junctions are found basal to the encircling adhesion bands of the zonulae adherentes and zonulae occludentes.[22,24]

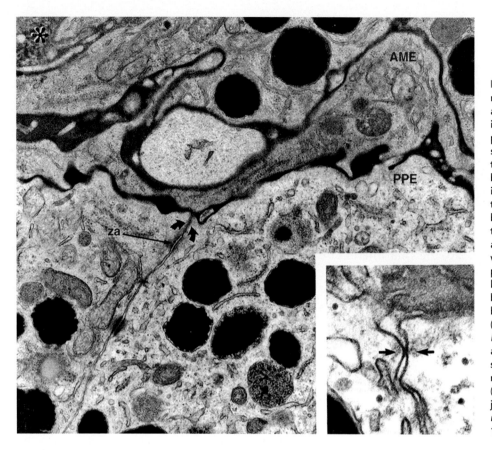

FIGURE 7.28 Transmission electron micrograph showing the adjoined apical surfaces of the iridial epithelia in a monkey iris. A black tracer for plasma protein diffusion fills the iris stroma (*asterisk*), having leaked from the fenestrated vessels of the ciliary body stroma and diffused into the iris stroma. The homogeneous black tracer permeates the intercellular cleft between adjacent anterior myoepithelial (AME) cells and between the apical surfaces between the AME with dark cytoplasm and posterior pigmented epithelial (PPE) cells with lighter cytoplasm. Passage of tracer between adjacent PPE cells is blocked by the presence of a zonula occludens (*curved arrows*). za, zonula adherens. *Inset*: A zonula occludens is identified as a series of contact points between specialized proteins embedded in the membranes of the adjoined PPE cells (*arrows*). (From Freddo T. Intercellular junctions of the iris epithelia in *Macaca mulatta. Invest Ophthalmol Vis Sci.* 1984;25:1094–1104.)

REFERENCES

1. Winn B, Whitaker D, Elliott DB, et al. Factors affecting light-adapted pupil size in normal human subjects. *Invest Ophthalmol Vis Sci.* 1994;35(3):1132–1137.
2. Freddo TF. Ultrastructure of the iris. *Microsc Res Tech.* 1996;33(5):369–389.
3. Prota G, Hu D, Vincensi MR, et al. Characterization of melanins in human irides and cultured uveal melanocytes from eyes of different colors. *Exp Eye Res.* 1998;67(3):293–299.
4. McCartney AC, Spalton DJ, Bull TB. Type IV melanosomes of the human albino iris. *Br J Ophthalmol.* 1985;69(7):537–541.
5. Eagle RC Jr. Iris pigmentation and pigmented lesions: an ultrastructural study. *Trans Am Ophthalmol Soc.* 1988;86:581–687.
6. Saenz RB. Primary care of infants and young children with down syndrome. *Am Fam Physician.* 1999;59:381–400.
7. Kiratli H. Head and neck: iris hamartomas. *Atlas Genet Cytogenet Oncol Haematol.* 2010;14(1):83–86.
8. Freddo TF. A contemporary concept of the blood–aqueous barrier. *Prog Retin Eye Res.* 2013;32:181–195.
9. Konstas A, Marshall G, Lee W. Immunocytochemical localisation of collagens (I–V) in the human iris. *Graefes Arch Clin Exp Ophthalmol.* 1990;228(1):180–186.
10. Rittig M, Lütjen-Drecoll E, Rauterberg J, et al. Type-VI collagen in the human iris and ciliary body. *Cell Tissue Res.* 1990;259(2):305–312.
11. McMenamin PG, Crewe J, Morrison S, et al. Immunomorphologic studies of macrophages and MHC class II-positive dendritic cells in the iris and ciliary body of the rat, mouse, and human eye. *Invest Ophthalmol Vis Sci.* 1994;35(8):3234–3250.
12. Wobmann PR, Fine BS. The clump cells of koganei: a light and electron microscopic study. *Am J Ophthalmol.* 1972;73(1):90–101.
13. Demeler U, Diekstall F, Kröncke W. Iris angiography of the anterior segment. *J Ophthalmic Photogr.* 1986;9(2):116–122.
14. Freddo TF, Raviola G. The homogeneous structure of blood vessels in the vascular tree of macaca mulatta iris. *Invest Ophthalmol Vis Sci.* 1982;22(3):279–291.
15. Gregersen E. The tubular tissue spaces surrounding the endothelial channels of the human iridie vessels. *Acta Ophthalmol.* 1959;37(3):199–208.
16. Freddo TF, Raviola G. Freeze-fracture analysis of the interendothelial junctions in the blood vessels of the iris in macaca mulatta. *Invest Ophthalmol Vis Sci.* 1982;23(2):154–167.
17. Freddo TF, Sacks-Wilner R. Interendothelial junctions of the rabbit iris vasculature in anterior uveitis. *Invest Ophthalmol Vis Sci.* 1989;30(6):1104–1111.
18. Laties AM. Ocular melanin and the adrenergic innervation to the eye. *Trans Am Ophthalmol Soc.* 1974;72:560–605.
19. Beynat J, Soichot P, Bidot S, et al. Iris heterochromia in acquired horner's syndrome. *J Fr Ophthalmol.* 2007;30(7):e19.
20. Pintor J. Autonomic nervous system: ophthalmic control. In: Squire LR, ed. *Encyclopedia of Neuroscience.* Oxford, UK: Academic Press; 2009:967–974.
21. Anderson JA, Malfroy B, Richard NR, et al. Substance P contracts the human iris sphincter: possible modulation by endogenous enkephalinase. *Regul Pept.* 1990;29(1):49–58.
22. Freddo TF. Intercellular junctions of the iris epithelia in macaca mulatta. *Invest Ophthalmol Vis Sci.* 1984;25(9):1094–1104.
23. Kincaid M. Pathology of diabetes mellitus. *Duanes Found Clin Ophthalmol.* 1996;2:1–14.
24. Freddo TF. A contemporary concept of the blood–aqueous barrier. *Prog Retin Eye Res.* 2013;32:181–195.

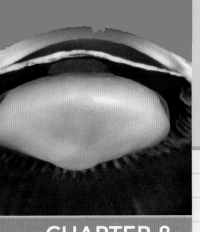

The Ciliary Body

CHAPTER 8

Overview

The ciliary body performs functions relating to aqueous production, aqueous outflow, and accommodation. It is the sole source of aqueous humor production and it also facilitates aqueous humor outflow to Schlemm's canal by contracting a group of smooth muscle fibers. As this group of smooth muscle fibers contracts, their tendons alter the conformation of the tissues of the conventional outflow pathway (described in **CHAPTER 9: ANATOMY OF THE AQUEOUS OUTFLOW PATHWAYS**) such that outflow of aqueous humor is enhanced and intraocular pressure decreases. The ciliary body also serves as part of the alternate pathway for aqueous humor outflow termed the uveoscleral pathway (also described in **CHAPTER 9: ANATOMY OF THE AQUEOUS OUTFLOW PATHWAYS**).

Near the posterior limit of the ciliary body, where it joins the sensory retina, at the ora serrata, the cells of its inner surface anchor the zonular fibers that suspend the crystalline lens in place behind the pupil. This same area also serves as the anterior limit of the attachment for the vitreous base, which is the firmest area of attachment of the vitreous body to the wall of the eye.

Through contraction of some of its smooth muscle fibers, the ciliary body also alters the tension on the zonular fibers that it anchors. Changing the tension on the zonules results in a change in the shape of the lens that shifts the focus of the eye from far to near in the process of accommodation.

Finally, there is some evidence that the ciliary body may play a role in the production and slow turnover of hyaluronic acid in the vitreous.[1,2]

Macroscopic and Clinical Anatomy of the Ciliary Body

The ciliary body forms the middle third of the uveal tract, situated between the iris root anteriorly and the retina and choroid posteriorly. The ora serrata is the abrupt juncture between the posterior margin of the ciliary body and the most peripheral portion of the retina. As the name implies, this juncture has a scalloped or serrated appearance grossly (**Fig. 8.1**). The anatomic details of this important transition and related structures are discussed in **CHAPTER 14: THE NEUROSENSORY RETINA**.

In the adult eye, the ciliary body extends posteriorly from the limbus approximately 7 mm on the temporal side and 6 mm on the nasal side of the eye.[3] There is, however, some variation in this dimension between eyes of different anteroposterior lengths.

The ciliary body is grossly subdivided into two portions, the pars plicata anteriorly and the pars plana posteriorly (**Fig. 8.1**). As its name implies, the inner surface of the pars plana is flat. The inner surface of the pars plicata exhibits 75 to 80 radially oriented, fin-like ridges, termed ciliary processes that form a ring around the equator of the crystalline lens (**Fig. 8.1**). Ciliary processes are divided into major and minor processes based upon their height.

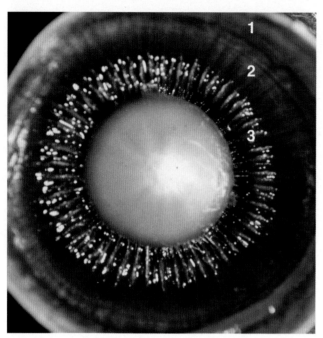

FIGURE 8.1 Macrophotograph of the interior of the anterior segment of the eye. The crystalline lens and surrounding ciliary body are evident, including the principal landmarks of the ora serrata (*1*) pars plana (*2*) and pars plicata (*3*). (From Freddo T, Gong H, Civan M. Anatomy of the ciliary body and outflow pathways. In: Tasman WS, Jaeger EA, eds. *Duane's Clinical Ophthalmology on CD-ROM*. Philadelphia, PA: Lippincott Williams and Wilkins; 2011.)

Major processes are approximately 1 mm high and minor processes approximately a third to a half millimeter in height (**Fig. 8.2**). It is the ciliary processes that secrete aqueous humor. **Figure 8.2** actually misrepresents the surface anatomy in vivo, because all of the zonular fibers have been removed from the surface of this specimen. In vivo, the entire surface of the pars plana, facing the posterior chamber (PC), is covered with a uniform carpet of zonular fibers that originate from anchoring points within the epithelium of the pars plana. As these fibers extend anteriorly and reach the ciliary processes of the pars plicata, they divide into packets and stack up in the

*The pars plana region of the ciliary body is much thinner and less vascularized than the pars plicata, making it the safest point of entry into the eye for surgical procedures, such as vitrectomies, that are performed on parts of the eye behind the crystalline lens (**Fig. 8.4**). To ensure that these entry points pass through the pars plana and not the pars plicata or the retina, measurements are commonly taken. As a general rule, the entry point(s) are made 4 mm behind the limbus in eyes with a natural lens (i.e., phakic) and 3.5 mm posterior to the limbus if there is a lens implant (pseudophakic) or no lens at all (aphakic).*

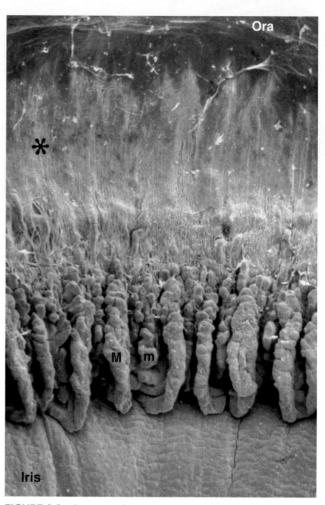

FIGURE 8.2 Scanning electron micrograph of the interior surface of the pars plana (*asterisk*) and pars plicata showing major (*M*) and minor (*m*) ciliary processes. In this micrograph the normally present carpet of zonular fibers covering the inner surface of the pars plana has been removed. (From Morrison JC, Van Buskirk EM, Freddo T. Anatomy, microcirculation and ultrastructure of the ciliary body. In: Ritch R, Shields MB, Krupin T, eds. *The Glaucomas*. St Louis, MO: CV Mosby; 1989.)

valleys between the adjacent ciliary processes en route to the surface of the lens. This leaves only the tips of each process exposed to the PC (**Fig. 8.3**).

Layers of the Ciliary Body

- In coronal sections of the ciliary body (**Fig. 8.5**) the following layers are identifiable beneath the sclera, in both the pars plicata and pars plana regions.
- The supraciliary space
- The ciliary muscle
- The ciliary body stroma
- The ciliary epithelium
  - Pigmented ciliary epithelium
  - Nonpigmented ciliary epithelium

Two layers of the ciliary epithelium line the entire inner surface of the ciliary body. In the pars plicata region, which

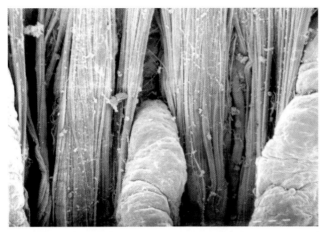

FIGURE 8.3 High magnification scanning electron micrograph of the posterior edge of the ciliary processes at the junction between the pars plana **(top)** and the pars plicata **(below)**. Note the way in which the zonular fibers on the inner surface of the pars plana are channeled into valleys between the ridges of adjacent ciliary processes. (From Freddo T, Gong H, Civan M. Anatomy of the ciliary body and outflow pathways. In: Tasman WS, Jaeger EA, eds. *Duane's Clinical Ophthalmology on CD-ROM*. Philadelphia, PA: Lippincott Williams and Wilkins; 2011.)

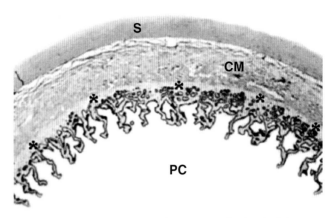

FIGURE 8.5 Coronal section of the eye at the level of the pars plicata with crystalline lens removed. Visible are the sclera (S), ciliary muscle (CM), ciliary body stroma (*asterisks*), the ciliary processes, and the posterior chamber (PC), where the lens would normally reside. The separation between the inner surface of the sclera (S) and the outer surface of the CM is an artifact but corresponds to the location of the supraciliary space in vivo.

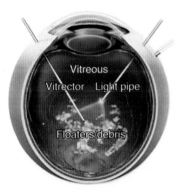

FIGURE 8.4 Diagrammatic representation of the portals of entry for vitrector and light pipe in surgery to remove the vitreous humor. Note that the portals enter the eye through the pars plana region of the ciliary body, posterior to the lens. (Courtesy of Modern Eye Hospital & Research Center, Nellore, India. Dr. PL Rao, Founder.)

But the supraciliary and suprachoroidal spaces are actually one continuous space, a space that is clinically important as part of the uveoscleral pathway for aqueous outflow (discussed in **CHAPTER 9: ANATOMY OF THE AQUEOUS OUTFLOW PATHWAYS**).

Meridional sections of the ciliary body provide a different perspective on the various layers (**Fig. 8.6**). All of the layers of the ciliary body remain evident and should be compared with the appearance of these same layers in the coronal section shown in **Figure 8.5**. As in **Figure 8.5**, the supraciliary space is artifactually distended. The separation of the ciliary body from the overlying sclera is a useful reminder that the only significant attachment points of the ciliary body to the sclera are at the points of origin and insertion of the ciliary muscle and where vessels and nerves passing into and out of the ciliary body pierce the sclera.

The continuity of the layers of the ciliary epithelium, with their counterparts lining the posterior surface of the iris, is evident in **Figure 8.6**, as is the continuity of the ciliary body stroma with the stroma of the iris at the iris root. The relationship between the ciliary body and the trabecular meshwork is also seen. The arrow in **Figure 8.6** identifies the lumen of the major arterial circle of the iris, which, despite its name, resides within the ciliary body.

Histology of the Layers of the Ciliary Body

THE CILIARY MUSCLE

Between the inner surface of the sclera and the ciliary body stroma is a layer of smooth muscle (**Figs. 8.5** and **8.6**). Three different fiber orientations are evident within this muscle in the pars plicata. These three sets of fibers

is shown in **Figure 8.5**, the cores of the ciliary processes projecting into the PC are filled with a fibrovascular stroma. This stroma extends out of each process to join a continuous layer of stroma that encircles the ciliary body (**Fig. 8.5**). External to the ring of ciliary body stroma is the ciliary muscle. Separating the external surface of the ciliary muscle from the inner surface of the sclera is a cleft that, in **Figure 8.5**, has been artificially widened by the shrinkage of the looser ciliary muscle tissue away from the denser sclera during tissue processing. This space is present in vivo but, under normal conditions, is narrow enough to be indiscernible. This potential space is referred to as the supraciliary space. This space undergoes a name change to the suprachoroidal space when the ciliary body transitions to the retina and choroid at the ora serrata.

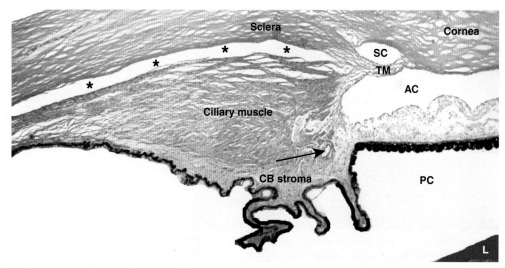

FIGURE 8.6 Meridional section of the ciliary body (CB) and its relationship to the anterior chamber, angle structures, and iris. The distention of the supraciliary space (*asterisks*) is an artifact of tissue processing. In the normal eye, in vivo, this is a potential space subtending no volume but represents the space through which uveoscleral outflow of aqueous humor passes. The lumen of the major circle of the iris is shown at the tip of the arrow. AC, anterior chamber; PC, posterior chamber; TM, trabecular meshwork; SC, Schlemm's canal; L, crystalline lens.

are the longitudinal bundle, the radial bundle, and the circular bundle (**Fig. 8.7**).

Longitudinal Bundle

The layer of smooth muscle closest to the sclera follows the contour of the inner surface of the sclera but is separated from the sclera by the supraciliary space. This layer is termed the longitudinal bundle. These fibers take origin from stellate processes anchored into the inner surface of the sclera in the pars plana region. These anchoring processes are called epichoroidal stars (**Fig. 8.7**). From these points of origin, the muscle fibers extend anteriorly to insert onto the posterior surface of the scleral spur (**Fig. 8.8**). As noted earlier, these two points of attachment of the longitudinal bundle are the only significant attachments of the ciliary body to the inner wall of the sclera.

Not all of the tendons of the longitudinal bundle end by attaching to the scleral spur. Some of these tendons extend anteriorly, beyond the lip of the scleral spur, through the meshwork, into the corneal stroma. Additional tendons make attachments to the trabecular meshwork and also make direct connections to the endothelium of the inner wall of Schlemm's canal. This complex of ciliary muscle tendons extending into the trabecular meshwork is referred to as the cribriform plexus. This plexus facilitates aqueous humor outflow when the ciliary muscle contracts and is described in full detail in **CHAPTER 9: ANATOMY OF THE AQUEOUS OUTFLOW PATHWAYS**.

Radial Bundle

Closer to the ciliary body stroma than the longitudinal bundle is the radial bundle. Like the longitudinal bundle, the radial bundle runs in a posteroanterior direction but as the fibers move anteriorly, these fibers bifurcate and run

an oblique path relative to the direction of the fibers in the longitudinal bundle (**Fig. 8.7**).

Circular Bundle

The innermost of the three smooth muscle layers runs like an encircling band or sphincter around the circumference of the ciliary body (**Fig. 8.7**). It is termed the circular bundle and functions principally in the process of accommodation. By contracting like a sphincter, the circular bundle decreases the diameter of the ciliary body around the lens, while the radial bundle creates a small anterior movement of the lens. Video of this contractile movement of the ciliary processes has been shown in vivo in primates following surgical removal of the iris.[4] (*This video can be accessed through the eBook bundled with this text.*) When the circular bundle contracts, the tonic tension on the zonular fibers is relaxed, allowing the lens to reflexively reconfigure to a more biconvex shape under the influence of its elastic capsule. The result is a change in focus from far to near, a process called accommodation. Our ability to accommodate decreases with age. This decrease results primarily from changes in the crystalline lens but partly from age-related fibrosis of the connective tissue of the ciliary body, which limits the contraction of the still functional ciliary muscle. This age-related loss of accommodative ability is termed presbyopia and it usually becomes clinically significant in the fifth decade, prompting the need for supplemental near vision corrections.

Innervation of the Ciliary Muscle

Large numbers of (parasympathetic) cholinergic nerve terminals, forming neuromuscular junctions, are present along ciliary muscle fibers.[5] Stimulation of the ciliary muscle by its parasympathetic inputs leads to rapid accommodation of

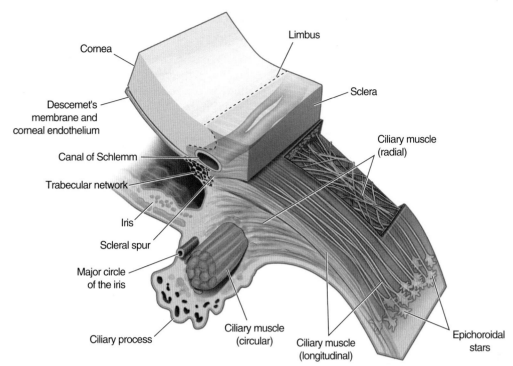

FIGURE 8.7 Sketch of the ciliary body and iris root, showing the orientation of the three bundles of the ciliary muscle from two perspectives. The limbal cornea and sclera are also shown. The trabecular meshwork is present as is Schlemm's canal. The three layers of the ciliary muscle are shown for comparison in meridional section and in progressive, stepwise dissection from the outer surface of the muscle. Closest to the sclera is the longitudinal bundle of the muscle. These smooth muscle fibers originate from epichoroidal stars that anchor these fibers into the inner surface of the sclera. These fibers end in insertions onto the posterior surface of the scleral spur and in the trabecular meshwork. Tendons of these fibers extend anteriorly into the corneal stroma and also extend into the trabecular meshwork, even making direct connections with the endothelial cells lining the inner wall of Schlemm's canal. Deeper than the longitudinal bundle is the "radial bundle," which exhibits wide bifurcations. In the perspective showing stepwise dissection **(upper right)**, bifurcations of these fibers are evident. Finally, the "circular bundle" is seen in cross section in the meridional perspective, in relation to the major circle of the iris.

the lens. The preganglionic parasympathetic fibers destined for the ciliary body leave the midbrain with the oculomotor nerve (CN III). En route to the orbit, CN III passes through the superior aspect of the lateral wall of the cavernous sinus. As the oculomotor nerve enters the orbit through the superior orbital fissure, it subdivides into superior and inferior divisions. The preganglionic parasympathetic fibers are carried into the inferior division and ultimately to its branch destined for the inferior oblique. En route to the muscle, the parasympathetic fibers leave the nerve via a communicating branch to the ciliary ganglion. In the ganglion, these preganglionic fibers synapse and the postganglionic fibers are conveyed to the eye on the short ciliary nerves, passing forward in the suprachoroidal and supraciliary spaces beneath the sclera, to reach the iris and the ciliary body (**SEE CHAPTER 3: OVERVIEW OF THE EYE**). It is clear that the ciliary muscle also receives sympathetic inputs. The postganglionic sympathetic fibers serving the ciliary body arise in the superior cervical ganglion and travel to the orbit as a plexus around the internal carotid artery and then the ophthalmic artery. These fibers finally traverse the ciliary ganglion without synapsing, to reach the eye as part of the long ciliary nerves.

Whether relaxation of accommodation is actively driven by these sympathetic inputs or is achieved primarily

through reduction in parasympathetic stimulation of the ciliary muscle is a matter of debate.[6–8] Most likely both are involved but either way, it is clear that adrenergic receptors do exist on ciliary muscle cells.[8]

THE CILIARY BODY STROMA

Internal to the ciliary muscle resides the ciliary body stroma, which is composed of a loose connective tissue matrix that supports the nerves and blood vessels traveling within it. The stroma is continuous with that of the iris at the iris root and with that of the choroid beyond the ora serrata. In the pars plicata, this connective tissue matrix extends into the core of each ciliary process (**Figs. 8.5** and **8.6**). Collagen types I, II, and VI have been reported in the ciliary body stroma, with type IV collagen present in the basement membranes of the ciliary epithelial layers.[9,10] With increasing age there is a progressive "hyalinization" of the stroma, which may contribute to presbyopia by restricting the contraction of the circular bundle of the ciliary muscle.

Anterior to the iris root, and posterior to the trabecular meshwork, the ciliary body stroma opens directly to the anterior chamber (**Figs. 8.6** and **8.8**). The surface of this portion of the stroma, facing the anterior chamber, can

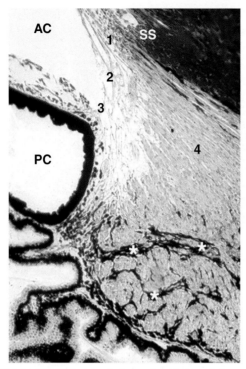

FIGURE 8.8 Light micrograph shows the relationship between the ciliary body and adjacent structures facing the anterior chamber (AC) and the posterior chamber (PC), including the scleral spur (SS), the trabecular meshwork (*1*) the ciliary body band (*2*) and the iris root (*3*). The ciliary muscle (*4*) and the pigmented, fibrovascular septae, separating the ciliary muscle fascicles of the circular bundle (*white asterisks*), are evident.

be seen clinically by gonioscopy and is referred to as the ciliary body band (SEE **CHAPTER 9: ANATOMY OF THE AQUEOUS OUTFLOW PATHWAYS**). Although most of the aqueous humor leaving the eye passes into the trabecular meshwork and then into Schlemm's canal, some of the aqueous humor from the anterior chamber enters the ciliary body stroma via the ciliary body band. This aqueous then passes through the pigmented fibrovascular connective tissue strands that are woven between the fascicles of the ciliary muscle as seen in **Figure 8.8**. Finally, this aqueous reaches the supraciliary and suprachoroidal space (**Figs. 8.5** and **8.6**). This pathway, called the uveoscleral outflow pathway, is described in greater detail in **CHAPTER 9: ANATOMY OF THE AQUEOUS OUTFLOW PATHWAYS**.

An appreciation of the fibrovascular matrix that interweaves with the smooth muscle fascicles of the ciliary body is important. It appears that the principal anatomic correlate for the documented increase in uveoscleral outflow produced by topical prostaglandins, which are used in the treatment of glaucoma, is mediated through degradation of this connective tissue matrix, thus allowing for enhanced outflow of aqueous humor along this route.[11]

Blood Supply

Within the ciliary body stroma are the principal blood vessels of this tissue. Two anastomotic vascular circles are created in the ciliary body. Both are discontinuous. One of these is formed within the ciliary muscle near the junction between the pars plicata and pars plana and is termed the intramuscular circle. This circle receives contributions primarily from the perforating branches of the anterior ciliary arteries, with smaller contributions from the two, long posterior ciliary arteries. This circle gives rise to the microvasculature of the posterior portion of the ciliary muscle and sends important recurrent vessels posteriorly to provide the blood supply for the anterior portion of the choroid (**Fig. 8.9**).

The second circle is the major circle of the iris, which despite its name, commonly resides just lateral to the root of the iris, within the ciliary body stroma (**Fig. 8.6**). In some cases, at various points in its circular route, this vessel may meander into the iris root, making it visible near the iris surface using a gonioscope. The major circle of the iris receives the bulk of the blood from the long posterior ciliary arteries, with smaller contributions, especially at the 12- and 6-o'clock positions, from the perforating branches of the anterior ciliary arteries (**Fig. 8.9**).

The microvasculature derived from the major circle of the iris provides for the metabolic needs of the anterior ciliary muscle with one set of vessels, and provides the reservoir of fluid and ions required for the production of aqueous humor with a different set (**Fig. 8.10**). A portion of the anterior portion of the ciliary muscle drains to the anterior ciliary veins. The remainder of the blood serving the anterior uveal tissues is drained posteriorly to the vortex veins.

The different sets of vessels serving each ciliary process arise from opposite surfaces of the major circle of the iris and are called the anterior and posterior arterioles (**Fig. 8.10**).[12] The anterior arterioles supply the large diameter marginal capillaries that run along the tip of each process. Using scanning electron microscopy, several investigators have observed constrictions in the afferent arterioles of the ciliary processes that may serve as points of regulation of blood flow under autonomic control.[12–15]

The posterior arterioles supply smaller caliber capillaries that run less deeply within each process (**Fig. 8.10**). The direction of blood flow in both of these systems is from anterior to posterior, toward the choroid, ultimately leaving the eye via the vortex veins. The capillaries derived from the posterior arterioles, which serve the ciliary muscle, are nonfenestrated and do not leak plasma proteins under normal conditions.

By contrast, the large diameter marginal capillaries derived from the anterior arteriole lack continuous tight junctions and are lined by fenestrated endothelial cells (**Fig. 8.11**). Using tracers for plasma protein leakage such

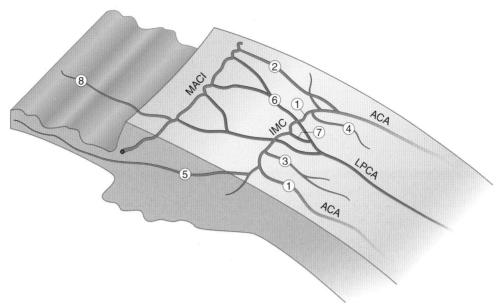

FIGURE 8.9 This sketch demonstrates the contributions of the anterior ciliary arteries (ACA) and the long posterior ciliary arteries (LPCA) to the two vascular circles that provide the blood supply of the ciliary body. The intramuscular circle (IMC) receives contributions principally from the perforating branches of the ACA that arise from the blood supplies of the rectus muscles. The major arterial circle of the iris (MACI) despite its name, resides in the ciliary body stroma, beyond the iris root. The MACI receives contributions principally from the lateral and medial LPCA, with smaller contributions, especially at 12- and 6-o'clock, from the ACA. (*1*) Branches from ACA forming the IMC. (*2*) Branch from ACA to MACI (principally seen at 12- and 6-o'clock). (*3*) Branch to posterior portion of ciliary muscle. (*4*) Recurrent artery serving choroid anterior to the equator of the eye. (*5*) Radial iris artery originating from IMC. (*6*) Primary branches from LPCA contributing to the MACI. (*7*) Branch from LPCA to IMC. (*8*) Radial iris artery from MACI. (Modified from Streeten B. The ciliary body. In: Tasman WS, Jaeger EA, eds. *Duane's Foundations of Clinical Ophthalmology on CD-ROM.* Philadelphia, PA: Lippincott, Williams & Wilkins; 2006.)

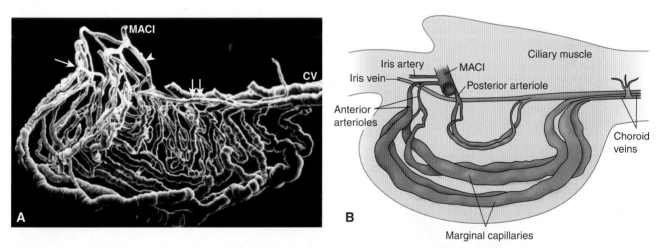

FIGURE 8.10 A: Scanning electron micrograph of the microvasculature of a single ciliary process. The major arterial circle of the iris (MACI—*arrowhead*) gives rise to anterior (*single arrow*) and posterior (*double arrow*) arterioles, both of which drain to choroidal veins (CV). **B:** Sketch of the vascular pattern depicted in A. The anterior arteriole serves the large, fenestrated, marginal capillaries near the tips of the process and the posterior arteriole serves the smaller, nonfenestrated vessels in the interior of the process. (Modified from Morrison JC, Van Buskirk EM, Freddo T. Anatomy, microcirculation and ultrastructure of the ciliary body. In: Ritch R, Shields MB, Krupin T, eds. *The Glaucomas.* St Louis, MO: CV Mosby; 1989.)

as horseradish peroxidase, the capillaries of the ciliary body stroma are seen to be very permeable to macromolecules as well as ions and fluid (**Fig. 8.11**).[16] Therefore, these capillaries, unlike those in the iris, are limited in their capacity to serve as a selective permeability barrier. That barrier function is therefore provided by the ciliary epithelium.

THE CILIARY EPITHELIUM

Two layers of epithelial cells cover the entire inner surface of the ciliary body, both the pars plicata and the pars plana. The layers are named for their relative content of melanin pigment and are readily distinguished in a cross section

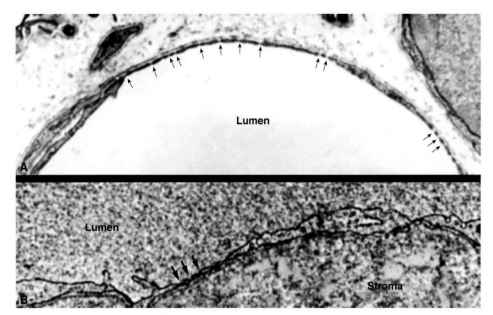

FIGURE 8.11   A: Transmission electron micrograph of marginal capillary shows multiple fenestrations (*arrows*) in the capillary endothelium. **B:** Transmission electron micrograph of a fenestrated capillary from the ciliary body of a monkey eye. Following intravenous injection of the tracer, horseradish peroxidase, granular tracer particles are seen both within and outside the lumen, having leaked through the vessel wall via fenestrations (*arrows*). The tracer that has left the vessel lumen decorates the connective tissue elements of the surrounding stroma. (From Morrison JC, Van Buskirk EM, Freddo T. Anatomy, microcirculation and ultrastructure of the ciliary body. In: Ritch R, Shields MB, Krupin T, eds. *The Glaucomas*. St Louis, MO: CV Mosby; 1989.)

of a ciliary process (**Fig. 8.12**). The layer closest to the posterior chamber (PC) is free of pigment and is termed the nonpigmented ciliary epithelium. The layer closest to the ciliary body stroma is termed the pigmented ciliary epithelium for its content of pigmented melanosomes. The nonpigmented ciliary epithelium is continuous with the posterior pigmented epithelium of the iris anteriorly and with the neurosensory retina posteriorly at the ora serrata (**Fig. 8.13**). The pigmented ciliary epithelium continues anteriorly as the anterior myoepithelium of the iris and posteriorly as the pigment epithelium of the retina. The double layer of epithelium covering the ciliary body, like the double layer of epithelium on the posterior surface of

the iris, actually represents two simple epithelia joined at their apical surfaces following the invagination of the optic cup during embryogenesis. With the apical surfaces of these two epithelial layers joined together, the basement membrane of the nonpigmented ciliary epithelium faces

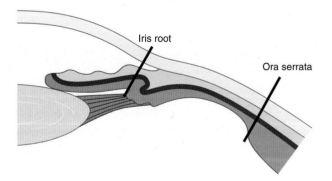

	Iris	Ciliary body	Retina
Outer layer	Anterior myoepithelium	Pigmented ciliary epithelium	Retinal pigment epithelium
Inner layer	Posterior pigmented epithelium	Nonpigmented ciliary epithelium	Neurosensory retina

FIGURE 8.13   Sketch and table show the continuity between derivatives of the outer and inner layers of the embryonic optic cup and the variable morphology that is produced in the iris, ciliary body, and retina. The pupil margin, where the anterior myoepithelium and posterior pigmented epithelium of the iris are joined, represents the adult vestige of the anterior rim of the optic cup.

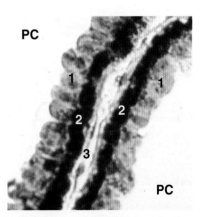

FIGURE 8.12   Light micrograph of lightly stained cross section of a ciliary process showing the nonpigmented ciliary epithelium (*1*), pigmented ciliary epithelium (*2*), and fibrovascular stroma in the core of the ciliary process. PC, posterior chamber.

the PC and that of the pigmented ciliary epithelium faces the ciliary body stroma.

The morphology of the ciliary epithelium varies along the surface of the ciliary body, from simple cuboidal to simple columnar, in accord with the different demands placed upon it in various locations.[17] From regional analyses, it appears that it is primarily the epithelia at the tips of the ciliary processes in the pars plicata that are involved in the production of aqueous humor. Recall that only the tips of each process project above the stacks of zonular fibers filling the valleys between processes. The ciliary processes are innervated by adrenergic (sympathetic) fibers. Beta-adrenergic stimulation leads to an increase in aqueous humor production, while alpha-2 adrenergic stimulation reduces aqueous production.[18] Logically, topical beta-adrenergic blocking agents and alpha-2 agonists have proven useful in inhibiting aqueous humor production and reducing intraocular pressure in glaucoma.[19]

Immunoelectron microscopic studies have clearly documented that Na-K-ATPase activity and carbonic anhydrase activity are found in the epithelium of the ciliary processes. Both of these enzymes are central to the production of aqueous humor and one of them, carbonic anhydrase, (seen localized to nonpigmented ciliary epithelial cell membranes by immunoelectron microscopy) (Fig. 8.14, arrows) is regularly targeted for pharmacologic inhibition to reduce intraocular pressure in glaucoma.[20,21]

The intercellular junctions of the ciliary epithelial layers are critically important to both the production of aqueous humor and to the maintenance of the pristine physiologic environment of the PC, one that is essentially devoid of plasma-derived proteins. Foremost among these junctions, and found only between the apico-lateral surfaces of the nonpigmented cells, are junctional complexes that completely encircle each nonpigmented cell and attach it to all of the cells that surround it. These complexes are composed of a zonula occludens (tight junction) and zonula adherens. The adherens junctions hold the nonpigmented cells to their neighbors around their entire circumference and the tight junctions prevent passive diffusion of plasma-derived macromolecules from the ciliary body stroma into the aqueous humor of the PC, via the intercellular spaces between the cells (**Fig. 8.15**). These tight junctions form a part of the blood–aqueous barrier that is described below.

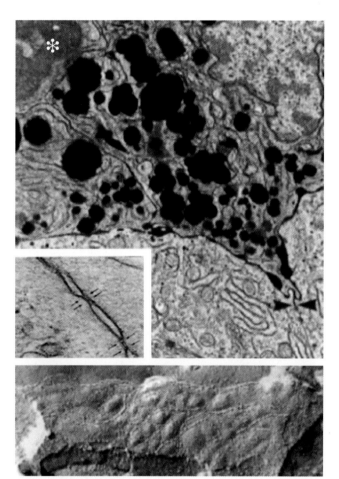

FIGURE 8.15 Transmission electron micrograph of ciliary epithelium of monkey eye, following intravenous injection of the protein tracer, horseradish peroxidase (HRP). Gray-black, granular HRP fills the ciliary body stroma (*asterisk*) and permeates the intercellular cleft between adjacent pigmented ciliary epithelial cells. Oval and round black cytoplasmic structures are melanin granules in the pigmented ciliary epithelium. The tracer is also seen as a black line separating the apposed apical surfaces of the pigmented and nonpigmented cell layers. The tracer is prevented from continuing toward the posterior chamber, between adjacent nonpigmented ciliary epithelial cells, by tight junctions joining the apico-lateral surfaces of the nonpigmented cells (*double arrowheads*). *Inset:* Higher magnification shows the cross-sectional appearance of the tight junction, with its multiple points of fusion between membrane-bound proteins in the membranes of the adjoined cells (*arrows*). The figure below shows the freeze fracture appearance of the tight junction, displaying the multiple branching and anastomosing strands of junctional proteins that join the cell membranes of adjacent nonpigmented ciliary epithelial cells. (From Morrison JC, Van Buskirk EM, Freddo T. Anatomy, microcirculation and ultrastructure of the ciliary body. In: Ritch R, Shields MB, Krupin T, eds. *The Glaucomas.* St Louis: CV Mosby, 1989.)

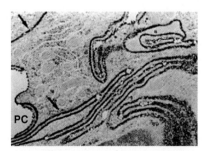

FIGURE 8.14 Immunohistochemical staining of carbonic anhydrase in ciliary epithelium (*arrows*). PC, posterior chamber. (From Lütjen-Drecoll E, Lönnerholm G, Eichorn M. Carbonic anhydrase distribution in the human and monkey eye by light and electron microscopy. *Graefes Arch Clin Exp Ophthalmol.* 1983.)

In order for aqueous to be produced in a coordinated fashion, the two layers of the ciliary epithelium must function as a syncytium to move ions from the ciliary body stroma into the nonpigmented ciliary epithelial cells from which they are secreted.[16] The pigmented epithelial cells first take in these various ions from the ciliary body stroma, via a system of regulated ports and channels.[22] To reach the nonpigmented cells, however, movement of ions between the layers occurs through gap junctions that bridge the adjoined apical surfaces of the pigmented and nonpigmented epithelial cells.

Additional gap junctions along the lateral surfaces of the nonpigmented and pigmented ciliary epithelial cells serve to coordinate aqueous production by providing conduits for electrotonic and metabolic messaging between cells. Also joining these cells are desmosomes, which serve to "spot-weld" the cell membranes together without interfering with production and secretion of aqueous humor into the narrow clefts between nonpigmented cells. A summary of the various intercellular junctions found in the two layers of the ciliary epithelium is presented in **Figure 8.16**.

The Anatomic Basis of the Blood–Aqueous Barrier in the Ciliary Body

Despite estimates of the plasma protein concentration in the ciliary body stroma being as high as 74% of that found in plasma, the plasma-derived protein content of aqueous humor in the anterior chamber is less than 1% of that found in plasma.[23,24] Proteins create turbidity, which scatters light, degrading the optical efficiency of the eye. The nonspecific entry of plasma-derived proteins

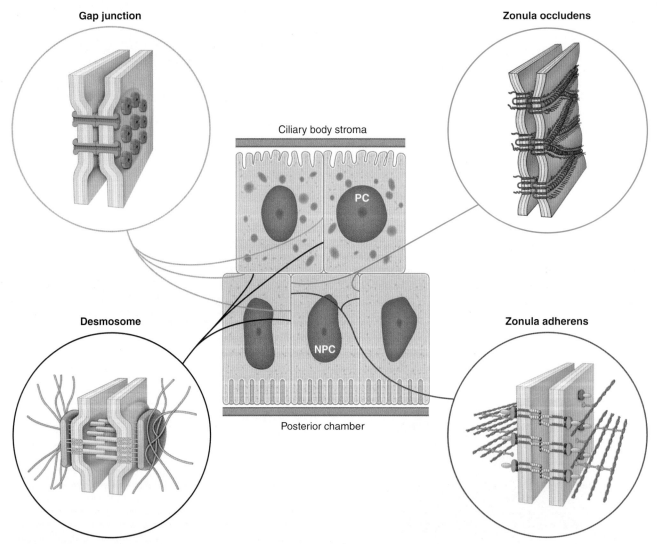

FIGURE 8.16 Four main types of intercellular junctions are found within and between the pigmented (PC) and non-pigmented ciliary (NPC) epithelial cells. Recall that these two epithelial layers are arranged apex to apex. Surrounding the apico-lateral surfaces of the NPCs, a junctional complex is formed, including a zonula occludens and zonula adherens. Adjoining the lateral surface of the PC and the NPC epithelial cells, numerous gap junctions and desmosomes are found. These same types of junctions join the apical surfaces of the PC and NPC epithelial cell layers.

such as albumin can bring with it unwanted or harmful growth factors, and other plasma components or antigens deleterious to the pristine environment required within the eye. To prevent this, and to ensure that potential antigens in the bloodstream are prevented from reaching the PC, the lens, vitreous, and retina, a selective anatomic barrier is positioned between the bloodstream and the aqueous humor. In the iris, this barrier is created by the tight junctions of the vascular endothelium.[25] But as noted earlier, the microvasculature of the ciliary body stroma is composed of fenestrated capillaries that readily leak fluids, ions, and plasma proteins in order to provide the reservoir from which the ciliary epithelium secretes aqueous humor. To ensure that the protein-laden fluid in the ciliary body stroma and the composition of the aqueous humor remain different, a barrier to macromolecular diffusion is interposed between the ciliary body stroma and the PC by the ciliary epithelium.[26]

Plasma proteins leaked into the ciliary body stoma, from its fenestrated capillaries, diffuse freely through the stroma to the ciliary epithelium where they easily diffuse between adjacent pigmented ciliary epithelial cells, filling the intercellular clefts (**Fig. 8.15**). Upon reaching the interface between the juxtaposed apical surfaces of the pigmented and nonpigmented layers, these proteins are again able to freely permeate the intercellular cleft between these cell layers. But, when this protein attempts to diffuse along the intercellular clefts between adjacent nonpigmented ciliary epithelial cells, progress toward the PC is blocked by an apico-lateral junctional complex, composed of a zonula occludens (tight junction) and zonula adherens (**Fig. 8.15**).[27]

Although this epithelial barrier prevents the passive diffusion of plasma-derived proteins and other macromolecules

from entering the PC, the ciliary body stroma is open to the anterior chamber at the ciliary body band (**Figs. 8.6** and **8.8**). Via this route, plasma proteins and other macromolecules leaked into the ciliary body stroma by its fenestrated capillaries have access to the iris stroma and the anterior chamber but not the PC (**Fig. 8.17**). This diffusional pathway from the ciliary body stroma to the anterior chamber, bypassing the PC is limited, but represents the route of entry for the plasma-derived protein measured in normal aqueous humor.[28] And it is the one-way valve created by apposition of the pupil to the anterior lens capsule, combined with the tight junctions between posterior pigmented epithelial cells of the iris, that prevent the protein-containing aqueous from the anterior chamber from reaching the PC.

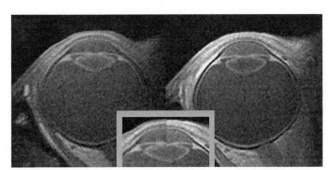

FIGURE 8.17 A pair of T1-weighted magnetic resonance images (MRI) of the same living human eye are shown before and after injection of an intravenous contrast agent that mimics the diffusional behavior of plasma proteins. Before injection of the contrast agent **(left)** note that both the anterior chamber and posterior chamber appear dark. But 90 minutes after introduction of the intravenous contrast agent **(right)**, note that the ciliary body is enhanced (*whiter*) and the contrast agent has entered and lightened the appearance of the anterior chamber but not the posterior chamber. A split-field comparison of the before and after images appears in the *inset*. (Reproduced from Freddo TF, Patz S, Arshanskiy Y. Pilocarpine's effects on the blood-aqueous barrier of the human eye as assessed by high-resolution, contrast magnetic resonance imaging. *Exp Eye Res.* 82:458–464, 2006.)

REFERENCES

1. Lütjen-Drecoll E. Histochemical and immunohistochemical localisation of hyaluronan and hyaluronan synthase in the anterior eye segment. *Basic Asp Glaucoma Res III*. 1993:53–66.
2. Haddad A, de Almeida JC, Laicine EM, et al. The origin of the intrinsic glycoproteins of the rabbit vitreous body: an immunohistochemical and autoradiographic study. *Exp Eye Res*. 1990;50(5):555–561.
3. Straatsma BR, Landers MB, Kreiger AE. The ora serrata in the adult human eye. *Arch Ophthalmol*. 1968;80(1):3–20.
4. Neider MW, Crawford K, Kaufman PL, et al. In vivo videography of the rhesus monkey accommodative apparatus: age-related loss of ciliary muscle response to central stimulation. *Arch Ophthalmol*. 1990;108(1):69–74.
5. Ruskell G. Innervation of the anterior segment of the eye. In: *Basic Aspects of Glaucoma Research*. Stuttgart, Germany: FK Schattauer Verlag; 1982:49.
6. Tornqvist G. The relative importance of the parasympathetic and sympathetic nervous systems for accommodation in monkeys. *Invest Ophthalmol*. 1967;6(6):612–617.
7. Hubbard WC, Robinson JC, Schmidt K, et al. Superior cervical ganglionectomy in monkeys: effects on refraction and intraocular pressure. *Exp Eye Res*. 1999;68(5):637–639.
8. Chen JC, Schmid KL, Brown B. The autonomic control of accommodation and implications for human myopia development: a review. *Ophthalmic Physiol Opt*. 2003;23(5):401–422.
9. Rittig M, Lütjen-Drecoll E, Rauterberg J, et al. Type-VI collagen in the human iris and ciliary body. *Cell Tissue Res*. 1990;259(2):305–312.
10. Marshall GE, Konstas A, Abraham S, et al. Extracellular matrix in aged human ciliary body: an immunoelectron microscope study. *Invest Ophthalmol Vis Sci*. 1992;33(8):2546–2560.
11. Lütjen-Drecoll E, Tamm E. Morphological study of the anterior segment of cynomolgus monkey eyes following treatment with prostaglandin F2α. *Exp Eye Res*. 1988;47(5):761–769.
12. Morrison JC, Van Buskirk EM. Ciliary process microvasculature of the primate eye. *Am J Ophthalmol*. 1984;97(3):372–383.
13. Funk R, Rohen JW. SEM studies of the functional morphology of the ciliary process vasculature in the cynomolgus monkey: reactions after application of epinephrine. *Exp Eye Res*. 1988;47(4):653–663.
14. Funk R, Rohen J. Scanning electron microscopic study on the vasculature of the human anterior eye segment, especially with respect to the ciliary processes. *Exp Eye Res*. 1990;51(6):651–661.
15. Funk R, Rohen JW. Functional morphology of the vasculature in the anterior eye segment. In: Lutjen-Drecoll E, Rohen JW, eds. *Basic Aspects of Glaucoma Research: Functional Morphology of the Vasculature in the Anterior Eye Segment*. Vol 2. Stuttgart, Germany: Schattauer; 1990:7–171.

16. Raviola G, Raviola E. Intercellular junctions in the ciliary epithelium. *Invest Ophthalmol Vis Sci.* 1978;17(10):958–981.

17. Tamm ER, Lütjen-Drecoll E. Ciliary body. *Microsc Res Tech.* 1996;33(5):390–439.

18. Nathanson JA. Adrenergic regulation of intraocular pressure: identification of beta 2-adrenergic-stimulated adenylate cyclase in ciliary process epithelium. *Proc Natl Acad Sci U S A.* 1980;77(12):7420–7424.

19. Sears M. Catecholamines in relation to the eye. In: Astwood E, Greep R, eds. *Handbook of Physiology—Endocrinology VI.* Washington, DC: American Physiological Society; 1975:553–590.

20. Flugel C, Lutjen-Drecoll E. Incidence and distribution of Na+ K+ ATPase in the ciliary body epithelium in the rabbit. *Fortschr Ophthalmol.* 1988;85(1):46–49.

21. Lütjen-Drecoll E, Lönnerholm G, Eichhorn M. Carbonic anhydrase distribution in the human and monkey eye by light and electron microscopy. *Graefes Arch Clin Exp Ophthalmol.* 1983;220(6):285–291.

22. Freddo T, Civan M, Gong H. Anatomy and pathophysiology of aqueous production and outflow. In: Albert DM, Jakobiec FA, eds. *Albert and Jakobiec's Principles and Practice of Ophthalmology.* 3rd ed. Philadelphia, PA: Elsevier Saunders; 2008.

23. Bill A. The blood-aqueous barrier. *Trans Ophthalmol Soc U K.* 1986;105(pt 2):149–155.

24. Tripathi RC, Millard CB, Tripathi BJ. Protein composition of human aqueous humor: SDS-PAGE analysis of surgical and post-mortem samples. *Exp Eye Res.* 1989;48(1):117–130.

25. Freddo TF, Raviola G. Freeze-fracture analysis of the interendothelial junctions in the blood vessels of the iris in macaca mulatta. *Invest Ophthalmol Vis Sci.* 1982;23(2):154–167.

26. Raviola G. The structural basis of the blood-ocular barriers. *Exp Eye Res.* 1977;25:27–63.

27. Freddo TF. Intercellular junctions of the ciliary epithelium in anterior uveitis. *Invest Ophthalmol Vis Sci.* 1987;28(2):320–329.

28. Freddo TF. A contemporary concept of the blood–aqueous barrier. *Prog Retin Eye Res.* 2013;32:181–195.

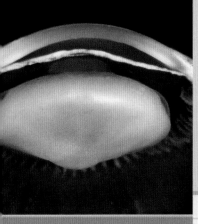

Anatomy of the Aqueous Outflow Pathways

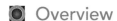 Overview

Aqueous humor, the clear nutritive fluid that sustains the avascular cornea, lens, and trabecular meshwork is produced by the ciliary body and secreted into the posterior chamber of the eye at a rate of 2.4 ± 0.6 μL per minute in adults aged 20 to 83 years.[1] Unable to diffuse through the iris, aqueous flows through the pupil into the anterior chamber where it circulates in a convection current driven by the temperature difference between the warm iris and the cornea, which is cooler because of its exposure to air. Rising along the warm surface of the iris and falling along the inner surface of the cornea, as it exchanges nutrients for waste products, aqueous flows out of the eye through two principal pathways. In the normal eye, most of the aqueous humor leaving the eye does so through the trabecular meshwork and a system of channels that meander through the thickness of the sclera to the episcleral venous system.[2] This system is known to be pressure dependent and is called the conventional or trabecular outflow pathway. The remainder passes into the connective tissues of the ciliary body, near the root of the iris, moving to the supraciliary space and then through the sclera. This is called the uveoscleral outflow pathway and it is regarded to be much less pressure dependent.[2]

The anatomy of each of these pathways is considered in this chapter (**Fig. 9.1**).

The Conventional or Trabecular Outflow Pathway

MACROSCOPIC AND CLINICAL ANATOMY OF THE TRABECULAR MESHWORK

The cells of the trabecular meshwork, along with macrophages, filter particulates such as pigment, in order to keep the outflow pathways free of extracellular debris. The trabecular meshwork also elaborates and maintains an extensive extracellular matrix that has an influence on aqueous humor outflow. Overall, the outflow system creates a resistance to the bulk flow of aqueous humor down a pressure gradient, from the anterior chamber to the bloodstream of the episclera. This resistance to outflow, in the face of continued aqueous production, creates a backpressure within the eye (intraocular pressure) that maintains the shape of the eye while still allowing for the continuous production and drainage of nutritive aqueous humor. The range of daytime intraocular pressures found in normal young adults is 12 to 21 mm Hg above ambient atmospheric pressure and increases by 1 mm Hg per decade after[3] the age of 40.

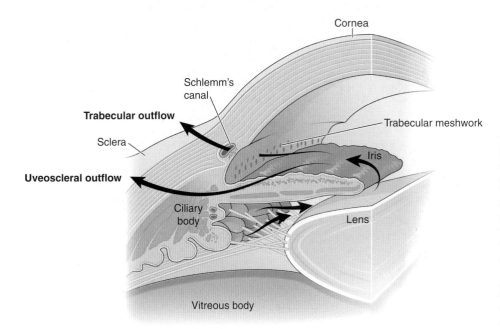

FIGURE 9.1 Sketch shows the pathways of aqueous flow, beginning with secretion into the posterior chamber, and flow through the pupil into the anterior chamber. Aqueous humor then leaves the eye by passing through one of two principal pathways. In the conventional outflow pathway, aqueous traverses the trabecular meshwork, to enter Schlemm's canal, which then drains to the episcleral venous system. In the uveoscleral outflow pathway, aqueous enters the ciliary body near the iris root and eventually traverses the sclera to be absorbed by orbital vessels.

The trabecular meshwork is positioned between the anterior chamber of the eye and the circumferentially oriented Schlemm's canal that lies just internal to the sclera (**Fig. 9.2**). Both the trabecular meshwork and the canal of Schlemm reside within the internal scleral sulcus (SEE **CHAPTER 6: THE SCLERA, EPISCLERA, AND TENON'S CAPSULE**).

In meridional sections, the trabecular meshwork appears as a triangular wedge of avascular tissue encircling the anterior chamber angle. The apex of this triangle is attached to the most posterior lamellae of the corneal stroma and to Schwalbe's line, the name given to the peripheral edge of Descemet's membrane (**Figs. 9.2** and **9.3**). Expanding from this apex posteriorly, the trabecular meshwork attaches

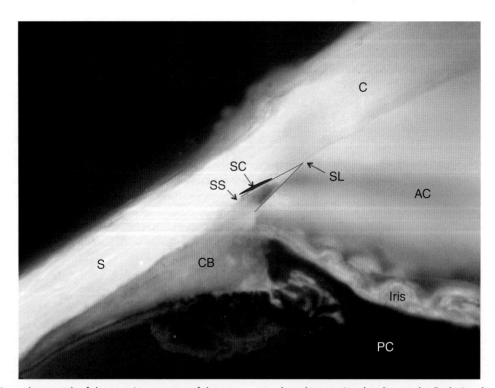

FIGURE 9.2 Macrophotograph of the anterior segment of the eye, centered on the anterior chamber angle. *Red triangle* outlines the position of the trabecular meshwork extending from Schwalbe's line (the edge of Descemet's membrane of the cornea—SL) to the scleral spur (SS). Note that Schlemm's canal (SC—shown in *blue*) does not extend all the way from the SS to SL. Also note that only the posterior portion of the trabecular meshwork, directly beneath SC, is pigmented. AC, anterior chamber; PC, posterior chamber; S, sclera; C, cornea; CB, ciliary body.

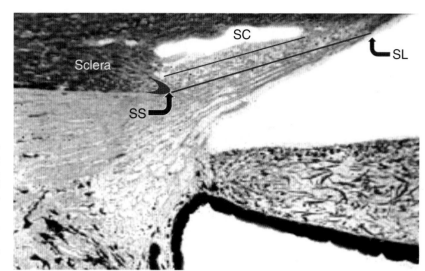

FIGURE 9.3 Light micrograph centered on the anterior chamber angle shows trabecular meshwork and Schlemm's canal (SC) in relation to Schwalbe's line (SL) and the scleral spur (SS). The portion of the trabecular meshwork between the anterior chamber and the *red line* is the uveal meshwork. The portion between the *red and blue lines* is the corneoscleral meshwork and the portion between the *blue line* and SC is the juxtacanalicular or cribriform meshwork.

to the sclera and to the stromas of the ciliary body and the iris root (**Figs. 9.2** and **9.3**).

Projecting into the base of this triangle is a shelf-like lip of sclera termed the scleral spur (**Figs. 9.2** and **9.3**). An imaginary line drawn from the scleral spur to Schwalbe's line separates the trabecular meshwork into two of its major parts (**Fig. 9.3**, red line). The portion of the trabecular meshwork closer to the anterior chamber than this imaginary line is called the uveal meshwork because it extends from Schwalbe's line to the stromas of the ciliary body and iris (i.e., anterior uvea). The meshwork lying just external to the imaginary line connects to the anterior surface of the scleral spur. This portion of the meshwork, extending from Schwalbe's line and the most posterior lamellae of the corneal stroma, to the scleral spur, is termed the corneoscleral meshwork.

Situated between the deepest trabeculae of the corneoscleral meshwork and Schlemm's canal is a narrow strip of loose, cellular connective tissue, called the juxtacanalicular connective tissue (JCT) (**Fig. 9.3**, area between blue line and endothelial lining of Schlemm's canal). It is within this thin portion of the trabecular meshwork where most investigators believe that the majority of aqueous humor outflow resistance resides. How this resistance is created, and its precise anatomical basis, remain uncertain. Recent reviews on this subject are available.[4] Equally uncertain are the source(s) and location(s) of the added resistance that leads to elevation of intraocular pressure in primary open-angle glaucoma.

With conventional clinical instruments such as a slit-lamp, the angle tissues cannot be viewed directly, since they are obscured by the overlying perilimbal sclera. These tissues can be viewed indirectly however, with the use of a goniolens or gonioprism, in a procedure called gonioscopy (**Fig. 9.4**). Both devices provide a view of the angle from a perspective equivalent to the view of

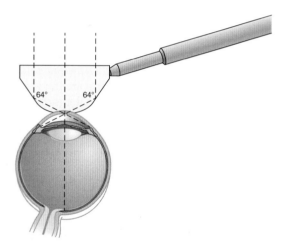

FIGURE 9.4 Schematic diagram of the light path utilized in a gonioprism in order to visualize the structures of the anterior chamber. Goniolenses are also available. They rely upon tilted mirrors, rather than a prism to redirect the light in a similar fashion.

a tiny observer standing in the pupil, as though it was a "manhole," with the observer's head in the anterior chamber, viewing the horizon. In the distance, the observer sees where the arcing dome of the cornea descends from overhead to meet the flat plane of the iris in the anterior chamber angle (**Fig. 9.5**).

As a clinician, one must be able to seamlessly visualize the anatomy of the angle as seen from two perspectives—one view is that obtained from meridional sections and the other is the view obtained through a gonioscope.

Figures 9.2 and **9.3** show the angle structures in macroscopic and microscopic meridional sections. **Figure 9.6** shows a macrophotograph of the angle of a monkey eye from a perspective equivalent to a gonioscopic view. In **Figure 9.6**, Schlemm's canal is filled with blood, revealing its position relative to the transparent trabecular meshwork that overlies

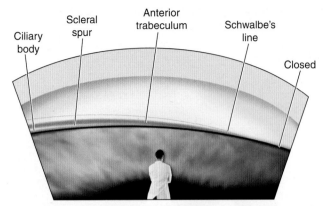

FIGURE 9.5 View of the structures of the anterior chamber angle from the perspective provided by a gonioprism or goniolens. The sketch depicts the appearance of progressively more closed anterior chamber angle approaches from left to right.

 Anterior displacement of Schwalbe's line can occur as an isolated developmental anomaly, with no complications. When this occurs it is called posterior embryotoxon (Fig. 9.7A). In such cases, however, one must determine whether there are also unusually large numbers of iris processes (Fig. 9.7B). Broad and numerous iris processes suggest Axenfeld–Rieger syndrome, a developmental anomaly that manifests a spectrum of iris and anterior chamber angle malformations and is often associated with glaucoma.[5]

it. Blood does not normally fill Schlemm's canal but has been introduced to more readily see the position of the canal. One can see the tan-gray line corresponding to Schwalbe's line, and below that, the trabecular meshwork overlying the blood-filled Schlemm's canal. Below Schlemm's canal, the line of lighter coloration given by the scleral spur is evident, as seen through the overlying, but transparent, meshwork. Finally, below the scleral spur, the dark coloration given by the pigment in the ciliary body stroma is seen. This lowest "layer" of the outflow tissues, as seen from the gonioscopic perspective, is referred to as the ciliary body band.

Another anatomic feature of the anterior chamber angle is the presence of stalks or narrow bands of pigmented tissue arising from the peripheral iris to meet the trabecular meshwork, as in the center of **Figure 9.6**. These stalks of tissue are called iris processes. They are embryologic remnants of anterior chamber development. In small numbers, they are a normal finding, assuming that Schwalbe's line is in its proper anatomic location.

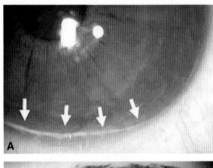
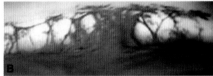

FIGURE 9.7 **A:** Anterior displacement of Schwalbe's line, known as posterior embryotoxon when seen as a solitary finding. **B:** Numerous abnormal, slender and broad iris processes typical of Axenfeld-Rieger syndrome as seen by gonioscopy. (From Tümer Z, Bach-Holm D. Axenfeld–Rieger syndrome and spectrum of *PITX2* and *FOXC1* mutations. European Journal of Human Genetics. 17: 2009, 1527–1539.)

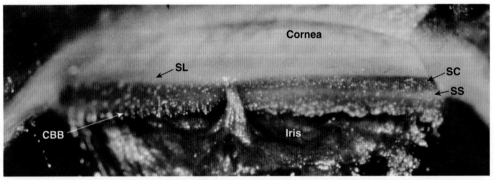

FIGURE 9.6 Macrophotograph of anterior chamber angle of a monkey eye shows Schwalbe's line (SL), a blood-filled Schlemm's canal (SC), the scleral spur (SS) and the ciliary body band (CBB) that merges with the anterior surface of the iris. Realize that all of these structures are being viewed through the transparent trabecular meshwork that overlies all three layers, extending from Schwalbe's line to the root of the iris. The stalk in the middle of the photo, rising from the iris root and inserting into the trabecular meshwork, is a normal anatomic variant termed an iris process. (From Freddo T. Anatomy and physiology related to aqueous humor production and outflow. In: Fingeret M, Lewis T, eds. *Primary Care of the Glaucomas*, Chapter 3. Stamford, CT: Appleton and Lange, 1993.)

Unfortunately, if one compares the macroscopic view of the angle shown in **Figure 9.6**, with the photograph of the normal angle of an older individual as seen through a goniolens in **Figure 9.8**, an important discrepancy arises. In **Figure 9.6**, four landmarks are identifiable. Beginning from top to bottom, they are Schwalbe's line, the trabecular meshwork (overlying the blood-filled canal of Schlemm), the scleral spur, and finally the ciliary body band. In **Figure 9.8**, however, five alternating dark and light bands are seen.

What does the goniophotograph reveal that is not seen in the macrophotograph? What the macrophotograph does not reveal is the variable distribution of phagocystosed pigment that is often found within portions of the trabecular meshwork in the older but normal human eye.

In the goniophotograph in **Figure 9.8**, from top to bottom, one sees a variegated and lightly pigmented line at the top, a lighter strip below it, a darker strip below that, and then another lighter and then a darker strip, below that. **Figure 9.9** shows the angle structures from both the meridional and gonioscopic perspectives simultaneously. Overlaid onto the gonioscopic perspective of **Figure 9.9** is a series of five dark and light lines corresponding to the locations of the five darker and lighter strips in the goniophotograph (**Fig. 9.8**). What is revealed is that the portion of the trabecular meshwork between Schwalbe's line and the scleral spur is not of uniform color. Why?

With increasing age, pigment is gradually accumulated within the cells of the trabecular meshwork, but

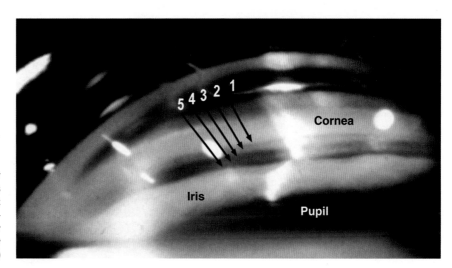

FIGURE 9.8 Goniophotograph of an older normal individual with an open angle shows five "layers" of alternating dark and light bands. (*1*) Schwalbe's line; (*2*) the anterior trabecular meshwork; (*3*) the posterior trabecular meshwork; (*4*) the scleral spur; (*5*) the ciliary body band. (Courtesy of Dr. Rodney Gutner.)

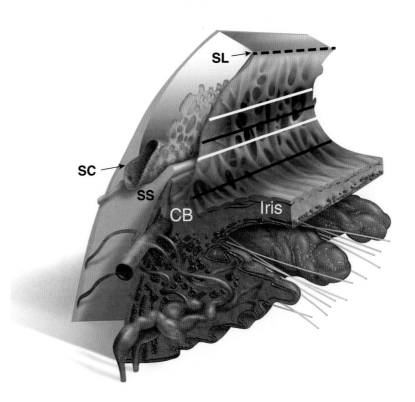

FIGURE 9.9 Sketch showing the anatomic relations of the gonioscopic landmarks representing the five dark and light bands seen in Figure 9.8. The *upper dashed line* at the top corresponds to the area of Schwalbe's line (SL). Below SL, the region surrounding the *upper white line* corresponds to the anterior trabecular meshwork, which does not lead directly to Schlemm's canal (SC). The *upper solid black line* corresponds to the posterior trabecular meshwork, which does lead directly to SC. The *lower white line* corresponds to the edge of the scleral spur (SS). The *lowest black line* corresponds to the ciliary body band (CB).

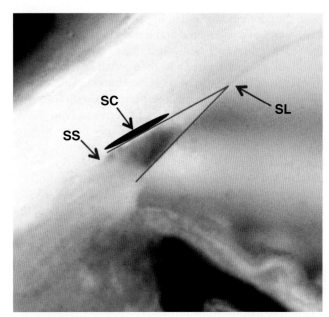

FIGURE 9.10 Macrophotograph of anterior chamber angle shows triangular outline of the entire trabecular meshwork in *red*, extending from Schwalbe's line (SL) to the scleral spur (SS). Note that Schlemm's canal (SC) does not extend all of the way from the SS to SL. Only the posterior meshwork, leading directly to SC, exhibits significant amounts of pigment.

its distribution is nonuniform. Schlemm's canal does not extend all the way from the scleral spur to Schwalbe's line (**Fig. 9.10**). Thus, the anterior portion of the trabecular meshwork, the portion between Schwalbe's line and the anterior edge of Schlemm's canal in **Figures 9.9** and **9.10**, does not lead directly to Schlemm's canal. As a result, this portion of the meshwork, called the anterior meshwork, sees less flow and accumulates less pigment than the posterior meshwork. The posterior trabecular meshwork is defined as that portion directly overlying the lumen of Schlemm's canal and corresponds to the posterior, pigmented portion of the meshwork within the red triangle in **Figure 9.10**.

In histologic sections of older normal eyes, the demarcation between the anterior and posterior portions of the meshwork can be dramatic. In **Figure 9.11**, the vertical black line corresponds to the anterior-most limit of Schlemm's canal. Note that there is virtually no pigment within the anterior meshwork to the right of the black line. Beyond the foundational anatomy provided here, a rich archive of goniophotographs, goniovideos, and tutorials on mastering gonioscopic anatomy and pathology are available at www.gonioscopy.org.

Architecture of the Uveal and Corneoscleral Meshwork

The basic architecture of the uveal and corneoscleral meshwork is similar. Both are composed of branching and anastomosing avascular beams, containing a collagen and elastin core (**Fig. 9.12**). This core is surrounded by a basement membrane that is produced by the single layer of endothelial cells that wrap the outside of each beam. The histologic details of these structures are detailed below. Near Schwalbe's line, where the meshwork and the cornea merge, the collagen within the cores of the beams is continuous

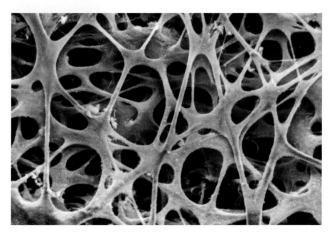

FIGURE 9.12 Scanning electron micrograph showing an en face view of the uveal face of the trabecular meshwork. The endothelial cell-lined, branching, and anastomosing beams of the uveal portion of the trabecular meshwork are evident. (Modified from Freddo TF, Patterson MM, Scott DR, et al. Influence of mercurial sulfhydryl agents on aqueous outflow pathways in enucleated eyes. *Invest Ophthalmol Vis Sci.* 25:278–285, 1984.)

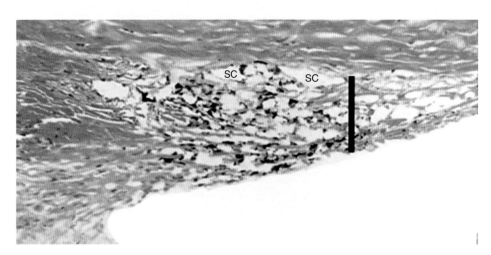

FIGURE 9.11 Light micrograph of the trabecular meshwork in an older but normal eye. The location of the anterior limit of Schlemm's canal (SC) corresponds to the position of the *vertical black line*. Note the abrupt difference in the distribution of pigment within the posterior meshwork that leads directly to SC (*left of the black line*) compared with the portion of the anterior meshwork shown to the right of the black line.

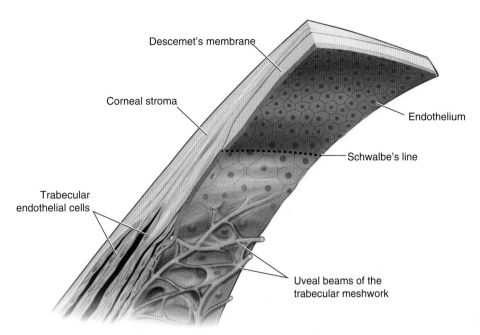

FIGURE 9.13 Artist's rendering of transition zone from the inner surface of the cornea into the trabecular meshwork. The single layer of corneal endothelium transitions beyond the peripheral edge of Descemet's membrane (Schwalbe's line) to become the single layer of trabecular endothelial cells that wrap the uveal and corneoscleral beams of the trabecular meshwork. The transition area likely harbors a shared population of stem cells capable of limited repopulation of both cell types. (Modified from Hogan MJ, Alvarado JA, Weddell JE. *Histology of the Human Eye.* Philadelphia, PA: WB Saunders; 1971:177.)

with the deepest layers of the corneal stroma. At this same location, the trabecular endothelium becomes continuous with the endothelium of the cornea (**Fig. 9.13**).[6]

Clearly, in the uveal meshwork facing the anterior chamber, shown in **Figure 9.12**, there are ample open spaces, 25 to 75 μm in size. These provide for unimpeded aqueous flow. The basic structure of the corneoscleral meshwork is similar to that of the uveal meshwork, including beams with a central, avascular core of collagen and elastic fibers, enveloped in a thin endothelium. The openings in the corneoscleral meshwork are, however, smaller. The open spaces between the corneoscleral beams are estimated to range from 2 to 15 μm. This gives the layers of the corneoscleral meshwork an en face appearance more aptly described as perforated sheets when compared to the uveal meshwork. Despite the progressive narrowing in the spaces available for flow, as one progresses from the uveal to the corneoscleral meshwork, the general consensus is that neither of these regions of the trabecular meshwork has narrow enough passages to contribute significant resistance to outflow.[4]

HISTOLOGY OF THE TRABECULAR MESHWORK

The Trabecular Beams

A section through a representative trabecular beam is shown in **Figure 9.14**. Within the cores of the trabecular beams, collagen types I and III predominate, whereas type V collagen fibrils link these core collagen fibers to the basement membranes of the endothelial cells that envelop each beam.[7] With increasing age, the so-called "wide-spacing collagen," principally composed of type VI collagen, is also found (see **Fig. 9.14**).[8,9] The collagen fibrils within the cores of the uveal and corneoscleral beams are associated with chondroitin sulfate, dermatan sulfate, and possibly keratan sulfate proteoglycans. In the adult eye, heparan sulfate is also found in small amounts within the beams, but it is associated primarily with the basal lamina.[10–13] The elastic fibers within the cores of the beams have an amorphous core of elastin surround by a microfibrillar sheath component that increases in thickness with age.[14]

The trabecular endothelial cells wrap the entire surface of each uveal and corneoscleral beam in a single, thin layer of cells (**Fig. 9.14**). These cells produce a continuous basement membrane on their basal surface. The basement membrane is composed principally of type IV collagen, laminin, fibronectin, and heparan sulfate proteoglycan.[10,11,15]

Trabecular endothelial cells commonly overlap their neighboring cells at their edges, creating a long interendothelial cleft. Although these cells are joined to each other with gap junctions, they are not joined by tight junctions (zonulae occludentes).[16] As such, the cores of the beams are permeable to fluid, ions, and even proteins.[17]

The trabecular endothelial cells are moderately phagocytic.[18] As noted earlier, the amount of pigment phagocytosed by these cells is generally proportional to the amount of aqueous flow in any part of the meshwork. The trabecular endothelial cells, assisted by wandering macrophages, keep the open spaces of the meshwork clear of potentially clogging

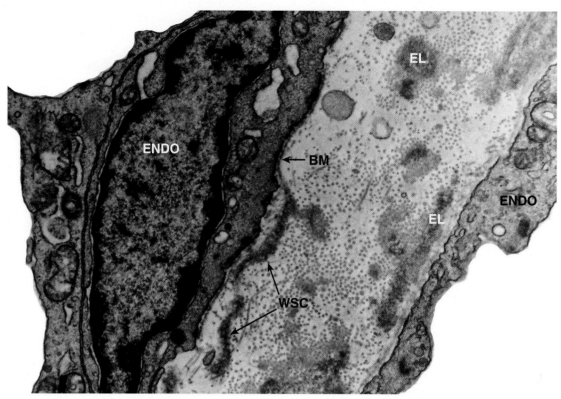

FIGURE 9.14 Transmission electron micrograph shows cross section through a trabecular beam. The beam is surrounded by a continuous wrapping of endothelial cells (ENDO) resting on a basement membrane (BM) that separates the endothelium from the core of the beam. The beam is composed of collagen fibers and elastic fibers (EL). In older eyes, there is also appearance of wide-spacing collagen (WSC). (From Freddo T. Anatomy and Physiology Related to Aqueous Humor Production and Outflow. In: Fingeret M, Lewis T, eds. *Primary Care of the Glaucomas*, Chapter 3. Stamford, CT: Appleton and Lange, 1993.)

debris. But, phagocytosis would seem to be at some long-term cost to the meshwork. As is the case with the corneal endothelium, with which the trabecular endothelium is continuous, trabecular endothelial cell number decreases with age.[19–21] Whether this progressive loss contributes to the development of glaucoma remains uncertain.

Despite the age-related loss of the endothelial cell populations in both the cornea and the trabecular meshwork, there is increasing evidence of a stem cell population in the transition zone between the endothelium of the cornea and that of the trabecular meshwork (**Fig. 9.13**). Raviola first identified a population of unusual cells in this transition zone in monkey eyes, which she called Schwalbe's line cells.[22] Cells from this region of the monkey eye, similar to those reported by Raviola, have since been shown to exhibit characteristics of stem cells.[23] Cells with demonstrated potential to differentiate into functional trabecular meshwork cells have most recently been isolated from this same transition area in human eyes.[24,25] While it is clear that under homeostatic conditions this nidus of putative stem cells does not ensure against progressive, age-related endothelial cell loss of either corneal or trabecular endothelial cells, they can be triggered to undergo mitotic division following laser trabeculoplasty, as part of a wound healing response. Hence, they could, in the future, be a

useful resource for repopulating damaged or diseased corneal endothelium and trabecular meshwork.[26,27]

The Juxtacanalicular Region

The portion of the trabecular meshwork between the outermost corneoscleral beams and Schlemm's canal has a fundamentally different architecture from that of the uveal and corneoscleral meshwork. The juxtacanalicular connective tissue (JCT) region, also known as the cribriform meshwork, is an open connective tissue matrix in which fibroblast-like cells, rather than endothelial cells, are found (**Fig. 9.15A**). The cells of the JCT region generally lack a basement membrane and do not exhibit a clear apical and basal surface as do the cells lining the trabecular beams.

JCT cells contact each other but also extend long, thin cell processes that attach with mushroom-shaped pads, directly to the endothelial cells lining the inner wall of Schlemm's canal (**Fig. 9.15A**). As such, the JCT cells can allow for some distention of the juxtacanalicular meshwork, beneath Schlemm's canal, without losing their connections to the endothelial cells lining the inner wall of the canal.[28,29]

The extracellular matrix of the JCT region exhibits collagen types I, III, IV, V, and VI (but not type II).[8] Also present are elastin, laminin, fibronectin, and glycosaminoglycans,

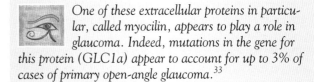

One of these extracellular proteins in particular, called myocilin, appears to play a role in glaucoma. Indeed, mutations in the gene for this protein (GLC1a) appear to account for up to 3% of cases of primary open-angle glaucoma.[33]

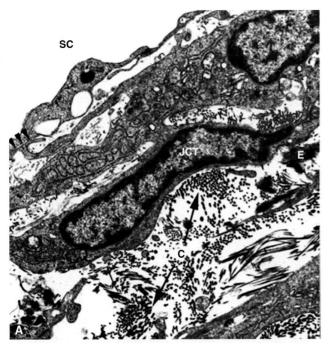

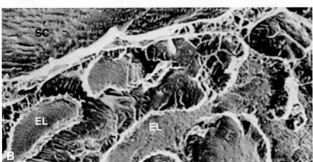

FIGURE 9.15 **A:** Transmission electron micrograph of the juxtacanalicular connective tissue (i.e., cribriform) region of the trabecular meshwork and the inner wall of Schlemm's canal (SC). Note the absence of delineated trabecular beams. Instead, an open connective tissue matrix of collagen (C) and elastic fibers (E) is present, along with fibroblast-like juxtacanalicular (JCT) cells that extend pad-like extensions connecting them to the inner wall of the SC (*triple arrowheads*). (From Freddo T. Anatomy and Physiology Related to Aqueous Humor Production and Outflow. In: Fingeret M, Lewis T, eds. *Primary Care of the Glaucomas*, Chapter 3. Stamford, CT: Appleton and Lange, 1993.) **B:** Quick-freeze, deep-etch micrograph showing more extensive extracellular matrix revealed using this method, compared with standard transmission electron microscopy shown above. SC, Schlemm's canal; EL, elastic fibers embedded in a filamentous matrix of collagen. (Modified from Gong H, Ruberti J, Overby D, et al. A new view of the human trabecular meshwork using quick-freeze, deep-etch electron microscopy. *Exp Eye Res.* 2002;75:347–358.)

particularly chondroitin sulfate, dermatan sulfate, and hyaluronic acid.[11,30] A regulable system of matrix metalloproteinases and their inhibitors is also present in the trabecular meshwork. These remain interesting prospects for contributing to and regulating outflow resistance.[31] Extensive reviews presenting greater detail on the extracellular matrix of the trabecular meshwork, and its possible regulatory role in aqueous outflow, are available.[12,32]

Unfortunately, using conventional methods the non-collagenous elements of this matrix generally collapse, or are dissolved during preparation of tissues for microscopic studies. As a result, using these methods, the amount of apparently open space for aqueous flow in the JCT region appears greater than actually exists. Thus, the contribution of this matrix to the anatomy of the trabecular meshwork is easily overlooked or underestimated, despite its critical relevance to the function of this tissue.

More representative images of the real ultrastructure of the JCT region have recently been obtained using a method called "quick-freeze-deep etch" that preserves a greater part of the extracellular matrix for examination at the ultrastructural level.[34] Using this technique, a much more elaborate and extensive extracellular matrix was seen filling the "open spaces" of the JCT region than has been seen using conventional methods (**Fig. 9.15B**).

Despite the enhanced matrix visibility, however, openings nearly a micron in size are still seen in the JCT region, an amount of apparently open space still deemed to be too great to account for a significant fraction of outflow resistance.[34] Most likely, even this method leaves some of the microanatomy of the JCT matrix unseen, but these images provide confirmation that views of the JCT region, as seen using conventional microscopic methods, provide an incomplete picture of the microanatomy. This inability to fully visualize the microanatomy of the apparently open space in the JCT region continues to hamper efforts to find anatomic correlates for aqueous outflow resistance in the normal and glaucomatous eye.

With increasing age, and particularly in eyes with glaucoma, there is an increase in the amount and density of extracellular matrix in the JCT region, even using conventional microscopic methods. There is also an accumulation of so-called "plaque material" surrounding the tendons of the cribriform plexus that extend into the JCT region.[14] Whether these changes play a role in the increasing outflow resistance seen with age, or in glaucoma, remains uncertain.

Schlemm's Canal

Schlemm's canal is an endothelial cell-lined channel that runs circumferentially around the eye, parallel to the limbus. It receives all of the aqueous humor that leaves the eye through the conventional (trabecular) outflow pathway. Because of its elongated, but relatively flattened profile in meridional sections, the canal is traditionally described as having an inner wall, with the basal surface of its endothelium facing the JCT region of the meshwork, and an outer wall, with the basal surface of this endothelium facing the adjacent sclera (**Fig. 9.16**). In human eyes it is common for Schlemm's canal to be bifid at various points in its circumference. At these locations, the canal splits into two parallel channels for a short distance and then anastomoses to a single lumen again.

> *The dimensions of Schlemm's canal have been shown to vary among populations. Importantly, eyes with glaucoma have been shown to exhibit significantly smaller dimensions of Schlemm's canal compared to age-matched normal eyes. Calculations have suggested that this one factor could account for nearly half of added resistance to aqueous humor outflow that distinguishes normal and glaucomatous eyes.*[35]

From the JCT region, aqueous humor must traverse the inner wall of Schlemm's canal. How aqueous humor traverses the endothelium of Schlemm's canal remains one of the enigmatic problems of ocular anatomy. The wall of Schlemm's canal is lined by a continuous endothelium. The endothelium of the inner wall exhibits unusual features including a discontinuous basement membrane and structures termed "giant vacuoles" (**Fig. 9.17**). Giant vacuoles appear to be pressure-dependent deformations of the inner wall. They are not found unless the anterior chamber tissues are chemically fixed under conditions

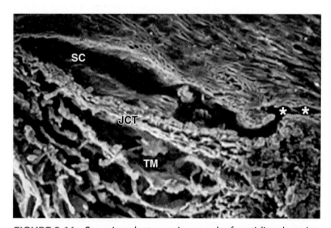

FIGURE 9.16 Scanning electron micrograph of meridional section of the anterior chamber angle shows the open beam structure of the uveal and corneoscleral trabecular meshwork (TM) and the more compacted tissues of the juxtacanalicular (JCT) region. The lumen of Schlemm's canal (SC) is also seen. Note the exit of an external collector channel (*double asterisks*) from the lumen of Schlemm's canal (SC). (From Freddo T. Anatomy and Physiology Related to Aqueous Humor Production and Outflow. In: Fingeret M, Lewis T, eds. *Primary Care of the Glaucomas*. Stamford, CT: Appleton and Lange, 1993.)

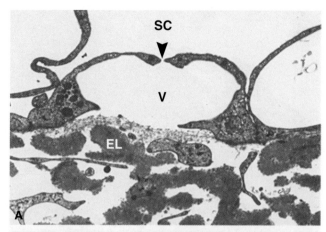

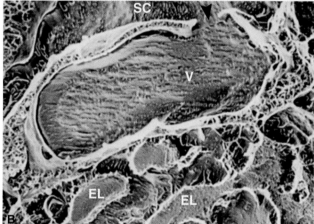

FIGURE 9.17   A: Transmission electron micrograph of juxtacanalicular region of the meshwork with elastic fibers (EL) and the lumen of Schlemm's canal (SC). Within the inner wall of SC, a giant vacuole (V) is present. Note that the lumen of the giant vacuole is continuous with the lumen of SC via a pore (*arrowhead*). **B:** Quick-freeze, deep-etch electron micrograph showing an equivalent area of juxtacanalicular region with EL and the lumen of SC including a pore (*arrowhead*) connecting the contents of a giant vacuole (V) with the lumen of the canal. Note the greater density and complexity of extracellular matrix visible using this method. (From Gong H, Ruberti J, Overby D, et al. A new view of the human trabecular meshwork using quick-freeze, deep-etch electron microscopy. *Exp Eye Res.* 75:347–358, 2002.)

of flow and pressure.[36] An enucleated eye that is simply placed into a jar of chemical fixative will rarely exhibit giant vacuoles when examined microscopically. These giant vacuoles are not unique to the trabecular meshwork but are also seen in the endothelial lining of the arachnoid villi of the brain that are responsible for reabsorption of the cerebrospinal fluid.[37]

It appears that giant vacuoles of Schlemm's canal represent focal bullous detachments of the inner wall endothelium that billow into the lumen of the canal. At some point, an opening or pore is produced in the wall of the stretched vacuole. Pore formation is likely preceded by an intermediate stage, exhibiting a focal thinning of the endothelial cell, which looks somewhat like a fenestration in a permeable capillary.[38] These fenestra-like structures in the inner wall of Schlemm's canal are termed "diaphragmed minipores."[39] Opening of these pores appears to allow for the aliquot of aqueous humor within the vacuole to enter Schlemm's canal. In this process, it is likely that some of the basement membrane under the vacuole is swept into the canal with the aliquot of aqueous, thus accounting for the discontinuities in the basement membrane.

Exactly how pores form and whether they contribute to outflow resistance remains uncertain, but two different sets of pores have been described based upon their location in scanning electron micrographs of the inner wall. They are termed I-pores and B-pores (**Fig. 9.18**).[40] I-pores appear to be transcellular and represent small openings created through the thickness of an entire cell, from one membrane to the other. B-pores are openings seen at the overlapping borders between endothelial cells of the inner wall. Their presence would infer a paracellular rather than a transcellular route for aqueous passage across the wall of Schlemm's canal.

The endothelial cells lining Schlemm's canal are joined by tight junctions and gap junctions. By freeze-fracture, the tight junctions have been shown to exhibit variable complexity (**Fig. 9.19**).[16] It has been demonstrated that with elevation of intraocular pressure, the overlap between inner wall endothelial cells decreases and the number of tight junctional strands forming these junctions reduces and may open focally.[41] Junctional simplification usually correlates with increased permeability. Focal reductions in tight junction strand number to zero could represent the anatomic basis of the B-pore found at the interendothelial cell border.

The Distal Outflow Pathways Beyond Schlemm's Canal

Aqueous humor from Schlemm's canal ultimately drains into the venous system of the episclera and then leaves the orbit via the ophthalmic veins. Approximately 30 external collector channels lead from the outer wall of Schlemm's canal, through the sclera and toward the vessels of the episclera in each eye (**Figs. 9.20** and **9.21**). External collector channels have been shown to exhibit smooth muscle actin, implying that these vessels could constrict and in doing so influence outflow.[42]

From the external collector channels, aqueous passes into a tortuous system of vessels within the thickness of the sclera, termed the deep scleral plexus. This plexus leads, in turn, to the more superficial intrascleral venous plexus, finally reaching the surface of the sclera to join the episcleral veins (**Fig. 9.22**). Through this tortuous route, the aqueous and blood are mixed.

In approximately 10% of eyes, however, a small number of unique vessels termed aqueous veins (of Ascher) bypass this tortuous pathway and connect directly from Schlemm's canal to the episcleral veins.[42] Although their significance remains unknown, these unique vessels are readily identified clinically near the limbus, at the 3 or 9 o'clock position. Because the aqueous humor and blood within them have

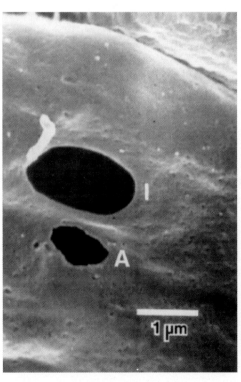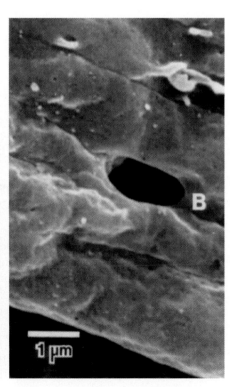

FIGURE 9.18 Scanning electron micrographs of en face views of the inner wall of Schlemm's canal. The figure on the left demonstrates an intracellular pore (*I*) and the rough, irregular edge of an artifactual break in the inner wall (**A**). The figure on the right shows a border-pore (**B**), clearly arising at the border between adjacent inner wall cells. (From Ethier CR, Coloma FM, Sit AJ, et al. Two pore types in the inner-wall endothelium of Schlemm's canal. *Invest Ophthalmol Vis Sci.* 1998;39:2041–2048.)

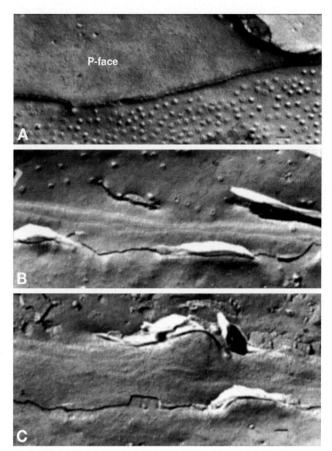

FIGURE 9.19   Freeze-fracture electron micrographs, showing the varied complexity of tight junctional strands joining adjacent cells within the inner wall of Schlemm's canal. **A:** Single strand running along the ridge at the edge of the P-face of the plasma membrane. **B:** Two parallel strands. **C:** More complex array of junctional strands showing 3 to 5 branching and anastomosing strands of junctional particles. The complexity of these junctions in the inner wall of Schlemm's canal simplies with increasing pressure. (From Ye W, Gong H, Sit A, et al. Interendothelial junctions in normal human Schlemm's canal respond to changes in pressure. *Invest Ophthalmol Vis Sci.* 1997;38:2460.)

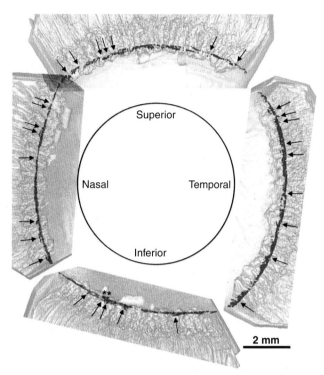

FIGURE 9.20   Composite microcomputed tomogram shows a coronal view of the lumen of Schlemm's canal (*magenta circle*) and the departure points of the 29 collector channels in this eye (*arrows*). (From Hann CR, Bentley MD, Vercnocke A, et al. Imaging the aqueous humor outflow pathway in human eyes by three-dimensional micro-computed tomography (3D micro-CT). *Exp Eye Res.* 2011;92:104–111.)

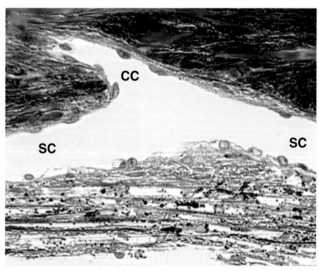

FIGURE 9.21   Light micrograph showing the exit of an external collector channel (CC) from the lumen of Schlemm's canal (SC). (Courtesy of Dr. Haiyan Gong.)

yet to mix, a laminar flow of blood and aqueous is readily visible as a central clear channel of aqueous humor surrounded by peripheral streams of blood (**Fig. 9.23**).

AQUEOUS OUTFLOW IS NOT UNIFORM AROUND THE CIRCUMFERENCE OF THE EYE

Areas of the trabecular meshwork around the circumference of the anterior chamber vary regarding the amount of flow that they carry and these areas can shift location over time.[43] It has been shown that regions of the trabecular meshwork containing the greatest amount of pigment (and therefore receiving the most flow) are localized to areas of the posterior meshwork corresponding to the locations of the collector channels.[44] Indeed, there are even regional variations in the expression of certain of the extracellular matrix components, such as versican.[45] As such, it is not appropriate to assume that aqueous humor is leaving all parts of the trabecular meshwork uniformly, around its entire circumference.

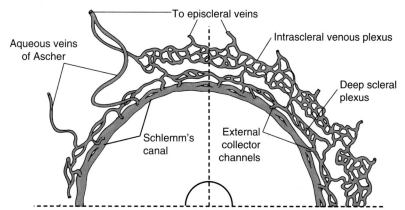

FIGURE 9.22   Composite sketch of outflow channels extending from Schlemm's canal, through the thickness of the sclera, to the episcleral veins. Note that in several locations, Schlemm's canal is bifid, splitting into two parallel canals before again merging into a single canal. On the right, the external collector channels are visible and their connections to the deep scleral plexus and intrascleral venous plexus are also shown. On the left, the departures of external collector channels are also seen and aqueous veins (of Ascher) are shown. Clinically, these are most readily seen near the limbus at the 3 and 9 o'clock positions, when present. Both the intrascleral plexus of vessels on the right and the aqueous veins (of Ascher) on the left, join the episcleral veins. (Modified from Hogan MJ, Alvarado JA, Weddell JE. *Histology of the Human Eye*. Philadelphia, PA: WB Saunders; 1971:140.)

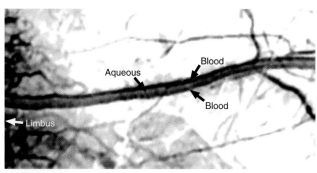

FIGURE 9.23   High magnification black and white clinical photo near the limbus at the 3 o'clock position shows an aqueous vein of Ascher. These are easily recognized by their trilaminar appearance in which the peripheral blood columns are separated by a central column of clear aqueous humor.

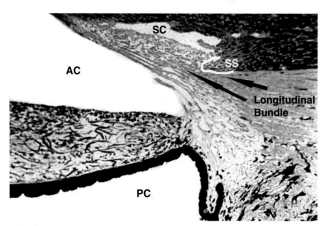

FIGURE 9.24   Light micrograph of anterior chamber angle shows some tendons of the longitudinal bundle of the ciliary muscle attaching the scleral spur (SS)—(*short arrow*). Additional tendons from the longitudinal bundle (*long arrow*) clearly bypass the SS where they make connections into the trabecular meshwork and to the inner wall of Schlemm's canal (SC). Still additional fine tendons pass directly through the meshwork to blend with stroma of the peripheral cornea. AC, anterior chamber; PC, posterior chamber.

Anatomic Relationships between the Ciliary Muscle and the Structures of the Outflow Pathways

As noted in **CHAPTER 8: THE CILIARY BODY**, the longitudinal portion of the ciliary muscle makes functionally important anatomic connections onto the scleral spur and into the trabecular meshwork as well.

Some of the tendons of the longitudinal bundle make direct connections to the posterior surface of the scleral spur (**Fig. 9.24**). When these muscle fibers contract, their tendons pull the scleral spur inward and posteriorly. In doing so, the trabeculae of the corneoscleral meshwork and the JCT region that are attached to the opposite surface of the scleral spur are fanned apart, increasing the facility of aqueous outflow.[46,47] Recent evidence suggests that eyes with glaucoma have a shorter scleral spur and this may decrease the ability of the ciliary muscle to produce its full effect on outflow through contraction.[48]

Additional studies have suggested that the scleral spur is more complex than a simple outcropping from the inner surface of the sclera. In the scleral spur, a unique population of cells is found. Like ciliary muscle cells, these cells express smooth muscle actin, but unlike ciliary muscle cells, they do not express desmin.[49] These cells are innervated and interconnected by gap junctions.[50] Their function is unclear at this time but their orientation is parallel to the circular bundle of the ciliary muscle rather than the longitudinal bundle.[51]

Also present around the entire circumference of the scleral spur are club-shaped nerve endings derived from myelinated nerves. The ultrastructure of these nerve endings bears a strong resemblance to the end-bulbs of mechanoreceptors elsewhere in the body. The scleral spur would be a logical place to position mechanoreceptors, as part of a proprioceptive feedback loop to regulate outflow, but further studies of these nerve endings will be required to determine if such a feedback loop truly exists.[52]

THE CRIBRIFORM PLEXUS AND THE SCLERAL SPUR

Two additional sets of tendons, from muscle fibers of the longitudinal bundle, have been described; both of these bypass the scleral spur. These tendons are referred to as the cribriform plexus.[53] One of these sets of tendons extends through the trabecular meshwork, inserting into the periphery of the posterior corneal stroma. The function of these tendons remains uncertain, beyond keeping the ciliary body and trabecular meshwork under passive tension for stability.

The second set of tendons that bypass the scleral spur make connections in the corneoscleral and juxtacanalicular meshwork (**Fig. 9.25**). Some of these fibrils even make direct elastin-containing connections to the endothelial cells of the inner wall of Schlemm's canal (**Fig. 9.26**).[54] These tendons exert tonic tension on the inner wall of Schlemm's canal, resisting collapse of Schlemm's canal when intraocular pressure is elevated.[55]

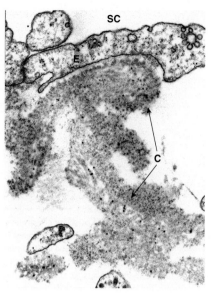

FIGURE 9.26   Electron micrograph of an elastic connecting fibril (C) of the cribriform plexus making contact with an endothelial cell (E) lining the inner wall of Schlemm's canal (SC). (From Gong H, Trinkaus-Randall V, Freddo TF, et al. Ultrastructural immunocytochemical localization of elastin in normal human trabecular meshwork. *Curr Eye Res.* 1989;8(10):1071–1082.)

Anatomy of the Uveoscleral Outflow Pathway

In the young human eye, most studies calculate that up to 40% of the total outflow of aqueous humor occurs via an alternate pathway known as the "unconventional" or uveoscleral outflow pathway.[2,56,57] This percentage decreases with age.[58] It is also known that contraction of the ciliary muscle, as occurs with the cholinergic drug pilocarpine, reduces uveoscleral flow significantly.[2] What determines whether aqueous humor will enter the trabecular outflow pathway or the uveoscleral pathway is the position of the scleral spur.

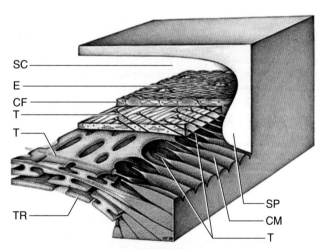

FIGURE 9.25   Sketch depicts connections of the cribriform plexus of tendons (T) from the smooth muscle fibers of the ciliary muscle (CM). These tendons extend past the scleral spur (SP) into the trabecular meshwork (TR) and send elastin connecting fibrils (CF) that contact the endothelium (E) of the inner wall of Schlemm's canal (SC). (From Lütjen-Drecoll E, Johannes W, Rohen JW. Functional Morphology of the Trabecular Meshwork. In: Tasman WS, Jaeger EA, eds. *Duane's Foundations of Clinical Ophthalmology on CD-ROM.* Philadelphia, PA: Lippincott Williams & Wilkins; 2006.)

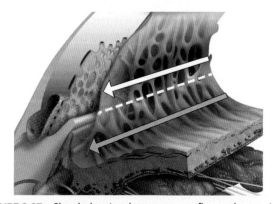

FIGURE 9.27   Sketch showing the aqueous outflow pathways. Aqueous humor leaving the anterior chamber above the scleral spur (*white arrow*) leaves the eye via the trabecular meshwork and Schlemm's canal. Aqueous humor leaving the eye below the scleral spur (*gray arrow*) enters the ciliary body and the uveoscleral outflow pathway. (Modified from Hogan MJ, Alvardo JA, Weddell JE. *Histology of the Human Eye.* Philadelphia, PA: WB Saunders; 1971:137.)

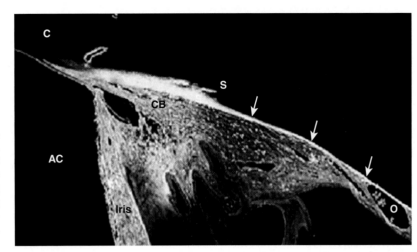

FIGURE 9.28 Light micrograph of the outflow pathways following anterior chamber (AC) perfusion with fluorescent tracer shows migration of the tracer into the ciliary body (CB) and further movement posteriorly toward the ora serrata (O) along the supraciliary space (*arrows*), just beneath the sclera (S). Cornea (C). (From Tripathi RC. Uveoscleral drainage of aqueous humor. *Exp Eye Res.* 1977;25(suppl):305–308.)

As aqueous humor enters the uveal face of trabecular meshwork, aqueous humor that flows "above" the scleral spur as seen gonioscopically will continue to Schlemm's canal and the conventional outflow pathway (white arrow) (**Fig. 9.27**). That which passes "below" the scleral spur (gray arrow) passes into the ciliary body and the uveoscleral outflow pathway. Upon entering the open stromal face of the ciliary body near the iris root, aqueous humor passes through the connective tissue fascicles that interweave with the smooth muscle fibers of the ciliary muscle.

It appears that the connective tissue fascicles that interweave with the bundles of smooth muscle fibers in the ciliary muscle are very important anatomic features of the uveoscleral outflow pathway. One of the most common medications used to lower intraocular pressure in glaucoma is one of a group of prostaglandins. Studies in monkeys indicate that one of the morphologic changes induced by these medications is to degrade this connective tissue matrix, thus enhancing passage of aqueous humor along the uveoscleral pathway.[59]

Ultimately, the fluid passing through the connective tissue bundles of the ciliary muscle reaches the inner surface of the sclera. As detailed in **CHAPTER 8: THE CILIARY BODY**, a potential space separates the longitudinal bundle of the ciliary muscle from the inner surface of the sclera. Through this space, called the supraciliary space and its continuation as the suprachoroidal space, aqueous moves posteriorly as shown in **Fig. 9.28**. Along this pathway, aqueous humor leaves the eye by either diffusing through the sclera (uveoscleral) or by diffusing through the scleral emissaria for the vortex veins (uveo-vortex) flow.[2] Whether the uveoscleral outflow pathway demonstrates the regional variability exhibited by the conventional outflow system remains unexplored.

REFERENCES

1. Brubaker RF. Measurement of aqueous flow by fluorophotometry. In: Ritch R, Shields MB, Krupin T, eds. *The Glaucomas.* St Louis, MO: Mosby; 1989:337–344.
2. Bill A, Phillips CI. Uveoscleral drainage of aqueous humour in human eyes. *Exp Eye Res.* 1971;12(3):275–281.
3. Martin XD. Normal intraocular pressure in man. *Ophthalmologica.* 1992;205(2):57–63.
4. Freddo T, Johnson M. Aqueous humor dynamics I: measurement methods and animal studies. In: Civan M, Benos D, Simon S, eds. *The Eye's Aqueous Humor.* Cambridge, MA: Academic Press; 2008.
5. Tümer Z, Bach-Holm D. Axenfeld–Rieger syndrome and spectrum of PITX2 and FOXC1 mutations. *Eur J Hum Genet.* 2009;17(12):1527–1539.
6. Dua HS, Faraj LA, Branch MJ, et al. The collagen matrix of the human trabecular meshwork is an extension of the novel pre-descemet's layer (Dua's layer). *Br J Ophthalmol.* 2014;98(5):691–697.
7. Marshall GE, Konstas AG, Lee WR. Immunogold ultrastructural localization of collagens in the aged human outflow system. *Ophthalmology.* 1991;98(5):692–700.
8. Lütjen-Drecoll E, Rittig M, Rauterberg J, et al. Immunomicroscopical study of type VI collagen in the trabecular meshwork of normal and glaucomatous eyes. *Exp Eye Res.* 1989;48(1):139–147.
9. Koudouna E, Young RD, Ueno M, et al. Three-dimensional architecture of collagen type VI in the human trabecular meshwork. *Mol Vis.* 2014;20:638.
10. Tawara A, Varner HH, Hollyfield JG. Distribution and characterization of sulfated proteoglycans in the human trabecular tissue. *Invest Ophthalmol Vis Sci.* 1989;30(10):2215–2231.
11. Gong H, Freddo TF, Johnson M. Age-related changes of sulfated proteoglycans in the normal human trabecular meshwork. *Exp Eye Res.* 1992;55(5):691–709.
12. Acott TS, Kelley MJ. Extracellular matrix in the trabecular meshwork. *Exp Eye Res.* 2008;86(4):543–561.
13. Johnson DH, Knepper PA. Microscale analysis of the glycosaminoglycans of human trabecular meshwork: a study in perfusion cultured eyes. *J Glaucoma.* 1994;3(1):58–69.
14. Lütjen-Drecoll E, Futa R, Rohen JW. Ultrahistochemical studies on tangential sections of the trabecular meshwork in normal and glaucomatous eyes. *Invest Ophthalmol Vis Sci.* 1981;21:563–573.
15. Marshall GE, Konstas AG, Lee WR. Immunogold localization of type IV collagen and laminin in the aging human outflow system. *Exp Eye Res.* 1990;51(6):691–699.
16. Bhatt K, Gong H, Freddo TF. Freeze-fracture studies of interendothelial junctions in the angle of the human eye. *Invest Ophthalmol Vis Sci.* 1995;36(7):1379–1389.
17. Melamed S, Freddo TF, Epstein DL. Use of cationized ferritin to trace aqueous humor outflow in the monkey eye. *Exp Eye Res.* 1986;43(2):273–278.

18. Rohen JW, van der Zypen E. The phagocytic activity of the trabecular meshwork endothelium. *Albrecht von Graefes Arch Klin Exp Ophthalmol.* 1968;175(2):143–160.

19. Alvarado J, Murphy C, Polansky J, et al. Age-related changes in trabecular meshwork cellularity. *Invest Ophthalmol Vis Sci.* 1981;21(5):714–727.

20. Grierson I, Howes RC. Age-related depletion of the cell population in the human trabecular meshwork. *Eye.* 1987;1(2):204–210.

21. Liton PB, Challa P, Stinnett S, et al. Cellular senescence in the glaucomatous outflow pathway. *Exp Gerontol.* 2005;40(8):745–748.

22. Raviola G. Schwalbe line's cells: a new cell type in the trabecular meshwork of *Macaca mulatta. Invest Ophthalmol Vis Sci.* 1982;22(1):45–56.

23. Braunger BM, Ademoglu B, Koschade SE, et al. Identification of adult stem cells in Schwalbe's line region of the primate Eye. *Invest Ophthalmol Vis Sci.* 2014;55(11):7499–7507.

24. Du Y, Roh DS, Mann MM, et al. Multipotent stem cells from trabecular meshwork become phagocytic TM cells. *Invest Ophthalmol Vis Sci.* 2012;53(3):1566–1575.

25. Yu WY, Sheridan C, Grierson I, et al. Progenitors for the corneal endothelium and trabecular meshwork: a potential source for personalized stem cell therapy in corneal endothelial diseases and glaucoma. *J Biomed Biotechnol.* 2011;2011:412743.

26. Kelley MJ, Rose AY, Keller KE, et al. Stem cells in the trabecular meshwork: present and future promises. *Exp Eye Res.* 2009;88(4):747–751.

27. Sun Y, Williams A, Waisbourd M, et al. Stem cell therapy for glaucoma: science or snake oil? *Surv Ophthalmol.* 2015;60(2):93–105.

28. Gong H, Tripathi RC, Tripathi BJ. Morphology of the aqueous outflow pathway. *Microsc Res Tech.* 1996;33(4):336–367.

29. Tripathi RC. Pressure-dependency of the aqueous outflow. *Am J Ophthalmol.* 1973;76(3):402–403.

30. Murphy CG, Yun AJ, Newsome DA, et al. Localization of extracellular proteins of the human trabecular meshwork by indirect immunofluorescence. *Am J Ophthalmol.* 1987;104(1):33–43.

31. Alexander JP, Samples JR, Van Buskirk EM, et al. Expression of matrix metalloproteinases and inhibitor by human trabecular meshwork. *Invest Ophthalmol Vis Sci.* 1991;32(1):172–180.

32. Keller KE, Aga M, Bradley JM, et al. Extracellular matrix turnover and outflow resistance. *Exp Eye Res.* 2009;88(4):676–682.

33. Alward WL, Fingert JH, Coote MA, et al. Clinical features associated with mutations in the chromosome 1 open-angle glaucoma gene (GLC1A). *N Engl J Med.* 1998;338(15):1022–1027.

34. Gong H, Ruberti J, Overby D, et al. A new view of the human trabecular meshwork using quick-freeze, deep-etch electron microscopy. *Exp Eye Res.* 2002;75(3):347–358.

35. Allingham RR, de Kater AW, Ethier RC. Schlemm's canal and primary open angle glaucoma: correlation between Schlemm's canal dimensions and outflow facility. *Exp Eye Res.* 1996;62(1):101–110.

36. Grierson I, Lee WR. Pressure-induced changes in the ultrastructure of the endothelium lining Schlemm's canal. *Am J Ophthalmol.* 1975;80(5):863–884.

37. Yamashima T. Functional ultrastructure of cerebrospinal fluid drainage channels in human arachnoid villi. *Neurosurgery.* 1988;22(4):633–641.

38. Bill A, Maepea O. Mechanisms and routes of aqueous humor drainage. In: Albert DM, Jakobiec FA, eds. *Principles and Practices of Ophthalmology Basic Sciences.* Vol I. Philadelphia, PA: WB Saunders. 1994:206–226.

39. Tamm ER, Lütjen-Drecoll E. Ciliary body. *Microsc Res Tech.* 1996;33(5): 390–439.

40. Ethier CR, Coloma FM, Sit AJ, et al. Two pore types in the inner-wall endothelium of Schlemm's canal. *Invest Ophthalmol Vis Sci.* 1998;39:2041–2048.

41. Ye W, Gong H, Sit A, et al. Interendothelial junctions in normal human Schlemm's canal respond to changes in pressure. *Invest Ophthalmol Vis Sci.* 1997;38(12):2460–2468.

42. de Kater AW, Shahsafaei A, Epstein DL. Localization of smooth muscle and nonmuscle actin isoforms in the human aqueous outflow pathway. *Invest Ophthalmol Vis Sci.* 1992;33(2):424–429.

43. Vranka JA, Bradley JM, Yang YF, et al. Mapping molecular differences and extracellular matrix gene expression in segmental outflow pathways of the human ocular trabecular meshwork. *PLoS One.* 2015;10(3):e0122483.

44. Hann CR, Fautsch MP. Preferential fluid flow in the human trabecular meshwork near collector channels. *Invest Ophthalmol Vis Sci.* 2009;50(4):1692–1697.

45. Keller KE, Bradley JM, Vranka JA, et al. Segmental versican expression in the trabecular meshwork and involvement in outflow facility. *Invest Ophthalmol Vis Sci.* 2011;52(8):5049–5057.

46. Lütjen-Drecoll E, Tamm E, Kaufman PL. Age-related loss of morphologic responses to pilocarpine in rhesus monkey ciliary muscle. *Arch Ophthalmol.* 1988;106(11):1591–1598.

47. Grierson I, Lee WR, Abraham S. Effects of pilocarpine on the morphology of the human outflow apparatus. *Br J Ophthalmol.* 1978;62(5):302–313.

48. Swain DL, Ho J, Lai J, et al. Shorter scleral spur in eyes with primary open-angle glaucoma. *Invest Ophthalmol Vis Sci.* 2015;56(3):1638–1648.

49. Tamm E, Flügel C, Stefani FH, et al. Contractile cells in the human scleral spur. *Exp Eye Res.* 1992;54(4):531–543.

50. Tamm ER, Koch TA, Mayer B, et al. Innervation of myofibroblast-like scleral spur cells in human monkey eyes. *Invest Ophthalmol Vis Sci.* 1995;36(8):1633–1644.

51. Tamm ER. The trabecular meshwork outflow pathways: structural and functional aspects. *Exp Eye Res.* 2009;88(4):648–655.

52. Tamm ER, Flügel C, Stefani FH, et al. Nerve endings with structural characteristics of mechanoreceptors in the human scleral spur. *Invest Ophthalmol Vis Sci.* 1994;35(3):1157–1166.

53. Rohen JW, Futa R, Lütjen-Drecoll E. The fine structure of the cribriform meshwork in normal and glaucomatous eyes as seen in tangential sections. *Invest Ophthalmol Vis Sci.* 1981;21(4):574–585.

54. Gong HY, Trinkaus-Randall V, Freddo TF. Ultrastructural immunocytochemical localization of elastin in normal human trabecular meshwork. *Curr Eye Res.* 1989;8(10):1071–1081.

55. Kaufman PL, Barany EH. Loss of acute pilocarpine effect on outflow facility following surgical disinsertion and retrodisplacement of the ciliary muscle from the scleral spur in the cynomolgus monkey. *Invest Ophthalmol.* 1976;15(10):793–807.

56. Townsend DJ, Brubaker RF. Immediate effect of epinephrine on aqueous formation in the normal human eye as measured by fluorophotometry. *Invest Ophthalmol Vis Sci.* 1980;19(3):256–266.

57. Toris CB, Yablonski ME, Wang YL, et al. Aqueous humor dynamics in the aging human eye. *Am J Ophthalmol.* 1999;127(4):407–412.

58. Alm A, Nilsson SF. Uveoscleral outflow—a review. *Exp Eye Res.* 2009;88(4):760–768.

59. Lütjen-Drecoll E, Tamm E. Morphological study of the anterior segment of cynomolgus monkey eyes following treatment with prostaglandin F2 alpha. *Exp Eye Res.* 1988;47(5):761–769.

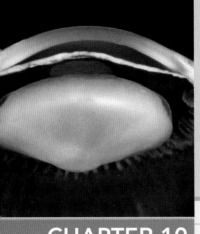

Crystalline Lens and Zonules

Overview

The crystalline lens is avascular, biconvex, and receives no innervation or lymphatic supply (**Fig. 10.1**). While it is not the major optical element in the eye, it has the unique ability to allow its shape and configuration to be changed in milliseconds, thereby shifting the focus of the eye from far to near. This process, called accommodation, is produced by contraction of the ciliary muscle and mediated through zonular fibers, which are filamentous connections from the ciliary body to the anterior, posterior, and equatorial lens surfaces (**Fig. 10.2**).

In addition to its optical functions, the lens provides mechanical support for the iris and, together with the pupillary margin, forms an important one-way valve, permitting flow of aqueous humor from the posterior chamber forward, but not in the reverse direction (**Fig. 10.1**).

Macroscopic and Clinical Anatomy of the Crystalline Lens

Although the cornea nearly reaches its adult diameter at birth, the diameter of the lens increases significantly with age. At birth, the diameter of the unaccommodated lens averages 6 to 6.5 mm, but by age 65, the diameter increases to an average of 9 to 9.5 mm. The average anterior-posterior lens thickness also increases with age, from an average of 3.5 to 4 mm at birth, to 4.5 to 5 mm after age 65.[1] The lens continues to grow throughout life. As the lens grows and expands, its capacity to change shape diminishes, contributing to an age-related loss of accommodative power. This loss of accommodation, termed presbyopia, becomes clinically significant for most patients in their fifth decade, requiring supplemental optical power in order to see clearly at near.

As with the cornea, it is common for asymmetry in the vertical and horizontal curvatures of the lens to produce astigmatism. Unlike the cornea, however, the lens more commonly manifests more optical power horizontally than vertically, a pattern of astigmatism referred to as "against the rule."

Finally, because the pupillary margin rests on the anterior lens surface, the age-related increase in lens thickness tends to push the central portion of the iris forward, giving it a more convex configuration in older individuals. Commensurate with this change, the volume of the anterior chamber is reduced, and the root of the iris is tilted forward. As the iris root tilts forward, toward the outflow pathways of the trabecular meshwork, this increases the risk that pupillary dilation might impede aqueous outflow and acutely elevate intraocular pressure.

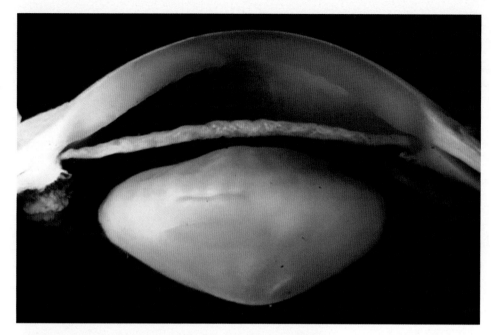

FIGURE 10.1 Macrophotograph of the anterior segment of the eye shows relationships between the arcing dome of the cornea, the iris, pars plicata region of the ciliary body, and a large, older crystalline lens. To avoid cutting through the lens, this is a paraxial cut through the eye. As such, the pupil is not seen. (Courtesy of Mission for Vision and Dr. Ben Glasgow [missionforvision.org].)

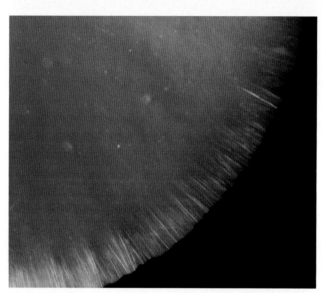

FIGURE 10.2   Clinical photograph showing a sector of the anterior surface of the crystalline lens, including the attachment of the zonular fibers to the lens periphery. (Courtesy Dr. Daniel Roberts.)

CLINICAL ANATOMY OF THE LENS CAPSULE

The lens is surrounded by a capsule that exhibits elasticity, but does not contain elastin. It is the lens capsule that anchors the zonular fibers extending from the ciliary body (Fig. 10.2). When viewed with the slit-lamp, using oblique illumination, the anterior capsular surface of the lens has a "beaten metal" appearance, occasionally described as "peau d'orange" for its similarity to the dimpled appearance of an orange peel (Fig. 10.3). In some individuals, an array of starfish-shaped melanocytes can be seen on the anterior lens capsule. These are referred to as epicapsular stars and they are a normal but uncommon variant (Fig. 10.4). They are a minor embryologic remnant of

the tunica vasculosa lentis, the pigmented, fibrovascular membrane that intimately surrounds the lens during early prenatal development and is then resorbed before birth (SEE CHAPTER 16: EMBRYOLOGY OF THE EYE AND ORBIT).

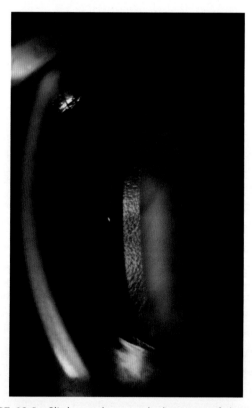

FIGURE 10.3   Slit-lamp photograph shows arc of the corneal curvature at left and a strip of the anterior surface of the lens through a dilated pupil. Note the beaten metal or "peau d'orange" appearance of the anterior surface of the lens. (Courtesy of Dr. Daniel Roberts.)

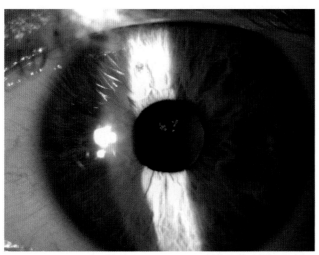

FIGURE 10.4 Slit-lamp photograph shows clusters of pigmented cells, remnants of the embryologic tunica vasculosa lentis, on the anterior surface of the crystalline lens. These are termed epicapsular stars. (Courtesy of Dr. Michelle Steenbakkers.)

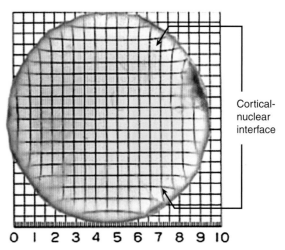

Cortical-nuclear interface

FIGURE 10.6 Macrophotograph of ex vivo normal crystalline lens shows transparent lens with clear periphery (cortex) and yellowish but transparent nucleus. (From Taylor VL, Al-Ghoul KJ, Lane CW, et al. Morphology of the normal human lens. *Invest Ophthalmol Vis Sci.* 1996;37:1396–1410.)

*The anterior lens capsule must be incised during cataract surgery (capsulorrhexis) in order to remove the cataractous lens material before proceeding with implantation of the artificial lens. In some cases, it can be very difficult to visualize the capsule and distinguish it from the underlying lens cortex. To assist in visualizing the capsule, a vital dye called trypan blue can be used to temporarily stain the capsule in vivo. This dye does not pass through the capsule and thus the underlying cortex can be readily distinguished from the capsule once the anterior capsule is incised and reflected (*Fig. 10.5*).[2,3]*

On the posterior surface of the lens, through a dilated pupil, a partial or complete gray-white ring, approximately 5 to 8 mm in diameter, is discernable in many adult eyes. This ring, called Egger's line, is the peripheral edge of Wieger's ligament (i.e., ligamentum hyaloideocapsulare), which attaches the anterior vitreous face to the posterior capsule of the lens. These are described in greater detail in **CHAPTER 11: THE VITREOUS.**

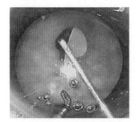

FIGURE 10.5 Intraoperative photograph of Trypan blue-stained lens capsule that has been incised and reflected to reveal the underlying cataractous lens material. (From Perrone DM. Argentinean flag sign is most common complication for intumescent cataracts. *Ocul Surg News US Ed.* 2000.)

CLINICAL ANATOMY OF THE LENS FIBERS

From a clinical standpoint, the lens fiber mass is divided into an inner nucleus and an outer cortex. In the noncataractous adult lens, the nucleus is seen to have a slight yellow coloration compared with the cortex, but both remain transparent[4] (**Fig. 10.6**).

  *When the lens nucleus and cortex are viewed as separate anatomic units, as in the yellow and white portions of the cross section depicted (*Fig. 10.7*), it becomes clear that the nucleus of the lens is thicker in its center than at its edges, making it a convergent lens (i.e., a plus lens). If the cortex is viewed in isolation, however, one notes that its edges are thicker than its center, making it a divergent lens (a minus lens). As patients develop age-related cataractous changes, these may cause changes in refractive error. If the older patient presents with a need for more minus power, this suggests the changes are primarily in the nucleus, causing it to have developed more plus power.[5] Conversely, if the patient demonstrates a need for plus power, the changes are more likely in the cortex, causing it to have developed more minus power.[6] Finally, changes in astigmatism are found more commonly with cortical changes than with changes in the nucleus of the lens.[7]*

Histology

LENS CAPSULE

The capsule of the lens is actually a basal lamina of variable thickness (**Fig. 10.8**). Like all true basement membranes, it

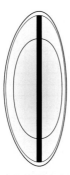

FIGURE 10.7 Sketch of sagittal cut through the crystalline lens with clear cortex and yellowish nucleus. Note that the nucleus has the structure of a biconvex lens, but the anterior and posterior segments of the cortex are thicker on their edges than at their centers.

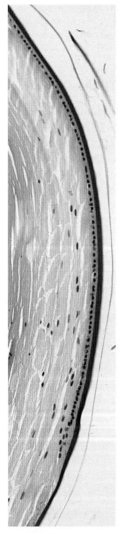

FIGURE 10.8 Light micrograph of equatorial region of the lens (anterior lens surface at top). The micrograph shows the variable thickness of the periodic acid-Schiff (PAS+) dark pink lens capsule and the single layer of lens epithelial cells inside the capsule that terminates just posterior to the lens equator. Note that as lens fibers form and become embedded deeper in the lens, the nuclei of the fibers become smaller and ultimately disappear. Outside of the lens capsule, irregular lengths of zonular fibers are also seen.

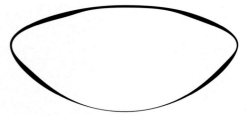

FIGURE 10.9 Diagram showing the changes in thickness of the lens capsule around its circumference. Anterior at top.

stains positively with periodic acid–Schiff reagents (PAS+) giving histologic sections of the capsule a dark magenta hue (see **Fig. 10.8**). Unlike most basement membranes, the turnover rate of its molecular constituents is very slow, on the order of months to years.[8] This molecular stability contributes to the ability of the capsule to remain intact decades after cataract surgery, during which the epithelial cells and lens fibers that sustained it have been removed, and the "bag" (i.e., the capsule) remains behind to contain the implanted prosthetic lens.

Lens capsule thickness changes with age. The capsule at the anterior pole increases in thickness with age, from an average of 11 to 15 µm. The thickest area of the capsule is the area just anterior to the lens equator. It thickens with age as well, from an average of 13.5 to 16 µm. The equatorial capsular thickness averages approximately 7 µm and varies little with age. The thinnest area of the capsule (3.5 to 4 µm) is the posterior pole. There is disagreement as to whether the posterior capsule thins, thickens slightly, or remains the same with age.[9,10] The normal pattern of variation in thickness of the lens capsule, around its circumference, is depicted in **Figure 10.9**.

The anterior lens capsule is secreted by the underlying lens epithelium and, posteriorly, by the surface lens fibers. It is composed principally of laminin and type IV collagen,[2,11–13] plus heparan sulfate proteoglycans, primarily perlecan.[11,14]

Although indiscernible clinically or by light microscopy, in the normal eye, the lens capsule is actually a laminated structure. The lamination can be seen in the normal lens by electron microscopy, at least until 45 to 50 years of age.[15]

During early embryologic development, the entire surface of the lens inside the capsule is covered by a single

In certain conditions, the laminated structure of the lens capsule can reveal itself clinically. One classical example is true exfoliation of the lens capsule, in which chronic exposure to infrared wavelengths leads to delamination of the lens capsule—termed true exfoliation. In **Figure 10.10***, note the delamination of the lens capsule.[16–18]*

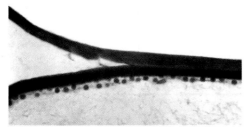

FIGURE 10.10 Black and white photomicrograph showing delamination of the lens capsule in true exfoliation of the lens. (From Karp CL, Fazio JR, Culbertson WW, et al. True exfoliation of the lens capsule. *Arch Ophthalmol.* 1999;117(8):1078–1080.)

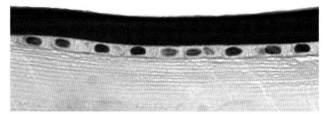

FIGURE 10.11 High magnification light micrograph of the crystalline lens shows the uniform appearance of the lens capsule. Beneath the capsule, the single layer of cuboidal lens epithelial cells is seen and beneath the epithelium, several layers of thin, cortical lens fibers are evident. The lens capsule is the basement membrane of the lens epithelium. Thus, the apical surfaces of the lens epithelial cells face the underlying lens fiber mass.

layer of cuboidal epithelial cells. Later in development, however, the supply of epithelial cells posterior to the equator is lost as they differentiate into primary lens fibers. In doing so, the embryonic nucleus of the lens is created. Thus, in the postnatal lens, only the anterior two-thirds of the lens exhibits a layer of epithelial cells beneath the lens capsule. With no epithelium on most of the posterior half of the lens, and minimal secretion and turnover of basement membrane components by the posterior lens fibers throughout postnatal life, it is not surprising that the thinnest area of the capsule is the posterior pole.[19]

LENS EPITHELIAL CELLS

The apical surfaces of the cuboidal lens epithelial cells face inward toward the lens fiber mass (**Fig. 10.11**). Their basal surfaces lie along the interior surface of the lens capsule, which is the basement membrane they have produced. Lens epithelial cell density appears to be greater in women than in men.[20] In the postnatal lens, epithelial cells undergo mitosis beneath the region where the lens capsule is thickest, anterior to the lens equator. Daughter cells of this division migrate posteriorly and differentiate into lens fibers, posterior to the equator of the lens.

The lens epithelial cells are remarkable among continuously replicating human epithelia for there is no known tumor derived from this epithelium. Given that this epithelium is constantly subjected to toxic oxidative by-products and DNA-damaging ultraviolet light, this epithelium is intensely studied by cancer biologists, to understand how it manages to avoid undergoing malignant transformation.[21]

LENS FIBER MASS

The interior of the lens is composed entirely of thin, band-shaped, hexagonal lens fibers, each one derived from a single epithelial cell, with very little extracellular space between them. Layer upon layer of these fibers is added to the outside of the existing fiber mass, but always beneath

the anterior epithelium and the lens capsule, in the same way that new rings of growth are added to a tree beneath its covering of bark (**Figs. 10.11** and **10.12**). The most superficial fibers are those formed most recently and, in the adult lens, these fibers represent the cortex.

The portion of the lens identified clinically as the nucleus has defined subsets that are named for developmental stages (**Fig. 10.13**). Most of these are not reliably discernable clinically. These subsets of the nucleus, from oldest to youngest, include the following.

The Embryonic Nucleus

The embryonic nucleus is composed of the fibers derived from the epithelial cells that originally lined the posterior half of the developing lens in utero. This supply of epithelial cells is completely depleted during this process, explaining

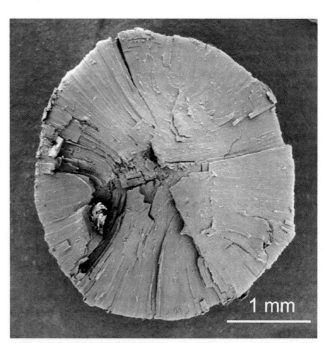

FIGURE 10.12 Scanning electron micrograph of excised lens fiber mass of the nucleus showing orientation and layers of lens fibers. (Courtesy of Dr. Elizabeth Wyles.)

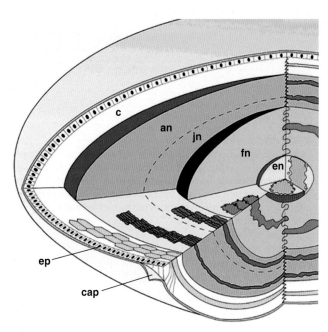

FIGURE 10.13 Diagram of an adult crystalline lens showing defined regions of the lens mass. The regions are drawn to scale except for the embryonic nucleus (en), which is enlarged to show detail. Surrounding regions include the fetal nucleus (fn), juvenile nucleus (jn), and adult nucleus (an). Enveloping these regions of the lens nucleus are the lens cortex (c), the lens epithelium (ep), and the lens capsule (cap). (From Taylor VL, Al-Ghoul KJ, Lane CW, et al. Morphology of the normal human lens. *Invest Ophthalmol Vis Sci.* 1996;37:1396–1410.)

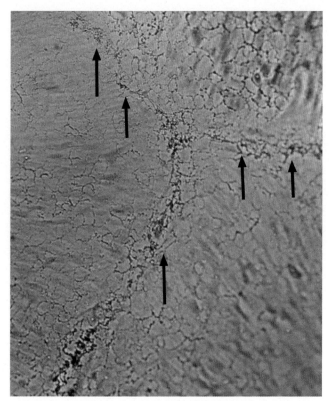

FIGURE 10.14 Light micrograph of the lens fiber mass showing the histologic appearance of a Y suture (*arrows*).

the absence of epithelial cells on the posterior half of the postpartum lens.

The Fetal Nucleus

The fetal nucleus is composed of secondary lens fibers, which are the first fibers resulting from division and differentiation of anterior lens epithelial cells. These are also formed in utero. It is this group of fibers that, with their pattern of fiber-to-fiber attachments anteriorly and posteriorly, create the clinically discernable Y sutures.

The Juvenile Nucleus

The juvenile nucleus is composed of the fibers formed between birth and puberty.

The Adult Nucleus

The adult nucleus forms after puberty. As fibers are packed deeper and deeper into the lens fiber mass, their nuclei gradually disappear. The histologic border between the lens cortex and the adult nucleus is most often defined as the point at which nuclei are no longer discernable in the lens fibers.[4]

The arrangement of individual fibers within the lens fiber mass is critical, since irregularities in structure create opacities. Years ago, it was thought that each lens fiber was

widest at its middle and tapered to a point at each end like a kayak. That has since been shown not to be the case.[22] The fibers that come closest to this shape are the primary lens fibers at the very center of the lens. These earliest fibers run an arcuate course from anterior to posterior, to converge on a single point at each end. But, as the size of the lens expands, more fibers are required in order to cover the expanding surface area. These much greater numbers of fibers still need attachment sites for their anterior and posterior ends, but there is no way to accommodate this greater number of fibers at a single point in the front and the back of the lens fiber mass.

For this greater number of fibers to attach to each other, the pattern of lens fiber assembly changes. The single points of attachment at the anterior and posterior poles of the fetal lens give way to lines of attachment, radiating toward the 10-, 2-, and 6-o'clock positions from these two single points. When seen histologically or clinically, these three radiating lines of fiber-to-fiber attachment, create two Y-shaped figures termed sutures (**Fig. 10.14**). The Y sutures are among the most prominent, clinically observable features of the lens, at least to middle age, when lens changes begin to obscure their visibility. The anterior Y suture is always upright and the posterior Y suture is always inverted (**Fig. 10.15**).

A major advantage of the packing arrangement of lens fibers and sutures is that it eliminates the need for each fiber to reach all the way from the anterior to the posterior pole

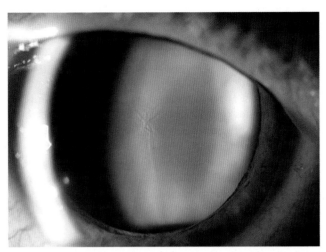

FIGURE 10.15 Clinical photograph shows the anterior Y suture of the lens in a young individual through a dilated pupil. (Courtesy of Dr. Daniel Roberts.)

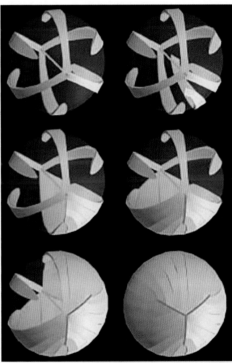

FIGURE 10.16 3D computer-assisted drawings showing key structural elements in the formation of Y sutures during fetal development. *Upper left*: After the primary fiber mass has been formed from the posterior epithelial cells (area surrounding *dark gold line*), six straight fibers define the limits of the Y suture. Three begin at the crux of the anterior Y suture and run to the three tips of the arms of the posterior Y suture and three run anteriorly from the crux of the posterior Y suture to the tips of the three arms of the anterior Y suture (*Upper right*). Filling between these sentinel fibers are S-shaped fibers (*middle left and right*). The ends of the S-shaped fibers abut and overlap to form suture branches (*gray lines*) that extend to confluence at the poles (*lower right and left*). The end result is an anterior Y suture that is upright and a posterior Y suture that is inverted (*lower right*). (From Kuszak JR, Costello MJ. Embryology and anatomy of human lenses. In: Tasman WS, Jaeger EA, eds. *Duane's Foundations of Clinical Ophthalmology on CD-ROM*. Philadelphia, PA: Lippincott, Williams & Wilkins; 2006.)

as the circumferential distance around the ever-growing lens increases. Instead, if a fiber begins at the crux of one of the Y sutures, it will run to the outermost tip of one of the arms of the Y suture on the opposite side, thus foreshortening the required length of its arcuate course (**Fig. 10.16**). Within each layer of fibers, termed growth shells, there are key fibers that attach to the very tips of the three arms and to the crux of each Y suture (**Fig. 10.16**). The remaining fibers of that shell fill in the remaining available space along the arms of the suture. In doing so, these latter fibers run a slightly S-shaped course compared to the arcing anteroposterior direction of the six cardinal fibers. The S-shaped fibers are not tapered to a point; they have squared ends, the breadth of which attaches to the squared end of another fiber along the line that is the suture.

As layer upon layer is added, the length of each arm of the Y extends further out, until the simple Y-shape is no longer complex enough for the much larger numbers of fibers to attach to one another. To meet this challenge, the sutural pattern becomes more complex, through progressive bifurcations of the arms of the suture, increasing to a six-branch star suture at the time of birth, and adding progressively more bifurcations thereafter (**Fig. 10.17**).

As new fibers are formed, older fibers are moved inward, toward the center of the lens, where they become progressively compacted, hardened, and brittle over the years. In histologic sections of paraffin-embedded older eyes, the brittleness of the lens nucleus sometimes results in pieces chipping out during sectioning (**Fig. 10.18**).

> *During phacoemulsification, a common method for removing cataractous lens material during surgery, hard and brittle lens nuclei must customarily be broken up or "chopped" before removal. This is necessary because the phacoemulsification tip operates by ultrasonic destruction, with the tip of the instrument vibrating at approximately 40,000 times per second. Delivering such energies to a solid brittle nucleus would be too destructive within the eye without first dividing the nucleus into smaller pieces.*

Because the lens is avascular, metabolic support, including oxygen, comes primarily from the aqueous humor. Not surprisingly, the oxygen levels are very low, compelling the lens to operate primarily via anaerobic metabolic pathways. In the absence of a blood supply, the ability to deliver metabolites and remove waste products into and out of the lens fiber mass is diffusion-limited, even with the assistance of numerous gap junctions/aquaporins to distribute small metabolites.

Thus, as the originally nucleated cells of the cortex just beneath the lens capsule differentiate into fibers, and begin to be displaced toward the lens center, the nuclei

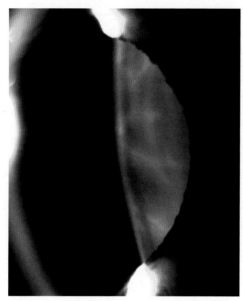

FIGURE 10.17   Clinical photograph shows slit beam section through an adult lens revealing portions of four bifurcating, radiating spokes of a more complex sutural pattern. (Courtesy of Dr. Elizabeth Wyles.)

are gradually lost (**Fig. 10.18**). Ghosts of nuclei remain evident initially, but as the fibers are buried deeper, into the adult nucleus, a fully differentiated, anucleate lens fiber, filled largely with specialized proteins called crystallins, remains.

To maintain optical clarity, the lens fibers must be held in a very tight and orderly array, even while the fiber mass, as a whole, is being continually reshaped by the elastic capsule during accommodation. In reshaping this mass, which is composed of thin, flat, hexagonally shaped fibers running an arcuate course, it would seem very easy for adjacent fibers to flex unevenly. If this occurred, gaps could develop between fibers. To ensure that adjacent fibers flex in unison, the membranes of the fibers, in their equatorial regions, interdigitate and some are provided with remarkable knob-like projections that are received into tightly fit pockets in the membrane of the adjoining cell, somewhat like Lego blocks (**Fig. 10.19**). In this way, the lens fiber mass flexes in unison when being reshaped by the lens capsule during accommodation, while the capsule also assists in ensuring a critically important smooth optical surface.

Within the lens, numerous gap junctions are found. In a solid, avascular tissue, gap junctions play a particularly important role in cell signaling and even movement of ions and metabolites into and out of the fiber mass. Gap junctions interconnect lens epithelial cells to other lens epithelial cells and lens fibers to one another. Gap junctions also connect lens fibers to the single row of lens epithelial cells found anteriorly at what is termed the "epithelial-fiber interface."[23,24] The junctional protein found in gap junctions between lens epithelial cells is predominantly connexin 43 (Cx43). In the lens fiber mass, the gap junction proteins include Cx46 and Cx50. In the lens cortex, where ball and socket connections are a common feature of the lens fibers, each ball and socket connection commonly exhibits gap junctions.[22] Point

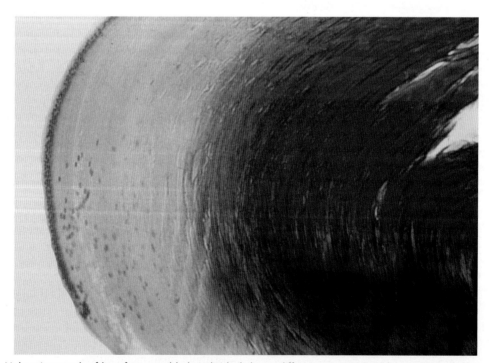

FIGURE 10.18   Light micrograph of lens from an elderly individual shows difference in staining characteristics between darker nucleus and lighter cortex. Due to the hard, brittle nature of the oldest lens fibers at the center of the lens, pieces have chipped out of the lens as it was sectioned for staining and microscopic examination. Note the gradual disappearance of lens fiber nuclei moving deeper into the lens fiber mass from the surface.

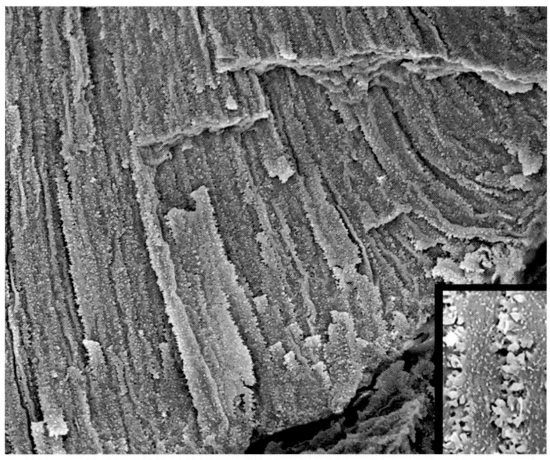

FIGURE 10.19 Scanning electron micrographs showing the surface morphology of cortical (*Main Figure*) and nuclear fibers (*Inset*). Cortical fibers are characterized by complex lateral interdigitations arising at the six corners of these flattened, hexagonally shaped fibers. In addition, small ball and socket-like interdigitations are found randomly on and within the lateral faces. *Inset*: By contrast, the lateral faces of nuclear fibers exhibit numerous furrowed membrane domains. (From Kuszak JR, Costello MJ. Embryology and anatomy of human lenses. In: Tasman WS, Jaeger EA, eds. *Duane's Foundations of Clinical Ophthalmology on CD-ROM*. Philadelphia, PA: Lippincott, Williams & Wilkins; 2006.)

mutations in the genes that encode for these connexins have been shown to be cataractogenic.[25,26]

The lens epithelial cells are also joined by desmosomes, but not tight junctions.[22] The apico-lateral membranes of lens epithelial cells do exhibit some linear arrays of junctional particles that some have referred to as "very leaky" tight junctions but the intercellular clefts between adjacent lens epithelial cells are freely permeable to macromolecular tracers.[27,28]

Macroscopic and Clinical Anatomy of the Zonules

The zonules originate primarily in the pars plana region of the ciliary body. At their points of origin, the zonular fibrils, ranging in diameter from 35 to 55 nm, pierce the basement membrane of the nonpigmented ciliary epithelium and anchor themselves by running a long, tangential path through the intercellular spaces between the cells of the nonpigmented layer.[29,30] Some zonules actually originate posterior to the ora serrata, inserting onto the surface of the peripheral retina. These fibers can be the source of traction that creates peripheral retinal tufts found in approximately 15% of adult eyes.[31]

From their anchor points within the ciliary epithelium, the zonular fibers run anteriorly as a continuous carpet covering the inner surface of the pars plana. As these fibers move forward and reach the pars plicata region of the ciliary body, some continue directly to the lens surface but most are channeled into the valleys between adjacent ciliary processes, making secondary attachments to the surface of the ciliary epithelium. From the ciliary body, the zonules vault across the posterior chamber in three major groups. One of them attaches to the lens capsule anterior to the equator (**Figs. 10.20** and **10.21**). A second group attaches posterior to the equator and a smaller third group of finer fibers attaches to the anterior and posterior margins of the lens equator.[32,33] In addition to these main packets of zonules, another group of vitreous zonules is also observed running as a chord length, traversing the

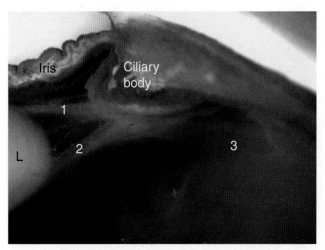

FIGURE 10.20 Meridional macrophotograph showing relationships between the iris, the lens (*L*), the ciliary body, and the principal packets of zonular fibers: (*1*) anterior (preequatorial) packet of zonules; (*2*) posterior (postequatorial) packet of zonules; (*3*) vitreous (hyaloid) zonules. The dark triangular space outlined by the anterior and posterior packets of zonules and the equator of the lens is the canal of Hannover. Two fine packets of equatorial zonules can be seen traversing this space. (Courtesy of Mission for Vision and Dr. Ben Glasgow [www.missionforvision.org].)

curved inner surface of the pars plana region of the ciliary body (**Fig. 10.20**).[34]

Between the main anterior and posterior zonular packets, a triangular channel is created that is traversed only by the zonules extending to the equator of the lens. The channel running between the anterior and posterior packets of zonules is termed the canal of Hannover (**Figs. 10.20** and **10.21**). Another anatomic space is created in the posterior chamber between the posterior packet of zonules and the hyaloid zonules. This space is most commonly termed the canal of Petit (**Fig. 10.21**).

 *There is a congenital anomaly termed "coloboma of the lens" in which an indentation is seen most commonly along the inferonasal edge of the lens for 2 to 3 clock hours when the pupil is dilated. In its most severe form, the entire inferior half of the lens is involved and the lens assumes an inverted teardrop shape (*SEE* **Chapter 16: Embryology of the Eye and Orbit**). In this latter form, there is commonly an associated defect in the inferior portion of the pupil. In fact, in all such cases, the lens is normal. The appearance is created because zonular fibers are not present in the indented areas and it is the zonules that pull the lens out to its circular form. The absence of zonules is the result of an unseen coloboma (i.e., neuroectodermal defect) in formation of the ciliary body in the affected areas.*

COMPOSITION OF THE ZONULES

Notwithstanding their elasticity, the zonules appear to contain no elastin, nor are they principally composed of collagen. They are sensitive to α-chymotrypsin but not to collagenase. The core proteins of these microfibrils, in postnatal eyes, have now been shown to be fibrillins, termed fibrillin-1 and fibrillin-2.[35,36] In addition, two microfibril-associated glycoproteins (MAGP-1 and MAGP-2) have been reported along with other components including proteoglycans.[37,38]

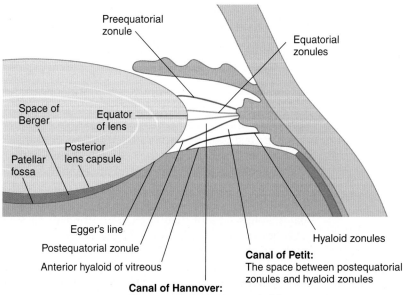

FIGURE 10.21 Sketch shows principal landmarks relating to the packets of zonules, the anterior vitreous face, and the surface of the crystalline lens.

Preequatorial zonule

Equatorial zonules

Space of Berger

Equator of lens

Posterior lens capsule

Patellar fossa

Egger's line

Postequatorial zonule

Anterior hyaloid of vitreous

Hyaloid zonules

Canal of Petit:
The space between postequatorial zonules and hyaloid zonules

Canal of Hannover:
The space between preequatorial and postequatorial zonules

Chapter 10 — Crystalline Lens and Zonules   **167**

CRYSTALLINE LENS AND ZONULES

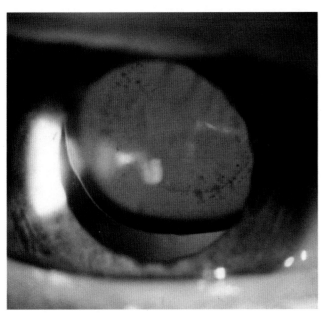

FIGURE 10.22 Clinical photograph shows superior dislocation (subluxation) of crystalline lens, following spontaneous lysis of inferior zonules in Marfan syndrome.

 Certain inherited conditions can give rise to defective zonules which can break, leading to partial dislocation of the lens (ectopia lentis). In Marfan syndrome, which is caused by a mutation on chromosome 15 (15q.21.1), fibrillin-1 is defective. This leads to zonular disruption and, most commonly, an upward dislocation of the lens (Fig. 10.22). Partial dislocation of the lens is termed subluxation, while complete dislocation is termed luxation. Some other conditions producing subluxation include Weill–Marchesani syndrome and homocystinuria. In these cases, the lens more commonly dislocates downward. Still other conditions, such as pseudoexfoliation syndrome, can weaken the zonules, increasing the risk of lens dislocation during cataract surgery.[39]

REFERENCES

1. Marshall J, Beaconsfield M, Rothery S. The anatomy and development of the human lens and zonules. *Trans Ophthalmol Soc U K.* 1982;102(pt 3):423–440.
2. Singh AJ, Sarodia UA, Brown L, et al. A histological analysis of lens capsules stained with trypan blue for capsulorrhexis in phacoemulsification cataract surgery. *Eye (Lond).* 2003;17(5):567–570.
3. Perrone DM. Argentinean flag sign is most common complication for intumescent cataracts. Ocular Surgery News, U S Edition. 2000. http://www.healio.com/ophthalmology/cataract-surgery/news/print/ocular-surgery-news/%7B33d6fae9-280c-4353-8abf-fd0c830975a8%7D/argentinean-flag-sign-is-most-common-complication-for-intumescent-cataracts. Accessed October 28, 2015.
4. Taylor VL, al-Ghoul KJ, Lane CW, et al. Morphology of the normal human lens. *Invest Ophthalmol Vis Sci.* 1996;37(7):1396–1410.
5. Brown NA, Hill AR. Cataract: the relation between myopia and cataract morphology. *Br J Ophthalmol.* 1987;71(6):405–414.
6. Planten JT, Kooijman AC, de Vries B, et al. Pathological-optic approach of cataract and lens. *Ophthalmologica.* 1978;176(6):331–334.
7. Pesudovs K, Elliott DB. Refractive error changes in cortical, nuclear, and posterior subcapsular cataracts. *Br J Ophthalmol.* 2003;87(8):964–967.
8. Haddad A, Bennett G. Synthesis of lens capsule and plasma membrane glycoproteins by lens epithelial cells and fibers in the rat. *Am J Anat.* 1988;183(3):212–225.
9. Krag S, Andreassen TT. Mechanical properties of the human posterior lens capsule. *Invest Ophthalmol Vis Sci.* 2003;44(2):691–696.
10. Barraquer RI, Michael R, Abreu R, et al. Human lens capsule thickness as a function of age and location along the sagittal lens perimeter. *Invest Ophthalmol Vis Sci.* 2006;47(5):2053–2060.
11. Cammarata PR, Cantu-Crouch D, Oakford L, et al. Macromolecular organization of bovine lens capsule. *Tissue Cell.* 1986;18(1):83–97.
12. Kohno T, Sorgente N, Ishibashi T, et al. Immunofluorescent studies of fibronectin and laminin in the human eye. *Invest Ophthalmol Vis Sci.* 1987;28(3):506–514.
13. Kelley PB, Sado Y, Duncan MK. Collagen IV in the developing lens capsule. *Matrix Biol.* 2002;21(5):415–423.
14. Rossi M, Morita H, Sormunen R, et al. Heparan sulfate chains of perlecan are indispensable in the lens capsule but not in the kidney. *EMBO J.* 2003;22(2):236–245.
15. Cavallotti C, Cerulli L. The laminated structure of the lens capsule decreases with age. In: *Age-Related Changes of the Human Eye.* Totowa, NJ: Humana Press; 2008:44–49.
16. Karp CL, Fazio JR, Culbertson WW, et al. True exfoliation of the lens capsule. *Arch Ophthalmol.* 1999;117(8):1078–1080.
17. Bahr GF. Electron microscopical studies on lamellar structure of crystalline capsule of the eye [in German]. *Albrecht Von Graefes Arch Ophthalmol.* 1954;155(6):635–638.
18. Cohen AI. The electron microscopy of the normal human lens. *Invest Ophthalmol.* 1965;4:433–446.
19. Brown NP, Bron AJ. Lens disorders: a clinical manual of cataract diagnosis. *Ophthalmic Lit.* 1996;1(49):64.
20. Guggenmoos-Holzmann I, Engel B, Henke V, et al. Cell density of human lens epithelium in women higher than in men. *Invest Ophthalmol Vis Sci.* 1989;30(2):330–332.
21. Seigel G, Kummer A. The enigma of lenticular oncology. *Digit J Ophthalmol.* 2002;7:1–6.
22. Kuszak J, Costello M. Embryology and anatomy of human lenses. In: Jaeger E, ed. *Duane's Ophthalmology.* CD-ROM Edition. Philadelphia, PA: Lippincott Williams & Wilkins; 1992.
23. Goodenough DA. The crystalline lens. A system networked by gap junctional intercellular communication. *Semin Cell Biol.* 1992;3(1):49–58.
24. Kuszak JR, Novak LA, Brown HG. An ultrastructural analysis of the epithelial-fiber interface (EFI) in primate lenses. *Exp Eye Res.* 1995;61(5):579–597.
25. Beyer EC, Ebihara L, Berthoud VM. Connexin mutants and cataracts. *Front Pharmacol.* 2013;4:43.
26. Lo W, Harding CV. Structure and distribution of gap junctions in lens epithelium and fiber cells. *Cell Tissue Res.* 1986;244(2):253–263.
27. Zampighi GA, Eskandari S, Kreman M. Epithelial organization of the mammalian lens. *Exp Eye Res.* 2000;71(4):415–435.
28. Rae JL, Stacey T. Lanthanum and procion yellow as extracellular markers in the crystalline lens of the rat. *Exp Eye Res.* 1979;28(1):1–21.
29. Streeten BW. The zonular insertion: a scanning electron microscopic study. *Invest Ophthalmol Vis Sci.* 1977;16(4):364–375.
30. Raviola G. The fine structure of the ciliary zonule and ciliary epithelium. with special regard to the organization and insertion of the zonular fibrils. *Invest Ophthalmol.* 1971;10(11):851–869.
31. Foos RY. Zonular traction tufts of the peripheral retina in cadaver eyes. *Arch Ophthalmol.* 1969;82(5):620–632.
32. Canals M, Costa-Vila J, Potau JM, et al. Scanning electron microscopy of the human zonule of the lens (zonula ciliaris). *Acta Anat (Basel).* 1996;157(4):309–314.

33. Mir S, Wheatley HM, Hussels IE, et al. A comparative histologic study of the fibrillin microfibrillar system in the lens capsule of normal subjects and subjects with Marfan Syndrome. *Invest Ophthalmol Vis Sci.* 1998;39(1):84–93.

34. Lutjen-Drecoll E, Kaufman PL, Wasielewski R, et al. Morphology and accommodative function of the vitreous zonule in human and monkey eyes. *Invest Ophthalmol Vis Sci.* 2010;51(3):1554–1564.

35. Ramirez F, Sakai LY, Dietz HC, et al. Fibrillin microfibrils: multi-purpose extracellular networks in organismal physiology. *Physiol Genomics.* 2004;19(2):151–154.

36. Zhang H, Apfelroth SD, Hu W, et al. Structure and expression of fibrillin-2, a novel microfibrillar component preferentially located in elastic matrices. *J Cell Biol.* 1994;124(5):855–863.

37. Gibson MA. Microfibril-associated glycoprotein-1 (MAGP-1) and other non-fibrillin macromolecules which may possess a functional association with the 10 nm microfibrils. *Madame Curie Biosci Database.* 2000.

38. Gibson MA, Finnis ML, Kumaratilake JS, et al. Microfibril-associated glycoprotein-2 (MAGP-2) is specifically associated with fibrillin-containing microfibrils but exhibits more restricted patterns of tissue localization and developmental expression than its structural relative MAGP-1. *J Histochem Cytochem.* 1998;46(8):871–886.

39. Ramachandra CJ, Mehta A, Guo KW, et al. Molecular pathogenesis of Marfan Syndrome. *Int J Cardiol.* 2015;187:585–591.

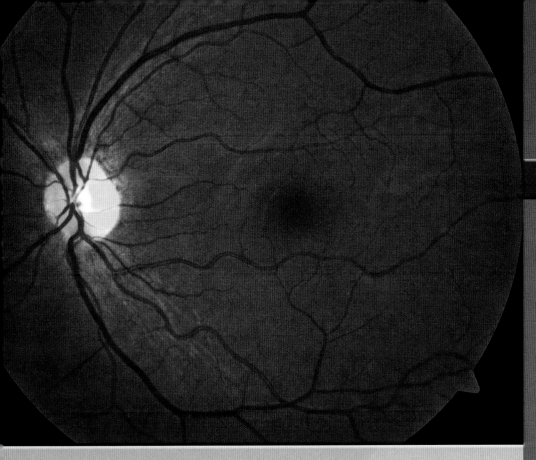

POSTERIOR SEGMENT
OF THE EYE

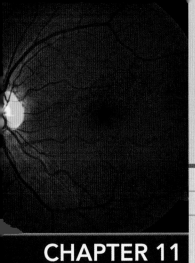

The Vitreous

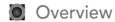 Overview

The vitreous body occupies approximately 75% to 80% of the total volume of the eye, filling the vitreous cavity between the lens and aqueous humor-filled posterior chamber, anteriorly, and the internal limiting membrane (ILM) of the retina, posteriorly. The vitreous is comprised of a clear core of viscoelastic gel (from Latin "vitrum," meaning glass) surrounded by an avascular, filamentous connective tissue envelope that encapsulates the gel and attaches the vitreous body to its surrounding ocular tissues **(Fig. 11.1)**. The vitreous gel in the adult emmetropic eye has an average volume of about 4.4 mL. The gel is two to three times more viscous than water, becoming more liquefied with age. Its refractive index is 1.335.[1,2] The vitreous provides structural support to the globe, retina, and lens. The semisolid nature of the gel matrix permits the vitreous to act as a shock absorber and to limit deformation of the delicate globe contents by blunt trauma.[3,4] The vitreous also plays an important role in modulating oxidative stress to the anterior segment of the eye, which is discussed in greater detail below.

Despite its biophysical complexity, the vitreous plays little, if any known biologically important, role in serving vision beyond its buffering capacity. The vitreous is removed routinely during intraocular surgery to permit

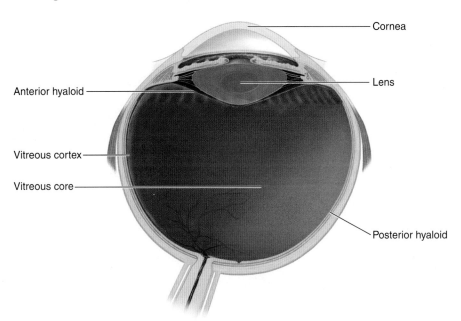

FIGURE 11.1 Cross-sectional view of the human eye depicting different substructures of the vitreous body. (From Tank PW, Gest TR, eds. *Lippincott Williams & Wilkins Atlas of Anatomy*. Philadelphia, PA: Wolters Kluwer; 2008.)

surgical access to the retina. The vitreous is replaced naturally by the aqueous humor, which fills the vitreous cavity once the anterior vitreous cortex has been resected. The aqueous-filled eye appears to sustain normal retinal function, and optical clarity without the formed vitreous.

Development of the Vitreous

The formation of the vitreous is described in detail in **CHAPTER 16: EMBRYOLOGY OF THE EYE AND ORBIT**. However, several important anatomic features of this unusual tissue require an embryologic context to understand fully and thus, an overview is provided here. Briefly, the vitreous body is of primarily neuroectodermal origin and develops in three stages, all of which make contributions to the final anatomy.

The primary vitreous is a syncytium through which a transient embryonic vascular bed develops to support the rapid growth and metabolic requirements of the lens during early development. The secondary vitreous is a Type II collagen and hyaluronate matrix that is secreted from the surface of the developing retina. As it grows, it compresses the primary vitreous inward, to the central axis of the vitreous body, surrounding the transient hyaloid artery that traverses the vitreous at that stage. The entire vitreous body is supported structurally by dense attachments, which straddle the anterior portion of the retina (the ora serrata) and the posterior region of the ciliary body. This area of attachment is known as the vitreous base.[5,6] The posterior surface of the vitreous is firmly adherent to the ILM of the retina in the region of the macula. This relationship and interface is an important source of vitreoretinal pathology. Later in development, the anterior portion of the vitreous, occupying the region between the ciliary body and the lens, condenses to form the tertiary vitreous, fine radially oriented fibrils connecting these two anterior structures. These fibers become the fibers of the lens zonules, which control focus and accommodation of the lens.

Macroscopic and Clinical Anatomy of the Vitreous

The vitreous body is attached to the other tissues of the eye by its surrounding envelope composed of a fine, filamentous matrix, termed variously the *hyaloid membrane* or *vitreous face*. Another term often used is the *vitreous cortex* but the term vitreous cortex includes both the hyaloid membrane and the outermost 100 to 200 μm of the vitreous gel (**Fig. 11.1**). The portion of the vitreous membrane that extends across the inside of the eye, parallel to the plane of the iris and posterior to the lens, is called the anterior vitreous face (also anterior hyaloid face). The portion that is attached to the inner surface of the retina and the edge of the optic nerve is termed the posterior vitreous face (also posterior hyaloid face). The division of the anterior and posterior faces occurs overlying the region of the ora serrata and is termed the vitreous base (**Fig. 11.2**). The attachments of these three main segments of the vitreous envelope are of clinical importance and are identified in **Figure 11.2** and described in detail below.

STRUCTURES RELATED TO THE ANTERIOR VITREOUS FACE

The principal attachment of the anterior vitreous face and its underlying cortex is termed the hyaloideocapsular ligament (also termed Wieger's ligament). This is a 1 to 2 mm

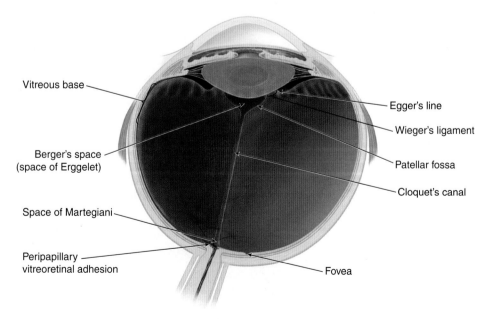

Vitreous base

Berger's space (space of Erggelet)

Space of Martegiani

Peripapillary vitreoretinal adhesion

Egger's line

Wieger's ligament

Patellar fossa

Cloquet's canal

Fovea

FIGURE 11.2 Vitreous anatomy and its sites of attachment: Berger's/Erggelet's space separating the anterior hyaloid face from the posterior lens capsule, within the limits of the hyaloideocapsular (Wieger's) ligament. The vitreous base, firmly adherent in the region of the pars plana and ora serrata, and attachment around the optic nerve are the other major attachments of the vitreous face. Cloquet's canal is the remnant of the primary vitreous and extends from the space of Martegiani overlying the optic nerve to Berger's space anteriorly. The patellar fossa is the portion of the anterior vitreous face within the confines of Wieger's ligament. (From Tank PW, Gest TR, eds. *Lippincott Williams & Wilkins Atlas of Anatomy*. Philadelphia, PA: Wolters Kluwer; 2008.)

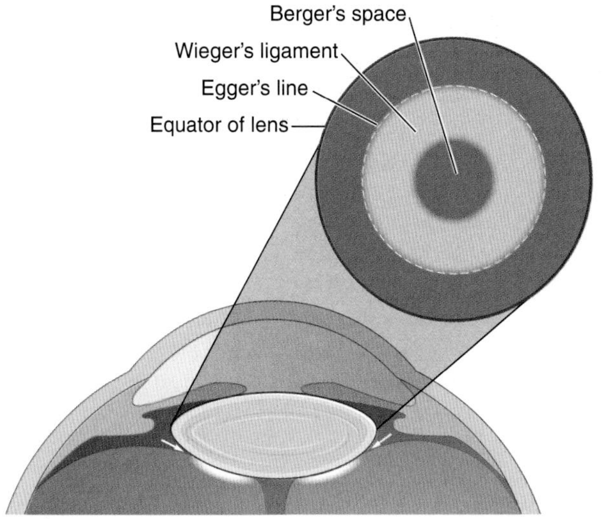

Berger's space
Wieger's ligament
Egger's line
Equator of lens

FIGURE 11.3 Drawing of the site of attachment of Wieger's ligament to the posterior lens capsule. The outer edge of Wieger's ligament is termed Egger's line.

wide ring of attachment of the anterior vitreous cortex to the posterior capsule of the lens (**Fig. 11.3**). The average diameter of Wieger's ligament is approximately 8 mm, in the adult eye. The peripheral edge of Wieger's ligament is termed Egger's line and this feature is visible in most adult eyes as an irregular, hazy ring on the posterior surface of the lens using a slit lamp biomicroscope. The orientation of the collagen fibrils of the hyaloideocapsular ligament is almost perpendicular to the lens capsule at Egger's line. In addition to the firm attachments of the anterior vitreous face to the posterior lens capsule, fine fibrillary remnants of the embryonic tertiary vitreous may connect the ciliary body to the anterior hyaloid membrane.

As the secondary vitreous is secreted, it compresses the primary vitreous and the remnants of the regressing hyaloid artery centrally, forming Cloquet's canal. The hyaloid vasculature is subsequently resorbed back to the surface of the optic nerve, leaving behind an S-shaped channel that runs from the posterior surface of the lens to the optic nerve. There are several additional anatomic landmarks related to the way in which Wieger's ligament attaches to the posterior surface of the lens. These include the patellar fossa of the anterior vitreous face and the retrolental space of Berger. The patellar fossa is the portion of the anterior vitreous face within the confines of Wieger's ligament. It is not attached to the lens. At this location, there is a potential space between the posterior lens capsule and the

The attachment of Wieger's ligament to the posterior lens capsule is very strong in children, nearly precluding removal of a congenital cataract without rupturing the anterior vitreous face in the days when the entire lens was removed. In older patients, the

attachment weakens significantly and often detaches making removal of the entire cataractous lens feasible. With modern intracapsular and phacoemulsification surgical methods, the lens capsule is left in situ and only the nuclear and cortical contents within the lens capsule are removed. Thus, in most modern cataract surgeries, this attachment between the lens capsule and the vitreous face is of less consequence to the outcome than it was in the past when the entire lens, including its capsule, had to be removed.

surface of the patellar fossa. This space is the retrolental space of Berger/Erggelet.

STRUCTURES RELATED TO THE POSTERIOR VITREOUS FACE

The posterior vitreous face makes fine, fibrillar attachments to the ILM of the retina (**Fig. 11.4**). Stronger attachments occur over the vessels in the macular region of the retina and around the edge of the optic nerve.[7] Remnants of the earliest stages of embryonic vitreous

As evidence of the stronger attachments of the posterior vitreous face to the macula and optic nerve, several examples of the vitreoretinal interface in pathologic conditions are shown in Figure 11.5. In younger patients, the posterior vitreous face is firmly attached to the ILM in the macula. An example of this firm attachment is shown in a patient who sustained a laser injury causing a hemorrhage in the left retina. The bleeding from the injury is sequestered between the ILM of the retina and the posterior hyaloid face, which can be seen to be tightly adherent to the macula. The firm attachment of the posterior vitreous face around the macula has not broken and thus the hemorrhage has been contained. However, distention of the posterior vitreous face has produced tension on the retina causing distortion of the ILM, which is evident as radial striae in the retina in the area surrounding the sequestered blood (Fig. 11.5A). Occasionally, firm attachments of the posterior hyaloid to the surface of the macula and in the retinal periphery are associated with mechanical distortion and forces that give rise to retinal injuries that manifest in a variety of ways. The firmer attachment of the posterior vitreous face to the macular region is clearly shown in the optical coherence tomography (OCT) image (Fig. 11.5B). The posterior vitreous face is detached from the retina except over the fovea, which has been distorted by the traction of the stronger vitreous attachment at this location.

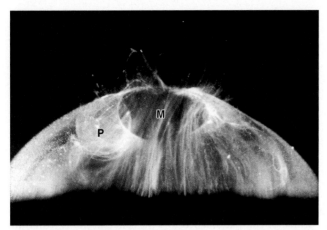

FIGURE 11.4 Vitreous fibers extending through holes in the prepapillary (*P*) and premacular (*M*) regions of the vitreous. These fibers are firmly attached to the internal limiting membrane over the macula. (From Sebag J, Balazs EA. Human vitreous fibers and vitreoretinal disease. *Trans Ophthalmol Soc UK*. 1985;104(pt 2): 123–128.)

 Because of the firm attachments of the vitreous body to its base overlying the peripheral retina, it is a common site of vitreoretinal pathology and the source of most rhegmatogenous ("rhegma," Greek for rent or rupture) retinal detachments. As the vitreous ages, it begins to separate from the retinal surface, but remains firmly attached at the posterior margin of the vitreous base. Traction in this area can create holes and tears in the retina, termed "horseshoe" tears, because of their shape. Horseshoe tears and the traction of the vitreous gel permit fluid to gain access to the subretinal space and commonly cause retinal detachment, a potentially blinding condition requiring surgical repair (**Fig. 11.7**).

development (**see Chapter 16: Embryology of the Eye and Orbit**) remain after the development of the eye is complete. These remnants (epipapillary gliosis) form the ring of attachment of the posterior vitreous face around the margin of the optic nerve, without attaching to the nerve itself. The space over the optic nerve head that is encompassed within this ring of attachment is the posterior terminus of Cloquet's canal, which extends through the vitreous from the optic nerve to the posterior surface of the lens via the space of Berger / Erggelet. The potential space over the optic nerve head is termed the space of Martegiani (**Fig. 11.3**).

The Vitreous Base

The vitreous base is the strongest attachment of the vitreous body to the wall of the eye. It is composed of dense collagen fibers creating a 3- to 4-mm-wide annular ring that straddles the ora serrata (the junction between the anterior limit of the retina and the pars plana portion of the ciliary body) (**Fig. 11.6**).[8] The vitreous base cannot be separated from its insertion except in rare cases of severe blunt trauma.

CHANGES IN THE VITREOUS WITH AGE

With increasing age, it is common for the posterior vitreous face to detach from the ILM of the retina. When this happens, the detached posterior vitreous face can be seen to sag forward and inferiorly during a clinical examination (**Fig. 11.8A**). In some instances, the ring of attachment to the margin of the optic nerve may remain intact, but in others, this ring detaches. In the latter case, a white fibrous ring is seen clinically, suspended anterior to the optic nerve. This finding is termed a Weiss ring (**Fig. 11.8B**). It is common for the traction at the edges of these vitreous detachments to tug on the retina, producing entoptic phenomena that patients report seeing "flashes of light." Condensations of degenerating vitreous collagen matrix also produce shadows upon the retina that patients describe as "floaters" in their visual field. Dilated retinal exams are in order in such cases to look for the detached posterior vitreous face and/or a Weiss ring to rule out the possibility that this traction has produced a retinal tear or rhegmatogenous retinal detachment.

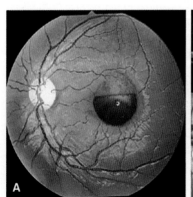
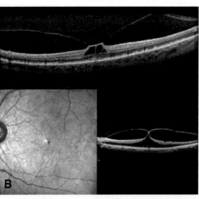

FIGURE 11.5 **A:** Fundus photograph of blood sequestered between the internal limiting membrane of the retina and the posterior hyaloid face. (From Shenoy R, Bialasiewicz AA, Bandara A, et al. Retinal damage from laser pointer misuse—case series from the military sector in Oman. *Middle East Afr J Ophthalmol.* 2015;22(3):399–403.) **B:** OCT images of the posterior vitreous face exerting traction over the fovea. Above, a plaque of traction is seen causing schisis of the inner retinal layers. Below, a focal point of traction in the fovea is seen en face (**left**) and in cross section (**right**). The focal vitreous attachment caused schisis in both the inner and outer retinal layers.

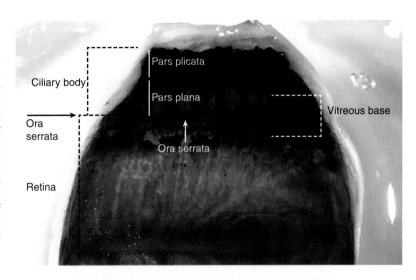

FIGURE 11.6 Sagittal section of the globe showing vitreous base anatomy. The vitreous base is a semitransparent substructure of the vitreous body located along the ora serrata (*white arrow*), which is the dividing line separating the ciliary body and retina (*along black dashed line indicated by black arrow*). The anterior border of the vitreous base extends over the pars plana of the ciliary body and the posterior border of the vitreous base extends 2 to 3 mm posterior to the ora serrata. The limits of the vitreous base are indicated by the area bracketed in white dashed lines. The pars plicata is the portion of ciliary body that contains the ciliary processes. (From Skeie JM, Mahajan, VB. Dissection of Human Vitreous Body Elements for Proteomic Analysis. *J Vis Exp.* 2011;47:e2455.)

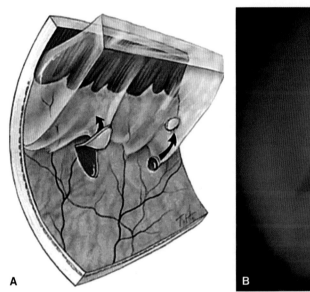

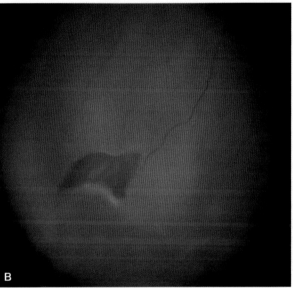

FIGURE 11.7 Drawing showing vitreous attachments (*arrows*) to a horseshoe tear and full thickness hole in the peripheral retina, creating a potential opening to the subretinal space (**A**). (From Connolly B, Regillo CD. In: Tasman WS, Jaeger EA, eds. Duane's Clinical Ophthalmology on CD-ROM. Philadelphia: Lippincott Williams and Wilkins, 2006.) Fundus photograph of a horseshoe tear in a patient with an underlying retinal detachment (**B**).

Appreciating the comparative strength and age-related changes in the degree of anatomic contact between the posterior vitreous cortex and the retina is essential. Vitreous detachments create traction on the retina and vitreous traction plays a central role in the pathogenesis and natural history of many important vision-threatening retinal diseases.[9–12]

Histology and Ultrastructure of the Vitreous Gel

The vitreous gel is composed primarily of water (~98% to 99%) that is bound within a hyaluronic acid (glycosaminoglycan) gel, supported by a matrix of glycoprotein-coated

In rhegmatogenous retinal detachments, particularly those associated with large tears or those that are chronic, retinal pigment epithelial (RPE) cells gain access to the vitreous cavity through the retinal opening. In such cases, the RPE cell can undergo an epithelial–mesenchymal transition. These cells become exposed to growth factors and inflammatory cytokines and begin to proliferate in the gel and on the surface of the retina to form contractile membranes. These membranes can exert significant mechanical force and traction on the relatively elastic retinal tissue and cause a tractional detachment of the retina. This condition, proliferative vitreoretinopathy (PVR), is the most common cause of failure of primary surgical repair of retinal detachments (Fig. 11.9).

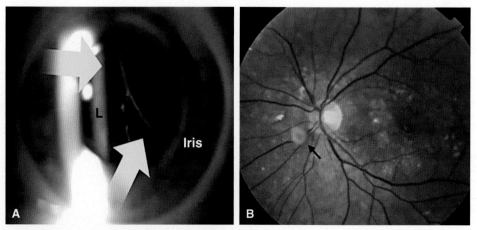

FIGURE 11.8   **A:** Slit lamp image of the vitreous showing collapse of the detached posterior vitreous face and vitreous gel (*yellow arrows*) behind the lens (*L*). **B:** Fundus photograph of a Weiss ring (*black arrow*) overlying the optic nerve in a patient with a posterior vitreous detachment and macular degeneration. (Courtesy of Dr. Michelle Steenbakkers.)

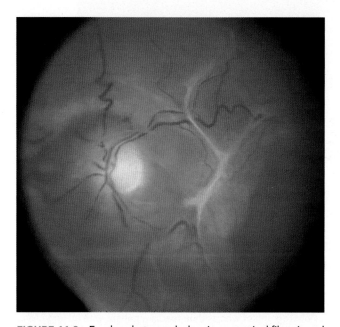

FIGURE 11.9   Fundus photograph showing preretinal fibrosis and a tractional retinal detachment of the left eye from scarring caused by proliferative vitreoretinopathy.

collagen fibrils approximately 6 to 16 nm in diameter. The most commonly identified proteoglycan is chondroitin sulfate.[8] Ninety percent of the vitreous collagen is Type II, organized into bundles, with smaller amounts of Types V/XI heterotrimers, and Type VI collagen. The Type II collagen fibrils are linked by thin connecting fibrils of Type IX collagen, whereas the surrounding hydrated matrix of hyaluronate keeps the fibrils separated (**Figs. 11.10** and **11.11**). This arrangement contributes to the transparency of this matrix and the hyaluronate coils give the vitreous its viscoelastic characteristics.[13,14] Other noncollagen structural proteins such as fibrillin-1 and opticin are also found. The structural proteins of the vitreous are found

more densely distributed in the vitreous cortex than in the central gel, as would be expected.

Additional proteins, glycoproteins, and amino acids are also found in the vitreous gel.[15] Most small molecules, like amino acids, are present in concentrations below that seen in plasma, but some, like ascorbate, are elevated, because of active transport mechanisms. As in the aqueous humor, elevated levels of ascorbate are presumed to play a role as oxygen and free-radical scavengers, antioxidants that protect the anterior segment and retina from oxidative stress coming from the highly vascularized choroid. The concentrations of smaller molecules are also essentially the same as those found in aqueous humor. This is not a surprise as the anterior vitreous face delimits the aqueous humor–filled posterior chamber and there is no diffusion barrier present at the aqueous/vitreous interface, in particular as the vitreous liquefies with aging.

There are very few cells in the central vitreous. A small complement of fibroblast-like cells is found in the vitreous cortex where the attachments of the vitreous to the retina are strongest. It is presumed that these cells participate in the very slow turnover of collagen in the gel. There is very little turnover of the other extracellular matrix components of the vitreous humor throughout adult life. There is, however, some evidence that the ciliary epithelium in the pars plana region of the ciliary body may contribute to the slow turnover of hyaluronate in the vitreous.[16,17] Additional vitreous cells, termed hyalocytes, are also found. Like the fibroblasts, these cells reside principally in the cortical region of the vitreous and are found in greatest numbers where the attachments of the posterior vitreous face are strongest (**Fig. 11.12**). Interestingly, hyalocytes are bone marrow–derived cells. They express the macrophage marker CD-64 (an Fc receptor) and are phagocytic, containing abundant lysosomes. They express S-100 proteins (commonly present in cells derived from the neural crest) but do not express proteins specific to retinal cell lineages

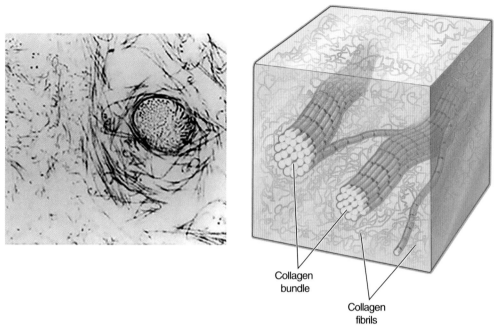

FIGURE 11.10 Electron micrograph and accompanying drawing of the microanatomy of collagen bundles and fibrils in the vitreous. The coiled material in the drawing represents the hyaluronic acid molecules. (From Sebag J. *The Vitreous: Structure, Function and Pathobiology.* New York, NY: Springer-Verlag; 1989.)

FIGURE 11.11 Scanning electron micrographs of the retinal surface in the posterior pole of the eye. The smooth internal limiting of the retina is seen (**A**) in contrast with the fibrillary collagen bundles and fibrils seen in the vitreous (**B**). (From Sebag J. *The Vitreous: Structure, Function and Pathobiology.* New York, NY: Springer-Verlag; 1989.)

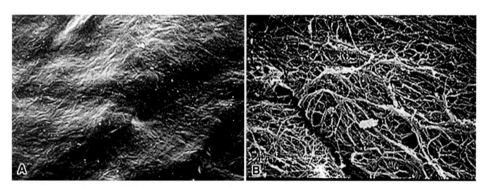

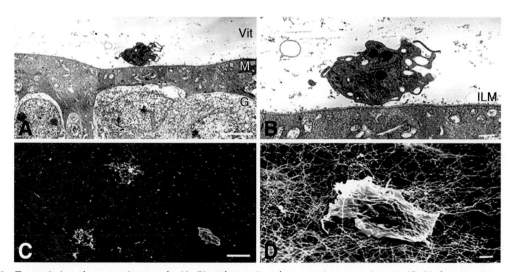

FIGURE 11.12 Transmission electron micrographs (**A, B**) and scanning electron microscopy images (**C, D**) showing vitreous hyalocytes at the internal limiting membrane (ILM) of the retina. M, Müller cell of internal limiting membrane; G, ganglion cell; Vit, vitreous. (From Qiao H, Hisatomi T, Sonoda K-H, et al. The characterization of hyalocytes: the origin, phenotype, and turnover. *Br J Ophthalmol* 2005;89:513–517.)

such as glial fibrillary acidic protein (Müller cells), or cellular retinaldehyde binding protein or cytokeratins (retinal pigment epithelium, RPE).[18,19] These cells have also been shown to be capable of synthesizing hyaluronate and they may contribute to a minimal turnover of the vitreous matrix. Hyalocytes have been shown to inhibit RPE cell proliferation and may help to prevent the development of PVR in the setting of retinal tears and detachments.[20]

Physical Chemistry of the Vitreous

The physical chemistry of the gel makes it highly viscous and sticky, resembling raw egg albumin in its characteristics and consistency (**Fig. 11.13**). Because the gel acts as a physiologic and metabolic buffer between the anterior segment of the eye and the retina, it also significantly limits the diffusion of topically applied drugs to the posterior segment.

The vitreous also provides a diffusion barrier to the movement of metabolites, cytokines, drugs, and components of the blood and aqueous which could adversely impact retinal function.[21–23] Similarly, it limits the anterior diffusion of oxygen from the choroid and retina, forward to the lens and other structures of the anterior segment of the eye that are potentially damaged by high levels of oxygen. This occurs in part through the barrier effect of the highly viscous gel and in part through the accumulation of ascorbate (vitamin C) in the vitreous gel, which acts to consume oxygen in an ascorbate-dependent chemical reaction.[24–26]

Although the retina and choroid are highly vascular and oxygenated tissues, the lens resides directly across the vitreous cavity and exists in a microenvironment that is only ~5% oxygen. Thus, the vitreous gel encompasses two very

distinct milieus with respect to oxygen concentrations and the low oxygen concentration behind the lens is maintained by the physiologic properties of the vitreous. Degeneration of the vitreous, either by age-related liquefaction ("syneresis") or by its removal during retinal surgery, increases the exposure of the anterior segment structures to higher oxygen levels coming from the choroid and retina both by decreasing vitreous ascorbate levels and by reducing oxygen consumption (**Fig. 11.14**). Thus, there are long-term consequences to the removal of the vitreous that may change the development and progression of pathologic conditions within the eye. In the absence of the natural diffusion barrier of the vitreous, oxygen delivery to the anterior segment, lens, and trabecular meshwork is significantly enhanced to tissues accustomed to functioning primarily via anaerobic metabolic pathways. Oxidative damage to proteins and lipids has been shown to increase the risk of formation of nuclear cataracts and the risk of glaucoma from oxidative damage to the trabecular meshwork.[27,28]

Degenerative Changes in the Vitreous Gel with Age

During the course of aging (and occurring at earlier ages in highly myopic eyes), the vitreous gel begins to liquefy through a process known as syneresis.[29,30] In this process, the water partitions from the hyaluronate complexes. Degeneration of the vitreous gel does not occur uniformly. Some areas liquefy earlier than others, resulting in the formation of optically empty pockets of liquefied vitreous, visible clinically as uniformly black lacunae. The liquefied gel in these lacunae coalesces with time and confers greater mobility of the vitreous body as a whole. This increased mobility can exert traction that is typically greatest just posterior to the vitreous base as described above. This traction is greatest in peripheral gaze and with lateral saccades.

Age-related partitioning of the water from the vitreous gel in syneresis is an important anatomic change. If there is a hole or tear in the retina, this fluid can access the subretinal spaces, leading to progressive retinal detachment. In the macular region, this liquid vitreous can gain access to the epiretinal/subcortical space via focal defects in the premacular vitreous cortex. With rotational eye movements, the liquid vitreous can dissect a plane between the vitreous cortex and the ILM of the retina. This results in cleavage and a posterior vitreous detachment (see **Fig. 11.8**). Conceptually, this can be modeled using a raw egg. If the egg is spun and stopped quickly, but then the finger used to the stop the rotation is quickly removed, the internal torque of the gelatinous albumin will start the egg spinning again. Similarly, the vitreous within the globe, having the same consistency, will continue to rotate after the eye stops, following an eye movement. This continued rotation of the vitreous within the eye can generate traction on the retina. This traction on the retina often gives rise to entoptic

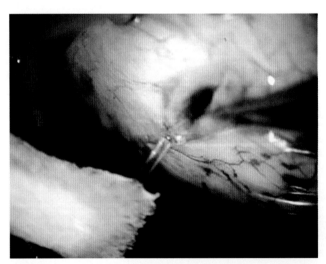

FIGURE 11.13 Intraoperative view of a scleral laceration (*dark opening*) showing the elastic nature of the prolapsed vitreous gel of the eye, extending to white swab at left.

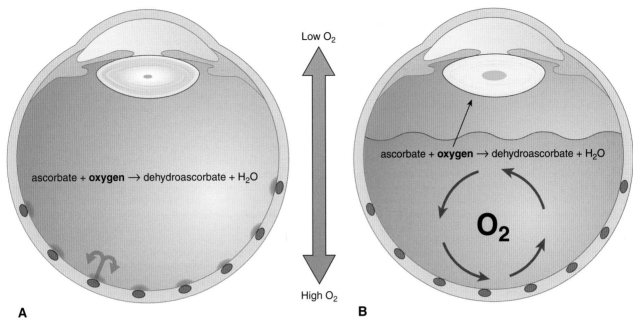

Low O$_2$

High O$_2$

ascorbate + **oxygen** → dehydroascorbate + H$_2$O

ascorbate + **oxygen** → dehydroascorbate + H$_2$O

A

B

FIGURE 11.14 **A:** Schematic demonstrating the oxygen and oxidant-buffering capacity of the vitreous gel and the changes that occur following vitrectomy. **B:** Removal of the vitreous gel permits oxygen from the choroid to permeate more easily to the anterior segment where it can cause cataract formation and glaucoma as a result of increased levels of oxidative stress.

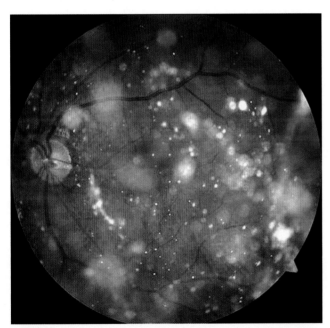

FIGURE 11.15 Asteroid hyalosis of the vitreous gel. Calcium oxalate and hydroxyphosphate precipitates in the vitreous present to the practitioner as glistening, refractile bodies within the gel. The patient is usually asymptomatic.

Degenerative changes in the vitreous gel are commonly associated with aging and occasionally with genetic conditions such as amyloidosis and inborn errors of collagen metabolism. Conditions such as Marfan syndrome, Ehlers–Danlos, and Wagner and Stickler's syndromes are associated with severe vitreous liquefaction when vitreoretinal adherence to the retina is strong. This association results in a high incidence of retinal tears and detachments in this group of patients.[31]

that precipitate in the vitreous as glistening, yellowish beads. These are easily seen on examination because of the refractile, sparkling appearance for which they are named, like asteroids in the night sky (**Fig. 11.15**). The deposits of asteroid hyalosis can be so dense as to virtually obscure the view of the retina. Despite this fact, the patient is commonly completely asymptomatic and visual acuity is unchanged.[33] In patients with severe asteroid hyalosis, the retina can be imaged through the vitreous opacities using fluorescein angiography.

REFERENCES

1. Girach A, Pakola S. Vitreomacular interface diseases: pathophysiology, diagnosis and future treatment options. *Expert Rev Ophthalmol.* 2012;7(4):311–323.
2. Locke JC, Morton WR. Further studies of the viscosity of aspirated human vitreous fluid: with special reference to its use in retinal detachment surgery. *Trans Am Ophthalmol Soc.* 1965;63:129–145.
3. Schepens CL, Neetens A. *The Vitreous and Vitreoretinal Interface.* New York, NY: Springer Science & Business Media; 1987.

phenomena causing the patient to see "flashes of light," typically when making quick lateral movements of the eyes.

One common form of degeneration that typically occurs unilaterally (75%) is asteroid hyalosis.[31,32] Asteroid hyalosis results from the formation of calcium oxalate monohydrate and calcium hydroxyphosphate soaps and phospholipids

4. Balazs EA, Denlinger J. The vitreous. In: Davson H, ed. *The Eye.* Vol IA. London, UK: Academic Press; 1984:533.

5. Balazs E, Denlinger J. The vitreous. In: Davson H, ed. *The Eye.* Vol IA. London, UK: Academic Press; 1972:32–42.

6. Hogan MJ, Alvarado JA, Weddell J. *Histology of the Human Eye: An Atlas and Textbook.* Philadelphia, PA: WB Saunders; 1971.

7. Sebag J, Balazs E. Morphology and ultrastructure of human vitreous fibers. *Invest Ophthalmol Vis Sci.* 1989;30(8):1867–1871.

8. Hogan MJ. The vitreous, its structure, and relation to the ciliary body and retina proctor award lecture. *Invest Ophthalmol Vis Sci.* 1963;2(5):418–445.

9. Streeten B. Disorders of the vitreous. In: Gamer A, Klintworth GK, eds. *Pathobiology of Ocular Disease—A Dynamic Approach.* New York, NY: Dekker; 1982(part B):1381–1419.

10. Sebag J, Balazs EA. Human vitreous fibres and vitreoretinal disease. *Trans Ophthalmol Soc UK.* 1985;104(pt 2):123–128.

11. Kakehashi A. Age-related changes in the premacular vitreous cortex. *Invest Ophthalmol Vis Sci.* 1996;37(3):2253–2253.

12. Foos RY. Vitreoretinal juncture; topographical variations. *Invest Ophthalmol.* 1972;11(10):801–808.

13. Sebag J. *The Vitreous: Structure, Function and Pathobiology.* New York, NY: Springer-Verlag; 1989.

14. Bishop PN. Structural macromolecules and supramolecular organisation of the vitreous gel. *Prog Retin Eye Res.* 2000;19(3):323–344.

15. Swann DA, Constable IJ. Vitreous structure I distribution of hyaluronate and protein. *Invest Ophthalmol.* 1972;11(3):159–163.

16. Halfter W, Sebag J, Cunningham E. Vitreoretinal interface and inner limiting membrane. In: Sebag J, ed. *Vitreous—In Health and Disease.* New York, NY: Springer; 2014:165–191.

17. Haddad A, De Almeida JC, Laicine EM, et al. The origin of the intrinsic glycoproteins of the rabbit vitreous body: an immunohistochemical and autoradiographic study. *Exp Eye Res.* 1990;50(5):555–561.

18. Lazarus HS, Hageman GS. In situ characterization of the human hyalocyte. *Arch Ophthalmol.* 1994;112(10):1356–1362.

19. Qiao H, Hisatomi T, Sonoda KH, et al. The characterisation of hyalocytes: the origin, phenotype, and turnover. *Br J Ophthalmol.* 2005;89(4):513–517.

20. Schonfeld CL. Hyalocytes inhibit retinal pigment epithelium cell proliferation in vitro. *Ger J Ophthalmol.* 1996;5(4):224–228.

21. Fatt I. Hydraulic flow conductivity of the vitreous gel. *Invest Ophthalmol Vis Sci.* 1977;16(6):565–568.

22. Scott JE. The chemical morphology of the vitreous. *Eye.* 1992;6(6):553–555.

23. Nickerson CS, Karageozian HL, Park J, et al. Internal tension: a novel hypothesis concerning the mechanical properties of the vitreous humor. *Macromol Symp.* 2005;227(1):183–190.

24. Holekamp NM, Shui YB, Beebe DC. Vitrectomy surgery increases oxygen exposure to the lens: a possible mechanism for nuclear cataract formation. *Am J Ophthalmol.* 2005;139(2):302–310.

25. Siegfried CJ, Shui Y, Holekamp NM, et al. Oxygen distribution in the human eye: relevance to the etiology of open-angle glaucoma after vitrectomy. *Invest Ophthalmol Vis Sci.* 2010;51(11):5731–5738.

26. Filas BA, Shui Y, Beebe DC. Computational model for oxygen transport and consumption in human vitreous. *Invest Ophthalmol Vis Sci.* 2013;54(10):6549–6559.

27. Shui Y, Holekamp NM, Kramer BC, et al. The gel state of the vitreous and ascorbate-dependent oxygen consumption: relationship to the etiology of nuclear cataracts. *Arch Ophthalmol.* 2009;127(4):475–482.

28. Beebe DC, Holekamp NM, Siegfried C, et al. Vitreoretinal influences on lens function and cataract. *Philos Trans R Soc Lond B Biol Sci.* 2011;366(1568):1293–1300.

29. Balazs EA, Denlinger JL. Aging changes in the vitreous. In: Sekuler R, Kline D, Dismukes K, eds. *Aging and Human Visual Function. Vol 2: Modern Aging Research.* New York, NY: Alan R Liss; 1982:45–57.

30. Jongebloed WL, Worst JE. The cisternal anatomy of the vitreous body. *Doc Ophthalmol.* 1987;67(1/2):183–196.

31. Snead MP, Yates JR. Clinical and molecular genetics of stickler syndrome. *J Med Genet.* 1999;36(5):353–359.

32. Mitchell P, Wang MY, Wang JJ. Asteroid hyalosis in an older population: the Blue Mountains Eye Study. *Ophthalmic Epidemiol.* 2003;10(5):331–335.

33. Kador PF, Wyman M. Asteroid hyalosis: pathogenesis and prospects for prevention. *Eye.* 2008;22(10):1278–1285.

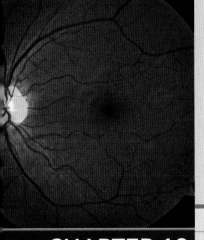

Choroid and Choroidal Circulation

Overview

The blood supply to the choroid is distinct from the more visible retinal circulation, and functionally provides critical nutrients and oxygen to the metabolically demanding photoreceptors and retinal pigment epithelium (RPE). To do this the choroid circulates ~500 to 2,000 mL of blood/min/100 g of tissue, rivaling the blood flow rate in the kidney.[1] Beyond meeting the high metabolic demand of the outer retina, one additional explanation for the high choroidal blood flow is to help regulate the temperature of the retina by serving as a heat sink. Photons that miss the photoreceptor discs are absorbed by the RPE and choroidal stromal melanocytes. The heat generated in this process is absorbed by the large volume of fast-moving choroidal blood and rapidly dissipated from the eye.[2]

Macroscopic and Clinical Anatomy of the Choroid and Choroidal Vasculature

The choroid (from "chorion," Greek for membrane) constitutes the posterior aspect of the uveal tract in the eye. It forms a dense vascular network between the inner surface of the sclera and the retina, which is continuous with the vasculature of the ciliary body, anterior to the ora serrata, and continues posteriorly to the optic nerve. It is composed of a spongy, layered system of progressively smaller blood vessels, residing within a pigmented, fibrocellular matrix.

The ophthalmic artery provides the blood supply to the choroid via branches of the posterior and anterior ciliary arteries (ACAs) (SEE CHAPTER 3: OVERVIEW OF THE EYE). Among its various branches, the ophthalmic artery gives rise to the large medial and lateral posterior ciliary arteries. Each posterior ciliary artery gives rise, in turn, to one long posterior ciliary artery (LPCA), and a variable number of short posterior ciliary arteries (SPCAs, ~15 to 20) (Fig. 12.1). Both contribute to the vascular supply of the choroid.

The SPCAs are divided into two groups termed paroptic and distal. The paroptic SPCAs enter the sclera as a ring around the optic nerve (~10 to 20 vessels).[3] Two additional clusters of vessels, termed the distal SPCAs, enter lateral and medial to the entry of the ring of paroptic vessels. The paroptic SPCAs contribute to the vascular supply of the optic nerve head, the peripapillary choroid, and anastomose with vessels of the pia mater, surrounding the optic nerve. It is the two clusters of distal SPCAs that ramify to supply most of the choroid posterior to the equator, including the choriocapillaris in this region (SEE CHAPTER 3: OVERVIEW OF THE EYE).

The two LPCAs, one medial and one lateral, enter the eye at a shallow angle, outside the ring of SPCAs. Once they have reached the inner surface of the sclera, they are clinically visible as they track anteriorly in the suprachoroid, along the horizontal equator of the eye (Fig. 12.2). The LPCAs anastomose with the ACAs in the ciliary body, forming the major arterial circle of the iris (Fig. 12.1). The ACAs arise as branches from the blood supplies of the four rectus muscles (Fig. 12.1). Recurrent branches from this anterior circulation supply the choroid anterior to the equator of the eye. Additional contributions come

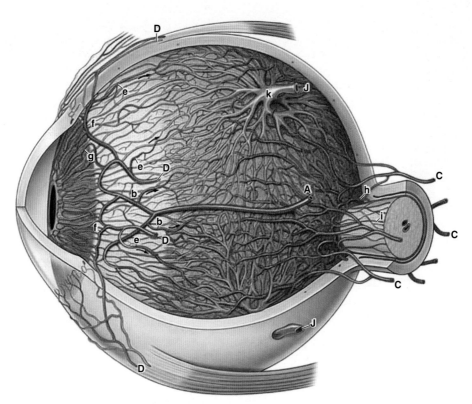

FIGURE 12.1 Drawing of the uveal blood supply. The blood supply of the choroid is derived from the long (LPCAs) and short posterior ciliary arteries (SPCAs). There are two LPCAs, one entering the uvea nasally and one temporally along the horizontal meridian of the eye (*A*). These two arteries give three to five branches (*b*) at the ora serrata. On the temporal side, branches from the LPCA pass directly back to supply the choroid anterior to the vertical equator (*b*). The SPCAs (two set of vessels termed *distal SPCAs*) enter the choroid lateral and medial optic nerve (*C*). They divide rather rapidly to form the posterior choriocapillaris that nourishes the retina as far anteriorly as the equator. This system of capillaries is continuous with recurrent vessels from the ciliary body that are derived from the LPCAs (*b*). The anterior ciliary arteries (*D*) pass forward from the rectus muscles then pierce the sclera to enter the ciliary body. Before joining the major circle of the iris, they give off 8 to 12 branches (*e*) that pass back through the ciliary muscle to join the anterior choriocapillaris. The major circle of the iris (*f*) lies in the pars plicata region of the ciliary body and sends branches posteriorly into the ciliary body as well as forward into the iris (*g*) and limbus. Some branches also join the episcleral system of vessels. The circle of Zinn–Haller (*h*) is formed by the paraoptic SPCAs that join pial branches (*i*). The circle lies in the sclera and furnishes part of the blood supply to the optic nerve and disc. These vessels also serve the pia mater surrounding the optic nerve (*i*). The vortex veins exit from the eye through the posterior sclera (*J*) after forming ampullae (*k*) in the deep choroid. (From Hogan MJ, Alvarado JA, Weddell JE, eds. *Histology of the Human Eye: An Atlas and Textbook.* Philadelphia, PA: WB Saunders; 1971:326.)

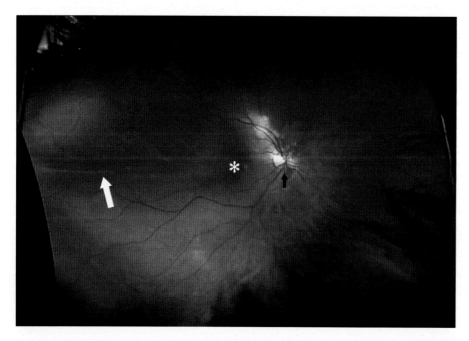

FIGURE 12.2 Wide-angle view of the retinal fundus showing one of the long posterior ciliary arteries (and nerve) entering the eye along the horizontal equator (*white arrow*). These vessels traverse the sclera at an oblique angle and once they reach the inner surface of the sclera, they are clinically visible as they track anteriorly in the suprachoroid. The optic nerve (*black arrow*) and macula (*asterisk*) are seen in the posterior pole. (Modified from Optos website. http://www.optos .com. 2016. Accessed January 18, 2017.)

from branches of the anterior and long posterior ciliary arteries, before they join the major circle of the iris. In addition, the temporal LPCA provides a recurrent branch that contributes to the blood supply of a wedge of choroid extending anteriorly from the point where the vessel emerges from its intrascleral emissary canal.[4,5] Additional details of

Due to the paucity of vessels traversing the sclera in the anterior choroid, the choroid is less firmly adherent to the sclera in this area. This lack of adherence creates the potential for significant accumulation of blood and fluid (hemorrhages/effusions) from disease or damaged choroidal vessels. This is particularly true for patients with hypertension and other vasculopathies. The absence of significant autoregulation of perfusion pressure in the choroid (see further discussion, below) puts the eye at risk of vision-threatening complications during surgery. The sudden decompression of the eye that occurs when the eye is entered during surgery is sometimes associated with the acute development of choroidal effusions and expulsive choroidal hemorrhage. A photographic montage of a choroidal effusion, based in the anterior periphery of the fundus, is shown (Fig. 12.3A). The posterior pole of the eye is normal in appearance but as one moves toward the temporal periphery, a large choroidal effusion is seen (right of dividing line in retinal photograph), bowing inward in that quadrant. The retina remains attached to the RPE and both bulge inward due to expansion of the choroid. Thus, this is a choroidal effusion not a retinal detachment. An axial MRI image of a choroidal effusion in the right eye of a patient is also shown, with opposing bullous separations of the retina from the wall

of the eye due to massive swelling of the choroidal tissue (Fig. 12.3B). Note the relatively more anterior location of the effusion in the temporal periphery. These bullous effusions are sometimes large enough to bring the opposing retinal surfaces together in the mid-vitreous cavity. Such cases are termed "kissing choroidals."

these vascular connections are presented in **CHAPTER 3: OVERVIEW OF THE EYE**.

Despite the entrance of the SPCAs around the optic nerve, the pattern of vascular filling in the choroid is not from back to front. The architecture of the arterial and venous circulation in the posterior choroid is lobular (**Fig. 12.4**).[6,7] The SPCAs pass through the choroidal stroma and branch widely to supply a central arteriolar branch for each lobule of the choriocapillaris. Each lobule receives arterial blood almost simultaneously from a vessel reaching it at its center. In this way, each individual lobule fills from its center to its periphery.

The lobules are functionally end arterioles with a segmental distribution.[8] The consequence of this pattern is the presence of watershed zones. Unlike most tissues, the arterial and venous vessels of the choroid do not parallel each other, except in the far periphery.[9] Rather, venous blood from each lobule is collected at the periphery of the adjoining lobules and drains rapidly through a dense plexus of low resistance venules that anastomose to form larger vessels closer to the sclera (in Sattler's and Haller's layers, discussed below). These veins ultimately converge on several ampullae, focal dilations of venous vessels that drain into the vortex veins. An average of seven ampullae are present per eye. This convergence of vessels toward an

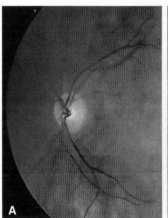
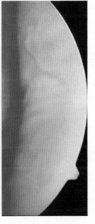
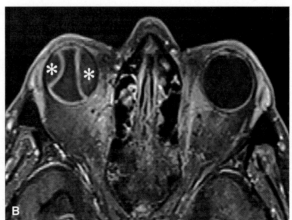

FIGURE 12.3   **A:** Photographic montage of a choroidal effusion, based in the anterior periphery is shown. The posterior pole of the eye is normal in appearance (left color image in **[A]**), but a large anterior choroidal effusion is seen bulging into the vitreous cavity on the right of the color image with a dark shadow at its edge. (Courtesy of Dr. Sarwat Salim. In Reddy AC, Salim S. Diagnosis and Management of Choroidal Effusions. *Eyenet*. 2012). **B:** An MRI image of a patient with multiple choroidal effusions in the right eye is also shown. There are opposing bullous effusions (*asterisks*). Note the relatively more anterior location of the effusion in the temporal periphery. (Case courtesy of Dr Charlie Chia-Tsong Hsu, Radiopaedia.org. From Chia-Tsong Hsu C. Ora serrata—retinal versus choroidal detachment. *Raidopaedia.org website.* http://radiopaedia.org/cases/ora-serrata-retinal-versus-choroidal-detachment. 2016. Accessed January 18, 2017.)

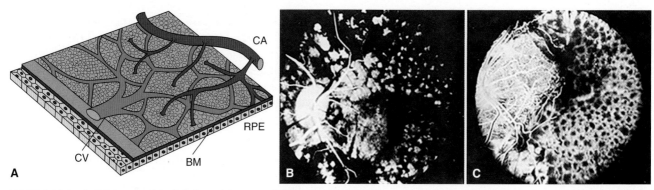

FIGURE 12.4 **A:** Schematic of the lobular architecture of the choroidal vessels and choriocapillaris **(left)** as seen from the choroidal side of Bruch's membrane (BM). Each lobule has a central filling choroidal arteriole (CA) and network of draining choroidal venules (CV); thus, each individual lobule fills from its center and drains from its periphery. (Modified from Alfaro DV, Kerrison JB. *Age-Related Macular Degeneration.* 2nd ed. Philadelphia, PA: Wolters Kluwer; 2014.) A fluorescein angiogram in a primate retina showing pattern of choroidal lobular arterial filling **(B)** and venous drainage **(C)** of the lobules. RPE, retinal pigment epithelium. (From Ryan SJ, ed. Retina. *Basic Science and Inherited Disease.* Vol 1. St. Louis: Mosby; 1994:78.)

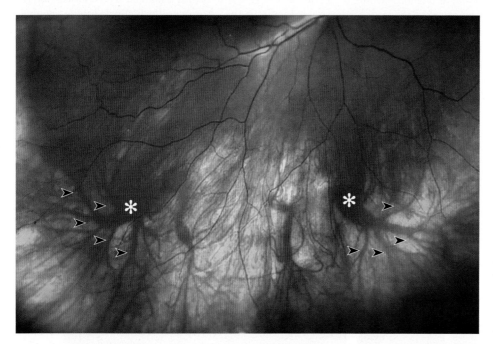

FIGURE 12.5 Wide-angle view of the retina showing some of the many branches of the choroidal veins (*arrowheads*) draining into the vortex veins (*asterisks*) in two quadrants of the fundus image. (Modified from Recognizing pathology, vortex veins and blonde fundus. Optos website. http://www.optos.com. 2016. Accessed January 19, 2017.)

ampulla exhibits a vorticeal pattern, giving the vortex veins their name **(Fig. 12.5)**. Usually four vortex veins exit the sclera posterior to the vertical equator, with one vortex vein from each quadrant of the eye, though there may be more.

 Common anatomic variants of the choroidal blood supply include cilioretinal arteries, which arise from the choroidal circulation but supply the circulation of the inner retina between the optic nerve and variable portions of the macula. These vessels typically arise near the temporal edge of the optic nerve (Fig. 12.6A). Such "aberrant" vessels can preserve central vision in what would otherwise be a blinding event, (e.g., in the case of an occlusion of the central retinal artery). The images in Figure 12.6B, left and right, show a central retinal artery occlusion of the right

eye. The almost totally infarcted retina in Figure 12.6B, left is milky in appearance (black arrow). However, due to the presence of two cilioretinal arteries (yellow arrow), a segment of the central and superior macula has preserved blood flow that includes the upper half of the fovea, and appears relatively normal. The fluorescein angiogram (Fig. 12.6B, right) demonstrates the preserved arterial blood flow provided to the central and superior macula in this patient (yellow arrow). The remainder of the retina is dark and non-perfused. Because of the cilioretinal artery, the portion of the retina between the optic nerve and the macula remains viable and a small wedge of good vision is preserved. Conversely, occlusion of cilioretinal arteries can cause central macular infarction in the absence of damage to the remaining retina.

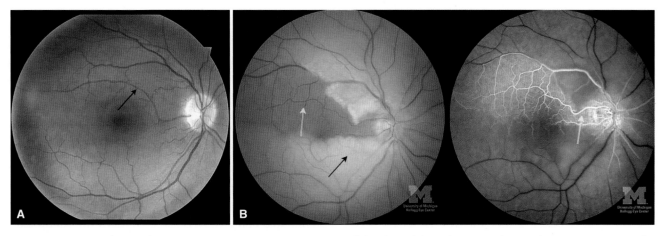

FIGURE 12.6   **A:** Cilioretinal arteries are common anatomic variants of the choroidal circulation. A cilioretinal artery is seen near the temporal margin of the optic nerve head (*arrow*), providing blood supply to the macular region. **B:** The images in the *left* and *right* show a central retinal artery occlusion of the right eye. The almost totally infarcted retina in the *left* figure is milky in appearance (*black arrow*). However, due to the presence of two cilioretinal arteries, a segment of the central and superior macula has preserved blood flow (*yellow arrow*). The fluorescein angiogram (*right*) demonstrates the preserved arterial blood flow provided to the macula in this patient (*yellow arrow*). (Courtesy of the University of Michigan Kellogg Eye Center Image Archive [Case 79] and RetinaDx website. http://kellogg.umich.edu/retinadx/retina_cases/79/photos.html. June 27, 2008. Accessed October 20, 2016.)

WATERSHED ZONES

From in vivo angiographic studies of choroidal vascular anatomy, it appears that the vascular fields served by each of the LPCAs do not freely anastomose. They instead behave as end arteries with little capacity for collateral flow between their respective vascular fields. These findings contrast with studies examining vascular casts in which free communication appears to occur.[10]

In **Figure 12.7** note the bright appearance of the temporal choroid, indicating that intravenously injected fluorescent dye is filling the portion of the choroid served by the lateral LPCA. In contrast, note the dark appearance of the choroid served by the nasal LPCA, indicating no blood flow in this portion of the choroid as a result of medial LPCA occlusion.[8] It is argued that if the choroidal vasculature was a freely anastomosing system of vessels, such significant differences in the anatomic distribution of blood flow should not occur. There is marked variability in the area and proportion of the choroid served by the lateral and medial LPCAs, but in almost all cases, perfusion of the entire choroid from only one of the LPCAs is not observed.

As an anatomic concept, the border between two non-anastomosing vascular fields is termed a "watershed zone." The functional significance of watershed zones is that tissues residing in these areas lie at the very end of the vascular fields that are served by each of the vessels that meet in that zone. As such, these tissues are at greatest risk of ischemic injury if blood flow is compromised in either vessel. The location of the watershed zone between lateral and medial LPCAs in the human eye is commonly a vertical band that can vary in location from temporal to the optic nerve head to a point nasal to the optic nerve.

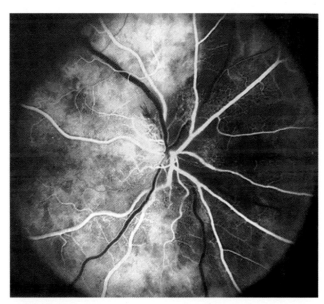

FIGURE 12.7   Watershed areas in the choroidal circulation. The temporal choroid, served by the temporal, long posterior ciliary artery (LPCA), is filled with fluorescent dye in this image. In contrast, the dark appearance of the choroid served by the medial LPCA demonstrates no blood flow as a result of medial LPCA occlusion. (From Hayreh SS. Interindividual variation in blood supply of the optic nerve. Its importance in various ischemic disorders of the optic nerve head, and glaucoma, low-tension glaucoma and allied disorders. *Doc Ophthalmol.* 1985;59:217–246.)

Alternatively, it may fall right through the optic nerve head. Note the vertical band of poor dye perfusion (vertical dark band) delineating the watershed zone, between the portions of the choroid served by the lateral and medial LPCAs, in an eye with limited perfusion of both vessels (**Fig. 12.8**).[11]

*Clinically, it is also apparent that there are few, if any, free anastomoses between the drainage fields of the vortex veins. Because of this, if there is obstruction of one vortex vein, blood draining from the quadrant of that vortex vein cannot readily shift its flow pattern to leave the eye from another of the vortex veins. This gives rise to choroidal effusions that appear localized to one quadrant or a portion of one quadrant (**Fig. 12.9**). Controversy remains on the extent to which the lack of anastomoses is absolute but the anatomic evidence supporting the independence of these zones is strong.*

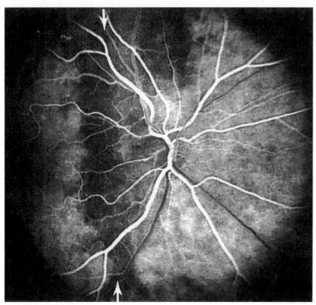

FIGURE 12.8 Watershed areas in the choroidal circulation. The location of the watershed zone between lateral and medial long posterior ciliary arteries in the human eye is commonly a vertical band. Note the vertical dark band of poor perfusion delineating the watershed zone in this eye in which there is limited perfusion by both vessels (*arrows*). (From Hayreh SS. In vivo choroidal circulation and its watershed zone. *Eye*. 1990;4:273–289.)

Histology of the Choroid

The choroid is highly vascular in nature and, as with the overlying retina, the choroid is thickest in the macular area (250 µm). The choroid thins significantly in its periphery (100 µm) and the overall thickness of the choroid declines with normal aging.[12,13] Because the purpose of the choroid is to deliver a large volume of fast-moving blood to a single layer of capillaries underlying the retina, vessels of different calibers reside in different layers. The largest vessels are those closest to the sclera. These progressively bifurcate into smaller vessels until they finally produce a uniform, single layer of capillaries beneath the RPE. Histologically, the choroid is traditionally divided into five layers based

largely upon the size of the vessels in each layer. It is important to appreciate that these various layers of vessels all reside within a pigmented connective tissue stromal matrix. From external to internal, these layers are:

- Suprachoroid (suprachoroidal space)
- Haller's layer of large vessels
- Sattler's layer of medium vessels
- Choriocapillaris
- Bruch's membrane

SUPRACHOROID

The suprachoroid is a potential space with a thin layer of pigmented connective tissue (~30 µm), internal to the lamina fusca, the pigmented and elastic inner layer of the sclera. It represents a transitional zone in which large vessels that have penetrated the sclera undergo rapid branching to give rise to the vessels of the choroidal stroma. The cells of the suprachoroid, like those of the lamina fusca, are primarily comprised of melanocytes, fibroblasts, and intrinsic, peripheral nervous system ganglion cells (primarily nitrous oxide [NO] and vasoactive intestinal peptide [VIP] signaling), embedded in a collagen and elastin fiber matrix. The choroid is most firmly attached to the sclera at the sites of entry of the SPCAs and the exit points of the vortex veins, posterior to the vertical equatorial of the eye. This explains the greater distensibility of the anterior choroid as mentioned earlier.

*The choroid is a pigmented tissue due to the presence of melanocytes in the choroidal stroma and lamina fusca of the sclera. Congenital, focal concentrations of pigmented cells, termed choroidal nevi, are commonly seen in clinical practice (4.6% to 7.9% in Caucasians). They should be noted, but they rarely cause complications or vision loss. Nonetheless, nevi must be monitored because they can undergo transformation into malignant choroidal melanomas even though the annual rate of malignant transformation of nevi is very low (~1 in 9,000 patients) (**Fig. 12.10**).[14] A common nevus (**A**) and choroidal melanoma (**B**) are shown. The difference in appearance between the flat, benign lesion and the three-dimensional mass of the melanoma is evident. Identifying transition of a nevus into melanoma can be more challenging.*

HALLER'S LAYER OF LARGE VESSELS AND SATTLER'S LAYER OF MEDIUM VESSELS

Internal to the suprachoroid are two major layers of vessels, both larger than capillaries. Closest to the sclera is Haller's layer of large vessels and between Haller's layer and the single layer of choroidal capillaries are the medium-sized vessels of Sattler's layer (**Fig. 12.11**). Haller's layer comprises the

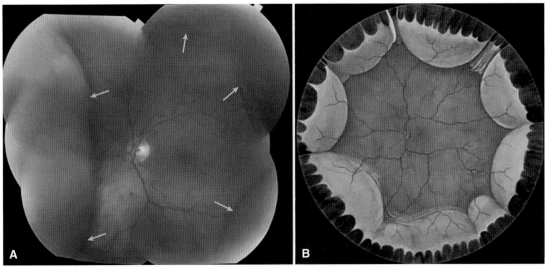

FIGURE 12.9 Absence of anastomoses between the drainage fields of the vortex veins. Blood draining from each vortex vein is restricted to that region and cannot readily drain to other quadrants to leave the eye via a different vortex vein. This gives rise to choroidal effusions that appear localized to one quadrant or a portion of one quadrant, with a scalloped appearance in retinal periphery (**A**, *arrows*). (From Choroidal Detachment. http://www.retinareference.com/. 2016. Accessed October 20, 2016.) An illustration showing the typical appearance of anterior choroidal effusions (**B**). **B:** Drawing of choroidal effusions resulting from reduced flow in vortex veins. (From Kanski J. Clinical Ophthalmology: A Systematic Approach. Philadelphia, PA: Elsevier, 2007.)

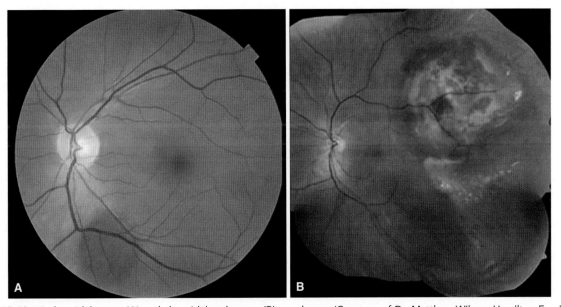

FIGURE 12.10 A choroidal nevus (**A**) and choroidal melanoma (**B**) are shown. (Courtesy of Dr. Matthew Wilson, Hamilton Eye Institute, Memphis, TN.)

large arteries traversing the suprachoroid, which quickly branch into the medium caliber vessels of Sattler's layer. The large veins that coalesce in a swirl pattern to converge on the ampullae of the vortex veins also reside in Haller's layer. Sattler's layer provides the feeding arterioles that terminate in the capillary lobules of the choriocapillaris (**Fig. 12.12**). The vascular walls of the larger vessels in the choroidal stroma are not fenestrated.

The stromal matrix surrounding the vascular elements of the choroid includes melanocytes, fibroblasts, mast cells, macrophages, and various cells of inflammatory lineage in a sparse collagenous matrix.[15] As with the suprachoroid, nerve fibers and neural ganglion cells are also present. Innervation of the choroid is discussed in detail later in this chapter.

CHORIOCAPILLARIS

The choriocapillaris is the functional capillary bed of the choroid, upon which the avascular outer retina, including the photoreceptors and RPE, are dependent. As noted

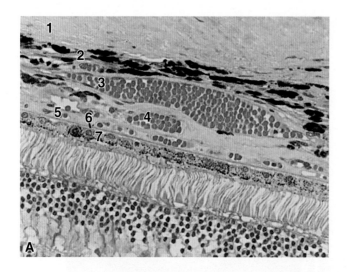

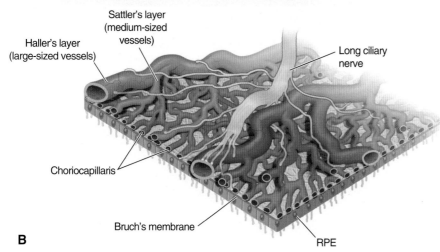

FIGURE 12.11 Vascular layers of the choroid. **A:** Histologic section (hematoxylin/eosin). (*1*) Sclera; (*2*) suprachoroid (lamina fusca) (note abundant melanocytes in the stroma of this layer and throughout the choroid); (*3*) large-sized vessel layer (Haller's layer); (*4*) medium-sized vessel layer (Sattler's layer); (*5*) choriocapillaris; (*6*) Bruch's membrane; (*7*) retinal pigment epithelium (RPE). **B:** 3D rendition of vascular layering in the choroid. RPE, retinal pigment epithelium. (**A:** © 2012 Ramírez JM, Salazar JJ, de Hoz R, Rojas B, Gallego BI, Ramírez AI, Triviño A. Choroidal vessel wall: hypercholesterolaemia-induced dysfunction and potential role of statins. Published in Haruo Sugi H, ed. Current Basic and Pathologic Approaches to the Function of Muscle Cells and Tissues—From Molecules to Humans under CC BY 3.0 license. Available from: http://dx.doi.org/10.57772/4779.)

earlier, the architecture of the choriocapillaris is arranged as lobules. These lobules are anatomically and functionally separate and form a mosaic of independently functioning neurovascular units served by the central arteriole of each lobule, arising in Sattler's layer. This arteriole is surrounded by a plexus of venules. The diameter of the lobules increases in size as one moves anteriorly, from the macula toward the equator. Vascular cast studies of the venous plexi suggest that the lobular anatomy converts to a more spindle-shaped, linear configuration and then a laddering pattern as one moves anteriorly, closer to the peripheral retina.[9] The low venous resistance draining the lobular and other configurations of the capillary plexi encourages rapid flow into and out of the draining venules. Note that the lobules of the choriocapillaris terminate at the margin of the optic nerve. Thus, the nerve does not receive any of its blood supply from the choriocapillaris and is dependent upon the paroptic SPCA circulation described above.

There are no anastomoses seen between adjacent lobules in the macular region, creating the potential for watershed areas at risk of ischemic injury to the overlying retina in this region. Whether the remainder of the choriocapillaris exhibits small, focal watershed areas remains uncertain. Mitigating against the potential negative impact of watershed areas of flow in the choriocapillaris is the fact that under normal conditions, blood flow far exceeds the amount required to meet the high metabolic requirements of the RPE and retinal photoreceptors. Additionally, the reduction in oxygen saturation between the arterial and venous sides of the choriocapillary beds is only a few percent, far less than the extraction of oxygen that occurs between the arterial and venous ends of capillaries in most other tissues. Thus, it would seem that the inherent risk of ischemia within the capillary beds in this highly oxygenated environment should be very low.

Histology and Ultrastructure of the Choriocapillaris

The capillaries of the choriocapillaris are among the largest in the body, measuring some 20 to 50 μm in diameter, thus allowing multiple red blood cells to pass simultaneously. By comparison, the luminal diameter of the average

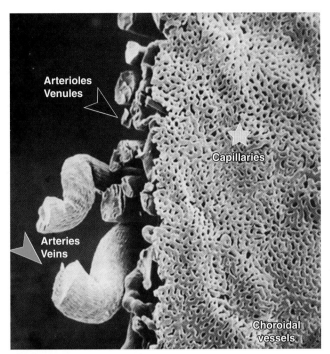

FIGURE 12.12 Corrosion cast of a cut face of the choroid seen by scanning electron microscopy. Image of the choroidal circulation showing the three vascular layers in the choroid: large-sized vessels of Haller's layer (*blue arrowhead*) and medium-sized vessels of choroid (*red arrowhead*) (Sattler's layer), and choriocapillaris that underlies Bruch's membrane and the retinal pigment epithelium (*yellow star*). (Modified from Zhang HR. Scanning electron-microscopic study of corrosion casts on retinal and choroidal angioarchitecture in man and animals. *Prog Ret Eye Res.* 1994;13:243–270.)

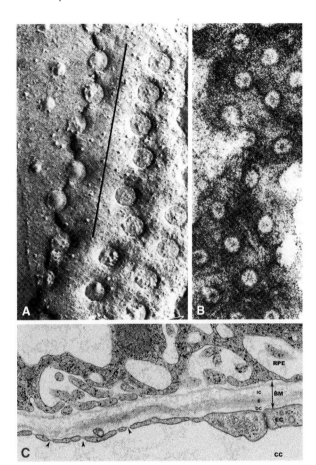

FIGURE 12.13 Fenestrated endothelium of a choroidal capillary. **A:** Freeze-fracture replica. Prominent diaphragms bridging the fenestrae show a smooth surface (**left of black line**). In the shadow area, small particles are present (**right of black line**). **B:** En-face thin section transmission electron micrograph showing central thickenings in the majority of diaphragms. **C:** Cross section transmission electron micrograph of interface between basal processes of retinal pigment epithelium (RPE) and fenestrations (*arrowheads*) of choriocapillary endothelium (EC). Separating the RPE and choriocapillary (CC) is Bruch's membrane (BM). Clearly evident are the inner (IC) and outer (OC) collagenous layers and the elastic layer (E). (**A,B:** From Reale ME. Fracture faces of fenestrations and junctions of endothelial cells in human choroidal vessels. *Invest Ophthalmol.* 1975;14(2):98–107. **C:** © 2012 Ramírez JM, Salazar JJ, de Hoz R, Rojas B, Gallego BI, Ramírez AI, Triviño A. Choroidal vessel wall: hypercholesterolaemia-induced dysfunction and potential role of statins. Published in Haruo Sugi H, ed. Current Basic and Pathologic Approaches to the Function of Muscle Cells and Tissues—From Molecules to Humans under CC BY 3.0 license. Available from: http://dx.doi.org/10.57772/47794.)

intraretinal capillary is approximately 6 μm (slightly smaller than the 7 μm average diameter of a red blood cell). These choriocapillaries are fenestrated, but not around their entire circumference.[16] Circular fenestra are present only on the surface facing Bruch's membrane where they are copiously distributed, except where endothelial cells overlap one another (**Fig. 12.13**). These 800 Å diameter fenestrations are closed by a very thin diaphragm and are readily observed with freeze-fracture and transmission electron microscopy (**Fig. 12.13**). This large complement of fenestrations permits the rapid diffusion of fluid, oxygen, glucose, and macromolecules into the choroidal stroma and Bruch's membrane, to provide adequate nutritional support to the metabolically active photoreceptors and adjacent RPE. But, as noted in **CHAPTER 13: THE RETINAL PIGMENT EPITHELIUM**, the macromolecules leaked through these fenestrations are prevented from nonspecific diffusion into the sensory retina by tight junctions that join the apico-lateral surfaces of the RPE cells.

BRUCH'S MEMBRANE

Bruch's membrane is a thin (~2 to 4 μm) compound basement membrane complex enveloping layers of collagen and elastin between the basement membranes of the

The fenestrations present in the walls of the choroidal capillaries permit the passive leakage of small molecules and even proteins from these vessels. This normal leakage is readily identified clinically following intravenous injection of fluorescent indocyanine green (ICG). The long wavelength fluorescent dye absorption and emission spectrum of ICG ranges from 600 to 950 nm. This absorption and fluorescence emission range creates an essentially transparent window through the RPE for viewing deeper biologic tissues in a way that fluorescein does not. Using ICG thus permits the clinical *visualization of the choroidal vasculature despite the over-lying layer of densely pigmented RPE cells (**Fig. 12.14**). This dye can also be used to probe the integrity of abnormal blood vessels arising from the choroid and seen growing under the macula to identify exudative ("wet") age-related macular degeneration.*

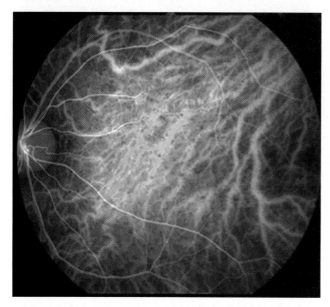

FIGURE 12.14 Indocyanine green angiography image of the choroidal vasculature. The independent retinal and choroidal circulations, with the thinner retinal vessels converging on the optic nerve head, are seen in the image.

choriocapillaris and that of the RPE. The ultrastructure of Bruch's membrane is comprised of five layers (**Figs. 12.13C** and **12.15**).

1. Basement membrane of choriocapillary endothelium
2. Outer collagenous layer
3. A discontinuous elastic layer
4. Inner collagenous layer
5. Basement membrane of the RPE

Choriocapillary endothelial cells do not form a uniform layer on the outer surface of Bruch's membrane. This creates windows for intercapillary columns of choroidal stroma to make direct attachments to Bruch's membrane, between the adjacent capillaries. As such, the surface of Bruch's membrane facing the choroidal capillaries is irregular. By contrast, the surface of Bruch's membrane facing the basal surface of the RPE cells is more uniform, providing for the attachment of the complex basal infoldings of the retinal pigment epithelial cells and for precise alignment of this tightly spaced monolayer of cells (**Fig. 12.15**).

Collagen fibrils within the inner and outer collagenous layers underlying the macula contain collagen types I, III, and V. Type IV and type VI collagens are present in the basement membrane of the choriocapillaris but appear to be absent from the basement membrane of the RPE, suggesting that they may play a specific role in anchoring the choriocapillaris. Type IV collagen is primarily responsible for the thickening of Bruch's membrane seen in age-related macular degeneration.[17,18] The inner and outer collagenous zones of Bruch's membrane are comprised of loosely organized collagen fibers, including types I, II, and V. These collagen fibers are surrounded by an extracellular matrix of proteoglycans and glycosaminoglycans, principally chondroitin and dermatan sulfates. The outer collagenous

The elastic layer of Bruch's membrane is very dense (and elastic) thus creating a strong and resilient structural barrier between the choroidal vessels and the overlying retina. As such it is

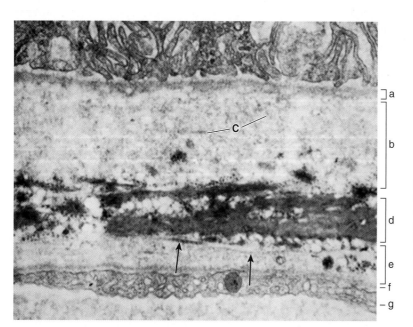

FIGURE 12.15 Electron micrograph of Bruch's membrane (BM). Basal processes of retinal pigment epithelial cell at top. (*a*) Basement membrane of retinal pigment epithelium (RPE); (*b*) anterior collagenous (C) layer; (*d*) elastic layer; (*e*) posterior collagenous layer; (*f*) basement membrane of choriocapillary endothelium; (*g*) choriocapillary endothelium. *Arrows* show integration of elastic fibers and collagen fibers. (From Hogan MJ, Alvarado JA, Weddell JE. *Histology of the Human Eye.* Philadelphia, PA: WB Saunders; 1971:333.)

remarkably effective in containing cellular infiltrates and tumors, inhibiting their access to the retina. Breaks in Bruch's membrane, from an array of causes, can predispose patients to the development of pathologic choroidal neovascularization, leading to the growth of aberrant blood vessels underneath the RPE and retina. Active secretion of angiogenic growth factors like vascular endothelial growth factor (VEGF) by the RPE help to maintain the choriocapillaris, but are balanced by anti-angiogenic growth factors such as pigment epithelial-derived factor, which sustain a homeostatic balance between physiologic vasculogenesis and pathologic angiogenesis. Breaks in Bruch's membrane alter this balance. As one example, breaks in Bruch's membrane that lead to abnormal growth of vessels from the choroid into the subretinal space occurs commonly in exudative ("wet") macular degeneration (Fig. 12.16). These new, leaky vessels can give rise to significant visual distortion and eventual vision loss. This same response can also occur in any condition in which defects in Bruch's membrane occur, including high myopia ("lacquer cracks" leading to a "Fuchs spot"), inherited defects in elastic tissue formation (Ehlers–Danlos and pseudoxanthoma elasticum), and traumatic injury to the membrane ("choroidal rupture"), to name a few.

layer is about half the thickness of the inner layer (0.7 vs. 1.5 μm). Between the inner and outer collagenous layers is an elastic layer, which is similar in thickness to the outer collagenous layer. This layer is comprised of layers of elastin fibers, which become more discontinuous near the anterior limit of this layer. This elastic layer extends from the edge of the optic nerve all the way to the pars plana.

◉ Innervation of the Choroid

Autoregulation is a reflexive physiologic process in which vessels automatically change their caliber to maintain flow, when the pressure difference between the inside and outside of the vessel is changed. Unlike the retinal vasculature in which blood flow is modulated by autoregulation, the choroidal blood flow is under autonomic control and is not believed to be autoregulated to any meaningful degree. The smooth muscle cells in the walls of the larger choroidal arteries (i.e., Haller's and Sattler's layers) exhibit dense innervation by both sympathetic and parasympathetic fibers. The choroidal circulation is controlled primarily by its sympathetic innervation and to a lesser degree by the parasympathetics.

The long and short ciliary nerves generally follow the paths of the long and SPCAs as they enter the eye. Upon

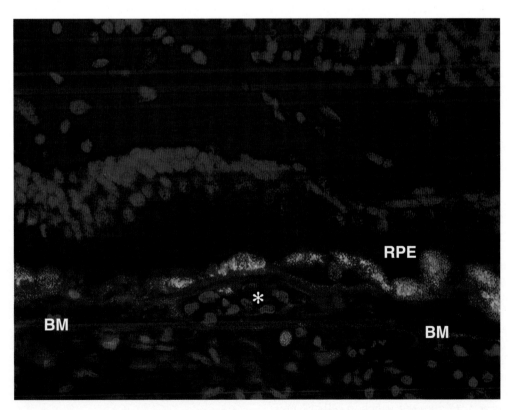

FIGURE 12.16 Pathologic choroidal neovascularization. An abnormal blood vessel from the choroid (*asterisk*) is seen between Bruch's membrane (BM) and the layer of retinal pigment epithelium (RPE) cells. This condition is associated with exudative ("wet") macular degeneration but can also be seen in other conditions such as retinal scarring and polypoidal choroidal vasculopathy. (From Milam A. *The Human Retina in Health and Disease Teaching Set.* © Scheie Eye Institute, University of Pennsylvania; 2016.)

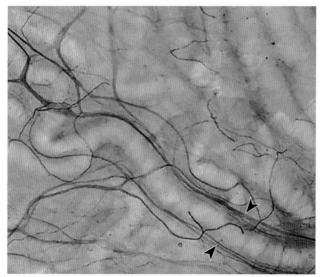

FIGURE 12.17 Human choroidal whole mount. Darkly stained nerve fibers attached to the choroidal vasculature (paravascular fibers) are seen lying parallel to the large arteries (*arrowheads*). The vessels are shown lighter than their surround due to their lack of blood and the more pigmented stroma surrounding each vessel. (From Triviño A, De Hoz R, Salazar JJ, et al. Distribution and organization of the nerve fiber and ganglion cells of the human choroid. *Anat Embryol (Berl)*. 2002;205:417–430.)

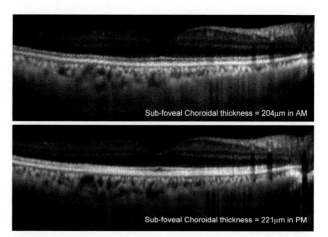

FIGURE 12.18 Optical coherence tomography image showing a diurnal rhythm to the thickness of the choroid in a normal patient. (From Toyokawa N, Kimura H, Fukomoto A, et al. Difference in morning and evening choroidal thickness in Japanese subjects with no chorioretinal disease. *Ophthalmic Surg Lasers Imaging*. 2012;43(2):109–114.)

traversing the thickness of the sclera, both sets of nerves enter the suprachoroidal space. From here they ramify, freely branching and anastomosing to form dense perivascular plexi (**Fig. 12.17**).[19] These plexi are formed at all levels of the choroidal stroma except for the choriocapillaris.[20] Neurovascular units are found on both vascular structures and nonvascular smooth muscle throughout the stroma.[21,22] Sympathetic stimulation causes choroidal vasoconstriction and a fall in intraocular pressure from a reduction in the ocular blood volume due to the stimulation of α-adrenergic receptors in the vascular smooth muscles.[23,24]

The postganglionic sympathetic fibers entering the choroid arise from the superior cervical ganglion. These noradrenergic neurons terminate on the blood vessels and mediate vasoconstriction. These fibers have also been shown to innervate nonvascular smooth muscle cells and intrinsic choroidal neurons (ICNs).[25] In mammals, the parasympathetic input to the choroid originates from the pterygopalatine ganglion and follows the same pathway as the fibers destined for the lacrimal gland (**SEE CHAPTER 1: THE ORBITS**) to reach the eye via the zygomatic branch of the maxillary division of the trigeminal nerve.[26]

ICNs are also found and are present mostly in the choroidal layers near the suprachoroid.[19] These fibers are predominantly cholinergic and are rich in the vasodilators vasoactive intestinal peptide (VIP) and nitric oxide (NO). As many as 2,500 nitrergic ganglion cells are present in the human choroid.[27] The functions of the ICNs remain unknown but their role in blood flow regulation is strongly suggested by their site of action (arterial walls)

and their secretion of the potent vasodilator, NO.[28,29] These neurons may be analogous to the intrinsic neurons in the enteric nervous system which function locally to integrate mechanical and thermal stimuli. They have also been suggested to act as intermediaries in the sympathetic system between the postganglionic neurons and smooth muscle in order to modulate their tone. Age-related decline in VIP-secreting neurons may play a role in dysregulation of choroidal blood flow seen with aging.[30]

There is an evolutionarily conserved diurnal rhythm to the thickness of the choroid (**Fig. 12.18**). Nonvascular smooth muscle cells in the choroidal stroma are thought to play a role in this diurnal variation and also in response to retinal defocus, which induces growth of the maturing choroid and sclera and has been proposed as a mechanism for refractive-induced myopia.[31–33] Acute changes in choroidal thickness also produce transient elevations of intraocular pressure. Animal models of refractive-induced myopia have shown that the process is under local control in the retina, that is, it does not require communication with the visual cortex.[34] The implication of these findings is that the choroid

 The thickness of the choroid has also been implicated in a new class of choroidal vascular diseases, termed pachychoroid spectrum disorders, which have been described in patients with features of central serous retinopathy and neovascular forms of macular degeneration.[35,36] These conditions are characterized by increased choroidal thickness on optical coherence tomography imaging (diffuse or focal), dilation of outer choroidal vessels, and attenuation and thinning of the choriocapillaris and the middle choroidal vessels overlying these dilated "pachyvessels."

is capable of producing growth-modulating molecules in response to visual input. Mechanisms regulating choroidal thickness and homeostatic control of refractive error will likely have an impact on understanding the causes of, and potential treatments for, myopia.

REFERENCES

1. Friedman E, Kopald HH, Smith TR, et al. Retinal and choroidal blood flow determined with krypton-85 anesthetized animals. *Invest Ophthalmol Vis Sci.* 1964;3(5):539–547.
2. Parver LM. Temperature modulating action of choroidal blood flow. *Eye.* 1991;5(2):181–185.
3. Hayreh SS. Posterior ciliary artery circulation in health and disease: the Weisenfeld Lecture. *Invest Ophthalmol Vis Sci.* 2004;45(3):749–757.
4. Weiter JJ, Ernest JT. Anatomy of the choroidal vasculature. *Am J Ophthalmol.* 1974;78(4):583–590.
5. Hayreh SS. The long posterior ciliary arteries. *Albrecht von Graefes Arch Klin Ophthalmol.* 1974;192(3):197–213.
6. Torczynski E, Tso MO. The architecture of the choriocapillaris at the posterior pole. *Am J Ophthalmol.* 1976;81(4):428–440.
7. Fryczkowski AW. Anatomical and functional choroidal lobuli. *Int Ophthalmol.* 1994;18(3):131–141.
8. Hayreh SS. Choroidal circulation in health and in acute vascular occlusion. *Int Ophthalmol.* 1976:157–170.
9. Yoneya S, Tso MO. Angioarchitecture of the human choroid. *Arch Ophthalmol.* 1987;105(5):681–687.
10. Araki M. Observations on the corrosion costs of the choriocapillaries [in Japanese]. *Nippon Ganka Gakkai Zasshi.* 1976;80(6):315–326.
11. Hayreh SS. In vivo choroidal circulation and its watershed zones. *Eye.* 1990;4(2):273–289.
12. Yoneya S, Tso MO, Shimizu K. Patterns of the choriocapillaris. *Int Ophthalmol.* 1983;6(2):95–99.
13. Ito YN, Mori K, Young-Duvall J, et al. Aging changes of the choroidal dye filling pattern in indocyanine green angiography of normal subjects. *Retina.* 2001;21(3):237–242.
14. Singh AD, Kalyani P, Topham A. Estimating the risk of malignant transformation of a choroidal nevus. *Ophthalmology.* 2005;112(10):1784–1789.
15. Bron A, Tripathi R, Tripathi B. *Wolff's Anatomy of the Eye and Orbit.* 8th ed. London: Chapman & Hall Medical; 1997.
16. Raviola G. The structural basis of the blood-ocular barriers. *Exp Eye Res.* 1977;25:27–63.
17. Marshall GE, Konstas AG, Reid GG, et al. Collagens in the aged human macula. *Graefe's Arch Clin Exp Ophthalmol.* 1994;232(3):133–140.
18. Sebastian R, Manuel J, Salazar Corral JJ, et al. Choroidal vessel wall: hypercholesterolaemia-induced dysfunction and potential role of statins. *InTech.* 2012. doi:10.5772/47794.
19. Castro-Correia J. Studies on the innervation of the uveal tract. *Ophthalmologica.* 1967;154(5):497–520.
20. Feeny L, Michael M. Electron microscopy of the human choroid, part I, II and III. *Am J Ophthalmol.* 1961;51:1057–1097.
21. Schrödl F, De Laet A, Tassignon M, et al. Intrinsic choroidal neurons in the human eye: projections, targets, and basic electrophysiological data. *Invest Ophthalmol Vis Sci.* 2003;44(9):3705–3712.
22. Schrödl F, Bergua A, Brehmer A, et al. Nonvascular smooth muscle as a main target for intrinsic choroid neurons in duck. *Exp Eye Res.* 1998;67:78.
23. Bill A, Sperber G. Control of retinal and choroidal blood flow. *Eye.* 1990;4(2):319–325.
24. Alm A, Bill A. Ocular and optic nerve blood flow at normal and increased intraocular pressures in monkeys (macaca irus): a study with radioactively labeled microspheres including flow determinations in brain and some other tissues. *Exp Eye Res.* 1973;15(1):15–29.
25. Triviño A, De Hoz R, Salazar JJ, et al. Distribution and organization of the nerve fiber and ganglion cells of the human choroid. *Anat Embryol.* 2002;205(5/6):417–430.
26. Ruskell G. Facial parasympathetic innervation of the choroidal blood-vessels in monkeys. *Exp Eye Res.* 1971;12(2):166–172.
27. Flügel C, Tamm ER, Mayer B, et al. Species differences in choroidal vasodilative innervation: evidence for specific intrinsic nitrergic and VIP-positive neurons in the human eye. *Invest Ophthalmol Vis Sci.* 1994;35(2):592–599.
28. Flügel-Koch C, May C, Lütjen-Drecoll E. Presence of a contractile cell network in the human choroid. *Ophthalmologica.* 1996;210(5):296–302.
29. Schrödl F, Schweigert M, Brehmer A, et al. Intrinsic neurons in the duck choroid are contacted by CGRP-immunoreactive nerve fibers: evidence for a local pre-central reflex arc in the eye. *Exp Eye Res.* 2001;72(2):137–146.
30. Jablonski MM, Iannaccone A, Reynolds DH, et al. Age-related decline in VIP-positive parasympathetic nerve fibers in the human submacular choroid. *Invest Ophthalmol Vis Sci.* 2007;48(2):479–485.
31. Brown JS, Flitcroft DI, Ying G, et al. In vivo human choroidal thickness measurements: evidence for diurnal fluctuations. *Invest Ophthalmol Vis Sci.* 2009;50(1):5–12.
32. Poukens V, Glasgow BJ, Demer JL. Nonvascular contractile cells in sclera and choroid of humans and monkeys. *Invest Ophthalmol Vis Sci.* 1998;39(10):1765–1774.
33. Toyokawa N, Kimura H, Fukomoto A, et al. Difference in morning and evening choroidal thickness in Japanese subjects with no chorioretinal disease. *Ophthalmic Surg Lasers Imaging.* 2012;43(2):109–114.
34. Marzani D, Wallman J. Growth of the two layers of the chick sclera is modulated reciprocally by visual conditions. *Invest Ophthalmol Vis Sci.* 1997;38(9):1726–1739.
35. Gallego-Pinazo R, Dolz-Marco R, Gómez-Ulla F, et al. Pachychoroid diseases of the macula. *Med Hypothesis Discov Innov Ophthalmol.* 2014;3(4):111–115.
36. Dansingani KK, Balaratnasingam C, Naysan J, et al. En face imaging of pachychoroid spectrum disorders with swept-source optical coherence tomography. *Retina.* 2016;36(3):499–516.

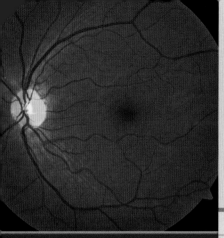

CHAPTER 13

The Retinal Pigment Epithelium

Overview

The retinal pigment epithelium (RPE) plays a central role in maintaining the health and function of the retina, especially the avascular outer retinal layers containing the photoreceptor cell bodies and inner and outer segments of these cells. Its functions include: (1) recycling and regeneration of visual pigment from the overlying rods and cones; (2) phagocytosis and digestion of the photoreceptor outer segment disc packets that are shed daily; (3) active transport of metabolites between the retina, subretinal space, and choriocapillaris; (4) absorption of stray light and heat in the retina by abundant melanin pigment granules; (5) secretion of the interphotoreceptor cell matrix; and (6) formation and maintenance of the outer blood–retinal barrier.

Histology of the Retinal Pigment Epithelium

The RPE is a confluent epithelial monolayer situated between the outer segments of the retinal photoreceptors and the choriocapillaris (**Fig. 13.1**). There are 4 to 6 million RPE cells in each eye. In an en face view, the RPE appears as a uniform array of hexagonal cells with centrally placed nuclei (**Fig. 13.2**). The cobblestone morphology of RPE cells differs between the macula and the retinal periphery

and this difference reflects important functional and protective features in the regional specialization of the RPE. As one moves away from the macula, toward the retinal periphery, the cells become larger, increasing in diameter from an average of 15 μm to approximately 60 μm. Also, toward the retinal periphery, RPE cells become flatter and less cuboidal. Despite these variations, the ratio of photoreceptor cells to RPE cells remains relatively constant. This layer of cells extends from the border of the optic nerve head to the ora serrata, where the RPE becomes continuous with the pigmented epithelium of the ciliary body (**Fig. 13.3**).

*Although the RPE is generally uniform in appearance, focal very dark areas of congenital hypertrophy of the retinal pigment epithelium (CHRPE) are a fairly common finding. CHRPE typically presents as a solitary lesion with sharp, scalloped edges that often develop central lacunae of retinal atrophy (**Fig. 13.4**). Heavily pigmented areas contain hypertrophic RPE cells whereas depigmented areas are atrophic with RPE cells containing cytoplasmic vacuoles and a few small melanosomes.[1,2] There is a known association between a form of CHRPE, typically multiple lesions with a "bear-track" appearance, and patients with Gardner syndrome, a familial intestinal polyposis that carries a high risk of colon cancer.*

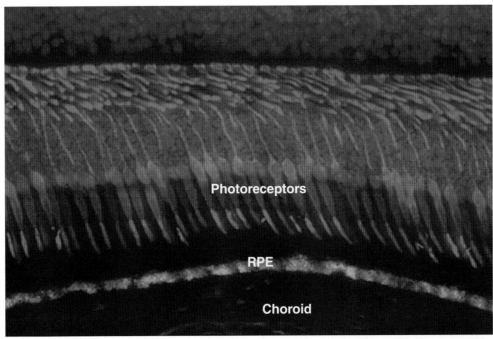

FIGURE 13.1   Confocal micrograph of the retina and retinal pigment epithelium (RPE). The photoreceptor cells overlie a monolayer of pigmented, autofluorescent RPE cells situated between the photoreceptors and the choroid. The dense melanin pigment in the unstained RPE cells is evident. (From Milam A. The Human Retina in Health and Disease Teaching Set. © Scheie Eye Institute, University of Pennsylvania. 2016.)

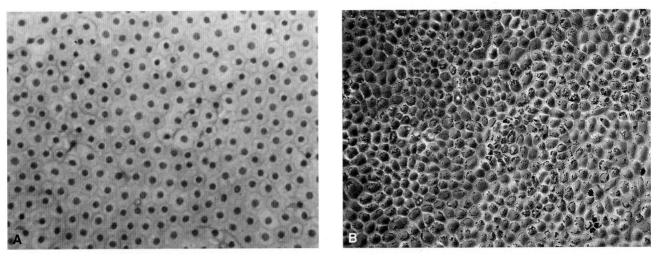

FIGURE 13.2   **A:** En face light micrograph of hexagonal array of retinal pigment epithelial cells. **B:** At lower magnification, a monolayer of RPE-derived cells is seen in tissue culture. The hexagonal shape, melanin granules, and tightly adherent growth characteristics are maintained in vitro. (Courtesy of Tim Blenkinsop and the Neural Stem Cell Institute, Rensselaer, NY.)

Polarized RPE Cell Anatomy and Function

The RPE cell is polarized, both in morphology and in function, and demonstrates highly specialized apical and basal membranes and differing cytoplasmic domains. The apical portion of these cells exhibits numerous, long microvilli and the apical cytoplasm exhibits numerous phagosomes, containing lamellar-appearing material that represents phagocytosed photoreceptor discs. Along the apico-lateral membrane of these cells a junctional complex is present, consisting of a zonula occludens, a zonula adherens, and numerous gap junctions. Desmosomes are also present along the lateral membrane, basal to the junctional complex. The central portion of the cytoplasm contains its round nucleus, numerous melanosomes, and lipofuscin granules. Lipofuscin is a yellowish, autofluorescent material that accumulates with age in lysosomes of neurons, retinal pigment epithelial cells, and cardiac myocytes.[3]

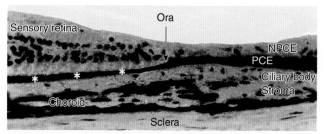

FIGURE 13.3   Light micrograph of the RPE cell layer in the region of the ora serrate (Ora). The RPE cell layer (*asterisks*) is contiguous with the pigmented ciliary epithelium (PCE) anterior to the ora serrata. The thinned cell layers of the neurosensory retina terminate at the ora and become continuous with the nonpigmented ciliary epithelium (NPCE).

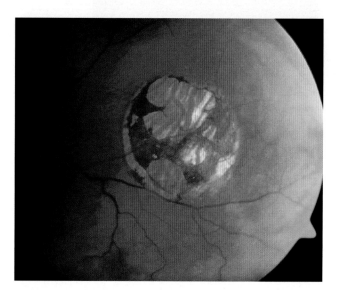

FIGURE 13.4   Congenital hypertrophy of the retinal pigment epithelium (CHRPE). The choroidal vasculature is visible beneath the areas of RPE atrophy.

The basal portion of the cell contains numerous residual bodies, the end stage of the phagocytic process, and the basal membrane is heavily convoluted. These features are described in greater detail below.

APICAL MEMBRANE SPECIALIZATIONS

On the apical surface of the RPE cells, there are ~4 µm long, vertically organized microvilli that interdigitate with the outer segments of both rod and cone photoreceptors (**Fig. 13.5**).[4,5] These microvilli are formed and maintained by a network of apical and circumferential bundles of actin filaments.[6] Microvilli are thought to form at the time of development of the photoreceptor cell outer segments, as the retinal and RPE neuroepithelia differentiate. The vertical alignment of the microvilli with the rod outer segments provides the close physical association required for photoreceptor disc shedding and uptake by the RPE,

and the milieu for the development and maintenance of the important interphotoreceptor matrix (IPM). This matrix of glycoproteins, cone matrix sheaths and rod matrix domains, which is discussed below, provides some physical attachments between the rod outer segments and apical microvilli of the RPE. These attachments serve to help adhere the retina to the RPE, either directly or through electrostatic forces. The tenacity of these attachments can be seen when an attempt is made to separate the retina from the RPE in a freshly harvested eye.[7,8]

The strength of the association between photoreceptors and the RPE is sufficient to create a source of shear stress in the outer retina when a blunt injury to the globe occurs. Deformation of the globe and lateral shearing forces disrupt the tight vertically oriented outer segments, which are normally aligned with the incident light reaching the macula. This anatomic disruption of the orientation gives rise to a reflection of light coming off of the macula (yellow arc surrounding the macula in the leftside of Fig. 13.6). This was originally termed "Berlin's edema" and was thought to be a swelling of the retina in response to the injury. Later, it was shown to be an injury-induced disruption of the rod outer segment orientation and dysfunction of the outer retinal barrier function provided by the RPE.[9,10] This trauma induced a sharp angle to occur between the inner and outer segments of the photoreceptor cells. The RPE response typically reflects the magnitude and severity of the shear injury and can range from mild with full recovery of vision, to severe, with massive pigment migration and scarring in the macula and significant loss of vision.

Notwithstanding the connections between RPE microvilli and photoreceptor outer segments, specialized intercellular junctions are not present between these tissues. As such, separations between the RPE and photoreceptor layer of the retina are more easily created in vivo than are separations between the intrinsic layers of the sensory retina (termed "schisis") or between the RPE and its basement membrane (pigment epithelial detachments).

It is in the plane of separation between RPE cells and photoreceptor outer segments that the clinical condition known as retinal detachment occurs. The black and white clinical photo in Fig. 13.7 reveals the darkened area of a serous retinal detachment with its edges marked by arrows. An optical coherence tomography (OCT) view, taken along the green line in the clinical photo, demonstrates the actual cleavage plane (asterisk) between the sensory retina and the underlying RPE layer. The RPE layer is indicated by the yellow arrows (Fig. 13.7).

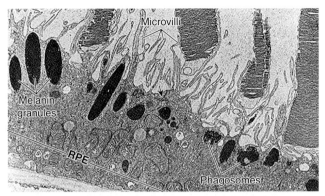

FIGURE 13.5 Electron micrograph of the interface between the apical microvilli of the RPE cells and the photoreceptor outer segments. Many thin microvilli extending from the apical cytoplasm are adherent with the outer segments and numerous phagosomes containing lamellar-appearing shed disc packets are seen. The oblong melanin granules are also preferentially seen in an apical distribution. RPE, retinal pigment epithelium. (Courtesy of Dr. Toichiro. In: Ross MH, Kaye GI, Pawlina W, eds. *Histology, A Text and Atlas.* 4th ed. Philadelphia: Lippincott Williams & Wilkins; 2003: 532–567.)

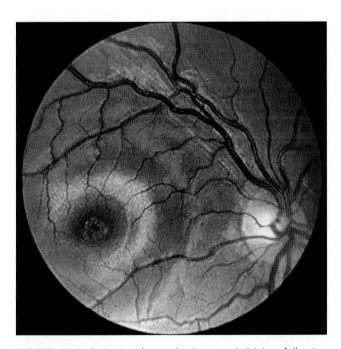

FIGURE 13.6 Patient with macular "commotio" injury following blunt trauma to the right eye.

Within the apical membranes of the RPE cells are an array of ion transporters, several of which are more commonly found in the basal or basolateral membranes of most other epithelia. These include the Na/K ATPase transporter pump. The Na/K ATPase transporter pump controls the flux of these two ions across the RPE cell to maintain the transmembrane electrical potential and the ionic content of the apical extracellular domain in the

region of the IPM. Other apical transport complexes in the RPE include a sodium bicarbonate cotransporter, Na/K/Cl cotransporter, and a Na/H anti-porter pump.[11] Joining adjacent RPE cells along their apico-lateral membranes are junctional complexes composed of a zonula occludens, zonula adherens, and both gap junctions and desmosomes.[12] The zonulae occludentes (i.e., tight junctions) serve three major functions in the RPE, they:

1. help maintain the polarity of the RPE cells,
2. maintain a transepithelial electrical potential, and
3. seal the intercellular cleft, preventing nonspecific diffusion of macromolecules from the choroid to the retina, between the cells of the RPE monolayer.

Maintaining Polarity

In order to preserve the ionic gradients and with them the passive centrifugal flow of water toward the choroid that maintains sensory retinal attachment, it is imperative that the various specialized intramembranous proteins representing ports, pumps, and receptors within the membrane are precluded from floating within the plasma membrane from the basal to the apical surface of the cell, or the reverse. By sealing the membrane leaflets of adjacent cells around the entire circumference of each cell, the tight junctions assure that the various receptors and pumps that distinguish the apical and basal membranes of the RPE cells remain in their proper membrane domains.[13–15]

Maintaining Transepithelial Potential

The tightness of the junctions between RPE cells is reflected in their transepithelial resistance. This transepithelial resistance creates an electrical potential across the RPE cell layer in both cultured cells and cells in vivo. The transepithelial potential gradient (~5 to 15 mV positive on the apical side of the membrane) provides an electrochemical force across the RPE layer, which assists in driving positively charged ions and enhances ion flux toward the choroid. However, the flux of important ions like Na^+, K^+, Cl^-, and bicarbonate is determined primarily by active transport via ion-specific pumps that are differentially distributed in either the apical and or basolateral membrane domains of the RPE cell.[16,17] These polarized pump functions provide the mechanism for the active, directed transport of ions across the RPE cell layer and the passive flow of water between the retina and choriocapillaris (**Fig. 13.8**).

Sealing the Intercellular Cleft

To maintain the pristine environment required for normal retinal function, a barrier to nonspecific diffusion of macromolecular components of the blood is essential. Within the sensory retina, this barrier is provided by the tight junctions that join the retinal vascular endothelial cells. This barrier exists at the level of the blood vessel wall. In the choroid, however, the capillaries are

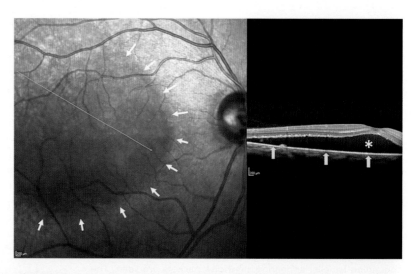

FIGURE 13.7 Neurosensory detachment of the retina in the posterior pole. In this image of a patient with central serous retinopathy, leakage of fluid under the retina has caused an exudative sensory retinal detachment in the macula (*white arrows, left*). OCT image (*right*), taken along green line of left image, shows that the separation occurs at the interface between the neurosensory retina and RPE (*yellow arrows*) as fluid accumulates underneath the sensory retina (*). The sensory retina and the RPE are derived from the inner and outer layers of the optic cup during development and a potential space remains between the two layers throughout life.

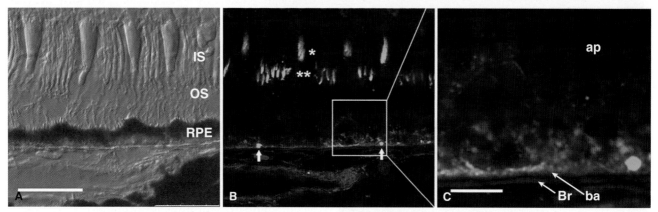

FIGURE 13.8 Micrographs demonstrating basal localization of a potassium pump in primate RPE cells. Immunofluorescence localization of KCNQ5 protein in monkey retina: subcellular localization of KCNQ5 in the distal retina: differential interference contrast (**A**) and confocal immunofluorescence image (**B, C**) of a cryosectioned neural retina-RPE-choroid from a monkey double-labeled with anti-KCNQ5 (*green*) and anti-CD29 (*red*) antibodies. Anti-KCNQ5 antibody labeled the inner plexiform layer (IPL) and outer plexiform layer (OPL), cone (*single asterisk*), and rod (*double asterisk*) photoreceptor inner segments (IS), and punctate structures near the RPE basal membrane (*block arrows*). Far right image (**C**) represents higher magnification of inset box in middle image showing scattered and focal (*arrows*) KCNQ5 distribution in the RPE at higher magnification. KCNQ5 immunolabeling is present near the basal membrane (ba) above Bruch's membrane (Br, *blue*). ap, apical membrane; IS, inner segments; OS, outer segments; RPE, retinal pigment epithelium. (Modified from Zhang X, Yang D, Hughes BA. KCNQ5/K(v)7.5 potassium channel expression and subcellular localization in primate retinal pigment epithelium and neural retina. *Am J Physiol Cell Physiol.* 2011;301(5):C1017–C1026.)

fenestrated and clearly cannot provide this barrier function. As such, the barrier function shifts to the RPE, much in the same way that the fenestrated capillaries of the ciliary body stroma require that the location of the blood–aqueous barrier shifts to the ciliary epithelium. The tight junctions of the retinal vasculature, discussed in detail in **CHAPTER 14: THE NEUROSENSORY RETINA**, are generally held to constitute the "inner" blood–retinal barrier. Those of the RPE are referred to as the "outer" blood–retinal barrier.[18,19]

As mentioned earlier, the RPE tight junctions are part of an apico-lateral junctional complex. In addition to the tight junction (zonula occludens) this complex is formed by a zonula adherens and multiple, focal gap junctions (**Fig. 13.9**). The zonula adherens forms a belt around the entire circumference of each cell, attaching the cell to all of its neighbors. The multiple gap junctions facilitate

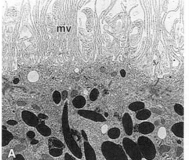
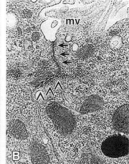

FIGURE 13.9 **A:** Electron micrograph of RPE cells showing well developed tight and adherens junctions, and abundant, long apical microvilli (*mv*). **B:** High magnification shows an intact junctional complex. Tight junction (*arrows*); zonula adherens junction (*arrowheads*). (Modified from Jin M, Ernesto Barron E, He S, et al. Regulation of RPE intercellular junction integrity and function by hepatocyte growth factor. *Invest Ophthalmol Vis Sci.* 2002;43:2782–2790.)

intercellular communication. The zonula occludens provides little adhesive strength and forms a branching and anastomosing belt of intramembranous particles, formed by proteins from the occludin family that are linked, on their cytoplasmic surface, to an encircling band of a protein known as ZO-1 (**Fig. 13.10**).[20] It is the zonula occludens (tight junction) that occludes the paracellular space, thus providing the barrier function. The tight junction constrains the flow of nutrients and metabolites, ions, drugs, and other components present in the blood from directly reaching the photoreceptors. Rather, they must pass by passive flow through Bruch's membrane and by regulated active transport through the RPE cell before they can reach the photoreceptors.[13–15]

 *Intravenous fluorescein angiography is used to assess the integrity of the blood–retinal barrier. In the images below (**Fig. 13.11**), from a patient with central serous chorioretinopathy, note that over most of the retina the fluorescence from the fluorescein that has leaked into the choroid from its fenestrated vessels is visible and has a ground glass appearance. This is due to the continuity of the RPE cell layer and intact tight junctions that contain the leakage within the choroid. However, in the macular region, the outer blood–retinal barrier has broken down, due to an abnormality in a focal region of the RPE. This functional break in the tight junctions between RPE cells permits the fluorescein dye from the choroidal vasculature to diffuse between the RPE cells in this region and detach the macula. A "smokestack" of leaking fluid and early filling of the space beneath the macular detachment is seen. The condition is idiopathic but may be associated with stress, and is exacerbated by the use of steroids.*

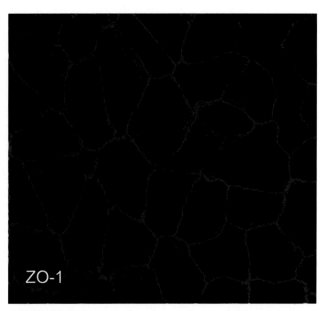

ZO-1

FIGURE 13.10   Immunofluorescence image of RPE cells in tissue culture with formation of zonula occludens (tight junctions) along the apico-lateral border between confluent cells. Junction-related ZO-1 protein staining identifies the location of the protein surrounding the circumference of every RPE cell.

Cytoplasmic Organelles and Inclusions

Along with the usual complement of organelles including mitochondria and endoplasmic reticulum, inclusions are commonly present in the cytoplasm of RPE cells. Among these are, of course, the melanosomes for which the RPE cells are named. Several other types of inclusions that generally reflect stages in the phagocytosis and catabolism of photoreceptor discs are also present.

BASAL MEMBRANE SPECIALIZATIONS

The basal membrane of the RPE cells is convoluted, with infoldings as deep as 1 μm (**Fig. 13.12**). As with the apical microvilli, these infoldings are created and maintained by an organization of cytoplasmic actin filaments. The basement membrane of the RPE, which forms an integral part of Bruch's membrane, exhibits type IV collagen and a proteoglycan-rich extracellular matrix including heparan sulfate and laminin.[21] This basement membrane functions to maintain RPE cell adherence to Bruch's membrane and may play a passive role in limiting diffusion of some plasma components diffusing toward the retina from the underlying fenestrated capillaries of the choroid. Basolateral membrane transporters include a Na-dependent lactate transporter and a Cl-bicarbonate exchanger.[11]

RPE MELANOSOMES

The RPE cell layer is the first to form pigment in the eye. The RPE cells are heavily pigmented, forming mature melanin pigment granules until about 2 years of age and then maintaining them in the post-mitotic RPE cell into adulthood. For reasons that are not yet understood, this early appearance of melanin plays a critical role in the normal differentiation and development of the retina, optic nerve, and the underlying choroid.[22,23]

Melanosomes of two shapes are present in RPE cells. Some are ovoid and some are spherical. Residing at the bases of the apical microvilli, the ovoid melanin pigment granules are oriented with their long axes parallel to the longitudinal axis of the microvilli. Spherical melanosomes tend to predominate toward the basal surface of the cell.

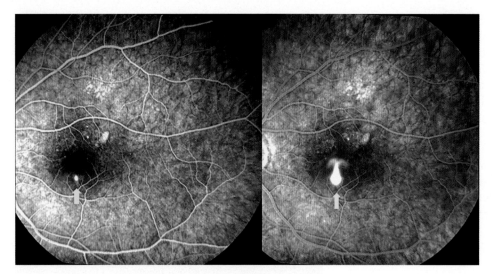

FIGURE 13.11 Fluorescein angiogram demonstrating loss of RPE barrier function in a patient with central serous chorioretinopathy. A small focus of leakage of dye through the RPE layer is seen (*yellow arrow, left*). Later in the study, the leaking dye persists, forming a classical "smoke-stack" (*yellow arrow, right*). Dye is also seen collecting at the margins of the neurosensory detachment.

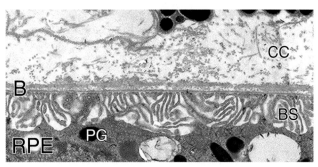

FIGURE 13.12 Electron micrograph showing Bruch's membrane (B), the RPE, a pigment granule (PG), the basal surface (BS) microvilli of the RPE, and the choroicapillary stroma (CC). (From Bruch's Membrane. Webvision website. http://webvision.med.utah.edu/. September 2015. Accessed March 21, 2017. Copyright © 2017 Webvision.)

The apical localization of the elongate pigment granules is maintained through interactions with the cytoskeletal actin filaments that also serve to support the apical microvilli. Melanosomes in lower vertebrates (fish, amphibians) actively migrate within the apical border and microvilli to provide a mobile pigment screen to shield the photoreceptors and RPE cells in response to light.[24] By contrast, however, the melanosomes concentrated in the apical microvilli in primates appear to be relatively static.

The overall darkness of the tissues in the posterior pole of the eye generally reflects the degree of pigmentation of the individual. But there are no racial differences in the density of melanin pigment in the RPE layver itself. Rather, the racial differences in the degree of overall pigmentation of the posterior poles of human eyes are principally influenced by the variable amounts of mesodermal and neural crest-derived melanocytes in the stroma of the choroid.

Three types of pigmented structures are found within RPE cells of all ages. The first of these are melanosomes containing melanin. The other two are lipofuscin and

granules representing complexes of melanin and lipofuscin.[25–27] With aging, there appears to be a progressive loss of melanosomes (~25% decrease in number) and an overall loss of the apical localization of these granules in the RPE cell. Total pigmentation within the cells may not decline however because the two other types of pigment granules, lipofuscin and melanofuscin complexes, increase with age. And it is known that with increasing age, RPE cells in the macular region contain more melanofuscin granules than RPE cells toward the retinal periphery.

The Roles of Melanin

Melanin plays several roles in the health of the retina and RPE. The ovoid-shaped melanin pigment granules that align with apical microvilli act to reduce light scatter by absorbing stray photons not absorbed by the photoreceptors.[28–30] They also act as a heat sink to reduce light-induced thermal damage to the retina. As elsewhere, including the skin, by absorbing photons not absorbed by photoreceptors, melanin also acts to protect the RPE cell DNA from photic damage and oxidative stress-induced cell death.[31–33]

Other protective functions attributed to the melanosomes of the RPE include serving as a free radical scavenger, an inhibitor of lipid peroxidation, and a nonenzymatic antioxidant within the cell.[34–37] Its antioxidant functions are supplemented by the ability of melanin to bind calcium and heavy metal ions that can play a role in oxidative processes in the cell, through ionic buffering.[38,39] Although these functions of melanin are all beneficial to the retina, melanin may also have a detrimental role by contributing to photochemical injuries produced by blue light. More evidence is needed but, at present, it appears more likely that lipofuscin is the detrimental RPE pigment in such cases.[40–43]

Genetic conditions like albinism and ocular albinism result from impaired tyrosinase enzyme activity that prevents or impairs the synthesis of melanin (Fig. 13.13). These conditions are associated not only with abnormal visual function due to aberrant light scatter within the eye and retina, but also with morphologic defects in fovea formation and with abnormal ganglion cell projections through the optic chiasm to the brain. The mechanisms by which the absence of melanin results in these major developmental abnormalities are not well understood.[44,45]

PHAGOSOMES AND LIPOFUSCIN GRANULES

Additional cytoplasmic inclusions commonly seen in RPE cells represent various stages in the process of phagocytosis and digestion of photopigment-containing membrane discs. The outer segments of the photoreceptor cells are composed almost exclusively of stacked membrane discs that are densely packed with rhodopsin or cone opsins the function of which is to transduce photons of light into an electrical signal.[46,47] The photoreceptor cell makes new membrane discs continuously, in the region of its inner segment (Fig. 13.14). These newly formed packets move progressively down the outer segment, toward the RPE, as new packets are formed behind them. To make room for new packets, the tip of the outer segment sheds aged, lipid-oxidized disc packets, which are phagocytosed by RPE cells. This ongoing process from disc formation to shedding takes approximately 11 days and permits active renewal

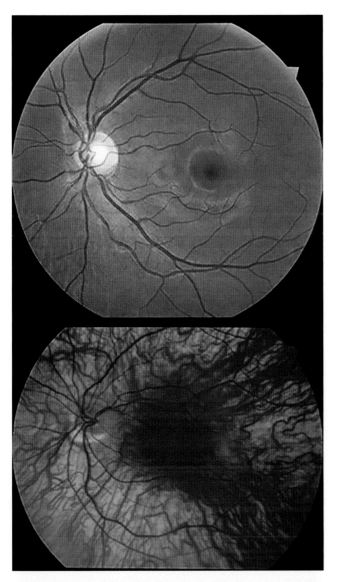

FIGURE 13.13 Fundus photographs of a retina with normal RPE and choroidal pigmentation **(top)** and a retina from a patient with ocular albinism with no pigmentation of the RPE or choroidal stroma. The choroidal vessels are easily seen through the RPE.

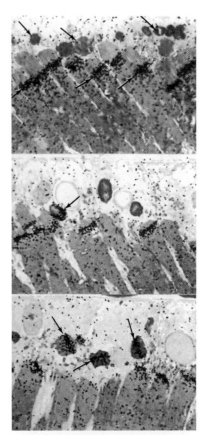

FIGURE 13.14 Autoradiograph of photoreceptor cell disc membrane shedding and renewal. *Black* particles represent incorporation of pulsed radioactivity into forming outer segment discs **(top)**. The newly formed packets (with their radioactivity) move progressively down the outer segment, toward the RPE, as new packets are formed behind them. The tip of the outer segment sheds aged, lipid-oxidized disc packets, which are phagocytosed by RPE cells (*arrows*). (Modified from Marmor MF, Wolfensberger TJ, eds. *The Retinal Pigment Epithelium.* New York: Oxford University Press; 1998:155.)

and recycling of photopigments for the photoreceptor, acting in concert with the RPE cell, which serves as its phagocytic partner. It is estimated that in humans ~4,000 disc packets are phagocytized and digested by each RPE cell every day, a significant catabolic and oxidative stress load for the RPE cells.[48,49]

Two forms of phagocytosis are seen in RPE cells. The minor one of these, micropinocytosis, occurs when ruffled cell membranes passively engulf and internalize material from the local extracellular environment. In contrast, the bulk of the phagocytosis in the RPE is receptor-mediated phagocytosis, which occurs as a result of specific and active interactions between the RPE cell membrane and the target disc packet being internalized. Transient pseudopodia form on the apical surface of the RPE cell in the regions of microvilli/outer segment interactions. Concurrently, the outer segment membrane releases the disc packet for uptake and digestion. The internalized photoreceptor disc packet is packaged in a phagosome (**Fig. 13.15**). Following production of the phagosome, it fuses with a lysosome, producing a secondary lysosome that is actively trafficked

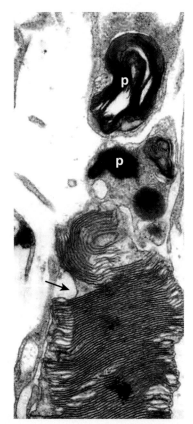

FIGURE 13.15 Electron micrograph of photoreceptor cell disc membrane shedding and phagocytosis by RPE cells. The disc packet is pinched off (*arrow*) by an active process and is trafficked to the lysosome in a membrane-bound phagosome (*p*) for digestion and recycling of components in the RPE cell. (Modified from Anderson DH, Fisher SK, Steinberg RH. Mammalian cones: disc shedding, phagocytosis, and renewal. *Invest Ophthalmol Vis Sci.* 1978;17(2):117–133.)

basally, utilizing a microtubule network. This network plays a direct role in mobilization of the phagosome and its fusion with lysosomes during autophagy.[50,51]

Adsorption and internalization of the phagosome by the RPE cell is an active, receptor-mediated process and is critical to the health of the photoreceptors. Defective phagocytosis is seen in patients with age-related macular degeneration (AMD) and in animal models in which a receptor is mutated: both result in retinal degeneration.[52,53]

Shedding of Photoreceptor Discs

There are two known environmental signals for outer segment disc shedding in humans. They are circadian rhythm and light cycling, with the latter of these playing the larger role in humans. In cold-blooded animals, such as amphibians, there is evidence that temperature may play a role as well, but this does not appear to be the case in mammals.[54] In the case of rod cells, which mediate scotopic vision, it is the onset of light that appears to be the initiating signal for shedding. In the case of cones, which mediate photopic vision, it is the onset of dark.[55,56] Artificially altering the light–dark cycle alters the pattern of disc shedding. For example, rod cells do not shed outer segments in a constant light environment. They require a period of dark adaptation to "prime" a new round of shedding when exposed to light. As such, the impact of constant light on the outer segment is to inhibit the shedding process. Outer segment growth continues under these conditions, leading to progressive elongation.

Pharmacologic studies of photoreceptor shedding have identified melatonin and dopamine as key regulators through a receptor-mediated process, at least in experimental animals.[57] The responsiveness to light identifies the photoreceptor cell as the driving force, but active interaction with the RPE cell is required to detach the disc packet.[58,59] Even at a young age, the process of digestion of all of the photoreceptor membrane phagocytosed by the RPE cells may remain incomplete. These remnants of incompletely digested residues of photoreceptor outer segment membrane discs remain in the RPE cytoplasm as visible inclusions termed lipofuscin granules.[60] Some lipofuscin granules are composed completely of lipofuscin while others form larger inclusions after fusing with melanin granules.

Lipofuscin

Lipofuscin is a heterogeneous, membrane-bound material composed of lipids, proteins, and additional compounds that exhibit spectral characteristics permitting its clinical and microscopic visualization by virtue of its intrinsic autofluorescence. This characteristic has made it very useful in the clinical assessment of the RPE by OCT methods. It has emerged as an important disease feature in AMD and other diseases of the retina and RPE in clinical practice. Like melanosomes, these deposits are electron-dense, making them a readily observable cytoplasmic inclusion by electron

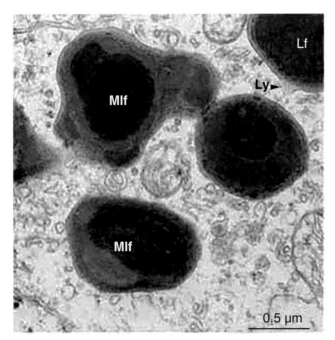

FIGURE 13.16 Complex granules resulting from interactions between melanosomes and various parts of the lysosomal system. Melanolipofuscin (Mlf) granules have a core of melanin and a cortex of lipofuscin material. The bleb (*Ly*) on the side of a lipofuscin granule (*Lf*) has been shown in other studies to contain lysosomal enzymes (×43,000). (From Grunwald GB. Structure and function of the retinal pigment epithelium. In: Tasman W, Jaeger EA, eds. *Duane's Ophthalmology on CD-ROM, 2006 Edition.* Philadelphia: Lippincott Williams & Wilkins; 2006.)

microscopy (**Fig. 13.16**). Indeed, by electron microscopy, one can distinguish inclusions of pure lipofuscin from those representing complexes with melanin granules. Inclusions of pure lipofuscin have a uniform medium electron density, whereas lipofuscin granules complexed with melanin show a more electron-dense melanin core, surrounded by the coating of less electron-dense lipofuscin.[61]

*Age-related dysfunction in the degradation of outer segment discs by the RPE phagosomes is the main source of clinically observable deposits called drusen. When occurring in the macular region, they are the hallmark of AMD. These membrane and lipoprotein-containing deposits collect between the RPE and Bruch's membrane and present as yellow/white, hard- or soft-appearing deposits in the macula in patients with the disease. These deposits have been shown to activate complement-mediated inflammation beneath the retina, contributing to the progression of the disease. The clinical appearance of drusen in the macular region and in histologic sections viewed by confocal microscopy are shown (**Fig. 13.17**). In addition to the formation of lipofuscin complexes, aging leads to the thickening of Bruch's membrane. These changes alter the flow of metabolites, oxygen, and growth factors between the choriocapillaris, the RPE and retina, and lead to the progression of AMD.*

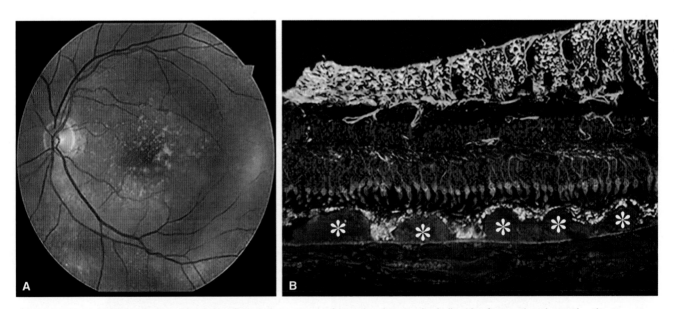

FIGURE 13.17 Fundus photograph of the clinical appearance of macular drusen, the hallmark of age-related macular degeneration. These membrane and lipoprotein-containing deposits collect between the RPE and Bruch's membrane and present as yellow/white, hard- or soft-appearing deposits **(A)**. Histologic sections viewed by confocal microscopy **(B)** are shown with large droplet-like deposits called drusen (*asterisks*) on Bruch's membrane (*light blue line*). Note the distortion of the photoreceptor outer segments and atrophy of the autofluorescent (*yellow*) RPE cells. (From Milam A. The Human Retina in Health and Disease Teaching Set. © Scheie Eye Institute, University of Pennsylvania. 2016.)

The healthy RPE shows a diffuse anatomic pattern of autofluorescence which is most intense adjacent to and surrounding the fovea. The autofluorescence in this region can increase with age as a consequence of age-related accumulation of additional lipofuscin in the RPE cells of this region. However, as the RPE cells become increasingly damaged, these cells begin to die off, leaving nummular areas of RPE cell loss in the central macula, termed geographic atrophy. Because the retinal photoreceptors are critically dependent upon the many functions of the RPE for their own health (oxygen and nutritional support, recycling of vitamin A, protection from photooxidative stress, etc.), as the RPE dies off, the overlying retina slowly degenerates, producing a disease called "dry" macular degeneration. A "wet" form may develop as well. The "wet" form is associated with the growth of abnormal choroidal blood vessels through defects that form in Bruch's membrane, leading to exudation, hemorrhage, and profound vision loss if left untreated.

*Reactive changes in the RPE, seen at the margins of lesions of geographic atrophy in AMD, lead to hyperfluorescence in the RPE cells adjacent to areas of atrophy. The hyperfluorescence suggests an enhanced accumulation of lipofuscin in these cells. Such cells are at risk of cell death as the geographic atrophy progresses (**Fig. 13.18**). These clinically apparent changes have been shown to correlate with AMD disease features and progression in recent clinical trials.[62,63]*

The Interphotoreceptor Matrix

There is an important extracellular matrix specialization between the RPE cells and the cones and rods of the macula. This glycosaminoglycan-rich substrate of cone matrix sheaths and rod matrix domains is termed the IPM. The IPM provides physical adhesions between the outer segments and apical microvilli of the RPE and serves to help mechanically adhere the retina to the RPE. In addition to its mechanical properties, the IPM also plays a critical role in maintaining the bidirectional passage of small molecules, proteins, and other factors required for the recycling of visual pigment, a key functional role of the RPE.[64,65]

This filamentous and fibrous matrix of water-soluble proteoglycans does not contain the collagen, fibronectin, or other elements commonly found as part of matrices produced by most epithelial cells.[8,66] The IPM is not a homogeneous matrix. There is molecular specialization of the IPM with respect to rods and cones. Cone matrix sheaths and rod domains are enriched with different types of glycoproteins and exhibit different lectin-binding domains. These all play a role in maintaining the specialized microenvironments required for the cone and rod photoreceptors, respectively (**Fig. 13.19**).[67] There is a light-evoked change in the distribution of 11-cis-retinal binding protein pools within the RPE cell and IPM. There is a more homogeneous distribution in dark-adapted retinas due to an increase in the solubility of RPE65, a 11-cis-retinal chaperone partner in the RPE cell.[68] As described above, the matrix of glycoproteins provides physical adhesions between the outer segments and apical microvilli of the RPE and serves to help adhere

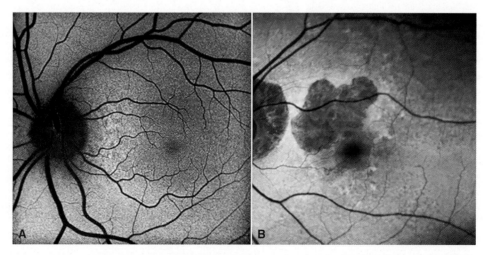

FIGURE 13.18 Optical coherence tomography autofluorescence images of the macula in a normal patient (**A**) and a patient with atrophic macular degeneration (**B**). The intrinsic autofluorescence of the healthy RPE has a ground glass appearance. The diseased retina shows geographic atrophy of the RPE (*dark areas*) and reactive hyperplasia and increased fluorescence in the surrounding cells. This characteristic has emerged as an important prognostic disease feature in clinical practice.

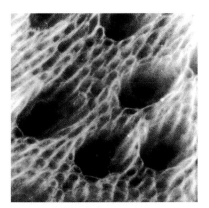

FIGURE 13.19 Scanning electron micrograph of the glycosamino-glycan-rich substrate of cone matrix sheaths (*large openings*) and rod matrix domains (*small openings*) of the interphotoreceptor matrix. (From Ryan SJ, ed. *Retina: Vol 1 Basic Science and Inherited Retinal Disease.* 2nd ed. St. Louis: Mosby; 1994:63, Originally published in Hollyfield JG, Rayborn ME, Landers RA, et al. Insoluble interphotoreceptor matrix domains surround rod photoreceptors in the human retina. *Exp Eye Res.* 1990;51(1):107–110.)

the retina to the RPE through direct mechanical forces and active fluid transport which generates hydrostatic forces (a functional suction) that maintain adherence. Enzymatic digestion of the proteoglycans of the IPM and removal of divalent cations have been shown to decrease the adhesion forces between the retina and RPE cell layers.[69] It has also been speculated that the filamentous nature of the IPM serves as a structural support to help maintain the regular alignment of the photoreceptors required to optimally trap photons for visual transduction.

Retinoid binding proteins in the IPM provide the mechanism for the transport and recycling of the photoactivated moiety of the rhodopsin molecule, which takes place in the RPE cell. The interphotoreceptor retinoid binding protein (IRBP) is secreted by the rod photoreceptor into the IPM and comprises the major protein of the IPM.[70,71] Other proteoglycans in the IPM appear to be secreted by retinal neurons, Müller cells, and the RPE. IRBP is involved in the bidirectional transport of photo-bleached visual pigment to the RPE for isomerization and the transport of 11-cis-retinaldehyde back to the photoreceptor cell. Several models of experimental autoimmune uveitis have been developed using sensitization to the IRBP molecule, suggesting that impaired immune privilege in the eye and exposure of the host immune system to IRBP may play a role in some ocular inflammatory diseases.[72]

REFERENCES

1. Buettner H. Congenital hypertrophy of the retinal pigment epithelium. *Am J Ophthalmol.* 1975;79:177–189.
2. Lloyd WC 3rd, Eagle RC Jr, Shields JA, et al. Congenital hypertrophy of the retinal pigment epithelium. Electron microscopic and morphometric observations. *Ophthalmology.* 1990;97:1052–1060.
3. Terman A, Brunk UT. Lipofuscin: mechanisms of formation and increase with age APMIS. 1998;106(2):265–276.
4. Nguyen-Legros J. Fine structure of the pigment epithelium in the vertebrate retina. *Int Rev Cytol Suppl.* 1978;(7):287–328.
5. Immel J, Negi A, Marmor MF. Acute changes in RPE apical morphology after retinal detachment in rabbit. A SEM study. *Invest Ophthalmol Vis Sci.* 1986;27(12):1770–1776.
6. Owaribe K. The cytoskeleton of retinal pigment epithelial cells. In: Osborne NN, Chader GJ, eds. *Progress in Retinal Research.* Vol 8. Oxford: Pergammon Press; 1988:23–49.
7. Hageman GS, Marmor MF, Yao XY, et al. The interphotoreceptor matrix mediates primate retinal adhesion. *Arch Ophthalmol.* 1995;113(5):655–660.
8. Hollyfield JG, Rayborn ME, Landers RA, et al. Insoluble interphotoreceptor matrix domains surround rod photoreceptors in the human retina. *Exp Eye Res.* 1990;51(1):107–110.
9. Sipperley JO, Quigley HA, Gass DM. Traumatic retinopathy in primates. The explanation of commotio retinae. *Arch Ophthalmol.* 1978;96(12):2267–2273.
10. Bunt-Milam AH, Black RA, Bensinger RE. Breakdown of the outer blood-retinal barrier in experimental commotio retinae. *Exp Eye Res.* 1986;43(3):397–412.
11. Reichhart N, Strauss O. Ion channels and transporters of the retinal pigment epithelium. *Exp Eye Res.* 2014;126:27–37.
12. Clark VM. The cell biology of the RPE. In: Adler R, Farber D, eds. *The Retina: A Model for Cell Biology.* Orlando: Academic Press; 1986:129–168.
13. Peyman GA, Bok D. Peroxidase diffusion in the normal and laser-coagulated primate retina. *Invest Ophthalmol.* 1972;11(1):35–45.
14. Gundersen D, Orlowski J, Rodriguez-Boulan E. Apical polarity of Na,K-ATPase in retinal pigment epithelium is linked to a reversal of the ankyrin-fodrin submembrane cytoskeleton. *J Cell Biol.* 1991;112(5):863–872.
15. Hudspeth AJ, Yee AG. The intercellular junctional complexes of retinal pigment epithelia. *Invest Ophthalmol.* 1973;12(5):354–365.
16. Rodriguez-Boulan E, Nelson WJ. Morphogenesis of the polarized epithelial cell phenotype. *Science.* 1989;245(4919):718–25.
17. Rodriguez-Boulan E, Powell SK. Polarity of epithelial and neuronal cells. *Annu Rev Cell Biol.* 1992;8:395–427.
18. Cuhna-Vaz JG. The blood-retinal barriers system. Basic concepts and clinical evaluation. *Exp Eye Res.* 2004;78:715–721.
19. Cunha-Vaz J, Bernardes R, Lobo C. Blood-retinal barrier. *Eur J Ophthalmol.* 2011;21(suppl 6):3–9.
20. Nevala H, Ylikomi T, Tähti H. Evaluation of the selected barrier properties of retinal pigment epithelial cell line ARPE-19 for an in-vitro blood-brain barrier model. *Hum Exp Toxicol.* 2008;27(10):741–749.
21. Bron AJ, Tripathi RC and Tripathi BJ. *Wolff's Anatomy of the Eye and Orbit,* Chapter 14. 8th ed. London: Chapman and Hall Medical; 1997:464.
22. Schraermeyer U, Peters S, Thumann G, et al. Melanin granules of retinal pigment epithelium are connected with the lysosomal degradation pathway. *Exp Eye Res.* 1999;68(2):237–245.
23. Dräger UC, Balkema GW. Does melanin do more than protect from light? *Neurosci Res Suppl.* 1987;6:S75–S86.
24. Femald RD. The optical system of fishes. Chapter 2. *The Visual System of Fish.* Eds: Douglas R, Djamgoz M. Chapman and Hall: London; 1990.
25. Feeney-Burns L, Hilderbrand ES, Eldridge S. Aging human RPE: morphometric analysis of macular, equatorial, and peripheral cells. *Invest Ophthalmol Vis Sci.* 1984;25(2):195–200.
26. Weiter JJ, Delori FC, Wing GL, Fitch KA. Retinal pigment epithelial lipofuscin and melanin and choroidal melanin in human eyes. *Invest Ophthalmol Vis Sci.* 1986 Feb;27(2):145–152.
27. Feeney-Burns L, Burns RP, Gao CL. Age-related macular changes in humans over 90 years old. *Am J Ophthalmol.* 1990;109(3):265–278.
28. Hogan MJ, Alvarado JA, Weddell JE. *Histology of the Human Eye.* Philadelphia: Saunders; 1971.
29. Feeney-Burns L. The pigments of the retinal pigment epithelium. *Curr Top Eye Res.* 1980;2:119–178.

30. Feeney-Burns L. The pigments of the retinal pigment epithelium. *Curr Top Eye Res.* 1980;2:119–178.

31. Birngruber R, Gabel VP. Thermal versus photochemical damage in the retina--thermal calculations for exposure limits. *Trans Ophthalmol Soc U K.* 1983;103(pt 4):422–427.

32. Seagle BL, Rezai KA, Gasyna EM, et al. Melanin photoprotection in the human retinal pigment epithelium and its correlation with light-induced cell apoptosis. *Proc Natl Acad Sci USA.* 2005;102(25):8978–8983.

33. Walls GL. *The Vertebrate Eye and Its Adaptive Radiation.* Vol 19. Bloomfield Hills, MI: Cranbrook Institute of Science Bulletin; 1942.

34. Sarna T and Swartz HM. Interactions of melanin with oxygen and related species. In: Scott G, ed. *Atmospheric Oxygen and Antioxidants.* Vol 3. Amsterdam: Elsevier Press; 1993:129–169.

35. Sarna T. Properties and function of the ocular melanin--a photobiophysical view. *J Photochem Photobiol B.* 1992;12(3):215–580.

36. Seagle BL, Rezai KA, Gasyna EM, et al. Time-resolved detection of melanin free radicals quenching reactive oxygen species. *J Am Chem Soc.* 2005;127(32):11220, 11221.

37. Dayhaw-Barker P. Retinal pigment epithelium melanin and ocular toxicity. *Int J Toxicol.* 2002;21(6):451–454.

38. Ostrovsky MA, Sakina NL, Dontsov AE. An antioxidative role of ocular screening pigments. *Vision Res.* 1987;27(6):893–899.

39. Rózanowska M, Bober A, Burke JM, et al. The role of retinal pigment epithelium melanin in photoinduced oxidation of ascorbate. *Photochem Photobiol.* 1997;65(3):472–490.

40. Ham WT Jr, Ruffolo JJ Jr, Mueller HA, et al. Histologic analysis of photochemical lesions produced in rhesus retina by short-wave-length light. *Invest Ophthalmol Vis Sci.* 1978;17(10):1029–1035.

41. Feeney L. Lipofuscin and melanin of human retinal pigment epithelium. Fluorescence, enzyme cytochemical, and ultrastructural studies. *Invest Ophthalmol Vis Sci.* 1978;17(7):583–600.

42. Mellerio J. Light effects on the retina. In: Albert DM, Jakobiec FA, eds. *Principles and Practice of Ophthalmology, Basic Sciences.* Philadelphia: Saunders; 1994:1326–1345.

43. Bok D. Retinal photoreceptor-pigment epithelium interactions. *Invest Ophthalmol Vis Sci.* 1985;26(12):1659–1694.

44. Guillery RW. Neural abnormalities of albinos. *Trends Neurosci.* 1986;9:364–367.

45. Jeffery G, Schütz G, Montoliu L. Correction of abnormal retinal pathways found with albinism by introduction of a functional tyrosinase gene in transgenic mice. *Dev Biol.* 1994;166(2):460–464.

46. LaVail MM. Rod outer segment disk shedding in rat retina: relationship to cyclic lighting. *Science.* 1976;194(4269):1071–1074.

47. Young RW, Bok D. Participation of the retinal pigment epithelium in the rod outer segment renewal process. *J Cell Biol.* 1969;42(2):392–403.

48. Young RW. The renewal of rod and cone outer segments in the rhesus monkey. *J Cell Biol.* 1971;49(2):303–318.

49. Young RW. The renewal of photoreceptor cell outer segments. *J Cell Biol.* 1967;33(1):61–72.

50. Hughes BA, Gallemore RP, Miller SS. Transport mechanisms in the retinal pigment epithelium. In: Marmor MF, Wolfensberger TJ, eds. *The Retinal Pigment Epithelium.* New York, Oxford University Press; 1998:103–134.

51. Frost LS, Mitchell CH, Boesze-Battaglia K. Autophagy in the eye: implications for ocular cell health. *Exp Eye Res.* 2014;124:56–66.

52. Swanson JA, Baer SC. Phagocytosis by zippers and triggers. *Trends Cell Biol.* 1995;5(3):89–93.

53. Bok D, Hall MO. The role of the pigment epithelium in the etiology of inherited retinal dystrophy in the rat. *J Cell Biol.* 1971;49(3):664–682.

54. Hollyfield JG, Besharse JC, Rayborn ME. Turnover of rod photoreceptor outer segments. I. Membrane addition and loss in relationship to temperature. *J Cell Biol.* 1977;75:490–506.

55. Bok D. Renewal of photoreceptor cells. *Methods Enzymol.* 1982;81:763–72.

56. Besharse JC. The daily light-dark cycle and rhythmic metabolism in the photoreceptor pigment epithelium complex. In: Osborne NN, Chader GJ Eds. *Progress in Retinal Research.* Vol 1. Oxford: Pergammon Press; 1982:81–124.

57. LaVail MM. Circadian nature of rod outer segment disc shedding in the rat. *Invest Ophthalmol Vis Sci.* 1980;19(4);407–411.

58. Matsumoto B, Defoe DM, Besharse JC. Membrane turnover in rod photoreceptors: ensheathment and phagocytosis of outer segment distal tips by pseudopodia of the retinal pigment epithelium. *Proc R Soc Lond B Biol Sci.* 1987;230(1260):339–354.

59. Williams DS, Fisher SK. Prevention of rod disk shedding by detachment from the retinal pigment epithelium. *Invest Ophthalmol Vis Sci.* 1987;28(1):184–187.

60. Katz ML, Drea CM, Eldred GE, et al. Influence of early photoreceptor degeneration on lipofuscin in the retinal pigment epithelium. *Exp Eye Res.* 1986;43(4):561–573.

61. Kennedy CJ, Rakoczy PE, Constable IJ. Lipofuscin of the retinal pigment epithelium: a review. *Eye.* 1995;9:763–771.

62. Schmidt-Erfurth U, Waldstein SM. A paradigm shift in imaging biomarkers in neovascular age-related macular degeneration. *Prog Retin Eye Res.* 2016;50:1–24.

63. Folgar FA, Yuan EL, Sevilla MB, et al; Age Related Eye Disease Study 2 Ancillary Spectral-Domain Optical Coherence Tomography Study Group. Drusen volume and retinal pigment epithelium abnormal thinning volume predict 2-year progression of age-related macular Degeneration. *Ophthalmology.* 2016;123(1):39–50.e1.

64. Adler AJ, Klucznik KM. Proteins and glycoproteins of the bovine interphotoreceptor matrix: composition and fractionation. *Exp Eye Res.* 1982;34(3):423–434.

65. Berman ER. An overview of the biochemistry of the interphotoreceptor matrix. In: Bridges, CD, Adler AJ, eds. *The IPM in Health and Disease.* New York: Alan R Liss; 1985:47–64.

66. Hageman GS, Johnson LV. Chondroitin 6-sulfate glycosaminoglycan is a major constituent of primate cone photoreceptor matrix sheaths. *Curr Eye Res.* 1987;6(4):639–646.

67. Johnson LV, Hageman GS, Blanks JC. Interphotoreceptor matrix domains ensheath vertebrate cone photoreceptor cells. *Invest Ophthalmol Vis Sci.* 1986;27(2):129–135.

68. Xue L, Gollapalli DR, Maiti P, et al. A palmitoylation switch mechanism in the regulation of the visual cycle. *Cell.* 2004;117(6):761–710.

69. Yao XY, Hageman GS, Marmor MF. Retinal adhesiveness is weakened by enzymatic modification of the interphotoreceptor matrix in vivo. *Invest Ophthalmol Vis Sci.* 1990;31(10):2051–2058.

70. Chader GJ. Interphotoreceptor retinoid-binding protein (IRBP): a model protein for molecular biological and clinically relevant studies. Friedenwald lecture. *Invest Ophthalmol Vis Sci.* 1989;30(1):7–22.

71. Okajima TI, Pepperberg DR, Ripps H, et al. Interphotoreceptor retinoid-binding protein: role in delivery of retinol to the pigment epithelium. *Exp Eye Res.* 1989;49(4):629–644.

72. Chen J, Qian H, Horai R, et al. Comparative analysis of induced vs. spontaneous models of autoimmune uveitis targeting the interphotoreceptor retinoid binding protein. *PLoS One.* 2013;8(8):e72161.

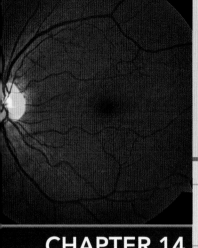

The Neurosensory Retina

CHAPTER 14

Overview

The retina (from the Latin "rete," for net) is classically comprised of the layers of neuronal and glial cells termed, the neurosensory retina, and a single layer of heavily pigmented epithelial cells termed the retinal pigment epithelium. Because of their unique complexities, we have chosen to discuss the neurosensory retina and the retinal pigment epithelium in separate chapters. The neurosensory retina is a highly specialized outgrowth of the brain that has evolved to capture photons of light, transduce that light into electrical signals, and initiate the processing of the resulting image. A complete understanding of how and why humans (and many other species) are able to see in such a rich fashion in ways that permit us to interact with our visual world, in all of its varied manifestations of luminance, color, motion, and dimensions is beyond the scope of this text. But an understanding of the fundamental anatomical complexity of this tissue is an essential first step. The purpose of this chapter is to provide the reader with a clinical overview of the anatomy and histology of the human retina and an overview of how it is functionally organized at the cellular level to play its role in processing visual input.

The neurosensory retina has a dual vascular supply. The inner half of the retina is served by an intraretinal vasculature, derived from the central retinal artery. The outer half of the retina receives its oxygen and nutrition from the choroidal circulation, conveyed to the retinal cells indirectly via the retinal pigment epithelium. Hence, the outer layers of the retinal tissue are avascular, relying upon the specialized functions of the retinal pigment epithelium to meet its high metabolic and oxygen demands. Additional material relevant to the development and function of the retina can also be found in **CHAPTER 12: CHOROID AND CHOROIDAL CIRCULATION, CHAPTER 13: THE RETINAL PIGMENT EPITHELIUM, CHAPTER 15: THE OPTIC NERVE AND VISUAL PATHWAYS**, and **CHAPTER 16: OCULAR EMBRYOLOGY**.

Macroscopic and Clinical Anatomy of the Retina

LANDMARKS OF THE OCULAR FUNDUS

The major landmarks visible in the normal retina (also termed ocular *fundus*) are shown. **Figure 14.1** provides a wide-angle view of the retina from nasal to temporal periphery and **Figure 14.2** provides a view limited to the posterior

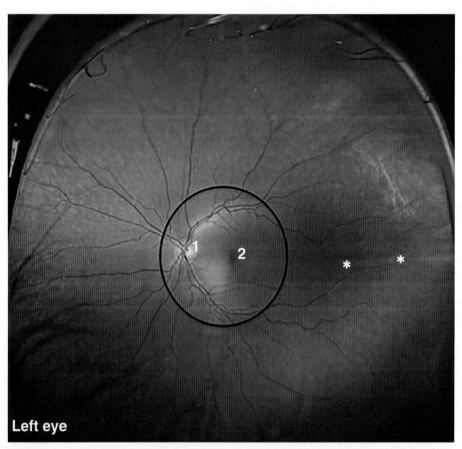

Left eye

FIGURE 14.1 Wide-angle view of the retina. The optic nerve (*1*) and macula (*2*) are seen in the posterior pole. The tracks of the long posterior ciliary artery and long ciliary nerve, in the periphery along the horizontal meridian, are also seen (*asterisks*). The *black circle* correlates with the standard fundus image of the posterior pole seen in Figure 14.2. (From Optos website. http://www.optos.com. 2016.)

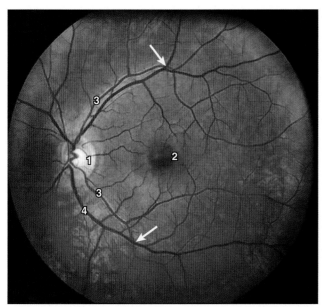

FIGURE 14.2 Standard fundus image of the posterior pole of the retina. The optic nerve (*1*) and macula (*2*) are noted. The major superior and inferior branches of the central retinal artery (*3*) and vein (*4*) are also shown. The first crossing points of the arterial and venous arcades (*arrows*) are often the site of visible arteriolar sclerotic changes in the retinal vasculature, manifest as compression of the veins by the overlying arteries ("A-V nicking").

pole, macula, and the optic nerve head. These images show the relationships between the retinal landmarks as seen in a normal left eye. The most obvious landmark is the optic nerve head (#1 in **Figs. 14.1** and **14.2**), which is made up of the retinal ganglion cell axons as they leave the eye to make their way to the brain. The figures also show the entrance and exit of the central retinal artery and central retinal vein. The optic nerve head is approximately 1.5 mm in horizontal diameter. This dimension, termed a "disc diameter," is commonly used as a size scale for describing both the size of a retinal lesion and its distance from the optic nerve along a specified clock hour. Temporal to the optic nerve head, a round, darker region is evident. This region represents the anatomical macula (#2 in **Figs. 14.1** and **14.2**). At its center is the fovea, a highly specialized portion of the retina that provides the best visual acuity. Details regarding the macula and fovea are presented later in this chapter.

The region of the retina encompassed within the area seen in **Fig. 14.2** is generally referred to as the posterior pole, although definitions of this term vary. It is this portion of the retina that is most commonly captured in a standard retinal photograph and is the maximum area of the retina readily visible using the direct ophthalmoscope with undilated pupils. It corresponds to the portion of the retina within the black circle in **Figure 14.1**. In addition to the optic nerve and macula, the posterior pole contains the major superior and inferior branches of the central retinal artery (3) and the central retinal vein (4). Also visible are the primary and secondary branch points of the retinal arteries and veins, and clinically important sites

where they cross each other (arrows, **Fig. 14.2**). Peripheral to the limits of the posterior pole, additional landmarks are more or less evident depending upon the intensity of pigmentation present in the choroid and retinal pigment epithelium (RPE). Some of these potentially visible landmarks of the retina are seen in **Figure 14.1**. These include the long posterior ciliary arteries and their accompanying long ciliary nerves. These have entered the sclera near the optic nerve head and traversed the thickness of the sclera at an oblique angle. Within the eye they are seen first as they emerge from their respective emissary scleral canals in the mid-periphery, along the horizontal meridian, near its intercept with the vertical equator of the eye. The temporal long posterior ciliary artery and long ciliary nerve are evident (**Fig. 14.1**, asterisks). Additional, potentially visible landmarks include short segments of the short ciliary nerves and, just anterior to the vertical equator of the eye, the coalescence of choroidal veins converging toward the ampullae of the vortex veins (SEE ALSO THE CHAPTER 12: CHOROID AND CHOROIDAL CIRCULATION). Peripheral to the ring of vortex vein ampullae, the retina continues to its anterior terminus called the ora serrata.

At the ora serrata, the retina merges with the posterior limit of the pars plana of the ciliary body. As its name implies, a portion of this ring exhibits a serrated appearance, but this is largely limited to the nasal side of the eye. On the temporal side of the eye, the ora is a relatively straight line. Where serrations exist, (**Fig. 14.3**) slender fingers of retinal tissue project anteriorly into the domain of the pars plana. These projections are termed dentate processes because they resemble sharp teeth. The portions of the pars plana enveloped between adjacent dentate processes are termed oral bays.[1]

Anatomical variants in the anatomy of the ora serrata can occur. In approximately 26% of eyes, at least one fold is present in the peripheral retina extending posteriorly from a dentate process. These are termed meridional folds (**Fig. 14.3**). In some cases, a dentate process extends forward as a ridge, to make direct connection with a ciliary process. These extensions are termed meridional complexes (**Fig. 14.3**). In still other cases, the tips of adjacent dentate processes will converge, partially or completely, enclosing a portion of the pars plana. These are termed enclosed ora bays (**Fig. 14.3**). While meridional folds and complexes can be associated with retinal breaks; partially or completely enclosed ora bays are not.

Also important regarding the anatomy of the ora is that the distribution of the vasculature derived from the central retinal artery does not reach all the way to the ora serrata (**Fig. 14.4**). This leaves the most peripheral portion of the retina with little vascular support, except for a greatly thinned choroid.

The absence of an intraretinal blood supply to the far peripheral retina, combined with an attenuated choroid, contribute to degenerative changes in the tissue. These common changes, termed microcystoid degeneration of

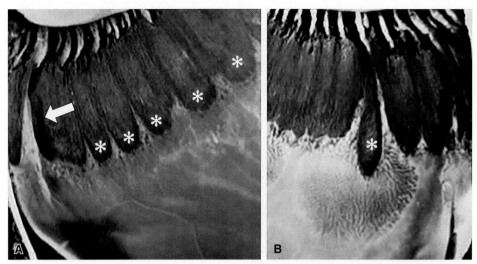

FIGURE 14.3   A: At the ora serrata on the nasal side of the eye, the scalloped appearance results from dentate processes and intervening ora bays (*asterisks*). In this specimen, a meridional complex is also seen, composed of an atypical dentate process (*arrow*), which aligns with and extends to a ciliary process above. The complex also has a meridional fold, which extends along the dentate process and posteriorly into the peripheral retina. **B:** Partially enclosed ora bay (*asterisk*). Posteriorly, the enlarged ora bay extends behind the general line of the ora serrata, and the retina shows a large arcuate area of typical cystoid degeneration. Anteriorly, the ora bay is embraced by two long dentate processes that converge toward (but do not meet in this case), a prominent ciliary process. On the temporal side of the eye, the prominent serrations for which the ora serrata is named, are either much less prominent or not present at all. (From Engstrom RE, Glasgow BJ, Foos RY, et al. Degenerative diseases of the peripheral retina. In: Tasman W, Jaeger EA, eds. *Duane's Ophthalmology on CD-Rom, 2006 Edition.* Philadelphia, PA: Lippincott Williams & Wilkins; 2006.)

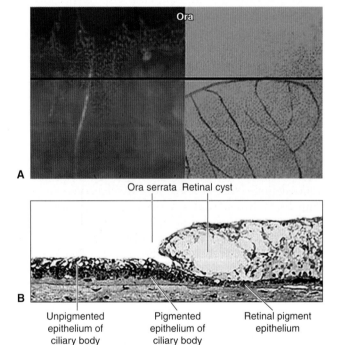

FIGURE 14.4   The ora serrata. The absence of an intraretinal blood supply to the most peripheral retina, combined with an attenuated choroid, contributes to degenerative changes, seen as microcystoid degeneration between black line and scalloped appearance of ora serrata **(A, left)**. The *black line* corresponds to the furthest extent of the capillary vessels derived from the central retinal artery. The vessels are more evident in a similar specimen **(A, right)**. Visible is the terminal arcade of the vasculature derived from the central retinal artery, which does not reach the ora serrata. The orange dots in the right-hand image are cone photoreceptor nuclei. The cystic changes in the top left image are seen in a histologic section of the far periphery of the retina at the ora **(B)**.

the retina, occur in the far periphery of the retina in virtually all individuals over 20 years of age **(Fig. 14.4)**. The clinical appearance of this cystoid degenerative change is clearly seen above the black line in **Figure 14.4A** (also visible in **Fig. 14.3B**). This line corresponds to the furthest extent of the retinal capillary bed in the image at right in **Figure 14.4A**. The orange dots on the right side of **Figure 14.4A** are the cone photoreceptor nuclei and the yellow represents the portion of the retina represented by rods. These cystic changes are seen in a histologic section of the far edge of the retina at the ora **(Fig. 14.4B)**.

Progressing from the posterior pole to the ora, the retina thins dramatically. In the posterior pole, excepting the regions of the central macula and fovea, the thickness of the sensory retina is approximately 250 μm. At the ora, the normal retina is less than a third of this thickness (80 μm) **(Fig. 14.5)**, making it understandable how vitreous traction and retinal atrophy can together lead to the formation of the holes and tears in the retinal periphery that can give rise to potentially blinding complications such as retinal detachment.[2] Overlying this peripheral portion of the retina and the most posterior portion of the pars plana is the vitreous base, the firmest site of attachment of the vitreous body to the wall of the eye **(SEE CHAPTER 11: THE VITREOUS)**.

Terminology Relating the Macula/ Fovea and Foveola

The terminology traditionally used to define the structures in the area of central vision in the posterior pole is confusing,

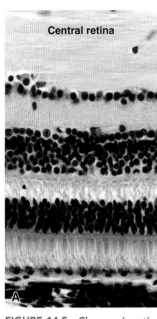

Central retina

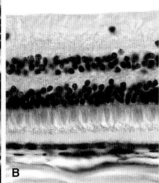

Peripheral retina

FIGURE 14.5   Changes in retinal thickness. Two sections through the central (**A**) and peripheral (**B**) regions of the retina, aligned at the retinal pigment epithelium. The peripheral retina is thinner and has only rare cell nuclei in the ganglion cell layer (the uppermost layer of nuclei). The number and density of cells in the inner and outer nuclear layers is also significantly reduced in the peripheral retina. (From King D. Comparison of peripheral and central retina. Sensorimotor Systems and Behavior unit [SSB] image index website. http://www.siumed.edu/~dking2/ssb/NM012b.htm. January 15, 2007. Accessed October 20, 2016.)

made worse by the fact that some of these terms are used differently by anatomists and clinicians. These terms are defined in **Figure 14.6**. We will limit ourselves to use of the terms macula, macula lutea, fovea, and foveola.

◉ Histology of the Retina

◉ Introduction to the Layers of the Neurosensory Retina

The term retina most commonly includes the single layer of retinal pigment epithelial cells and the nine neurosensory layers. A separate chapter is devoted to the RPE. Hence, this chapter is devoted to the neurosensory retina. The neurosensory retina is a highly structured, laminar, neural tissue that contains morphologically and functionally specialized anatomical features that serve to provide us with high-resolution visual acuity, broad dynamic visual range and function, and signal processing and integration of vision. The layers of the neurosensory retina include three principal layers of neuronal cell bodies, separated by two synaptic layers (**Fig. 14.7**). These layers are inverted relative to the pathway of light, and thus, except in the fovea, photons must transverse the inner vascularized retina to reach the light-sensitive photoreceptors residing in the deepest portion of the retina.

FIGURE 14.6   Relationship between the clinical and anatomical features of the macula. The anatomical macula is ~5.5 mm in diameter and is the region of the retina where the retinal ganglion cells layer is more than one cell thick. Clinically the area in the photograph is called the posterior pole. The fovea is ~1.5 mm in diameter and contains the xanthophyll pigment. Clinically this region is called the macula. The foveola is ~0.33 mm in diameter and is the central region of the retina within the foveal avascular zone (FAZ) containing only cone cells. Clinically this region is called the fovea. The umbo is the region of the foveal light reflex. (From Danny Hope and Macula of retina. Wikiwand website. http://www.wikiwand .com/en/Macula_of_retina. November 8, 2014. Accessed October 20, 2016.)

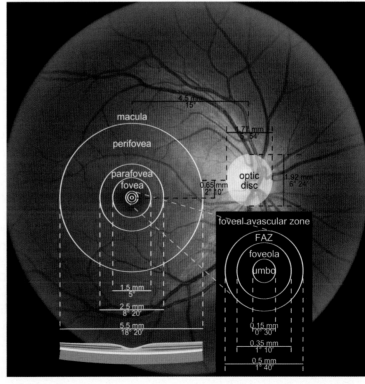

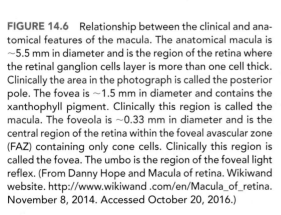

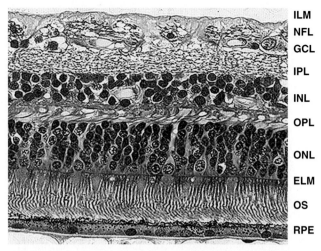

ILM
NFL
GCL
IPL
INL
OPL
ONL
ELM
OS
RPE

FIGURE 14.7 Cross section showing the 10 layers of the human retina. From inner to outer retina. ILM, internal limiting membrane; NFL, nerve fiber layer; GCL, retinal ganglion cell layer; IPL, inner plexiform layer; INL, inner nuclear layer; OPL, outer plexiform layer; ONL, outer nuclear layer; ELM, external limiting membrane; OS, photoreceptor inner and outer segments; RPE, retinal pigment epithelium. (From Milam A. *The Human Retina in Health and Disease Teaching Set.* © Scheie Eye Institute, University of Pennsylvania; 2016.)

The nine layers of the neurosensory retina (excluding the fovea described later), progressing from the RPE toward the vitreous are:

1. *Photoreceptor layer*: this layer contains the light-sensitive portions of the photoreceptor cells, divided into the photopigment-containing outer segments (OS), closest to the RPE and the inner segments (IS) containing most of the photoreceptor cell organelles. The inner and outer segments are connected only by a thin bridge of cytoplasm supported by a connecting cilium not visible at the light microscopic level.

2. *External limiting membrane*: this layer represents a linear array of zonulae adherentes junctions that surround the photoreceptors like a belt and attaches them around their entire circumference to their neighboring photoreceptor cells and adjacent Müller cells (glia).

3. *Outer nuclear layer*: this layer is comprised of the cell bodies (nuclei) of the photoreceptor cells.

4. *Outer plexiform layer*: this layer contains the interconnecting cell processes and synpases between the photoreceptor cells and those of the horizontal and bipolar cell interneurons.

   Note that all four of these outer retinal layers are largely defined by the different anatomical parts of the photoreceptor cells (rods and cones). And it is these four outermost layers that are devoid of blood vessels.

5. *Inner nuclear layer*: this layer is made up of the cell bodies of the bipolar cells and horizontal cells (both of which are located in the outer portion of this layer), together with the Müller cell nuclei and most of the amacrine cell nuclei, both of which are preferentially located in the inner portion of the layer. Retinal ganglion cells have occasionally been shown to be displaced into this layer.

6. *Inner plexiform layer*: this layer contains the connecting processes of the intermediate cells of the inner nuclear layer including the bipolar, amacrine and interplexiform cells and their connections to the dendrites of the retinal ganglion cells.

7. *Retinal ganglion cell layer*: this layer contains the cell bodies of the innermost layer of neurons in the retina, the retinal ganglion cells. A subclass of amacrine cell bodies may also be "displaced" into the ganglion cell layer.

8. *Nerve fiber layer*: this layer is composed of the retinal ganglion cell axons that run just beneath the internal limiting membrane of the retina. In addition, glial cells are present, some of which provide a support function and some of which function as phagocytic cells in the retina, as they do in the brain.

   Logically, as more axons from the peripheral to the central retina are gathered into this layer, the nerve fiber layer progressively thickens as it approaches the optic nerve head. It is these axons that converge to form the optic nerve. The axons continue to their synaptic connections in the brain; primarily in the lateral geniculate nucleus of the thalamus (**SEE CHAPTER 15: THE OPTIC NERVE AND VISUAL PATHWAYS**). However, not all fibers reach the thalamus. Some axons exit the optic tracts to synapse on other nuclei of the midbrain, specifically the superior colliculi, pretectum, and suprachiasmatic nucleus of the hypothalamus.

9. *Internal limiting membrane*: this surface-covering layer is formed by expanded "foot plates" of the elongated glial cells of the retina, the Müller cells. These foot plates blend together to form a continuous mosaic at the retinal surface that is the retinal interface with the posterior vitreous cortex, to which the internal limiting membrane of the retina is attached.

   The Müller cells forming this layer extend from their foot plates through nearly the entire neurosensory retina, terminating just external to the external limiting membrane of the retina, not quite reaching the RPE. As the major glial element of the retina, Müller cells have connections with all retinal neuron cell types. As described in detail later, they play a critical role in the maintenance of normal retinal structure and function, providing growth factors, components of the interphotoreceptor matrix, and trophic support to the retinal neurons (**Fig. 14.8**). The introduction of optical coherence tomography (OCT) imaging of the retina (and anterior segment) over the past two decades has revolutionized clinical practice. OCT is a medical imaging method that uses reflected light to capture high resolution, black and white (or false color) images of tissue, analogous to the way that ultrasound is used to visualize internal organs. OCT is the optical equivalent of an ultrasound in the eye. Because the ocular tissues are mostly transparent, until one gets to the RPE cell layer, OCT is able to provide an image of the retina with remarkable clarity and anatomical detail. A representative high resolution OCT image and its ability to non-invasively

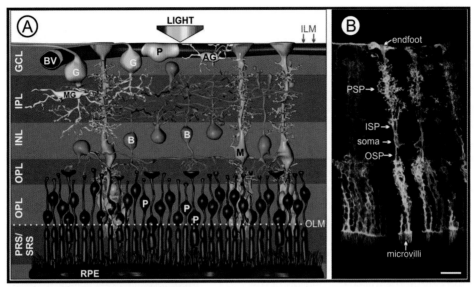

FIGURE 14.8   Müller cells in the vascularized retina. **(A)** Artist's view on the cellular composition of a vertebrate retina. The cell bodies of retinal neurons are arranged in three nuclear layers—the ganglion cell layer (GCL), the inner nuclear layer (INL), and the outer plexiform layer (ONL). The somata of the light-sensitive photoreceptors (P) are tightly packed in the latter and, thus, light has to pass all retinal layers to reach them. The synaptic contacts mediating the information transfer are located in the outer and inner plexiform layer (OPL, IPL). Aside from Müller cells (M, orange) as the main macroglial cells in the retina, there are astrocytes (AG, yellow) exclusively located in the nerve fiber layer and microglia (MG, the immuncompetent cells of the retina, green) residing in the plexiform layers. B, bipolar cell; BV, blood vessel; ILM, inner limiting membrane; OLM, outer limiting membrane; PRS, photoreceptor segments; RPE, retinal pigment epithelium; SRS, subretinal space. Modified from Retinal Glia. Reichenbach A, Bringmann A. Morgan and Claypool Life Sciences. 2015. **(B)** Highly specialized morphology of Müller cells in the mouse retina. ISP, inner stem process; OSP, outer stem process; PSP, perisynaptc processes. Scale bar, 20 μm.

show the layers of the retina, in vivo is compared with a histological section in **Figure 14.9**. Because this new technology brings the need to know ocular histology into the clinic on an everyday basis, a separate chapter on ocular anatomy as seen with OCT is included in this textbook (**See Chapter 17: Ocular Anatomy by Optical Coherence Tomography**).

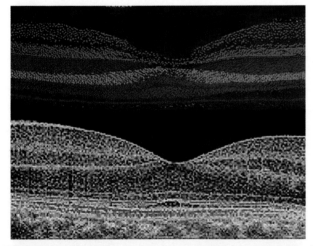

FIGURE 14.9   Comparison of histological section seen by confocal microscopy **(top)** and in vivo, optical coherence tomography (OCT) images of the retina **(bottom)**. OCT uses reflected light to capture high resolution images of retinal tissue with remarkable clarity and anatomical detail in vivo (**See Chapter 17: Ocular Anatomy by Optical Coherence Tomography**). (Top image from Milam A. *The Human Retina in Health and Disease Teaching Set.* © Scheie Eye Institute, University of Pennsylvania; 2016; Bottom image from Zeiss Cirrus OCT.)

Anatomical and Functional Details of Neurosensory Layers of the Retina

PHOTORECEPTOR CELLS

The photoreceptor cells of the human retina are of two principal types—rods and cones. Both cell types extend from the apicial surface of the retinal pigment epithelial cells to their synapses in the outer plexiform layer of the retina. The human retina contains approximately 125 million rods and 6.4 million cones.[3,4]

ROD PHOTORECEPTORS MEDIATE SCOTOPIC VISION

In order to maximize light perception under both very dim conditions of illumination as well as in bright light, the retina has evolved two separate but interconnected pathways to mediate perception. The dim-light pathway uses the rod photoreceptors and a variety of anatomical features to achieve maximal sensitivity, so that under ideal conditions, humans can perceive a single photon of light. These features include: (1) long, rod-shaped outer segments, OS containing hundreds of rhodopsin-containing membrane disks oriented orthogonal to the path of incoming light, to maximize chances that an incoming photon will be captured by the rhodopsin pigment, and (2) convergence of synaptic connections of groups of rod cells to a given second order neuron (bipolar cell) to amplify the signals obtained. The rod pathway primarily provides information about the *rate of photon capture* (i.e., overall illumination) with little discrimination of color. Because it is a convergent pathway (pooled input from regions of the retina), visual discrimination is reduced, resulting in the type of vision one experiences at dusk or at night (scotopic vision).

Rod cells contain the photopigment rhodopsin, which has an absorption peak at 498 nm. The sensitivity of rod cells to low luminance levels (dim light and night vision) and blue/green wavelength light (scotopic conditions) is high, but acuity from rod function is comparatively low. The relative density of rod cells in the nonmacular retina varies. The density of rod cell distribution increases as one moves away from the fovea and is greatest in regions that are eccentric to the fovea by approximately 18°. This is why stars in the night sky are most easily seen if one looks slightly off axis from the intended target. It is well established that there are no rod cells in the fovea, the portion of the retina that provides us with our highest resolution vision and color vision under conditions of bright illumination.[5,6]

CONES PHOTORECEPTORS MEDIATE PHOTOPIC VISION

Cone cells are widely distributed throughout the human retina, but they are the only photoreceptor type are found in the human foveola. A topographic map of cone cell density demonstrates this extreme regional localization relative to that of the rod cells as a function of eccentricity from the fovea (**Fig. 14.10**). To achieve this greater packing density in the foveal region, the cone OS in the fovea are elongated and extremely thin, looking more like slender rods than the conical shape found in the extrafoveal retina and for which these photoreceptors are named (**Figs. 14.11** and **14.12**). This modification in the morphology of cones in the foveal region allows them to achieve an average packing density of 200,000 cones per mm². This tighter packing density contributes to, but does not fully account for, the better spatial resolution found in this part of the retina.[5] About 30 cone cells or 28 rod cells interact with each RPE cell in their respective regions of their greatest density.[7]

Retinal cones, which mediate vision under conditions of bright light (photopic conditions) provide high acuity and contrast, and color sensitivity. In comparison to rods, cones have many fewer folded membrane disks in each outer segment and there are far fewer total numbers of cones (though they are concentrated in the fovea and much sparser in the remainder of the retina). In the fovea, one cone cell synapses with a given second order bipolar cell, so there is less signal convergence but much higher acuity. Each cone outer segment contains one of the three types of photopigments that maximally absorb in either the red, green, or blue portion of the visible light spectrum. Information sent from cones to bipolar cells is "computed" as the relative input contributions from these three types of color-specific cones.

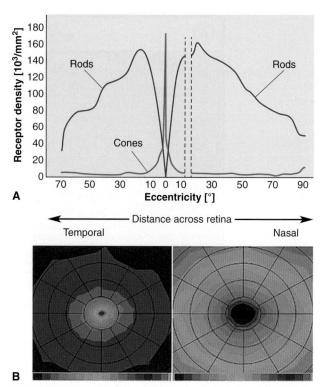

FIGURE 14.10 **A:** Cross section and topographic maps of the density of cone and rod photoreceptors across the retina. **B:** The cone density is greatest in the small central island of the fovea (**left**), whereas the rod cells are entirely absent from the fovea (**right, black center**) but are otherwise distributed throughout the retina. The site of greatest rod density is a concentric ring ~18° eccentric from the central fovea (**blue ring, right**) ([A] modified from Østerberg G. Topography of the layer of rods and cones in the human retina. *Acta Ophthal.* 1935;(suppl 6):1–103. [B] from Curcio CA, Sloan KR, Kalina RE, et al. Human photoreceptor topography. *J Comp Neurol.* 1990;292:497–523.)

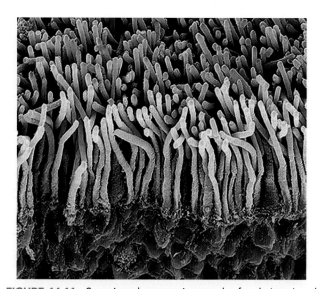

FIGURE 14.11 Scanning electron micrograph of rods (*grey*) and cones (*purple*) showing the different shapes for which each photoreceptor type is named (false color image). The photoreceptor cell nuclei are seen at the bottom of the image (brown). (Image from Steve Gschmeissner and Science Photo Library website. http://www .sciencephoto.com. Accessed October 20, 2016.)

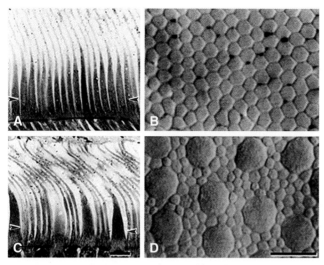

FIGURE 14.12 Comparison of vertical histologic **(A, C)** and en face optical **(B, D)** sections through photoreceptors in the fovea **(A, B)** and near periphery **(C, D)** of human retina. *Arrowheads* in **(A)** and **(C)** indicate approximate level through the ellipsoid portion of photoreceptor inner segments where photographs **(B, D)** are taken. All profiles in **(B)** are cones; large profiles in **(D)** are the cones and small intervening profiles are rods. *Bars = 10 μm.* (From Curcio CA, Sloan KR, Kalina RE, et al. Human photoreceptor topography. *J Comp Neurol.* 1990;292:497–523.)

There are three main types of cones, which are characterized by the absorption spectrum of the cell's opsin molecule; L-cones ("long wavelength" red-spectrum light; 564 nm), M-cones, which are unique to primates ("middle wavelength" green spectrum light; 534 nm), and S-cones ("short wavelength" blue spectrum light; 420 nm) (**Fig. 14.13**).[8,9] The majority of cones in the fovea are L-cones and M-cones. S-cones are present in smaller numbers and, importantly, are absent from the foveola. Together, the three color-spectrum sensitive opsins provide the basis for our color perception and vision, termed "trichromacy."

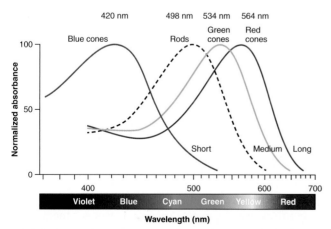

FIGURE 14.13 Absorption spectra of cone and rod photoreceptors in the human retina. (From Bowmaker JK, Dartnall HJA. Visual pigments of rods and cones in a human retina. *J Physiol.* 1980;298:501–511.)

It is a common misperception that the three different wavelength sensitivities of cone cells in the retina act like the red:green:blue pixels on a television screen to convey color information to the brain. This is not the case. Rather, the response of a particular cone cell to light is a function of the wavelength of light, its intensity, the angle of incidence of the photon with the long axis of the photoreceptor and the cone cell's sensitivity spectrum. By comparing the differential signals received from two (or all three) types of cones, the brain can determine both the intensity and the color of the light.[10–12] The three different types of wavelength-sensitive cone cells act in concert to convey a broad spectrum of color information. The L- and M-cones together mediate red-green color sensitivity and discrimination (the R-G "channel"). Blue-yellow sensitivity is provided by S-cones (the B-Y "channel"). Perceived overall luminance is primarily the sum of the L- and M-cone signals. Thus, simultaneous combinations of cone cell responses mediate trichromatic visual perception. It is estimated that the human retina can distinguish up to 10 million different colors.[13]

*The term "color blindness" is generally a misnomer. Most patients who are color-blind have a genetic defect in one cone opsin and are therefore "anomalous trichromats" (also termed deuteranomalous) (i.e., they see a broad spectrum of colors but the colors in a specific range of wavelengths are muted or desaturated). They may also be "deuteranopic" where one cone opsin is absent and a portion of the color spectrum is missing. In anomalous trichromats a mutation of the opsin protein changes the peak of the light wavelength sensitivity, diminishing the range of colors that can be distinguished from each other (**Fig. 14.14**).[14] Protanomaly is reduced sensitivity to red light, deuteranomaly is reduced sensitivity to green light, and tritanomaly (rarest) is reduced sensitivity to blue light. Deuteranomlous vision is the most common form of inherited color blindness, usually occurring in males, because it is X-linked. About 5% of males are deuteranomalous trichromats. A very rare congenital condition called achromatopsia (also termed rod monochromacy) is associated with absence of cone cell function altogether and complete blindness to color. These patients also have severely reduced vision (~20/200), photophobia, and nystagmus due to the absence of foveal function and its intrinsic acuity. In addition to these congenital color vision anomalies, certain diseases (and medications) can give rise to acquired color vision defects. In general, outer retinal diseases and media changes (such as cataract) result in blue-yellow color defects; while diseases of the inner retina, optic nerve, visual pathway, and visual cortex will result in acquired red-green defects. This concept is commonly termed Kollner's rule.[15,16]*

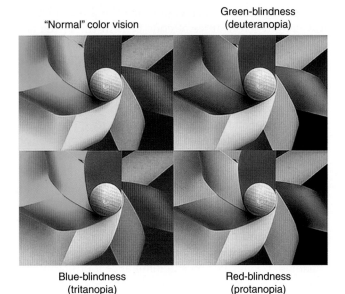

"Normal" color vision

Green-blindness
(deuteranopia)

Blue-blindness
(tritanopia)

Red-blindness
(protanopia)

FIGURE 14.14 Simulations of the visual color perception associated with the three main trichromatic color deficiencies in humans; deuteranopia, protanopia, and tritanopia. (From Ahlmann J. Simulation of different color deficiencies, color blindness. Flickr website. https://www.flickr.com/photos/entirelysubjective/6146852926/. September 14, 2011. Accessed October 20, 2016.)

Photoreceptor Ultrastructure

The rods and cones have a generally similar structure but with some important morphologic distinctions, which are seen primarily at the ultrastructural level. Both are subdivided into an outer segment and an inner segment (Fig. 14.15). The outer segment contains the stacks of photopigment impregnated membrane. The inner segment contains the cell organelles. The portion of each cell containing the organelles is further subdivided into an ellipsoid and myoid region, with the ellipsoid region being closest to the outer segment. These are described in more detail, below, including the external limiting membrane.

The nuclei of the photoreceptor cells constitute the outer nuclear layer of the retina and the synaptic connections of these cells (termed spherules in rods and pedicles in cones) reach the outer plexiform layer. In this way, the various parts of the photoreceptor cell contribute virtually all of the avascular, outer layers of the retina except for the RPE. These include the photoreceptor layer, the external limiting membrane, the outer nuclear layer, and a portion of the outer plexiform layer.

The Outer Segment

Light is absorbed by one of the opsin photopigments (present in color-specific cones) or by rhodopsin (in rod cells); both of which reside within layers of stacked cell membranes in the outer segment of their respective photoreceptors. These photosensitive membranes are formed continuously by the inner segment of the photoreceptor cells as an elaboration

of the plasma membrane that becomes highly enfolded and then compacted to form the outer segment (Fig. 14.16). In rod photoreceptors, these enfolded membranes fuse to form closed, bilayered disks that are stacked very tightly and encased by, but separate from, the plasma membrane throughout the length of the rod outer segment—like stacks of pita bread encased in a cellophane wrapper. In cones, the enfolded membranes result from tight folding of the plasma membrane of the cell itself, resembling a collapsed accordion. In both rods and cones, the addition of new photopigment containing leaflets/disks at the base of the outer segment is balanced by the active shedding of an equivalent amount of membrane from the apical tip of the outer segment, resulting in a continual replacement of photopigment.

The distal tip of the photoreceptor is surrounded by retinal pigment epithelial cells, which phagocytose and degrade the shed tips, catabolizing their molecular assemblies, recycling them through the process of autophagy, and excreting waste through Bruch's membrane to the underlying choriocapillaris for removal from the eye.[17–19]

In humans, disk shedding is controlled by circadian rhythms and the light/dark cycle. In the case of rod photoreceptors, which mediate *scotopic* (low light) vision, shedding is triggered at light onset. In the case of cone cells, which mediate *photopic* (bright light) vision, shedding is triggered at light offset.[20] Intrinsically photosensitive retinal ganglion cells that contain the photopigment melanopsin are also present in the human retina and are discussed below in the context of the circadian rhythm.

The Inner Segment

The inner segment of the photoreceptor cell functions as the principal site of cellular metabolic and synthetic activity and thus contains organelles that support these functions including mitochondria, the Golgi apparatus and rough endoplasmic reticulum. The inner segment is ultrastructurally subdivided into a myoid region and an ellipsoid region, as mentioned earlier. The myoid region is the portion of the inner segment closest to the external limiting membrane and the cell nucleus, in which the rough endoplasmic reticulum and Golgi apparatus are found. The ellipsoid region is continuous with the myoid region and extends to the junction between the outer and inner segments of the photoreceptor cells (see Fig. 14.15). The ellipsoid region contains principally mitochondria, with cones having larger numbers of mitochondria that are also larger in size than those in rods. The mitochondria provide the metabolic energy required to continuously synthesize the outer segment membrane leaflets and to recycle the photopigment and proteins required for the process of visual transduction. Connecting the inner and outer segments of the photoreceptor cells

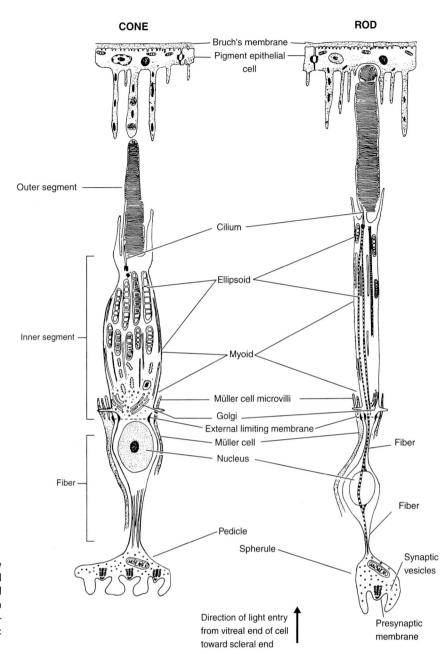

CONE **ROD**

Bruch's membrane
Pigment epithelial cell
Outer segment
Cilium
Ellipsoid
Inner segment
Myoid
Müller cell microvilli
Golgi
External limiting membrane
Müller cell
Nucleus
Fiber
Fiber
Fiber
Pedicle
Spherule
Synaptic vesicles
Presynaptic membrane
Direction of light entry from vitreal end of cell toward scleral end

FIGURE 14.15 Comparative sketches show the principal anatomic subdivisions of rod and cone type photoreceptor cells. (Modified from and courtesy of Dr. B. Borwein. In: Enoch JM, Tobey FL, eds. *Springer Series in Optical Sciences.* Vol 23. Heidelberg, Germany: Springer-Verlag; 1981.)

is a very narrow isthmus of cytoplasm containing a single cilium (**Figs. 14.16** and **14.17**). This cilium is anchored to a modified centriole and basal body found in the ellipsoid region of the outer segment. Within the core of each cilium, the typical ring of nine microtubule doublets is found (**Fig. 14.17**); however, the central doublet that characterizes motile cilia is not present.

EXTERNAL LIMITING MEMBRANE OF THE RETINA

Both photoreceptor cell types and the adjacent Müller glial cells (discussed below) are radially oriented in the retina

and tightly packed together. This tight packing is ensured by the external limiting membrane. At the light microscopic level, this appears to be a continuous line crossing the photoreceptor cells, just external to the photoreceptor cell nuclei. This line is particularly well demarcated in OCT images of the retina (**Fig. 14.18**).

At the ultrastructural level, however, this line is seen to be discontinuous and actually represents a linear array of zonulae adherentes junctions that join each photoreceptor to its surrounding photoreceptors and the intervening Müller glial cells around their entire circumference (**Fig. 14.19**). Unlike zonulae occludentes that prevent intercellular diffusion of macromolecules, zonulae adherentes function

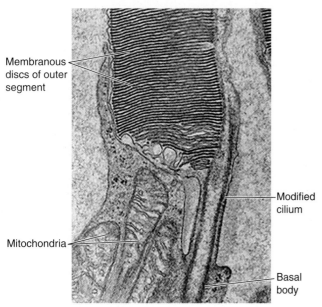

Membranous discs of outer segment

Modified cilium

Mitochondria

Basal body

FIGURE 14.16 Junction of the inner and outer segments of a rod photoreceptor. The connecting cilium and basal body of the inner segment are seen. The formation of the membrane disc packets is evident at the base of the outer segment and the tightly associated mitochondria of the ellipsoid region providing energy for membrane protein synthesis. (Transmission electron microscope; ×45,000.) (From Krause WJ, Cutts JH. *Concise Text of Histology*. Baltimore, MD: Williams & Wilkins; 1981.)

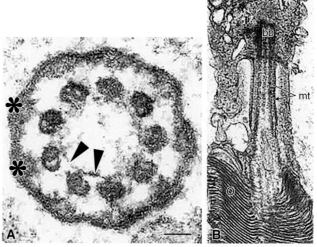

FIGURE 14.17 Electron micrographs of the connecting cilium of human photoreceptors. **A:** Cross section of a cilium shows nine doublets of microtubules forming a ring characteristic of sensory (non-motile) cilia. The microtubules are interconnected by nexin links (*arrowheads*) and joined to the surface membrane by Y-shaped linkers (*asterisks*). Bar = 0.04 μm. **B:** Longitudinal section of cilium. Microtubules (mt) stacks of membrane discs in the outer segment (*O*), and basal body (bb) in the inner segment (*I*). Bar = 0.15 μm. (From Milam A, Smith JE, John SK. Anatomy and cell biology of the human retina. In: Tasman W, Jaeger EA, eds. *Duane's Ophthalmology on CD-Rom, 2006 Edition*. Philadelphia, PA: Lippincott Williams & Wilkins; 2006.)

in intercellular adhesion, in this case, ensuring that each photoreceptor always maintains its same physical position relative to its neighbors. This is important because each photoreceptor is wired to represent a particular position in visual space. If you indent your eye by pushing on the upper lid, note that although things are distorted, everything that you see moves together, without shifting the relative positions of the parts of the scene. Without the external limiting membrane, photoreceptor cells could possibly change their positions relative to their neighbors and rearrange the relative positions of parts of a scene.

OUTER NUCLEAR LAYER

The cell bodies and nuclei of both types of photoreceptor cells constitute the outer nuclear layer of the retina. This layer is about 8 to 10 cells thick and is similar in appearance across the retina except for the foveal and

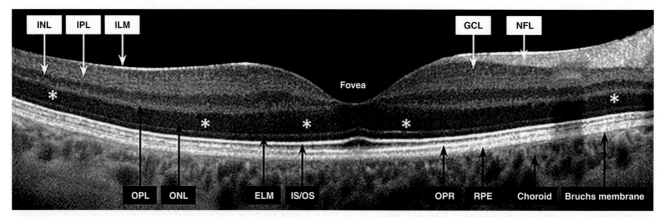

FIGURE 14.18 High resolution spectral-domain OCT of the human retina including the fovea. *Asterisks* show that the outer nuclear layer is about the same thickness throughout the posterior pole. ELM, external limiting membrane; GCL, retinal ganglion cell layer; ILM, internal limiting membrane; INL, inner nuclear layer; IPL, inner plexiform layer; IS/OS, photoreceptor inner and outer segments; NFL, nerve fiber layer; ONL, outer nuclear layer; OPL, outer plexiform layer; OPR, outer segment RPE complex; RPE, retinal pigment epithelium. (From www.hoacls.org.)

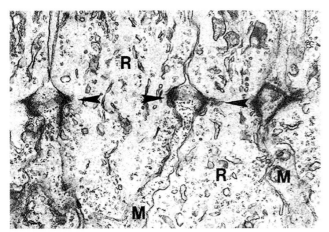

FIGURE 14.19 Transmission electron micrograph shows that the external limiting membrane is formed by zonulae adherentes junctions. The continuous row of junctions (*arrowheads*) between photoreceptors (*R*) and Müller cells (*M*) forms the external limiting membrane. (From Park S. The anatomy and the cell biology of the retina. In: Tasman W, Jaeger EA, eds. *Duane's Ophthalmology on CD-Rom, 2006 Edition.* Philadelphia, PA: Lippincott Williams & Wilkins; 2006.)

parafoveal regions. In non-foveal regions of the retina, a given photoreceptor nucleus is located internal to, and in line with, its inner and outer segments. However, in the cone-rich foveola, the outer nuclear layer is splayed radially, so that cone OS are more directly exposed to incoming light without interference from any overlying retina cell body elements. The radial displacement of foveal cone

nuclei causes a slight bulge in the retinal thickness in the parafoveal region. The ratio of cones to rods varies across the remainder of the retina, with rods outnumbering cones as one moves further out into the retinal periphery.

OUTER PLEXIFORM LAYER

Rod and cone cells synapse with bipolar and horizontal cells in the outer plexiform layer and, except in the fovea where they are displaced, photoreceptors communicate with second order neurons with which they are vertically aligned in the light path.[21,22] Rod synaptic terminals are called spherules and comprise (1) the presynaptic structures of the rod, including a presynaptic ribbon and large aggregates of synaptic vesicles and (2) a triad arrangement of postsynaptic elements usually including two laterally positioned processes from horizontal cells and one centrally positioned dendrite from a rod bipolar cell. Rod spherules are comprised of one triad that synapses with horizontal cells and rod bipolar cells, whereas cone synaptic terminals, called pedicles, contain several invaginating synapses with horizontal cells and cone bipolar cells. Cone pedicles also exhibit structures termed flat synapses (**Fig. 14.20**), contributed by a subset of cone bipolar cells termed "off" bipolar cells. Three processes from postsynaptic cells are arranged (indented or invaginated) in close association with a synaptic ribbon. A single cone cell makes contact with both types of bipolar cells. The central process is a bipolar cell dendrite with the two lateral processes being from horizontal cells.[23–26]

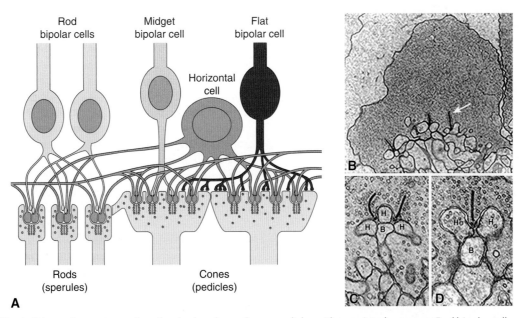

FIGURE 14.20 A: Schematic representation of rod spherules and cone pedicles with associated synapses. Rod bipolar cells, a midget cone bipolar cell, and a horizontal cell form invaginating synapses with the rods and cones. A flat cone bipolar cell forms flat synapses onto the cone pedicles. Gap junctions are also present between the rod spherules and cone pedicles. **B:** Electron micrograph of a cone's synaptic pedicle shown here from a turtle retina. An arrow points to a ribbon with a halo of synaptic vesicles. High power view of the invaginating complex in the turtle **(C)** and in the monkey (Macaca) retina **(D).** The lateral processes made by horizontal cells are usually empty (as in Image B) or occasionally contain scattered vesicles (as in Image C). H, horizontal cell lateral process; B, bipolar cell dendrite. ([A] from Hogan MJ, Alvarado JA, Weddell JE. *Histology of the Human Eye.* Philadelphia, PA: WB Saunders; 1971. [B–D] Courtesy of Elio Raviola, Harvard Medical School. In: Schwartz EA. Transport-mediated synapses in the retina. *Physiol Rev.* 2002;82(4):875–891.)

These complex synapses play an integral role in the intrinsic signal processing seen in the retina. All signaling in the retina prior to reaching the amacrine and retinal ganglion cell occurs through graded membrane potentials. It is only the amacrine and retinal ganglion cells (RGC) that appear to be capable of generating an action potential. The tightly integrated synapses of the outer plexiform layer bring the photoreceptor cells, the horizontal cells, and the bipolar cells together, permitting the integration and modulation of the signals coming from the rods and cones. With the exception of the foveal cones, there is a convergence of many cone inputs onto one bipolar cell, permitting the integration of signal from a broad array of photoreceptors stimulated by light (**Fig. 14.21**). The bipolar cell, located in the inner nuclear layer, receives some of its input directly from the photoreceptors. The input ranges from one cone cell in the fovea to thousands of rods in the peripheral retina. In addition, bipolar cells receive inhibitory input from horizontal cells. These

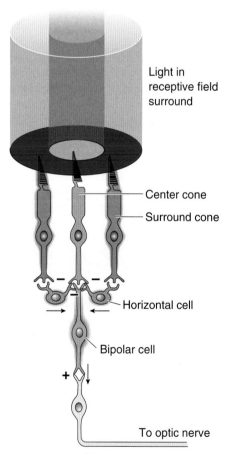

FIGURE 14.21 Receptive fields of retinal bipolar cells. The bipolar cell receives some of its input directly from photoreceptors, in addition to inhibitory input from horizontal cells. Thus, the receptive field of the bipolar cell has two signaling components: a central component directly from the photoreceptors and a surrounding component of information conveyed by the horizontal cells. (Modified from Bear MF, Connors BW, Paradiso MW. *Neuroscience*. 4th ed. Philadelphia, PA: Wolters Kluwer; 2015.)

horizontal cells receive their input from photoreceptors in the receptive field surrounding the central photoreceptors, which directly signal the bipolar cell. Thus, the receptive field of the bipolar cell has two signaling components: a central component directly from the photoreceptors and a surrounding component of information conveyed by the horizontal cells.

A given outer segment absorbs photons emitted from the area of the visual field in direct alignment with the outer segment's location in the retinal array and functions as a photon detector that monitors photon flux from a specific area of the visual field.[27] This assignment is defined as the cell's "receptive field", which has been measured experimentally, not just for photoreceptors but for all other retinal neurons that receive direct or indirect input from photoreceptors. Comparisons between the receptive fields of different neurons have helped to establish the functional circuitry of the retina. For example, the receptive field of a single rod is small, but because of the convergence of many rods onto a single bipolar cell, the receptive field of the bipolar cell will be larger and equal to the sum of the receptive fields of all rods signaling it. That signal is modulated by the horizontal cell, which provides feedback inhibition to many bipolar cells and functions to sharpen the edges of a receptive field.

INNER NUCLEAR LAYER

Within the inner nuclear layer are the cell bodies of five principal cell types that can be distinguished by immunohistochemical markers. These include; (1) horizontal cells and (2) bipolar cells, typically in the layers closest to the outer plexiform layer, and (3) Müller cells, (4) amacrine cells, and (5) interplexiform cells, closer to the inner plexiform layer. The inner nuclear layer is thicker in the macula than it is in the peripheral retina. This is due primarily to an increase in the density of cone bipolar cells and the organization of the horizontal and amacrine cells modulating pathway inputs from the dense foveal cones.

The intrinsic circuitry of the retina is complex. The synaptic connections among photoreceptors, bipolar cells, interneurons (including horizontal, amacrine and interplexiform cells), and RGCs permit significant amounts of summation and integration of visual information from the photoreceptors even before the visual information is relayed to the midbrain and visual cortex.[28] Visual information processing in the retina occurs through excitatory, inhibitory, and feedback connections. Parallel processing of visual stimuli in the retina permits integration of visual perception of both still and moving objects.[29,30] Parallel anatomical tracts in the brain convey complex visual information such as stereopsis, feature recognition, and others. Detailed discussions of our changing understanding of retinal microcircuits are best obtained from regularly updated and published review articles.

Bipolar Cells (On and Off)

Object recognition and movement detection are essential components of visual perception. Bipolar cell circuits function to enhance responses to any increase or decrease in light. Conversely they are largely nonresponsive when light levels are not changing. The information passed from bipolar cells to ganglion cells is highly filtered by horizontal cells to contain information about edges (contributing to perception of shapes or forms) and additionally filtered by bipolar cells to contain information about changing light levels (contributing to perception of movement and of light/dark).[31,32]

As the name implies, bipolar cells convey synaptic information from the retinal photoreceptors in the outer retina to the amacrine cells and ganglion cells in the inner retina.[32] Because the number of bipolar cells is far less than the number of photoreceptors, the bipolar cell functions to converge sensory input to improve sensitivity in the retinal periphery. However, with foveal cones there is a 1:1 relationship with bipolar cells (and RGCs), thus no similar convergence occurs in the fovea.[33] This anatomy contributes to the high visual acuity provided by the foveal cones. Bipolar cells convert a range of light inputs from the photoreceptors into "on" inputs or "off" inputs to the inner retina. These are the first higher order visual processing neurons in the retina, and thus exhibit behavior demonstrating the concept of "receptive fields", that is, they can respond to complex sensory inputs sent from an area of the retina, not just from an individual cell.[34,35]

There are two major types of cone-specific bipolar cells and 10 subclassifications; but there is just one type of rod-specific bipolar cell. The two functional types of cone-specific bipolar cells are "on" cone bipolar cells (which are stimulated when the light is turned on) and "off" cone bipolar cells (which are stimulated when the light is turned off). Both on and off bipolar cells have several morphologic variants.

Cone Bipolar Cells: The "on" cone bipolar cells have invaginating synapses in the cone pedicles and their axons are seen to terminate in the inner strata of the inner plexiform layer. The "off" bipolar cells have flat synapses and their axons terminate in the outer strata of the inner plexiform layer. Six (or seven types) of the cone bipolar cells are defined and synapse with many cone cells and three types synapse with a single cone cell (flat midget, invaginating midget). The bipolar cells are 'flat' (off) or 'invaginating' (on) or (depending on the morphology of the dendritic tips) either on the cell surface or penetrating the synaptic terminals.[35,36] The diffuse types of cone bipolar cells synapse with 5 to 10 L- and M-cone pedicles, and less commonly with S-cones. Each cone in the fovea has a synapse with only one "on" and one "off" midget bipolar cell.[21,37] The invaginating midget bipolar cells synapse in the inner strata of the inner plexiform layer along with

the other "on" bipolar cells. S-cones have a synapse with a subpopulation of "on" blue cone bipolar cells that also terminate in the inner strata.[38]

The midget bipolar cells directly connect one cone cell in the region of the fovea to one RGC and thus provide the conduit for one-to-one communication between the cones of the fovea and the brain. This high cell density and direct circuitry underlie the high resolving power and thus, visual acuity, obtained by the human fovea. It has been proposed that the direct circuitry from single cone cells provided by the midget bipolar cell was a necessary evolutionary precondition for the development of trichromatic vision in primates, since pooled signals to RGCs integrating cone inputs that are responsive to a spectrum of light wavelengths would not convey meaningful color information.[12]

Rod Bipolar Cells: The one type of rod bipolar cell in the human retina that functions as an "on" cell outnumbers the cone bipolar cells due to the much larger number of rods in the retina. Each rod bipolar cell receives synaptic input from 6 to 40 rod spherules (up to 40 in the peripheral retina).[38,39] The processes of each rod bipolar cell terminate in the inner portion of the inner plexiform layer. In contrast to cone bipolar cells, rod bipolar cells do not synapse directly with RGCs, but rather "hitch a ride" on cone bipolar-to-ganglion cell pathways (**Fig. 14.22**).[40,41] While the rod and cone photon collection systems are separate, it is too "expensive" for the retina to maintain separate synaptic pathways all the way from the retina to the brain. Instead, the rod and cone signals synapse on a designated bipolar cell and this cell has to handle both types of information. In general, low light information is blocked in bright light (since rods become saturated in bright light) and conversely, in low light, cones are inactive. Thus, bipolar cells are generally handling only rod or cone information at any given time.

Since the rod-driven circuit 'piggy-backs' onto cone-based circuitry at the bipolar cell level, this means that there are no distinct classes of ganglion cells dedicated specifically for rod-based scotopic vision.[38] Within this circuit, light stimulation of rods initiates a signal that culminates in cone 'ON' bipolar cell excitation and cone 'OFF' bipolar cell inhibition. Similarly, the converse occurs (cone 'ON' bipolar cell inhibition and cone 'OFF' bipolar cell excitation) upon exposure of the rod to darkness. This illustrates another unique feature of rod-based retinal circuits, as the signal splits into ON and OFF channels after it has been transmitted across two synapses (rods to rod bipolar cells and then to AII amacrine cells). In contrast, cone-driven signals separate into these parallel channels at the first synapse in the outer plexiform layer.

Bipolar cells in the retina function primarily as edge detectors, sensing light from "center-surround" receptive fields. The various morphologic types of bipolar cells also express different neurotransmitter receptors, and demonstrate

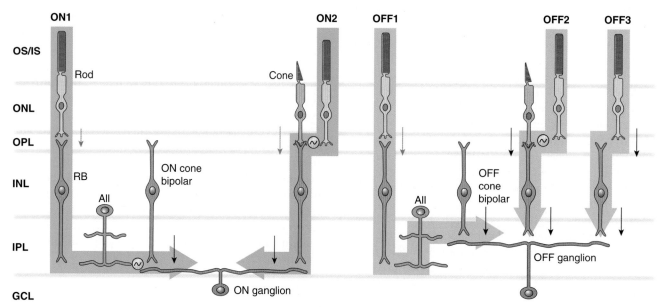

FIGURE 14.22 Schematic wiring diagram of the mammalian retina, showing the rod (scotopic) pathways. ON pathways **(left)**; OFF pathways **(right)**. Cone circuitry is indicated using just two cone photoreceptors; that in the left half is shown connecting via an ON cone bipolar cell to an ON ganglion cell; that in the right half is shown connecting via an OFF cone bipolar cell to an OFF ganglion cell. In contrast to cone bipolar cells, rod bipolar cells do not synapse directly with retinal ganglion cells, but rather "hitch a ride" on cone bipolar-to-ganglion cell pathways. RB, rod bipolar cell; GCL, retinal ganglion cell layer; INL, inner nuclear layer; IPL, inner plexiform layer; ONL, outer nuclear layer; OPL, outer plexiform layer; OS/IS, photoreceptor outer and inner segments. (Modified from Wässle H. Parallel processing in the mammalian retina. *Nat Rev Neurosci.* 2004;5:1–11 and Lamb TD. Evolution of vertebrate retinal photoreception. *Philos Trans R Soc Lond B Biol Sci.* 2009;364:2911–2924.)

different responses to light stimulation. The bipolar cells that respond to sustained light stimulation with an "off" signal synapse in the outer strata of the "off layer" of the inner plexiform layer, and those that respond to sustained light stimulation with an "on" signal synapse in the inner strata of the inner plexiform layer (IPL) (**Fig. 14.22**). These cells demonstrate two distinct electrophysiologic responses to light illumination, depolarization, or hyperpolarization. Bipolar cells that depolarize in response to light hitting their receptive field (and hyperpolarize to surround stimulation) synapse with ON-center ganglion cells. Conversely, bipolar cells that hyperpolarize in response to light hitting their receptive field (and depolarize to surround stimulation) synapse with OFF-center RGCs (**Fig. 14.23**).[38]

Horizontal Cells

Horizontal cells are inhibitory interneurons that modify information passed from photoreceptor synapses to bipolar cell dendrites.[42,43] As the name implies, their processes extend horizontally at the level of the outer plexiform layer, where they make reciprocal synapses with many adjacent photoreceptors. If input from a photoreceptor synapse activates a given horizontal cell process, the horizontal cell responds by sending inhibitory signals to all other surrounding photoreceptor synapses that it contacts. Likewise, if a horizontal cell process becomes inhibited, then it will excite all other photoreceptor synapses it contacts.

How can an inhibitory neuron have both excitatory and inhibitory effects? Recall that all retinal neurons (except amacrine and RGCs) operate with only graded potentials, not action potentials. This means that the amount of neurotransmitter released will be increased or decreased in an analog fashion depending on the state of depolarization. Thus a horizontal cell can inhibit surrounding photoreceptors by releasing relatively more inhibitory neurotransmitter gamma amino butyric acid (GABA) or they can excite (more correctly disinhibit) surrounding photoreceptors by releasing relatively less GABA.[44,45] Because of these reciprocal inhibitory/excitatory effects, horizontal cells essentially block or dampen much of the total information output of photoreceptor cells, but importantly allow information to pass only when the horizontal cell itself is partially excited by some of its connecting photoreceptors and partially inhibited by others and thus is silent. This occurs only when one patch of photoreceptors is exposed to light and the adjacent patch of photoreceptors is in the dark, i.e., when there is an edge of light falling on the retina. Horizontal cells are silenced in these regions under these conditions and allow visual information encoding the edge of light to pass to bipolar cells. Thus, they act as a type of spatial filter, an edge detection filter.

The horizontal cells detect "change" in visual input and play a major *inhibitory* feedback role via their lateral processes and input/output connections within photoreceptor triads, which integrate and modulate the output signals from the photoreceptors at the synaptic triad.

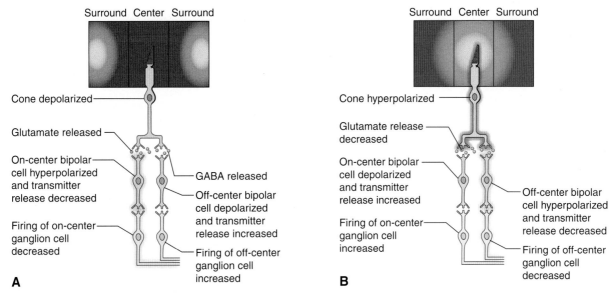

Surround Center Surround

Cone depolarized

Glutamate released

On-center bipolar cell hyperpolarized and transmitter release decreased

GABA released

Off-center bipolar cell depolarized and transmitter release increased

Firing of on-center ganglion cell decreased

Firing of off-center ganglion cell increased

A

Surround Center Surround

Cone hyperpolarized

Glutamate release decreased

On-center bipolar cell depolarized and transmitter release increased

Firing of on-center ganglion cell increased

Off-center bipolar cell hyperpolarized and transmitter release decreased

Firing of off-center ganglion cell decreased

B

FIGURE 14.23 Responses of retinal bipolar and ganglion cells to darkness and illumination in the receptive field center. **A:** Changes in the electrical activity of the photoreceptor and on-center and off-center bipolar and ganglion cells when the photoreceptor receptive field center is in the dark. **B:** Changes in the electrical activity of the photoreceptor and on-center and off-center bipolar and ganglion cells when the photoreceptor receptive field center is illuminated. (Modified from Siegel A, Sapru HN. *Essential Neuroscience.* 3rd ed. Philadelphia, PA: Wolters Kluwer; 2014.)

There are three different types of horizontal cells in the retina, H1, H2, and H3 cells (also termed HI, HII, HIII). Cells of each specific type form diffuse; laterally arranged plexi of interconnected cells throughout the retina, which communicate via gap junctions. H1 cells receive their inputs from L-cones and M-cones, and their axons terminate in rod cell spherules. H2 cells (smaller than H1 cells) are innervated by all cone subtypes. The axons of H2 cells communicate mainly with S-cones. H3 cells are unique to human retinas and are similar to H1 cells, but with broader and more asymmetric synaptic connections, however they do not appear to receive input from the S-cones.[25,35]

The gap junctions between horizontal cells create broader receptive fields than the individual dendritic trees of other retinal neurons. Horizontal cells function to deliver lateral inhibitory feedback by summing light-induced signals across the retina and subtracting it from the local photoreceptor signal (**Fig. 14.21**). Other possible mechanisms of action include direct or indirect modulation of photoreceptor glutamate release. Together with the synaptic connections of the amacrine cells in the IPL, the horizontal cell connections in the outer plexiform layer of the retina act as a local circuit to modulate and process visual information.

Amacrine Cells

There are more than 40 known subtypes of amacrine cells (*amacrine*—no axon), whose cell bodies make up the innermost strata of the inner nuclear layer, which are classified based on their dendrite morphology and stratification.[21,38]

Each cell type has a specific morphologic structure, laminar extension of synapses within the IPL, and dendritic field type. They are mostly inhibitory neurons but utilize numerous classes of inhibitory neurotransmitters (e.g., GABAergic, glycinergic, cholinergic, etc.). Like horizontal cells, the amacrine cells act as lateral inhibitory neurons and interact over long distances to modify the output of bipolar cells. The highly diverse population of amacrine cells have complex filtering properties, only some of which are understood.[46–48] One example is the directionally-sensitive class of amacrine cells that is activated only when an edge of light passes over their receptive fields in a given direction.[49] This directional selectivity is passed to ganglion cells and acts to further strengthen the perception of movement.

Amacrine connections can occur via gap junctions, with bipolar cells, ganglion cells, and other amacrine cells in the IPL (**Fig. 14.24**).[31,50–52] The amacrine cells serve to integrate visual input from the photoreceptors and influence signal processing at the level of contact between the bipolar and ganglion cells. Functionally, they play a role in signal processing by modulating image brightness and by integrating the sequential activation of neurons to detect motion. A convenient way to conceptualize their role is that they act to sense transience, that is, changes occurring in a changing input. They are described both morphologically and in the context of their receptive fields and interactions with the RGCs, to which they communicate this information.

Broadly, amacrine cells can be classified by their neurotransmitter (see below) or by the reach of their dendritic arbors (**Fig. 14.25**). The "narrow field" (e.g., *starburst* amacrine cell, ~75 μm), "medium field" (~175 μm), and

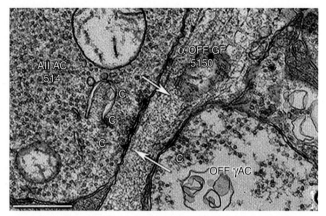

FIGURE 14.24 False color transmission electron micrograph of amacrine cell connections can occur via gap junctions with bipolar cells, ganglion cells, and other amacrine cells in the inner plexiform layer. AII cell (514) making a multi-projection conventional presynaptic specialization (C) targeting an OFF ganglion cell 5150 (arrow). (Modified from Marc RE, Anderson JR, Jones BW, et al. The AII amacrine cell connectome: a dense network hub. *Front Neural Circuits.* 2014;8:104.)

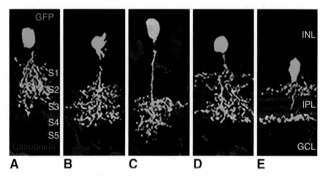

FIGURE 14.25 Different classes of amacrine cells based upon their dendritic arbors. **A:** Green fluorescent protein labeled dendritic trees of different types of amacrine cells are seen localized to specific substrata (S1–S5) or throughout the inner plexiform layer (IPL). Glycinergic amacrine cells expressing green fluorescent protein. **B:** Type 2 cell. **C:** Type 3 cell. **D:** Type 4 cell. **E:** Type 7 cell. **E:** A8 cell. GCL, retinal ganglion cell layer; INL, inner nuclear layer. (Modified from Wassle H, Heinze L, Ivanova E, et al. Glycinergic transmission in the mammalian retina. *Front Mol Neurosci.* 2009;2:6.)

"wide field" (~350 μm) type cells are based upon the size of their dendritic fields in the IPL. Dendritic trees of all types of cells are seen localized to the specific strata or throughout the inner plexiform layer.[52,53] The narrow field cells, as the name implies are narrowly branching cells within each of the different substrata of the IPL and function to vertically integrate visual signals coming from the photoreceptors and interneurons. Overlapping sectors of the dendritic trees of starburst amacrine cells also play a role as functional subunits, which detect movement and directional motion within larger ganglion cell receptive fields. Medium field and wide field amacrine cells are also thought to play a limited feedback role in vertical signal integration but their main

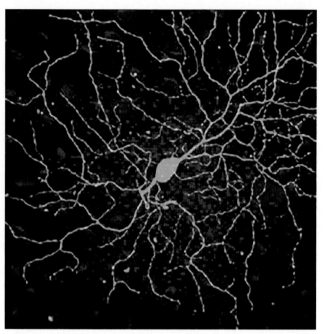

FIGURE 14.26 Flat-mounted retinal ganglion cell (RGC) (GFP-tagged in green) overlying a field of starburst amacrine cells (red), taken using a tri-channel confocal fluorescence microscope. DAPI-stained nuclei (in blue). The underlying field of amacrine cells all contribute to modulating the signal conveyed to the broad receptor field of the RGC above them. (Courtesy of Daniel O'Shea and the Princeton University Art of Science Competition.)

functions remain to be elucidated. The receptive fields of medium field amacrine cells are more similar to that of the RGCs they communicate with (~250 μm), and thus they are unlikely to act as functional subunits in the way that narrow field cells do. Wide field amacrine cells may aid in communicating between different layers of cells.

Amacrine cells are distributed in mosaic-like arrangements across the retina, ensuring that visual signals from all parts of the retinal photoreceptor network can be both vertically and laterally integrated (**Fig. 14.26**).[54,55] Amacrine cells also demonstrate two distinct electrophysiologic responses to light, sustained or transient responses. Transient response cells synapse with on–off RGCs (see below).

As described above, amacrine cells primarily secrete inhibitory neurotransmitters; 85% of these cells secrete the neurotransmitters gamma aminobutyric acid (GABA) or glycine.[56] Narrow field starburst amacrine cells secrete GABA. Wide field amacrine cells (of which there are ~30 different types) are GABAergic cells whose cell bodies are seen in the inner nuclear layer and which also make up a subset of amacrine cells "displaced" to the ganglion cell layer. Several types of GABAergic amacrine cells demonstrate paracrine function and release more than one type of neurotransmitter, including dopamine. Co-release of GABA and dopamine occurs in amacrine cells that diffusely modulate light and dark adaption and the circadian rhythm. The prototypical glycinergic cell (of which there are ~15 different types) is the

AII amacrine cell, which has a small and vertically oriented dendritic field. This cell functions to integrate synaptic input from rod-specific bipolar cells and laterally redistribute it to the cone bipolar cells, mediating signals from rod cells under scotopic vision conditions. Other neurotransmitters and neuromodulators are also secreted by some types of amacrine cells, including acetylcholine (excitatory), serotonin, small peptides, and nitric oxide.[57–59]

Interplexiform Cells

These cells reside at the inner border of the inner nuclear layer and, as the name implies, have synapses in both the inner and outer plexiform layers of the retina.[60,61] The synapses in the outer plexiform layer are presynaptic to both bipolar and horizontal cells. The synapses in the IPL are both pre- and postsynaptic. Unlike the vertical flow of information seen in the bipolar cells, the interplexiform cells are thought to convey the reciprocal flow of information from the inner retina to the outer retina. Interplexiform cells appear to use dopamine as their neurotransmitter.

INNER PLEXIFORM LAYER

The IPL is functionally laminar in nature, whereby the processes of functionally similar neurons terminate and synapse in spatially distinct strata of the IPL. The "off" bipolar cells synapse with the "off" RGCs in the outer strata of the IPL ("off layer") and the "on" bipolar cells synapse with the retinal "on" ganglion cells in the inner strata. But, there are combined "on-off" RGCs as well. These cells find synapses within both layers of the IPL. The IPL from a mouse retina is shown (**Fig. 14.27**). The dendritic trees of the amacrine cells and RGCs co-label in specific layers in this image (yellow bands) within the IPL.

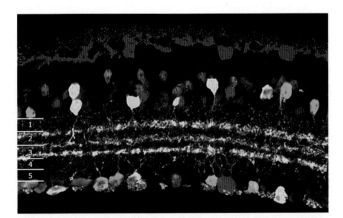

FIGURE 14.27   Five layers of stratification of the IPL of the retina. The labeled dendrites of amacrine and ganglion cells are confined to three narrow *yellow bands*, segregating four dark bands of reduced label. This shows that the inner plexiform layer is precisely stratified and within these strata different aspects of the light signal are processed. (From Wässle H. Parallel processing in the mammalian retina. *Nat Rev Neurosci.* 2004;5:747–757.)

GANGLION CELL LAYER

There are 750,000 to 1.5 million cells in the RGC layer. The RGC layer also contains a small percentage of "displaced" amacrine cell bodies.[47,62] This subpopulation of amacrine cells comprises only a small percentage of the nuclei in the ganglion cell layer centrally (~3%) but they make up the majority of cell bodies in this layer in the retinal periphery. The cell bodies of RGCs are among the largest in the retina and are up to 30 μm in diameter. The ganglion cell layer of the retina is only one cell thick in much of the retina. Indeed, progressing toward the retinal periphery, this single layer of cells is commonly discontinuous. By contrast, in the macular region, the ganglion cell layer is several cells thick.

More than 20 types of RGCs are known, based upon features of their physiology, function, and anatomical projections to the brain. Each projects a single axon into the nerve fiber layer of the retina, most continuing to its synapse in the lateral geniculate nucleus of the thalamus as part of the optic nerve. RGCs have either diffuse dendritic trees throughout the inner plexiform layer or more stratified dendritic trees that track in one or a few strata of the IPL.[63–66] There is an inverse relationship between the size of the dendritic tree and the RGC density. Based upon their projections and function, there are several classes of RGCs. The most common cell types in the primate retina are the midget ganglion cells (parvocellular or P cells, or beta cells) and the parasol cells (magnocellular or M cells, or alpha cells) (~70% to 80% of RGCs) (**Fig. 14.28**).[21,38,67–69] The midget ganglion cells synapse with midget bipolar cells and convey information from single cone cells as described above. Other types of ganglion cells include, for example, bistratified ganglion cells, delta ganglion cells, cells that project to the superior colliculus controlling saccadic eye movements and to the accessory optic nucleus of the brain, and melanopsin-containing intrinsically photosensitive ganglion cells.[70–73] The dendritic trees of these different RGC types stratify at different levels within the IPL where they synapse with specific bipolar cells and classes of amacrine cells. Together, they transduce light into as many as 20 different parallel processing pathways to the brain, which accounts for the complex aspects of visual discrimination.[74–76]

As with bipolar cells, the function of RGC in relaying visual signals is best understood through the concept of concentric center/surround "receptive fields."[73,77] Whereas the bipolar cell responds to the inputs of many photoreceptor cells (or one cone in the fovea), the RGC responds to the integrated input from many bipolar cells, thus further integrating the retinal signal. Its receptive field is similarly target shaped, with a central circular field surrounded by an annular field that responds to light in an antagonistic fashion (**Fig. 14.29**).[78–81] The center-surround organization of RGCs confers a form of signal compression termed "opponent processing." Local variations in luminance are

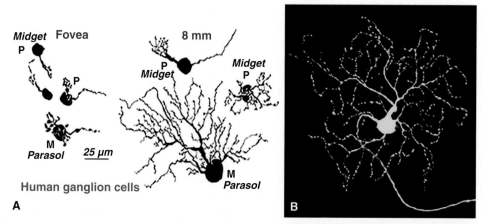

FIGURE 14.28 Morphology of retinal ganglion cells (RGCs). **A:** Drawings of parasol and midget ganglion cells from different regions of the retina. **B:** A micrograph of a RGC, with its central cell body from which branches spread out to receive messages from other retinal cells. The axon fiber that communicates via action potentials with the brain leaves the picture at (**lower right**). ([A] From Kolb H. Glial Cells of the Retina. Webvision website. Webvision website. http://webvision.med.utah.edu/. November 2013. Accessed March 21, 2017. Copyright © 2017 Webvision . [B] What is Glaucoma? In: Quigley HA. Glaucoma: What Every Patient Should Know. Wilmer Eye Institute and Glaucoma Center for Excellence of John Hopkins University School of Medicine website. http://www.hopkinsmedicine.org/wilmer/services/glaucoma /book/index.html. Accessed March 21, 2017. Copyright © 2011 Harry A. Quigley MD.)

detected by subtracting the surround signal from that of the center to minimize light signals common to both, which improves the dynamic range.

The magnocellular RGCs (M cells) are driven primarily by rod cell input and reflect the input of the on or off bipolar cells. The parvocellular RGCs (P cells) of the central retina receive their input from the cone bipolar cells. They have small, color responsive receptive fields, which serve to maintain the high resolution images transmitted by the foveal cones. Since the M cell signal is rod-based, these cells provide part of the neural basis for detection of luminance (the luminance "channel"); however, P cells must also play a role to contribute to the known achromatic spatial resolution of the luminance channel.

The P cells receive input from single L- or M-cones in the fovea through the midget bipolar cells.[81–83] Thus in the fovea, cone input must be a "center on" mechanism. This combination of single cone input to the center and mixed input in the surround receptive field assures that the center/surround fields of P cells serving the fovea are spectrally opponent, that is, their receptive fields will be selective for different chromatic signals (e.g., red inhibitory center and green excitatory surround) (**Fig. 14.29**, right). More complex ganglion cell receptive fields have also been described that transmit visual information including; direction-sensitive movement, linear and nonlinear light summation, transient light, and color summation (**Fig. 14.30**).[84]

Importantly, a small class of RGCs (~1%) contain photosensitive melanopsin and demonstrate intrinsic light responses (phototransduction) to provide an alternative input to the brain reflecting ambient light intensity.[72,73] These RGCs synapse in the suprachiasmatic nucleus of the hypothalamus and play a role in the maintenance of the circadian rhythm. They also have synapses in the olivary pretectal nucleus of the midbrain, which regulates pupillary responses, and are thought to play a role in the light induced regulation of melatonin secretion from the pineal gland.[85–89]

THE NERVE FIBER LAYER

The axons of the RGCs form the nerve fiber layer of the retina. These fibers are unmyelinated while coursing within the retina, since myelin is opaque and would obstruct the passage of light to the underlying photoreceptors. These ganglion cell axons collect into a bundled tract to exit the eye as the optic nerve, at which point these axons acquire a myelin sheath provided by oligodendrocytes. These fibers constitute the collective synaptic output of the retina and convey the integrated visual signal from the retina to the brain.

As these fibers course toward the optic nerve, their pathway follows a consistent pattern in all eyes. An imaginary line drawn through the optic nerve and the center of the fovea defines a landmark known as the horizontal raphe (**Fig. 14.31**). The axons of the ganglion cells do not cross the raphe in passing from their ganglion cell soma to the optic nerve (**Fig. 14.31**). Those fibers coming from superior, inferior, and nasal quadrants send their axons directly toward the margin of the optic nerve, following a curvilinear path. However, those axons travelling from ganglion cells in the temporal retinal periphery, both above and below the horizontal raphe, must arch around the bulge in the fiber pattern created by the large number of fibers coming from the tightly packed photoreceptors in the fovea and surrounding macular region (**Fig. 14.31**). This large number of axons, creating the bulge in the pattern of the temporal nerve fiber layer, runs from the macular region to the temporal edge of the optic nerve head and is termed the papillomacular (PM) bundle. As more fibers are added to the nerve fiber layer, from the retinal periphery

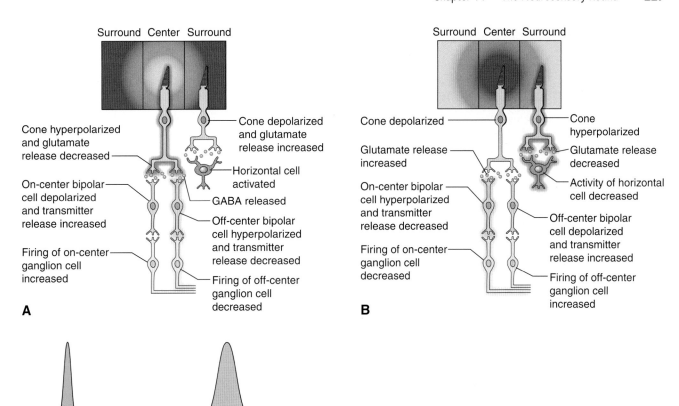

A

Surround Center Surround

Cone hyperpolarized and glutamate release decreased

Cone depolarized and glutamate release increased

Horizontal cell activated

GABA released

On-center bipolar cell depolarized and transmitter release increased

Off-center bipolar cell hyperpolarized and transmitter release decreased

Firing of on-center ganglion cell increased

Firing of off-center ganglion cell decreased

B

Surround Center Surround

Cone depolarized

Cone hyperpolarized

Glutamate release increased

Glutamate release decreased

Activity of horizontal cell decreased

On-center bipolar cell hyperpolarized and transmitter release decreased

Off-center bipolar cell depolarized and transmitter release increased

Firing of on-center ganglion cell decreased

Firing of off-center ganglion cell increased

C

FIGURE 14.29 Retinal ganglion cell receptive fields. **Top:** Some synapses connect ON-center bipolar cells to ON-center ganglion cells **(A)**, while others **(B)** connect OFF-center bipolar cells to OFF-center ganglion cells. The accentuation of contrasts by the center-surround receptive fields of the bipolar cells is thereby preserved and passed on to the ganglion cells, and ultimately to the visual cortex. **(C, left)** Midget ganglion cells serving foveal vision are connected to *single red* **(top)** or *green* **(bottom)** cones via midget bipolars (represented by the *red* and *green arrows*). Blue cones are absent in the fovea. The surrounds of the bipolar cells are nonselectively connected to both red and green cones. Consequently, the ganglion cell receptive fields are automatically spectrally opponent with red or green centers and yellow surrounds. The two ganglion cells illustrated are both on-center, but off-center varieties also exist. Beyond perifoveal regions **(C, right)**, RGCs are connected to 15 to 30 cones via multiple midget bipolar cells. If these connections are random, the spectral composition of the center signal would be expected to be shifted toward yellow and the spectral opponency of the receptive field reduced. **Bottom:** However, the combination of patchy *red* and *green* distributions and elliptical receptive field centers makes it possible for cone purity of the center signal, and thus the spectral opponency of the receptive field, to be retained.

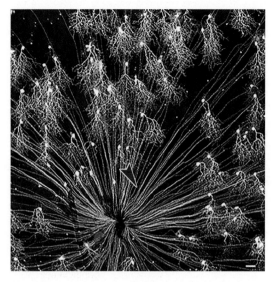

FIGURE 14.30 Micrograph of motion sensitive retinal ganglion cells in the rodent retina. The direction of motion is shown (*red arrowhead*) relative to the orientation of the cells. (From Kim IJ, Zhang Y, Yamagata M, et al. Molecular identification of a retinal cell type that responds to upward motion. *Nature.* 2008;452(7186): 478–482.)

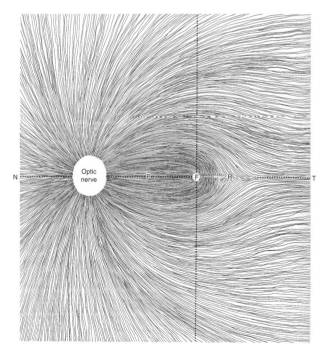

FIGURE 14.31 Topography of the retinal nerve fiber layer in the retina. Note that on the temporal side, the nerve fibers pass around the region of the fovea (*F*) to reach the optic nerve. On the nasal side, the fibers run a relatively straight course to the optic nerve. Fibers from the fovea pass directly to the temporal edge of the disc via the papillomacular bundle (*P*). Dashed line from nasal (N) to temporal (T) corresponds to the horizontal raphe (*R*), the division between the superior and inferior retinal ganglion cell fiber axons coursing to the nerve. (Modified from Visual Field. StudyBlue website. https://www.studyblue.com. April 12, 2013. Accessed October 20, 2016.)

toward the optic nerve head, the nerve fiber layer thickens, forming thick radial bundles at the disc margin, which are greatest superiorly and inferiorly.

Strict adherence to the pattern described above is critical because throughout the visual pathway from the retina to the visual cortex, specific locations in visual space maintain their relationship with other locations. This is termed retinotopic projection and is discussed in greater detail in **CHAPTER 15: THE OPTIC NERVE AND VISUAL PATHWAYS.** Axons from RGCs residing nasal to a virtual vertical line passing through the fovea, cross the midline at the optic chiasm to make connections in the contralateral side of the brain. Conversely, axons from the retinal periphery, temporal to the fovea, remain uncrossed as they travel to communicate with the visual cortex of the brain. Some functional overlap of the vertical distribution of ganglion cells serving the region of the fovea is also seen.

 Retinal nerve fibers, especially those of the papillomacular bundle, are easily seen clinically, where they traverse toward the optic nerve head in an arcuate fashion that parallels the large retinal vessels (Fig. 14.32A). It is important to appreciate these striations clinically because as ganglion cells are lost, in conditions such as glaucoma, the striations become less well seen. Three-dimensional imaging and analysis of the retinal nerve fiber layer (RNFL) is now a routine part of the clinical care of glaucoma, using spectral-domain optical coherence tomography (SD-OCT) and scanning laser polarimetry (which uses polarized light to measure the thickness of the RNFL). These methods provide quantitative and longitudinal measurements of the distribution pattern of RNFL defects in patients as well as statistical comparisons to standardized patient cohorts. These methods provide numerous metrics including; RNFL distribution, average RNFL thickness, and changes over time. An example of a RNFL thickness and thickness deviation map is shown (Fig. 14.32B).

GLIAL CELLS OF THE RETINA

Müller Cells

The Müller cells traverse almost the full thickness of the retina and have been shown to play diverse and critical roles in both retinal development and retinal function. The specialized basement membrane and the footplates of the Müller cells form the internal limiting membrane of the retina internally and the specialized microvillous junctions of the Müller cells (fiber basket of Schultze) interact with the external limiting membrane at the level of the photoreceptor IS externally (**Fig. 14.33**). The Müller cell processes envelop the photoreceptors and interneurons throughout the retina, where they provide critical structural

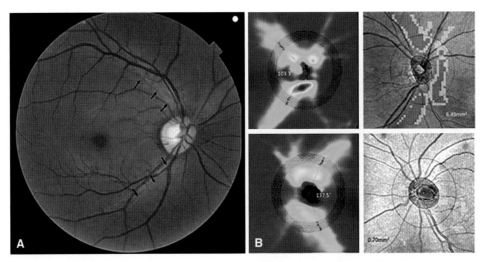

FIGURE 14.32 **A:** Retinal nerve fibers passing along the vascular arcades to reach the optic disc **(left)**. The birefringent RNFL of the healthy retina is seen (*arrows*) **(right)**. **B:** RNFL thickness maps **(left panel)** and the retina; nerve fiber layer (RNFL) thickness deviation maps **(right panel)** of two myopic eyes. Two areas of abnormal RNFL measurements (in *yellow* and *red* in the thickness deviation map) are seen on clinical assessment of the NFL. Nerve fiber layer (NFL) thickness is a critical parameter monitored in patients with glaucoma. (From Kai-Shun Leung C, Yu M, Weinreb RN, et al. Retinal nerve fiber layer imaging with spectral-domain optical coherence tomography: interpreting the rnfl maps in healthy myopic eyes. *Invest Ophthalmol Vis Sci.* 2012;53:7194–2000.)

and trophic support to the retinal neurons via the secretion of growth and neurotrophic factors, regulation of the ionic (K+) and neurotransmitter content of the extracellular milieu (in particular GABA and acetylcholine), local glucose metabolism, phagocytosis, and modulation of pH and CO_2 levels.[90] The photoreceptors and interneurons are surrounded by Müller cell processes throughout the retina, which also serves to electrically insulate these neurons in the absence of myelin. More recently, in guinea pig retina, they have been shown to act as a fiberoptic channel for light to reach the outer retina; however, similar function of Müller cells in the primate retina has not yet been demonstrated.[91]

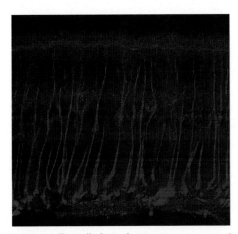

FIGURE 14.33 Müller cell glia in the mouse, seen spanning almost the entire thickness of the retina from the retinal interface with the vitreous **(bottom)** to the external limiting membrane of the retina **(bright line near top of image)**. (From Nicolás Cuenca of the Department of Physiology, Genetics and Microbiology at the University of Alicante. Glilal Cells. http://www.retinalmicroscopy.com/glial.html. 2008. Accessed October 20, 2016.)

In fish and amphibians, Müller cells express stem cell markers and serve as progenitors of retinal neurons after injury through asymmetric, self-renewing division. This stem cell capacity appears to be retained in the mammalian retina only to a very limited degree, but it is the focus of active research as a potential approach to retinal stem cell therapy and regrowth.[92–94]

Astrocytes

The glial astrocytes in the retina are strongly associated with the retinal vasculature and located almost exclusively in the nerve fiber layer, and prelaminar portion of the optic nerve, with smaller numbers of cells also seen in the ganglion cell layer (**Fig. 14.34**).[95] These cells are capable of secreting growth factors and play a significant role in ion homeostasis.

Microglia

The microglia of the retina are stellate-appearing blood-derived cells that serve as the macrophages of the central nervous system and retina. Like astrocytes, they reside near the retinal vessels and the vascular beds derived from the central retinal artery that are found between the ganglion cell and nerve fiber layers and between the outer plexiform and inner nuclear layers (**Fig. 14.35**). They are mobile and phagocytic and become activated under conditions of retinal tissue injury where they digest and remove damaged cells and debris. They also participate in antigen presentation for T-cell immune function. Microglia are absent from the fovea where there are no intraretinal vessels.

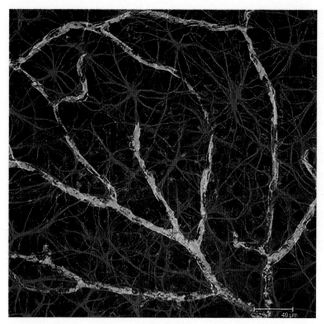

FIGURE 14.34 Dense network of astrocytes (*red*) seen in a micrograph of the rat retina among ganglion cells (*blue*) and associated blood vessels (*green*). Oblong nuclei of vascular endothelial cells within the vessels appear light blue. (Courtesy of Laura Fernandez-Sanchez and Nicolas Cuenca. In: Kolb H. Glial Cells of the Retina. Webvision website. Webvision website. http://webvision.med.utah.edu/. November 2013. Accessed March 21, 2017. Copyright © 2017 Webvision.)

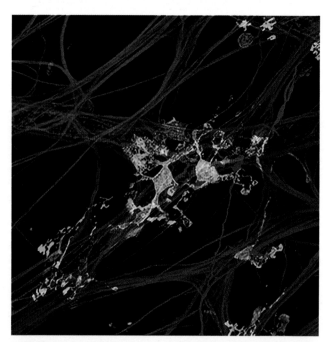

FIGURE 14.35 Microglia seen in a wholemount human retina preparation, triple labeled with fluorescent antibodies that stain blood vessels (*blue*), astrocytes (*red*) and microglia (*green*). (Courtesy of Scott McLeod from Jerry Lutty's Lab. In Kolb H. Glial Cells of the Retina. Webvision website. http://webvision.med.utah.edu/. November 2013. Accessed March 21, 2017. Copyright © 2017 Webvision.)

⦿ Histology of the Macula and Macula Lutea

The macula can be histologically defined as that portion of the retina in which the ganglion cell layer is more than one cell thick and as the portion of the retina in which the orientation of the fibers in the outer plexiform layer is more horizontal than vertical (i.e., the nerve fiber layer of Henle, **Fig. 14.36**). As noted earlier, a direct correspondence between this histologic definition and the generally darker area temporal to the optic disc that is commonly referred to clinically as the macula is not possible.

Within the macula, as anatomically defined above, is a smaller area in which the retinal tissue is highly enriched with the carotenoid pigments, lutein and zeaxanthin, for which specialized transport mechanisms exist (**Fig. 14.37**).[96,97] These pigments are distributed principally in the outer nuclear and outer plexiform layers and contribute to the darker appearance of the macular area of the retina seen clinically. The area of the macula in which this pigment is present is approximately 3 to 5 mm in diameter and is traditionally termed the macula lutea. Luteal pigment acts as a spectral filter and is believed to help protect the foveal cones from blue light induced photo-oxidative stress.

 Nutritional deficiencies of these luteal pigments in the diets of elderly patients, combined with other factors may underlie, in part, susceptibility to age-related macular degeneration. In clinical practice, it is routine to recommend particular over-the-counter dietary supplements containing lutein, zeaxanthin, zinc, and anti-oxidant vitamins in a particular combination. This combination was shown to reduce the risk of disease progression in patients with moderate to advanced macular degeneration. These particular combinations were proven to have efficacy in a series of National Eye Institute-funded clinical trials known as the Age-Related Eye Disease Studies (AREDS and AREDS2) and others.[98–100]

⦿ Histology of the Fovea and Foveola

THE FOVEA AND FOVEOLA

At the center of the macula are the fovea and its central foveola where our highest-resolution acuity resides. All of the photoreceptor cells in this portion of the retina are cones, anatomically modified to pack more densely. As such these cones look long and slender like rods rather than having the cone shape for which these photoreceptors are named. The fovea is approximately 1.5 mm in diameter and functionally represents the central 5° of the visual

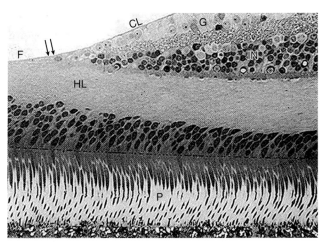

FIGURE 14.36 Histologic section of the region demarcating the border of the fovea. The retinal ganglion cells (G) are seen displaced away from the foveal cones. The synaptic connections are made by the fibers in Henle's layer (HL), which lies almost perpendicular to the path of the light and is the anatomical equivalent of the outer plexiform layer in this region. Clivus (CL) is seen sloping toward the edge of the foveola (F, *arrows*). IN, inner nuclear layer; P, photoreceptors. (From Tripathi RC, Tripathi BJ. In: Davson H, ed. *The Eye.* New York, NY: Academic Press; 1984.)

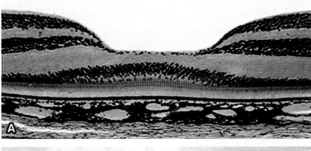

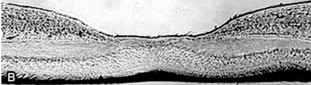

FIGURE 14.37 **A:** Standard histological section of the macular region for comparison with unstained section (**B**), showing distribution of yellow luteal pigment in the retinal layers. The retinal tissue of the macula lutea is highly enriched with the carotenoid pigments, lutein and zeaxanthin, which are thought to act as spectral filters to reduce blue light-induced photo-oxidative stress photo-oxidative stress in the macula. (From Snodderly DM, Auran JD, Delori FC. The macular pigment. II. Spatial distribution in primate retina. *Invest Ophthal Vis Sci.* 1984;25:674–685.)

field. Central retinal artery-derived capillaries are excluded from the central 0.75 mm of the fovea, creating what is termed the "foveal avascular zone." At the center of the fovea is the foveola, which is 0.1 to 0.3 mm in diameter and lies slightly below the horizontal raphe. The foveola is only 0.13 mm in thickness and functionally represents the central 1° of the visual field.

The fovea is much thinner than the surrounding retina. It forms an anatomical depression in the cross section of the central retina that is comprised almost exclusively of the layers of the neurosensory retina represented by the cone photoreceptor cells, plus the internal limiting membrane of the retina. Anatomically, the slopes of this focal depression are referred to as the clivus. The base of this depression, the foveola, is devoid of all retinal cell bodies except those of the photoreceptor cells and contains only the OS of red and green cone cells. It is here that all of our maximal visual acuity resides. It is from this point that we define up, down, left, and right in visual space.

In younger individuals, the surface of the retina, including the fovea, is quite reflective. When examining young to middle-aged individuals with various illuminated instruments it is common to see a bright dot of light located precisely at the center of the fovea, known as the umbo. This is termed the foveal reflex (Fig. 14.38). Its existence is due to the shape of the fovea, which creates the equivalent of a concave mirror, reflecting parallel rays of light toward a focal point just anterior to the retinal surface in the posterior vitreous cortex. Swelling or distortion of foveal tissue from macular edema or retinal traction can reduce the concavity of its surface, resulting in the loss of this foveal reflex.

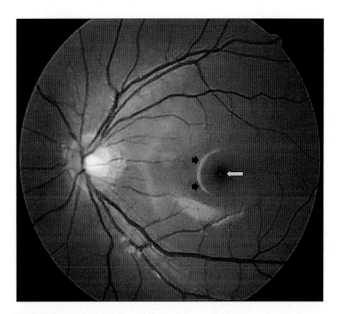

FIGURE 14.38 The foveal light reflex off of the umbo is shown (*yellow arrow*). Reflections from the ILM (*black arrowheads*) are also commonly seen in younger patients, giving the young retina a generally reflective sheen.

As in the nonmacular retina, the photoreceptors of the fovea connect in turn to bipolar cells and then ganglion cells but these connections have migrated laterally during postnatal development to exclude them, and the vascular supply of the inner retinal layers, from the light path. The margin of the foveal depression is where the retina is thickest (~250 μm), due to the displacement of the ganglion cells and inner and outer nuclear layers away from the foveola. It is the outer edge of this thickened area that has created the arcuate reflection of light designated by the black arrows in **Figure 14.38**. This accounts for the variation in thickness of the ganglion cell layer in the macula. This lateral displacement shifts the orientation of the fibers in the outer plexiform layer of the retina from parallel to the incoming light to nearly perpendicular to the light path.

◉ The Retinal Circulation

The sole arterial supply to the inner retina is from the central retinal artery, a branch of the ophthalmic artery (itself a branch of the internal carotid artery) that enters the eye through the center of the optic nerve. The artery lies immediately adjacent and nasal to the central retinal vein as they enter (and exit) from the center of the optic nerve head, to branch within the sensory retina (**Fig. 14.39**). The average diameter of the central retinal artery at the optic nerve head is approximately 100 μm. The normal vein is commonly 1.5 times larger in diameter. Because

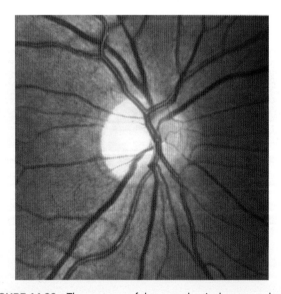

FIGURE 14.39 The anatomy of the central retinal artery and vein. The artery typically lies immediately adjacent and nasal to the central retinal vein as they enter (and exit) from the center of the optic nerve head, to branch within the sensory retina. The retinal arteries show evidence of their muscular walls as a white stripe down the center of the vessel. Retinal veins lack this feature. The average diameter of the central retinal artery (arteriole) at the optic nerve is approximately 100 μm.

intraocular pressure is often near the pressure in the central retinal vein it is not uncommon to see a pulse in the central retinal vein at the optic nerve head. In most cases this is normal. However, a pulse in the central retinal artery is always abnormal and suggests either an unusually high intraocular pressure or systemic vascular disease.

MAJOR RETINAL VESSELS

The major branches of the central retinal artery divide into superior and inferior circulatory trees with temporal and nasal trunks feeding the four major quadrants of the retina. The nasal arteries leave the nerve head in a relatively straight line, whereas, the temporal branches exit above and below the optic nerve head, arching around the macula as they course temporally. These vessels are commonly referred to as the superior and inferior arcades. The retinal arterioles are associated with retinal astrocytes and with the footplates of the Müller cells that form the internal limiting membrane of the retina. As they exit the optic nerve, the larger branches of the retinal circulation lie just beneath the internal limiting membrane, within the nerve fiber layer. Here, near the retinal surface, there are weak attachments between the vessels and posterior hyaloid (vitreous) face.

Notwithstanding its name, the central retinal artery, except near its origin from the ophthalmic artery, meets the histologic criteria of an arteriole, not an artery. Like the short posterior ciliary arteries, the central retinal artery has several layers of smooth muscle in its tunica media. But unlike the short posterior ciliary arteries that serve the choroid and optic nerve head, the central retinal artery does not have an elastic lamina. The arterial and venous vessels generally follow parallel paths of distribution and are readily distinguished by the fact that the venous blood is darker red in appearance and in normal young eyes, the venous vessels are larger in diameter in a ratio of approximately 4/3. An additional distinguishing feature is that the smooth muscle coat in the wall of the arterioles gives rise to a reflective white strip down the center of these vessels in vivo; this is less evident in the veins (**Fig. 14.39**).

With increasing age, arteriolar sclerotic changes occur, increasing the thickness of the arteriolar walls. As this process ensues, the ratio between the diameters of the arteriolar and venular vessels approaches 1:1. The arterioles and venules commonly cross as they branch in the retina; however, arterioles never cross arterioles and venules never cross venules. Importantly, at these crossing points, the arterioles and venules share a common tunica adventitia, thus binding them tightly together. This relationship can be a source of problems in patients with arteriolar sclerotic changes. At these crossing points, focal compression of the venule by the expanding and hardening arteriole can give rise to venous occlusions affecting the distal retina and capillary bed.

The portions of the retinal circulation arising from the superior and inferior arcades are effectively independent of each other and generally respect a virtual line passing through the optic nerve and fovea. The retinal vasculature is an end-arterial system and connections between superior and inferior vascular beds occur only indirectly through the capillary beds in the macula. When venous occlusions occur in the retina, these small capillary vessels remodel and form shunts, which convey blood from the occluded venous bed to the patent venous bed in the other hemisphere (**Fig. 14.40**).

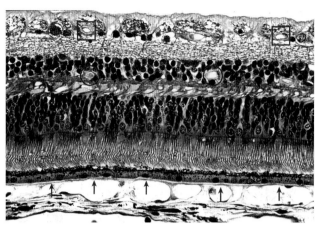

FIGURE 14.41 The capillary beds of the retinal circulation. Two restricted layers of capillaries are found within the inner retina. The most superficial of these is found within the ganglion cell layer (*red squares*). The deeper capillary bed is found at the junction between the inner nuclear and outer plexiform layers (*red circles*). Tight junctions joining the endothelial cells of these vessels form the inner blood-retinal barrier. The outer blood-retinal barrier is provided by the tight junctions of the RPE layer. The outer barrier prevents leakage from the choriocapillaris (*arrows*) into the retina. (Courtesy of Scheie Eye Institute and Park SS. The anatomy of cell biology of the retina. In: Tasman W, Jaeger EA, eds. *Duane's Ophthalmology on CD-Rom, 2006 Edition.* Philadelphia, PA: Lippincott Williams & Wilkins; 2006.)

○ Histology of the Retinal Vessels

RETINAL CAPILLARIES

The capillary beds of the retinal circulation are not uniformly distributed within the tissue. Instead, two restricted layers of capillaries are found within the inner retina. The most superficial of these is found within the ganglion cell layer. The deeper capillary bed is found at the junction between the inner nuclear and outer plexiform layers (**Fig. 14.41**). The retinal layers deeper than the outer plexiform layer are dependent upon the choroidal vasculature for their metabolic needs. Thus, it is principally the photoreceptor cells and their supporting glia that are dependent upon the choroidal vasculature. The smaller branches of the major retinal arterioles run perpendicular to their origin in the posterior pole and exhibit more dichotomous branching anterior to the vertical equator of the eye. Retinal arterioles also maintain a capillary-free-zone adjacent to them. Neither

of these features is seen in the corresponding retinal venules (**Fig. 14.42**). Retinal arterioles and venules are both lined by a continuous endothelium. This endothelium elaborates a complex basement membrane that includes collagen types I, III, IV, and V, plus fibronectin, laminin, and heparan sulfate proteoglycan core protein. The basal lamina secreted by the endothelial cells contains collagen types IV and V, laminin, and heparan sulfate proteoglycan core protein.[101–103]

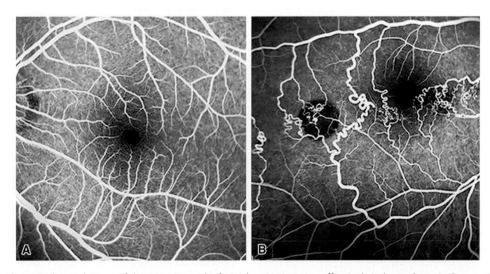

FIGURE 14.40 The retinal vasculatures of the superior and inferior hemiretinae are effectively independent. **A:** Connections between the superior and inferior vascular beds of the retina occur only through the small capillary beds in the macula and periphery. **B:** When venous occlusions occur in the retina, these small capillary vessels remodel and form shunts, which convey blood from the occluded venous bed to the patent venous bed in the other hemisphere. Note that the vessels that remodel into vascular shunts have competent endothelial cell linings and do not leak fluorescein dye.

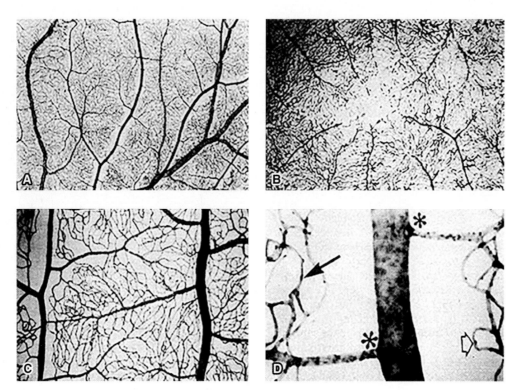

FIGURE 14.42   Trypsin digest preparation of the human retinal vasculature. The narrower channels, surrounded by capillary-free-zones, are arterioles (**A**). Capillary bed around the macula (**B**). There is a capillary-free zone in the center (the foveal avascular zone). **C:** Equatorial zone of the retina. The narrower arteriole on the left, exhibits a capillary-free zone. **D:** An arteriole gives off pre-capillary vessels (*asterisks*), which in turn give off capillaries (*arrow*). FAZ, foveal avascular zone. (Courtesy of Dr. Paul Henkind and Park SS. The anatomy of cell biology of the retina. In: Tasman W, Jaeger EA, eds. *Duane's Ophthalmology on CD-Rom, 2006 Edition.* Philadelphia, PA: Lippincott Williams & Wilkins; 2006.)

Knowing where the intraretinal vessels lie is useful in understanding the distribution of retinal hemorrhages and exudates. Those resulting from vascular changes in the large retinal vessels and the superficial capillary bed result in lesions that commonly overlie the large vessels, obstructing a view of their continuity (e.g., cotton-wool spots and striate hemorrhages). By contrast, hemorrhages and exudates resulting from vascular abnormalities in the deeper capillary bed result in hemorrhage and exudates that do not obscure the visible continuity of the large retinal vessels. Most of these deeper lesions begin in the outer plexiform layer (Fig. 14.43).

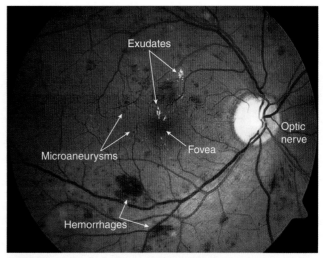

FIGURE 14.43   Locating retinal lesion depth based upon retinal anatomy. Hemorrhages and exudates resulting from vascular abnormalities in the deeper capillary bed cause deep lesions that do not obscure the visible continuity of the large retinal vessels. Most of these deeper lesions begin in the outer plexiform layer. Superficial lesions such as cotton wool spots and striate hemorrhages tend to obstruct the view of larger vessels, which run in this layer of the retina. Note how the upper, labeled hemorrhage obscures the visible continuity of the adjacent vessel.

In addition to the superficial and deep capillary beds, an additional plexus of vessels exists in the peripapillary retina at the level of the inner nuclear layer. This plexus is termed the radial peripapillary plexus (**Fig. 14.44**). Importantly, the radial peripapillary plexus surrounding the optic nerve head is composed of long straight radiating vessels with few interconnections. As such, the peripapillary retina has a diminished capacity

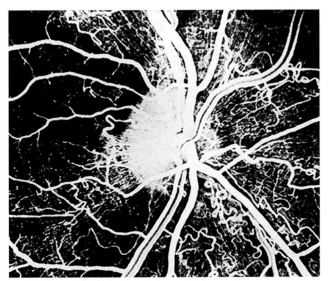

FIGURE 14.44 The radial peripapillary plexus of the optic nerve head is composed of straight radiating vessels with few interconnections. Therefore, the peripapillary retina has a diminished capacity for collateral flow relative to other retinal areas and is at greater risk of ischemic insults and injury. (From Henkind P. Radial peripapillary capillaries of the retina. I. Anatomy: human and comparative. *Br J Ophthalmol.* 1967;51:115–123.)

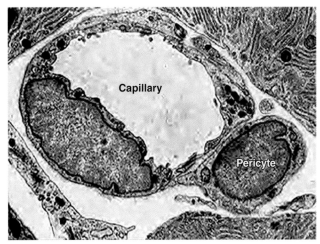

FIGURE 14.45 Pericyte, seen encased within the basement membrane of a retinal capillary. (Courtesy of Don W. Fawcett.)

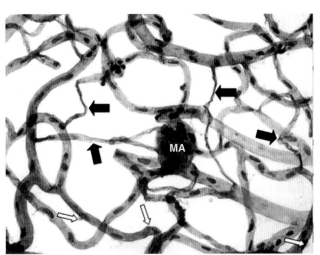

FIGURE 14.46 Diabetic microvascular changes in retinal capillaries (mouse model example). *Black arrows* are diabetes-induced degenerating capillaries. Pericyte ghosts are shown by *white arrows*, also shown is a capillary microaneurysm (MA). The nuclei of vascular endothelial cells appear elongate and within the vessel in these preparations. The nuclei of pericytes appear round and look as though they are stuck on the outside of the vessel. (From Kern TS, Tang J, Berkowitz BA. Validation of structural and functional lesions of diabetic retinopathy in mice. *Mol Vis.* 2010;16: 2121–2131.)

for collateral flow relative to other retinal areas.[104] The peripapillary retina not only has a relatively diminished capacity for collateral flow, but this blood supply must support a greater dependent tissue mass, as the nerve fiber layer thickens as it gets closer to the optic nerve. As such, a given degree of vascular occlusion is more likely to be of greater consequence in the peripapillary region than elsewhere in the retina.[105] This may explain why cotton-wool spots, fluffy, yellow-white retinal lesions resulting from microvascular occlusion and retinal ishcemia, occur more often in the peripapillary region than elsewhere in the retina.

The capillaries of the retina are small in diameter. Their intraluminal diameter averages only 6 μm, smaller than the average diameter of a red blood cell (7 μm). The tunica intima of retinal capillaries consists of a nonfenestrated endothelium joined by very complex tight junctions (zonulae occludentes). Gap junctions are also present between these endothelial cells. Under normal circumstances these capillaries do not leak macromolecules or intravenously injected sodium fluorescein dye.

Pericytes

Enveloped within the splits in the basal lamina of retinal vessels are cells called pericytes (**Fig. 14.45**). In whole mount preparations of retinal vessels the endothelial cell nuclei appear elongated and within the vessel. By contrast, in such preparations, pericytes appear to be rounded and nearer to the outer surface of the vessel (**Fig. 14.46**). In the normal retina, the number of endothelial cells and the

number of pericytes is roughly equal. The pericyte plays a critical role in maintaining the integrity of the endothelial cell wall and vessel patency.[106] Pericytes possess receptors for vasoactive peptides and thus are thought to have contractile function similar to the vascular smooth muscle and help to regulate capillary blood flow and perfusion.[107] In addition, they are believed to play a key role in transcellular transport (like the RPE) and thus are key players in regulating inner retinal vascular permeability.

In diabetic retinopathy, microvascular damage from oxidative and metabolic stress from hyperglycemia causes a preferential loss of pericytes.[105] The loss of these cells contributes a focal weakening in the wall of the vessel that can lead to formation of a microaneurysm, one of the hallmark clinical findings of this retinopathy (**Fig. 14.46**). The loss of pericytes seen in diabetes is associated with endothelial cell loss, capillary occlusion, and macular edema from breakdown of the blood-retinal barrier.

BLOOD SUPPLY TO THE MACULA

The smaller arterioles supplying blood flow to the macula arise directly from the central retinal artery, or as secondary branches that arise from the major arcades arching around the macula. In about a quarter of all patients, a cilioretinal artery arising from the choroidal circulation is also seen, providing blood to the central macula (**SEE CHAPTER 12: CHOROID AND CHOROIDAL CIRCULATION**).[108]

There is an important capillary-free zone in the central macula, surrounding the fovea and its central foveola (**Fig. 14.47A**). This capillary-free zone, approximately 450 to 600 μm in diameter, corresponds to the region of displacement of the inner retinal layers away from the foveola (**Fig. 14.47B**). This thinned portion of the retina within what is termed the foveal avascular zone (FAZ) obtains all of its metabolic support from the underlying choriocapillaris, mediated by the RPE.

REGULATION OF RETINAL BLOOD FLOW

Although the autonomic nervous system plays a major role in controlling the arterial blood flow throughout the body, including to the choroid and outer retina, the inner retinal circulation is an exception. Sympathetic nerves do not regulate intraretinal arterial blood flow; however, they have recently been shown to play a role in maintaining the integrity of the retinal endothelium and blood-retinal barrier in small animal models.[107] Rather, autoregulation of retinal blood flow occurs, causing vasoconstriction or vasodilation modulated by the arterial smooth muscle, in response to variations in perfusion pressure, the difference between the arterial pressure and the intraocular pressure. This smooth muscle autoregulatory mechanism maintains relatively constant blood flow to the inner retina as pressure changes. Tissue responses to metabolic and oxygenation demands have also been shown to directly affect the vascular tone and increase or decrease blood flow. The regulation of retinal blood flow differs between the outer retina (choroidal circulation) and inner retina (retinal circulation). Blood flow to the choroid is very high and effectively unregulated under normal physiologic conditions.

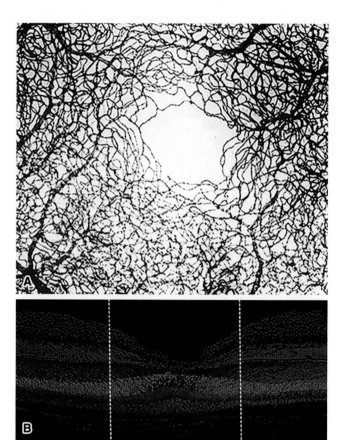

FIGURE 14.47 **A:** Comparison of the capillary-free zone of the fovea (foveal avascular zone) and foveola with a cross sectional confocal microscopic image. **B:** The absence of both the inner retinal layers and capillaries in the region of the fovea minimize light scatter and, together with densely packed and very slender cones permit a high level of visual acuity. (Courtesy of Scheie Eye Institute and Park SS. The anatomy of cell biology of the retina. In: Tasman W, Jaeger EA, eds. *Duane's Ophthalmology on CD-Rom, 2006 Edition*. Philadelphia, PA: Lippincott Williams & Wilkins; 2006.)

The Blood-Retinal Barrier

To maintain the unique extracellular environment required by the retina and to regulate the blood-borne metabolites that reach the retina, a barrier against non-specific diffusion of plasma components is present between the retinal blood supply and the sensory retina. Classically, the blood-retinal barrier is described in two parts, since the retina has a dual vascular supply. These are traditionally referred to as the outer blood-retinal barrier and the inner blood-retinal barrier.

The outer blood-retinal barrier prevents non-specific diffusion of plasma constituents from reaching the retina from the choriocapillaris. The fenestrated vessels of the choroidal capillaries leak fluid, ions and even plasma proteins into the choroidal stroma (**Fig. 14.48**). What prevents their non-specific entry into the retina is a barrier created by the RPE and the tight junctions that join the apico-lateral surfaces of these cells.[109,110]

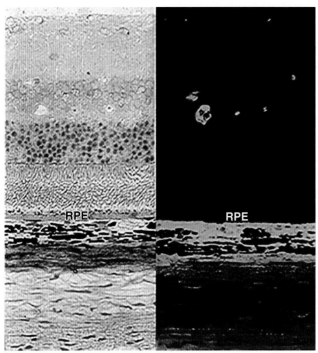

FIGURE 14.48 Light micrograph of normal rat retina **(left)**, and freeze dried preparation of adjacent section taken after injection of fluorescein, demonstrating the way in which the dye is contained within the lumen of retinal vessels by the tight junctions of the endothelial cells of the retinal circulation. Fluorescein freely leaks from the fenestrated choroidal capillaries, into the choroidal extravascular space, also staining the sclera. This material is prevented from non-specific entry into the sensory retina by tight junctions of the retinal pigment epithelium (RPE). (From The Normal Retina. In: Spalton DJ, Hitchings RA, Hunter PA, eds. *Atlas of Clinical Ophthalmology.* 3rd ed. Philadelphia, PA: Mosby; 2004.)

(Discussed in greater detail in **CHAPTER 13: THE RETINAL PIGMENT EPITHELIUM.**)

The inner blood-retinal barrier is established and maintained by the endothelial cells and pericytes in the capillaries of the retinal circulation. As detailed above, the vascular endothelial cells within the retina exhibit a continuous endothelium joined by complex zonulae occludentes that severely restrict paracellular flow of macromolecules (**Fig. 14.48**). As is also seen in the RPE, control of the flow of ions, nutrients, and proteins across the endothelial cell is regulated by their transport either across the cell (transcellular) via energy dependent ion channels, receptor mediated mechanisms, and endocytosis, or flow (primarily water and ions without transporters) between cells (paracellular) across intercellular clefts between the tight junctions. Paracellular flow between cells is driven primarily by osmotic and electrochemical gradients, and by electrostatic forces, similar to the RPE.[111–114] The extracellular matrix, glycoproteins, and proteoglycans surrounding the endothelial cells of the retinal capillaries assist in intercellular adherence of vascular endothelial cells. These modulate shear force and provide a stable platform for the tight junctions that occlude the intercellular clefts.

The retinal glia, astrocytes, and Müller cells, have also been shown to play a role in maintaining the integrity of the inner blood-retinal barrier. These cells are tightly associated with the capillaries (astrocytes in the ganglion cell layer and nerve) and provide both direct barrier function and trophic factors and cytokines, which can both positively and negatively affect the integrity of the endothelial cell (and RPE) tight junction barrier. Impaired arterial autoregulation and vascular tone in the retina is seen in a number of systemic diseases, in particular hypertension and diabetes mellitus and is also seen in the aging retina. Impaired autoregulation may lead to increased hydrostatic pressure in the retinal vasculature and may contribute to loss of blood-retinal barrier function by the endothelial cell tight junctions, pericytes, and glia. Both the outer and inner blood-retinal barriers prevent leakage of plasma constituents into the retina.

These barriers also prevent non-specific leakage of the intravenous dye, sodium fluorescein into the sensory retina (**Fig. 14.48**). Fluorescein angiography is routinely performed clinically to assess the integrity of the outer and inner blood-retinal barriers and is diagnostic of many retinal disease states, and microvascular pathology. In the normal retina, intravenously injected fluorescein does not leak from the intraretinal vasculature and is fully contained within the choroid by the RPE and its tight junctions.

REFERENCES

1. Spencer LM, Foos RY, Straatsma BR. Meridional folds, meridional complexes, and associated abnormalities of the peripheral retina. *Am J Ophthalmol.* 1970;70(5):697–714.
2. Engstrom RE, Glasgow BJ, Foos RY, et al. Degenerative diseases of the peripheral retina. In: Tasman W, Jaeger EA, eds. *Duane's Ophthalmology on CD-Rom, 2006 Edition.* Philadelphia, PA: Lippincott Williams & Wilkins; 2006.
3. Osterberg G. *Topography of the Layer of Rods and Cones in the Human Retina.* Copenhagen, Denmark: Nyt Nordisk Forlag; 1935.
4. Curcio CA, Sloan KR, Kalina RE, et al. Human photoreceptor topography. *J Comp Neurol.* 1990;292(4):497–523.
5. Curcio CA, Sloan KR, Packer O, et al. Distribution of cones in human and monkey retina: individual variability and radial asymmetry. *Science.* 1987;236:579–582.
6. Curcio CA, Allen KA, Sloan KR, et al. Distribution and morphology of human cone photoreceptors stained with anti-blue opsin. *J Comp Neurol.* 1991;312(4):610–624.
7. Rapaport DH, Rakic P, Yasamura D, et al. Genesis of the retinal pigment epithelium in the macaque monkey. *J Comp Neurol.* 1995;363(3):359–376.
8. Bowmaker JK, Dartnall H. Visual pigments of rods and cones in a human retina. *J Physiol (Lond).* 1980;298(1):501–511.
9. Ahnelt PK, Kolb H, Pflug R. Identification of a subtype of cone photoreceptor, likely to be blue sensitive, in the human retina. *J Comp Neurol.* 1987;255:18–34.
10. Kolb H, Lipetz LE. The anatomical basis for colour vision in the vertebrate retina. In: Gouras P, ed. *Vision and Visual Dysfunction: The Perception of Colour.* Vol 6. London, UK: Macmillan Press Ltd.; 1991:128–145.
11. Hofer H, Carroll J, Neitz J, et al. Organization of the human trichromatic cone mosaic. *J Neurosci.* 2005;25:9669–9679.
12. Gouras P, Zrenner E. Color coding in primate retina. *Vision Res.* 1981;21:1591–1598.

13. Wyszecki G. *Color*. Chicago, IL: World Book Inc; 2006.

14. Nathans J, Piantanida TP, Eddy RL, et al. Molecular genetics of inherited variation in human color vision. *Science*. 1986;232:203–210.

15. Köllner H. *Die Störungen des Farbensinnes. ihre klinische Bedeutung und ihre Diagnose*. Berlin, Germany: Karger; 1912.

16. Schwartz S. *Visual Perception: A Clinical Orientation*. New York, NY: McGraw Hill; 2004.

17. LaVail MM. Circadian nature of rod outer segment disc shedding in the rat. *Invest Ophthalmol Vis Sci*. 1980;19:407–411.

18. LaVail MM. Outer segment disc shedding and phagocytosis in the outer retina. *Trans Ophthalmol Soc U K*. 1983;103(pt 4):397–404.

19. Besharse JC, Defoe DM. Role of the retinal pigment epithelium in photoreceptor membrane turnover. In: Marmor MF, Wolfensberger TJ, eds. *The Retinal Pigment Epithelium*. Oxford, UK: Oxford University Press; 1998:152–172.

20. LaVail MM. Rod outer segment disc shedding in relation to cyclic lighting. *Exp Eye Res*. 1976;23:277–280.

21. Dowling JE. *The Retina: An Approachable Part of the Brain*. Cambridge, MA: Harvard University Press; 1987.

22. Kolb H, Nelson R. The organization of photoreceptor to bipolar synapses in the outer plexiform layer. In: Djamgoz MBA, Archer SN, Vallerga S, eds. *Neurobiology and Clinical Aspects of the Outer Retina*. Heidelberg, Germany: Springer; 1995:273–296.

23. Boycott B, Wässle H. Morphological classification of bipolar cells of the primate retina. *Eur J Neurosci*. 1991;3(11):1069–1088.

24. Kolb H, Linberg KA, Fisher SK. Neurons of the human retina: a golgi study. *J Comp Neurol*. 1992;318(2):147–187.

25. Ahnelt P, Kolb H. Horizontal cells and cone photoreceptors in human retina: a Golgi-electron microscopic study of spectral connectivity. *J Comp Neurol*. 1994;343:406–427.

26. Kolb H. Organization of the outer plexiform layer of the primate retina: electron microscopy of Golgi-impregnated cells. *Philos Trans R Soc Lond B Biol Sci*. 1970;258:261–283.

27. Li W, DeVries SH. Bipolar cell pathways for color and luminance vision in a dichromatic mammalian retina. *Nat Neurosci*. 2006;9(5):669–675.

28. Gollisch T, Meister M. Eye smarter than scientists believed: neural computations in circuits of the retina. *Neuron*. 2010;65(2):150–164.

29. Kim I, Zhang Y, Yamagata M, et al. Molecular identification of a retinal cell type that responds to upward motion. *Nature*. 2008;452(7186):478–482.

30. Vaney DI, Sivyer B, Taylor WR. Direction selectivity in the retina: symmetry and asymmetry in structure and function. *Nat Rev Neurosci*. 2012;13(3):194–208.

31. Dowling JE, Boycott BB. Organization of the primate retina: electron microscopy. *Proc R Soc Lond B Biol Sci*. 1966;166(1002):80–111.

32. Dowling JE. Organization of vertebrate retinas. *Invest Ophthalmol*. 1970;9(9):655–680.

33. Polyak SL. *The Retina*. Chicago, IL: University of Chicago Press; 1941.

34. Stell WK, Ishida AT, Lightfoot DO. Structural basis for on-and off-center responses in retinal bipolar cells. *Science*. 1977;198(4323):1269–1271.

35. Wässle H, Yamashita M, Greferath U, et al. The rod bipolar cell of the mammalian retina. *Vis Neurosci*. 1991;7(1/2):99–112.

36. De Robertis E, Franchi CM. Electron microscope observations on synaptic vesicles in synapses of the retinal rods and cones. *J Biophys Biochem Cytol*. 1956;2(3):307–318.

37. Haverkamp S, Grünert U, Wässle H. The cone pedicle, a complex synapse in the retina. *Neuron*. 2000;27(1):85–95.

38. Masland RH. The fundamental plan of the retina. *Nat Neurosci*. 2001;4:877–886.

39. Euler T, Masland RH. Light-evoked responses of bipolar cells in a mammalian retina. *J Neurophysiol*. 2000;83:1817–1829.

40. Vaney DI, Young HM, Gynther IC. The rod circuit in the rabbit retina. *Vis Neurosci*. 1991;7(1/2):141–154.

41. Famiglietti EV Jr, Kolb HA. Bistratified amacrine cell and synaptic circuitry in the inner plexiform layer of the retina. *Brain Res*. 1975;84:293–300.

42. Gallego A. Horizontal and amacrine cells in the mammal's retina. *Vision Res*. 1971;(suppl 3):33–50.

43. Kolb H, Mariani A, Gallego A. A second type of horizontal cell in the monkey retina. *J Comp Neurol*. 1980;189(1):31–44.

44. Vaney DI. Retinal neurons: cell types and coupled networks. *Prog Brain Res*. 2002;136:239–254.

45. Baldridge WH, Vaney DI, Weiler R. The modulation of intercellular coupling in the retina. *Semin Cell Dev Biol*. 1998;9(3):311–318.

46. Marc RE, Anderson JR, Jones BW, et al. The AII amacrine cell connectome: a dense network hub. *Neural Circuits Reveal*. 2015;26:32.

47. Kolb H. *Roles of Amacrine Cells. Webvision: The Organization of the Retina and Visual System*; 2007. http://webvision.med.utah.edu/book/part-iii-retinal-circuits/roles-of-amacrine-cells/

48. MacNeil MA, Masland RH. Extreme diversity among amacrine cells: implications for function. *Neuron*. 1998;20:971–982.

49. Euler T, Detwiler PB, Denk W. Directionally selective calcium signals in dendrites of starburst amacrine cells. *Nature*. 2002;418(6900):845–852.

50. Kolb H, Nelson R, Mariani A. Amacrine cells, bipolar cells and ganglion cells of the cat retina: a Golgi study. *Vision Res*. 1981;21:1081–1114.

51. Masland RH. Amacrine cells. *Trends Neurosci*. 1988;11:405–410.

52. Kolb H, Nelson R. Hyperpolarizing, small-field amacrine cells in cone pathways of cat retina. *J Comp Neurol*. 1996;371:415–436.

53. Vaney DI. The mosaic of amacrine cells in the mammalian retina. *Prog Retin Res*. 1990;9:49–100.

54. Bloomfield SA. Relationship between receptive and dendritic field size of amacrine cells in the rabbit retina. *J Neurophysiol*. 1992;68:711–725.

55. Strettoi E, Raviola E, Dacheux RF. Synaptic connections of the narrow-field, bistratified rod amacrine cell (AII) in the rabbit retina. *J Comp Neurol*. 1992;325:152–168.

56. Crooks J, Kolb H. Localization of GABA, glycine, glutamate and tyrosine hydroxylase in the human retina. *J Comp Neurol*. 1992;315:287–230.

57. Pourcho RG, Goebel DJ. Co-localization of substance P and GABA in amacrine cells of the cat retina. *Brain Res*. 1988;447:164–168.

58. Dacey DM. The dopaminergic amacrine cell. *J Comp Neurol*. 1990;301:461–489.

59. Zucker CL, Ehinger BE. Complexities of retina circuitry revealed by neurotransmitter receptor localization. In: Kolb H, Ripps H, Wu S, eds. *Concepts and Challenges in Retinal Biology: a Tribute to John E. Dowling*. Vol 131. Amsterdam, Netherlands: Elsevier. Progress in Brain Research; 2001:71–81.

60. Dowling JE, Ehinger B. The interplexiform cell system. I. Synapses of the dopaminergic neurons of the goldfish retina. *Proc R Soc Lond B Biol Sci*. 1978;201(1142):7–26.

61. Dowling JE, Boycott BB. Neural connections of the retina: fine structure of the inner plexiform layer. *Cold Spring Harb Symp Quant Biol*. 1965;30:393–402.

62. Perry VH, Walker M. Amacrine cells, displaced amacrine cells and interplexiform cells in the retina of the rat. *Proc R Soc Lond B Biol Sci*. 1980;208(1173):415–431.

63. Dacey DM, Petersen MR. Dendritic field size and morphology of midget and parasol ganglion cells of the human retina. *Proc Natl Acad Sci USA*. 1992;89(20):9666–9670.

64. Nelson R, Famiglietti EV, Kolb H. Intracellular staining reveals different levels of stratification for on-center and off-center ganglion cells in the cat retina. *J Neurophyiol*. 1978;41:427–483.

65. Perry VH, Silveira LC. Functional lamination in the ganglion cell layer of the macaque's retina. *Neuroscience*. 1988;25(1):217–223.

66. Perry VH, Silveira LC, Cowey A. Pathways mediating resolution in the primate retina. *Ciba Found Symp*. 1990;155:5–14.

67. Famiglietti EV, Kolb H. Structural basis of "On-" and "Off-" centre responses in retinal ganglion cells. *Science*. 1976;194:193–195.

68. Dacey DM. The mosaic of midget ganglion cells in the human retina. *J Neurosci*. 1993;13:5334–5355.

69. Watanabe M, Rodieck RW. Parasol and midget ganglion cells of the primate retina. *J Comp Neurol*. 1989;289(3):434–454.

70. Dacey DM. Morphology of a small-field bistratified ganglion cell type in the macaque and human retina. *Vis Neurosci.* 1993;10(6):1081–1098.

71. Rodieck RW, Watanabe M. Survey of the morphology of macaque retinal ganglion cells that project to the pretectum, superior colliculus, and parvicellular laminae of the lateral geniculate nucleus. *J Comp Neurol.* 1993;338(2):289–303.

72. Provencio I, Rodriguez IR, Jiang G, et al. A novel human opsin in the inner retina. *J Neurosci.* 2000;20(2):600–605.

73. Berson DM. Phototransduction in ganglion-cell photoreceptors. *Pflügers Arch.* 2007;454(5):849–855.

74. Neitz J, Neitz M. Colour vision: the wonder of hue. *Curr Biol.* 2008;26(18):R700–R702.

75. Stiles WS. Increment thresholds and the mechanisms of colour vision. *Doc Ophthalmol.* 1949;3:138–165.

76. Chatterjee S, Callaway EM. Parallel colour opponent pathways to primary visual cortex. *Nature.* 2003;426:668–671.

77. Lee BB. Neural models and physiological reality. *Vis Neurosci.* 2008;25:231–241.

78. Mullen KT, Kingdom FA. Differential distributions of red-green and blue-yellow cone opponency across the visual field. *Vis Neurosci.* 2002;19:109–118.

79. Kolb H. Anatomical pathways for color vision in the human retina. *Vis Neurosci.* 1991;7:61–74.

80. Yin L, Smith RG, Sterling P, et al. Physiology and morphology of Color-Opponent ganglion cells in a retina expressing a dual gradient of S and M opsins. *J Neurosci.* 2009;29:2706–2724.

81. Gouras P. The function of the midget system in primate color vision. *Vision Res.* 1971;(suppl 3):397–410.

82. Calkins DJ, Schein SJ, Tsukamoto Y, et al. M and L cones in macaque fovea connect to midget ganglion cells by different numbers of excitatory synapses. *Nature.* 1994;371:70–72.

83. Rodieck RW, Binmoeller KF, Dineen JT. Parasol and midget ganglion cells of the human retina. *J Comp Neurol.* 1985;233:115–132.

84. Taylor WR, He S, Levick WR, et al. Dendritic computation of direction selectivity by retinal ganglion cells. *Science.* 2000;289(5488):2347–2350.

85. Berson DM, Dunn FA, Takao M. Phototransduction by retinal ganglion cells that set the circadian clock. *Science.* 2002;295(5557):1070–1073.

86. Freedman MS, Lucas RJ, Soni B, et al. Regulation of mammalian circadian behavior by non-rod, non-cone, ocular photoreceptors. *Science.* 1999;284(5413):502–504.

87. Perry VH, Cowey A. Retinal ganglion cells that project to the superior colliculus and pretectum in the macaque monkey. *Neuroscience.* 1984;12:1125–1137.

88. Panda S, Nayak SK, Campo B, et al. Illumination of the melanopsin signaling pathway. *Science.* 2005;307(5709):600–604.

89. Arendt D. Evolution of eyes and photoreceptor cell types. *Int J Dev Biol.* 2003;47:563–571.

90. Chan-Ling T. Glial, neuronal and vascular interactions in the mammalian retina. *Prog Retin Eye Res.* 1994;13:357–389.

91. Franze K, Grosche J, Skatchkov SN, et al. Muller cells are living optical fibers in the vertebrate retina. *Proc Natl Acad Sci USA.* 2007;104(20):8287–8292.

92. Bernardos RL, Barthel LK, Meyers JR, et al. Late-stage neuronal progenitors in the retina are radial Muller glia that function as retinal stem cells. *J Neurosci.* 2007;27(26):7028–7040.

93. Giannelli SG, Demontis GC, Pertile G, et al. Adult human Müller glia cells are a highly efficient source of rod photoreceptors. *Stem Cells.* 2011;29(2):344–356.

94. Belecky-Adams TL, Chernoff EC, Wilson JM, et al. Reactive Muller glia as potential retinal progenitors. Rijeka, Croatia: INTECH Open Access Publisher; 2013.

95. Stone J, Dreher Z. Relationship between astrocytes, ganglion cells and vasculature of the retina. *J Comp Neurol.* 1987;255:35–49.

96. Bernstein PS, Li B, Vachali PP, et al. Lutein, zeaxanthin, and meso-zeaxanthin: the basic and clinical science underlying carotenoid-based nutritional interventions against ocular disease. *Prog Retin Eye Res.* 2016;50:34–66.

97. Snodderly DM, Auran JD, Delori FC. The macular pigment. II. Spatial distribution in primate retina. *Invest Ophthal Vis Sci.* 1984;25:674–685.

98. Age-Related Eye Disease Study Research Group. A randomized, placebo-controlled, clinical trial of high-dose supplementation with vitamins C and E, beta carotene, and zinc for age-related macular degeneration and vision loss: AREDS report no. 8. *Arch Ophthalmol.* 2001;119(10):1417–1436.

99. Meyers KJ, Johnson EJ, Bernstein PS, et al. Genetic determinants of macular pigments in women of the Carotenoids in Age-Related Eye Disease Study. *Invest Ophthalmol Vis Sci.* 2013;54(3):2333–2345.

100. Meyers KJ, Mares JA, Igo RP Jr, et al. Genetic evidence for role of carotenoids in age-related macular degeneration in the Carotenoids in Age-Related Eye Disease Study (CAREDS). *Invest Ophthalmol Vis Sci.* 2014;55(1):587–599.

101. Das A, Frank RN, Zhang NL, et al. Ultrastructural localization of extracellular matrix components in human retinal vessels and bruch's membrane. *Arch Ophthalmol.* 1990;108(3):421–429.

102. Kuwabara T, Cogan DG. Retinal vascular patterns: VI. Mural cells of the retinal capillaries. *Arch Ophthalmol.* 1963;69(4):492–502.

103. Sagaties M, Raviola G, Schaeffer S, et al. The structural basis of the inner blood-retina barrier in the eye of macaca mulatta. *Invest Ophthalmol Vis Sci.* 1987;28(12):2000–2014.

104. Henkind P. Symposium on glaucoma: joint meeting with the national society for the prevention of blindness: new observations on the radial peripapillary capillaries. *Invest Ophthalmol Vis Sci.* 1967;6(2):103.

105. Alm A, Bill A. Ocular and optic nerve blood flow at normal and increased intraocular pressures in monkeys (Macaca irus): a study with radioactively labelled microspheres including flow determinations in brain and some other tissues. *Exp Eye Res.* 1973;15:15–29.

106. Hammes HP, Lin J, Renner O, et al. Pericytes and the pathogenesis of diabetic retinopathy. *Diabetes.* 2002;51(10):3107–3112.

107. Wiley LA, Rupp GR, Steinle JJ. Sympathetic innervation regulates basement membrane thickening and pericyte number in rat retina. *Invest Ophthalmol Vis Sci.* 2005;46(2):744–748.

108. Hayreh SS. The cilio-retinal arteries. *Br J Ophthalmol.* 1963;47:71–89.

109. Rizzolo LJ. Polarity and the development of the outer blood-retinal barrier. *Histol Histopathol.* 1997;12:1057–1067.

110. Bok D. The retinal pigment epithelium: a versatile partner in vision. *J Cell Sci Suppl.* 1993;17:189–195.

111. Wimmers S, Karl MO, Strauss O. Ion channels in the RPE. *Prog Retin Eye Res.* 2007;26:263–301.

112. Hughes BA, Gallemore RP, Miller SS. Transport mechanisms in the retinal pigment epithelium. In: Marmor MF, Wolfensberger TJ, eds. *The Retinal Pigment Epithelium.* Oxford, UK: Oxford University Press; 1998:103–134.

113. Joseph DP, Miller SS. Apical and basal membrane ion transport mechanisms in bovine retinal pigment epithelium. *J Physiol.* 1991;435:439–463.

114. Strauss O. The retinal pigment epithelium in visual function. *Physiol Rev.* 2005;85:845–881.

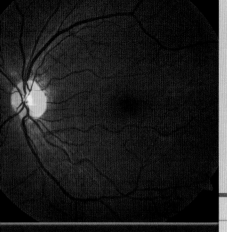

The Optic Nerve and Visual Pathways

CHAPTER 15

Overview

The optic nerves (cranial nerve II) are large, bundled tracts that convey the retinal ganglion cell (RGC) axons from each eye to the optic chiasm in the middle cranial fossa. The two optic nerves exchange fibers at the optic chiasm and are reassembled as the optic tracts that deliver these axons to their synaptic connections in the lateral geniculate nucleus of the thalamus. Postsynaptic fibers from the lateral geniculate nuclei comprise the optic radiations that relay visual input to the primary visual cortex in the occipital lobes of the brain. Some optic nerve fibers also diverge from the post-chiasmal portions of the nerves to make connections in the superior colliculi, the suprachiasmatic nuclei, and the pretectum. These fibers serve reflexive and circadian aspects of vision. Specifically, the superior colliculi control the orientation of head and saccadic eye movements, the pretectum controls pupillary functions and accommodative functions of the lens, and the suprachiasmatic nucleus of the hypothalamus plays a role in regulating circadian rhythms. The RGC axons are also accompanied by several glial cell types in the optic nerve including astrocytes, microglia, and, once the axons leave the globe, the oligodendrocytes that ensheath the axons in myelin to enhance nerve conduction velocity.

The optic nerve is anatomically and functionally complex and conveys the complete visual output of each eye. Bundles of axons from specific parts of the retina, each representing specific parts of the visual field, travel together. This provides what is termed retinotopic organization within the optic nerve. The organization of the RGC axons in the optic nerve changes as these fibers pass from the retina into the nerve itself and then exchange fibers at the optic chiasm to form the optic tracts. Even with such changes, a predictable pattern of retinotopic organization is preserved throughout the visual pathway. Thus, similar types of lesions (e.g., compressive) may have very different effects on the field of vision depending upon where the lesion impacts the nerve and the distal portions of the visual pathways. But in each case, knowledge of the predictable retinotopic pattern provides diagnostic cues as to the location of the lesion via the visual field changes that ensue. These patterns are detailed later in this chapter.

Structural aspects of the optic nerve head and its unique vascular supply also need to be clear to the clinician in order to understand the risk factors for, and manifestations of diseases of the optic nerve, in particular glaucoma and vascular diseases of the nerve and retina. Embryologic and racial variations in the appearance of the optic nerve are common and comprise a broad spectrum of normal and abnormal features, which must be understood in order to decide which features are abnormal and which features are simply anatomic variants. Finally, the organization of the optic nerves differs from the organization of the optic tract fibers; thus, knowing the basic anatomy of the optic tracts, the lateral geniculate nucleus, and the cortical pathways in the brain is also important to understanding the visual manifestations of diseases of the central nervous system and brain that have the potential to impact vision. These will be described in a basic overview in this chapter, but readers are encouraged to seek additional texts and reviews for a more thorough understanding of cortical processing aspects of vision.

Macroscopic and Clinical Anatomy of the Optic Nerve

The pathway of the optic nerve from the eye to the optic chiasm is continuous but is commonly described in segments pertaining to the spaces through which the nerve passes. Each of these segments has distinct clinical vulnerabilities. These segments (**Fig. 15.1**) include:

- Intrascleral, as it traverses the scleral coat of the globe (~1 mm),
- Intraconal (or intraorbital) as it passes through the extraocular muscle cone in the orbit to reach the orbital apex (~25 to 30mm),
- Intracanalicular, as it passes through the optic canal of the sphenoid bone (~9 mm),
- Intracranial, as it traverses the middle cranial fossa to reach the optic chiasm (~15 mm). These fibers decussate, reassembling as the optic tracts that continue to the lateral geniculate nuclei.

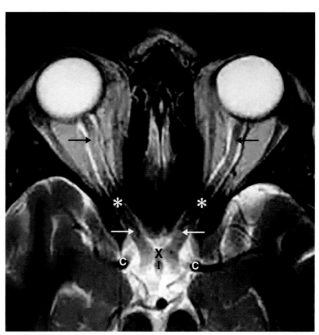

FIGURE 15.1 Normal imaging appearance of the optic nerves and chiasm. The optic nerves in their entirety are seen on this axial T2-weighted image. Clearly visible are the intraorbital (*black arrows*), intracanalicular (*white asterisks*), and intracranial segments of the optic nerves (*white arrows*). The MRI signal in the optic nerves matches that of the white matter in the brain. Also seen is the optic chiasm (*X*) and its relationship with the internal carotid arteries (*C*) and infundibulum of the pituitary gland (*I*). (From Sanelli P, Schaefer P, Loevner L, eds. *Neuroimaging: The Essentials*. Philadelphia, PA: Wolters Kluwer; 2015.)

> *The length of the optic nerve within the orbit (~25 mm) exceeds the distance from the posterior surface of the eye to the optic canal.* Thus, there is slack in the nerve, permitting free movement of the nerve without traction. By contrast, in its passage from the orbit through the optic canal of the sphenoid bone, the nerve is tightly adherent to the wall of the canal (**Fig. 15.1**). This tight association makes the nerve particularly vulnerable to shear injury from blunt trauma, fractures of the sphenoid bone, damage from bony erosion by a sphenoid sinusitis, or swelling of the optic nerve in this location. Principal vulnerabilities in the intracranial portion of the nerve result from compression by abnormalities of surrounding structures (pituitary tumors, carotid artery aneurysm, etc.).

THE OPTIC NERVE HEAD

The clinically visible optic nerve head (the optic papilla) usually appears as a vertically elongated oval with a horizontal diameter of approximately 1.5 mm. The position of the center of the optic nerve head is approximately 3 mm (i.e., two disc diameters) medial to, and slightly above, a horizontal meridian passing through the fovea (**Fig. 15.2**).

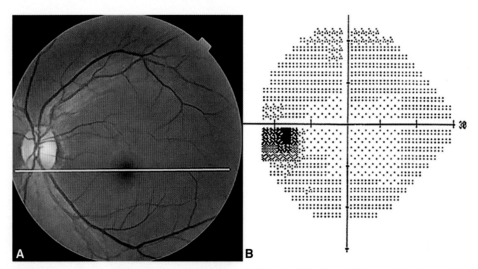

FIGURE 15.2   **A:** Fundus photograph of the optic nerve and macula, left eye. A horizontal line passing through the fovea (the point of fixation) typically passes inferior to the midline or just below the edge of the optic nerve (*yellow line*). **B:** The point of fixation in the visual field test (convergence of horizontal and vertical lines) projects to a position in visual space that is just superior to the physiologic blind spot created by the optic nerve (dark area at B).

This location projects to a position in visual space that is approximately 10° to 15° temporal to, and slightly below, a horizontal meridian passing through the point of fixation. Because the optic nerve head has no sensory cells, the optic nerve projects into the visual field as a blind spot. However the blind spots from each eye do not project to the same point in visual space, so they are not appreciated under normal binocular viewing conditions.

 The area of the optic nerve head and its horizontal diameter are referred to as the "disc area" and "disc diameter," respectively. This dimension is commonly used as a comparative measure for size and location when describing lesions in the posterior pole of the retina. For example, a typical clinical use of this dimension would be to describe the size and position of a retinal lesion as being "X disc diameters in size at Y disc diameters from the disc, along the Z o'clock meridian." These metrics are also used in the formal determination of "clinically significant macular edema," the criterion for performing laser treatment in patients with diabetic retinopathy and macular edema.

The optic nerve is comprised of between 750,000 and 1.5 million ganglion cell axons, with an average of ~1.1 million. The axons project from their cell bodies in the ganglion cell layer of the retina, into the overlying nerve fiber layer of the retina and then turn to become the optic nerve. From the peripheral retina, as more fibers are added, the nerve fiber layer of the retina thickens progressively toward the optic nerve head (**Fig. 15.3**). The false color

optical coherence tomography (OCT) image shows a cross section through the macula of a normal retina. The laminated structure of the retinal layers is evident, as is the foveal depression in the center of the image. The nerve fiber layer is seen as a progressively thickening layer of (red) tissue along the inner layer of the retina between the fovea and the optic nerve just beyond the right edge of the picture.

The normal optic nerve head varies in size, and thus, nerves with similar numbers of ganglion cell axons differ in clinical appearance from patient to patient. The fibers may fill the center of the nerve head completely, or they may form a neuroretinal rim of tissue that is displaced from the center of the nerve, forming a central depression or "cup" that appears more yellow in color than the orange/pink of the surrounding neuroretinal rim (**Fig. 15.4**). In general, a characteristic pattern of neuroretinal rim thickness is seen in each quadrant surrounding the cup. The neuroretinal rim of a normal disc is commonly thickest inferiorly (I). Next thickest is the superior (S) and then the nasal rim (N), with the thinnest portion being the temporal rim. Hence, a normal disc is said to follow the ISNT rule. Optic nerve atrophy, especially that which is associated with advancing glaucoma, tends to alter the rim asymmetrically, causing it to violate the ISNT rule.[1]

It is also routine to clinically estimate the percentage of the disc diameter that is occupied by the central excavation of the cup. This "cup-to-disc" C/D ratio is a commonly recorded clinical parameter.

Enlargement of the cup, especially vertical elongation, and notching of the rim are common, relatively early signs of glaucomatous optic atrophy. The median C/D ratio is ~0.3 but variations on this ratio that are still normal are quite common. Importantly, the C/D ratio rarely differs

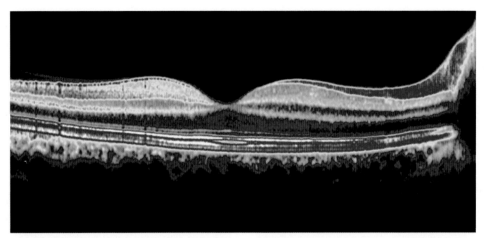

FIGURE 15.3   False color optical coherence tomography cross section image of the macula, foveal depression, and the nerve fiber layer (red superficial layer) as it approaches the optic nerve at far right. (Courtesy of Dr Jean-Michel Muratet and Optovue website. http://www .oct-optovue.com. October 17, 2008. Accessed October 20, 2016.)

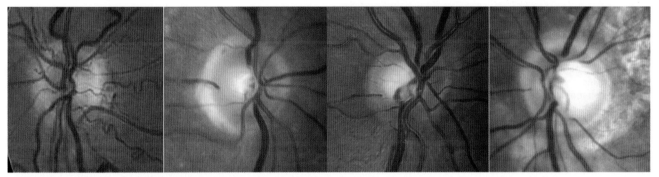

FIGURE 15.4   Photomontage of cup-to-disc (C/D) ratios seen in normal optic nerves. The C/D ratio describes the relationship between the physiologic depression in the center of the optic nerve head and the total optic disc diameter. The horizontal C/D ratios for the four nerves shown are approximately 0.0, 0.2, 0.35, and 0.6. Customarily, estimates of horizontal and vertical C/D are recorded separately.

between the two eyes by an amount greater than 0.1. Patients of African and Hispanic heritage generally have larger optic discs than Caucasians and Asians, and the shape of the optic nerve head is more commonly vertically oval. Women tend toward smaller optic nerve heads and smaller C/D ratios as well.[2]

Normal anatomic variants in the appearance of the optic disc can include the presence of a white crescent along the temporal edge of the disc or a pigmented crescent along the margin of the disc. In the former case, this results from the choroid and retinal pigment epithelium (RPE) having failed to reach the edge of the optic nerve, allowing visualization of the underlying sclera. In the latter case, a thickening of the RPE has occurred at the disc margin.

Understanding anatomic variants in peripapillary architecture is particularly important in the evaluation and assessment of disease progression in glaucoma. There are two distinct, somewhat concentric zones of atrophy adjacent to, and occasionally surrounding, the normal optic disc. This peripapillary atrophy is seen ophthalmoscopically and histologically as two distinct regions termed *zone alpha* and *zone beta*. The inner zone, beta, is an area at the peripheral edge of the scleral rim of Elshnig (see **Fig. 15.5**) in which the RPE and choriocapillaris are absent, but the underlying choroidal vasculature is intact. These areas of atrophy are predominately located temporally but can encircle the entire nerve. Areas of zone beta are more commonly seen in nerves with glaucoma, and the size of the area correlates with other features of the disease (e.g., visual field) and is used to help distinguish different types of open-angle glaucoma (**Fig. 15.5**).[3] Zone alpha atrophy is located peripheral to zone beta (if present) and is more common in normal eyes. It can contain areas of both hyper- and hypo-pigmentation and is associated with thinning of the underlying choriocapillaris. The areas of zone alpha and zone beta atrophy are distinct from the scleral crescents that are commonly seen in myopic patients. Peripapillary atrophy surrounding the optic nerve is a common finding in patients and represents a region adjacent to the optic nerve head in which there

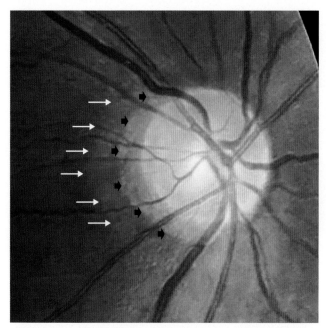

FIGURE 15.5 Peripapillary architecture. Two concentric zones of atrophy are seen adjacent to the optic disc termed zone alpha and zone beta. The inner, zone beta (*black arrowheads*) is an area in which the retinal pigment epithelium and choriocapillaris are absent, but the underlying choroidal vasculature is intact. Areas of zone beta are more commonly seen in nerves with glaucoma. The outer, zone alpha is peripheral to zone beta (if present) (*white arrows* in this image). It can be hyper- and hypo-pigmentation and is associated with thinning of the choriocapillaris.

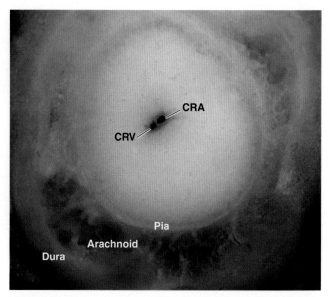

FIGURE 15.6 Gross anatomy of the optic nerve in cross section just posterior to the globe. The central retinal artery (CRA) and central retinal vein (CRV) run together in the axial portion of the nerve. The nerve is surrounded by the three concentric meningeal sheaths just like the brain. These include the tightly adherent pia mater, the loose trabecular arachnoid, and the thick dura mater. The yellowish color of the nerve results from its content of myelin.

is degeneration of all three layers of tissue internal to the sclera, the neural retina, the RPE, and the choroid. Peripapillary atrophy itself is not a risk factor for glaucoma; however, the atrophic area appears to be larger in eyes with open-angle glaucoma, compared to age-matched controls, making it an important anatomic parameter for routine clinical assessment.[4–7]

THE INTRACONAL OPTIC NERVE

After the optic nerve passes through the sclera, it becomes covered by all three layers of the meninges, including the dura, arachnoid, and the pia mater (**Fig. 15.6**). The subarachnoid space surrounding the nerve is continuous with that of the brain, and cerebral spinal fluid surrounds the optic nerve all the way up to the sclera. The dural covering of this fibrovascular meningeal sheath blends with the sclera around the optic nerve and with Tenon's capsule. The arachnoid layer, like that of the brain, forms a loose syncytium, whereas the pial layer is tightly adherent to the nerve. At the histologic level the pia extends fine fibrovascular septae into the nerve, dividing its axons into bundled fascicles and bringing with it fine vessels to provide blood flow to the substance of the nerve within the orbit.

 The subarachnoid space surrounding the optic nerve contains cerebrospinal fluid (CSF) and is continuous with the CSF compartments within and surrounding the brain. Chronically increased CSF pressure can restrict the blood flow to the optic nerve and interfere with axoplasmic flow, causing swelling of the optic nerve head, a condition called papilledema (Fig. 15.7). Papilledema can be the presenting sign of a space-occupying mass in the intracranial cavity that elevates intracranial pressure. More commonly in clinical practice, papilledema is caused by a condition known as pseudotumor cerebri (PTC), which presents with a history of headache with or without visual symptoms, commonly in overweight, young adult women. PTC is believed to result from intracranial venous hypertension and/or a defect in the reabsorption of the CSF by the arachnoid granulations, which normally return CSF to the venous circulation. The disease and diagnosis is established by confirmation of elevated intracranial pressure (measured by lumbar puncture) in the setting of a normal brain magnetic resonance imaging study.

Histology of the Optic Nerve Head

The optic nerve head is a complex neurovascular and connective tissue structure. It must physically support the ~1.1 million axons that are the confluence of the

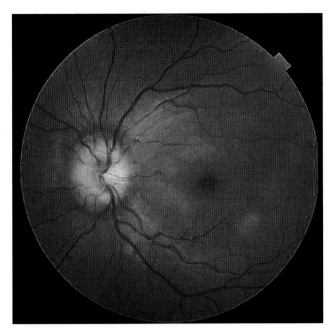

FIGURE 15.7 Papilledema. Chronically increased cerebrospinal fluid pressure can restrict the blood flow to the optic nerve and interfere with axoplasmic flow, causing swelling of the optic nerve head, termed papilledema. Note the blurred optic disc margins and elevation of the retinal vessels as they pass over the swollen nerve head.

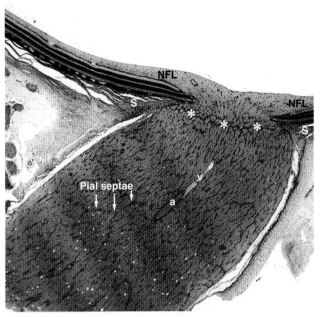

FIGURE 15.8 Light microscopy of the major histologic landmarks of the optic nerve head and their relationships with surrounding structures. The axons of the nerve pass the edges of the retinal pigment epithelium, Bruch's membrane, and the choroid. The nerve fibers then pass through the scleral canal (*S*) and the lamina cribrosa (*asterisks*). Posterior to the lamina cribrosa, each axon picks up a myelin sheath that doubles the diameter of the optic nerve at the point where it emerges from the sclera canal. Axons are gathered into bundles by septae representing fibrovascular extensions of pia mater into the substance of the nerve. The central retinal artery (*a*) and vein (*v*) are also seen. NFL, nerve fiber layer. (Modified from Takizawa P. Optic Nerve slide. Yale Histology Sensory Systems Lab website. http://medcell.med.yale.edu/histology/sensory_systems_lab /optic_nerve.php. Accessed March 21, 2017.)

nerve fiber layer of the retina as they transit past the surrounding choroid and then traverse the scleral canal. This support must be resilient to the force applied by the intraocular pressure over the surface of the nerve head and the force of the CSF pressure applied posteriorly around the circumference of the nerve. It must accommodate a complex microvasculature to nourish these axons and their supporting glial cells. Adding further to the complexity, in the 1 mm length of the intrascleral portion of the optic nerve, each axon becomes ensheathed in insulating layers of myelin produced by the oligodendrocytes, which doubles the diameter of the optic nerve from 1.5 to 3 mm in thickness over this short span.

The major histologic landmarks of the optic nerve head and its relationships with surrounding structures are shown in **Fig. 15.8**. Note that as the nerve fiber layer approaches the edge of the optic nerve head, the fibers must turn 90° and pass the edges of the RPE and Bruch's membrane. Passing posteriorly, the optic nerve borders the choroid before reaching the scleral canal, where the connective tissue support matrix of the lamina cribrosa interweaves with the axon bundles of the optic nerve. Finally, posterior to the lamina cribrosa, the optic nerve is also surrounded by an investing layer of pia mater on its outer surface that gives rise to fibrovascular pial septae that provide the microvascular supply for the core of the nerve. At the lamina cribrosa is where oligodendrocytes are first found. These invest each axon with a myelin sheath and, in doing so, double the diameter of the nerve.

The anterior extension of the subarachnoid space to where the nerve axons pierce the scleral coat is evident in **Fig. 15.8** as is the histologic connection between the dura mater and the posterior surface of the sclera.

GLIAL SUPPORTING CELLS IN THE OPTIC NERVE

There are three principal types of glial cells within the optic nerve—oligodendrocytes, microglia, and astrocytes. Myelin-producing oligodendrocytes are only present posterior to the lamina cribrosa. The microglia of the optic nerve, as elsewhere in the central nervous system, are the resident phagocytic cells and are found within both the axon bundles and the connective tissue of the pial septae.[8,9] Like macrophages, they act as antigen-presenting cells to the immune system. During development, they also play a significant role in eliminating RGCs that have not successfully made connections in the brain.

Two subtypes of astrocytes have been described in the optic nerve. Various sources list them as types 1 and 2 or types 1a and 1b. These subtypes are based upon differences in immunohistochemical staining characteristics.[10,11] Both cell types stain positively for glial fibrillary acidic protein (GFAP). Type 1 cells are found primarily at the edges of the lamina cribrosa and the glial limiting membrane surrounding the nerve. By contrast, type 2 astrocytes are found within the nerve. These astrocytes contribute to the glial columns separating the bundles of axons from the connective tissue pial septae and may interface with the microvasculature. The astrocytes of the optic nerve play an important role in regulating the ionic milieu by buffering extracellular K+ ions through active transport mechanisms in the nerve and by acting as a metabolic energy reservoir under conditions of stress.

◉ Zones of the Optic Nerve Head

The optic nerve head is commonly divided into four zones based upon structural differences in the nerve, its anatomic relationships, and the changes in vascular supply that support these zones. From anterior to posterior, these zones are:

- Superficial nerve fiber layer (anterior to Bruch's membrane)
- Prelaminar zone (between Bruch's membrane and the lamina cribrosa)
- Laminar zone
- Retrolaminar zone (posterior to the lamina cribrosa)

THE SUPERFICIAL NERVE FIBER LAYER

The superficial nerve fiber layer of the optic nerve head is composed of RGC axons as they turn posteriorly to enter the optic nerve head (**Fig.15.9**). The architectural assembly of these fibers retains the retinotopic organization of the RGCs in the retina. The surface of the optic nerve head is covered by the internal limiting membrane of Elschnig, which is formed by astrocytes (see **Fig. 15.10**). The internal limiting membrane of Elschnig is continuous with the internal limiting membrane of the retina that is provided by the Müller cells at the margins of the optic nerve head. This ring of transition corresponds roughly to the ring of attachment of the posterior vitreous face to the edges of the optic nerve. Over the optic nerve head, between the internal limiting membrane and the posterior vitreous face, is the space of Martegiani (**SEE CHAPTER 11: THE VITREOUS**). In the central portion of the optic nerve head, the internal limiting membrane is slightly thicker, owing to the presence of additional astrocytes that persist after the resorption of the hyaloid artery and vein during embryogenesis. This thickened portion of the internal limiting membrane is termed the central meniscus of Kuhnt (see **Fig.15.10**).

PRELAMINAR ZONE

The principal features of the prelaminar portion of the optic nerve head arise from the relationship between the edges of the optic nerve and the surrounding sensory retina, RPE, Bruch's membrane, choroid, and the innermost lamellae of the sclera (**Fig. 15.9**). After the neuroectoderm-derived axons pass posteriorly, through these layers, they are insulated from direct contact with the surrounding connective tissues by layers of astrocytes. The portion of this astrocytic ring of separation between the prelaminar portion of the optic nerve and the adjacent sensory retina is the intermediary tissue of Kuhnt (**Fig.15.10**). Continuation of this astrocytic ring posteriorly separates the prelaminar portion of the optic nerve from the adjacent choroid and innermost lamellae of the surrounding sclera. This portion of the astrocytic ring is termed the border tissue of Jacoby (**Fig. 15.10**).

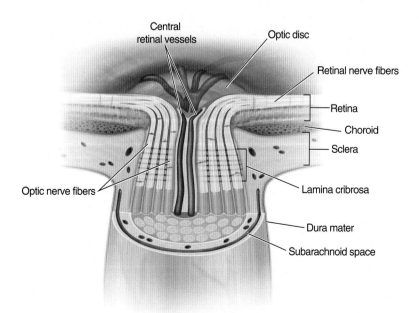

FIGURE 15.9 The anatomy of the optic nerve head.

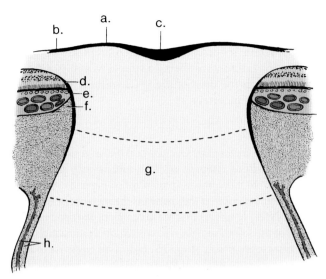

FIGURE 15.10   Supportive structures of the optic nerve head: internal limiting membrane of Elschnig (*a*) continuous with the internal limiting membrane of the retina (*b*), central meniscus of Kuhnt (*c*), intermediary tissue of Kuhnt (*d*), border tissue of Jacoby (*e*), border tissue of Elschnig (*f*), lamina cribrosa (*g*), and meningeal sheaths (*h*). (Modified from Allingham RR, Damji KF, Freedman SF, et al. *Shields Textbook of Glaucoma.* 6th ed. Philadelphia, PA: Wolters Kluwer; 2010.)

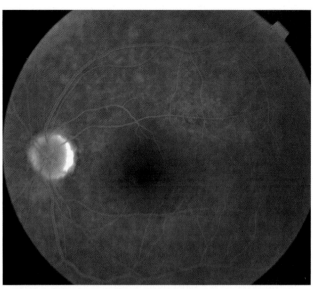

FIGURE 15.11   Late images from fluorescein angiogram study showing staining of the optic nerve head.

 Of clinical importance, the border tissues of Kuhnt and Jacoby do not represent a permeability barrier surrounding the optic nerve head. As such, following intravenous injection of sodium fluorescein, it is normal to observe a time-related fluorescent staining of the optic nerve head. This fluorescence results from diffusion of fluorescein that has leaked from the fenestrated choroidal capillaries. Because this diffusion takes time, the fluorescence within the normal optic nerve head is most readily apparent in later phases of the angiographic imaging sequence, at a time after the fluorescein has traversed the retinal circulation and been diluted in the systemic circulation (Fig. 15.11).

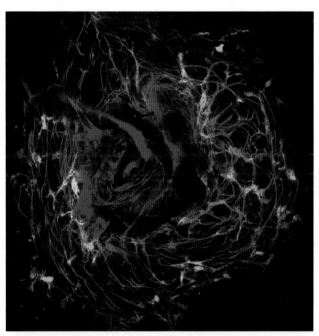

FIGURE 15.12   Optic nerve head of a normal mouse retina displaying the "glial tubes" formed by the astrocytic network (red anti-GFAP antibody stains astrocytes). Anti-GFP (*green*) and anti-collagen IV (*blue*) were used to determine the numbers of astrocytes and relative locations in relation to blood vessels. (From Gabriel Luna and Steve Fisher/Geoff Lewis's Retinal Cell Biology Lab, UC Santa Barbara Neuroscience Research Institute, 2016. In: Optic Nerve Head. Webvision website. Webvision website. http://webvision.med.utah.edu/. December 2011. Accessed March 21, 2017. Copyright © 2017 Webvision.)

In addition to the glial border tissues of Kuhnt and Jacoby, the innermost lamellae of the sclera surrounding the nerve project anteriorly in some eyes. In doing so, this lip of scleral tissue may intervene between the peripheral margins of the nerve and the posterior layers of the choroid. In cases, where the innermost aspect of the scleral rim projects forward in this way, this ring of scleral tissue is termed the border tissue of Elschnig (Fig. 15.10).

LAMINAR ZONE

As can be seen in the prelaminar portion of the optic nerve head, the axons are collected into bundles, separated from each other by a layer of astrocytes (Fig. 15.12). These intervening layers of astrocytes also provide a conduit for

the entrance of the microvasculature serving this portion of the nerve. Upon reaching the lamina cribrosa, however, these astrocytic bundles are further divided into fascicles of nerve fibers interwoven with a fibrovascular matrix of collagens, elastin, and a sparse complement of fibroblasts that are collectively termed the lamina cribrosa.

STRUCTURE OF THE LAMINA CRIBROSA

The scleral opening through which the ganglion cell axons pass to reach the orbital section of the nerve is supported by a complex web of fibrovascular tissue that separates and supports the bundles of axons and their surrounding astrocytes. In addition, it provides a conduit for the microvasculature supplying this portion of the optic nerve head to extend from the surrounding pia mater, into the core of the nerve. As seen, the lamina cribrosa is composed of a system of trabeculae that surround openings through which the bundles of axons and the central retinal vein and artery pass (**Fig. 15.13**). It has been shown that these openings are generally larger superiorly and inferiorly, suggesting that less support for the axon bundles may be present at these sites.[12] This may contribute to the tendency of the axons in these areas to be preferentially damaged when intraocular pressure is elevated in glaucoma.

The trabeculae of the lamina cribrosa consist of a core of elastin interwoven with a matrix of collagen types I and III, which are associated with type IV collagen and laminin.[13,14] The type IV collagen appears to arise from both the astroglial cells and connective tissue fibroblasts within the trabeculae. By contrast, in the surrounding sclera to which the trabeculae of the lamina cribrosa are attached, there is almost no elastin, it is 90% type I collagen by weight. In addition, collagen types III, IV, V, VI, VIII, XII, and XIII have been reported in small quantities.[15-19] Comparing the matrix composition of the lamina cribrosa and the sclera, it becomes clear that a simplistic notion of the lamina cribrosa just being a simple weaving of scleral fibers through the mass of the ~1.1 million axons of the optic nerve is incorrect.

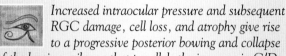

Increased intraocular pressure and subsequent RGC damage, cell loss, and atrophy give rise to a progressive posterior bowing and collapse of the lamina cribrosa that parallels the increase in C/D ratio. Note, however, that the anatomy of the optic nerve head at the scleral margin remains relatively unchanged as the disease progresses (Fig. 15.14). This gives rise to the "bean pot" appearance of the excavated optic nerve head seen in many patients with advanced glaucomatous cupping of the optic nerve.

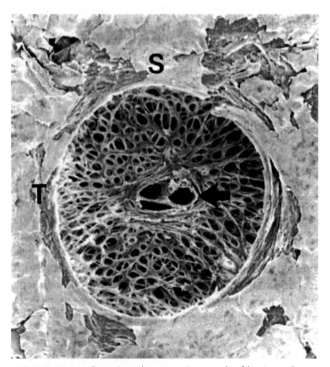

FIGURE 15.13 Scanning electron micrograph of lamina cribrosa showing openings for central retinal vessels (*black arrow*) and surrounding fenestra of lamina for passage of axon bundles. Note larger size of fenestra in superior and inferior quadrants. S, superior; T, temporal. (From Allingham RR, Damji KF, Freedman SF, et al. *Shields Textbook of Glaucoma.* 6th ed. Philadelphia, PA: Wolters Kluwer; 2010.)

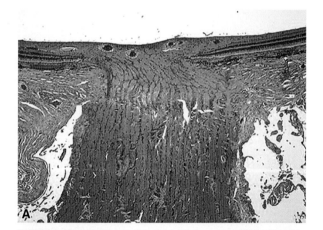
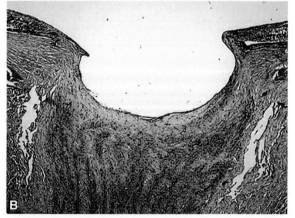

FIGURE 15.14 H&E-stained sections of optic nerves. **A:** Histologic section of normal optic nerve. **B:** Optic nerve from advanced glaucoma. The anatomy of the optic nerve head at the scleral margin remains largely unchanged, giving rise to a "bean pot" appearing excavation of the optic nerve as the disease progresses. (From Rhee DJ, ed. *Color Atlas and Synopsis of Clinical Ophthalmology—Wills Eye Institute—Glaucoma.* 2nd ed. Philadelphia, PA: Wolters Kluwer; 2012.)

RETROLAMINAR ZONE

The posterior margin of the lamina cribrosa is the point in the visual pathway where oligodendrocytes begin to envelop each axon. The oligodendrocytes provide a myelin sheath and nodes of Ranvier, which dramatically accelerate the signal transmission rate over that possible in the retina and prelaminar and laminar portions of the optic nerve. The wrapping of each axon in its myelinated envelope doubles the diameter of each fiber (**Fig. 15.15**). This in turn doubles the diameter of the optic nerve overall, from 1.5 mm at the optic nerve head to 3 mm at its exit from the scleral canal. Embryologically, the myelination of the optic nerve occurs late in development and proceeds from the brain to the eye. In a small number of individuals, the process of myelination of the optic nerve fails to stop at the lamina cribrosa. In such cases, myelin may continue onto the fibers of the nerve fiber layer of the retina (see Figure 16.50 in **CHAPTER 16: EMBRYOLOGY OF THE EYE AND ORBIT**).

The retrolaminar zone of the optic nerve head technically lies within the intraconal (intraorbital) part of the optic nerve and is the first portion of the optic nerve surrounded by a meningeal covering of dura mater, arachnoid, and pia mater. In the retrolaminar portion of the optic nerve, the fascicles of nerve fibers are separated by vascularized septae derived from the pial covering that tightly invests the exterior surface of the optic nerve (**Fig. 15.16**). As elsewhere, an astroglial covering separates the bundles of axons from the fibrovascular pial septae that surround them.

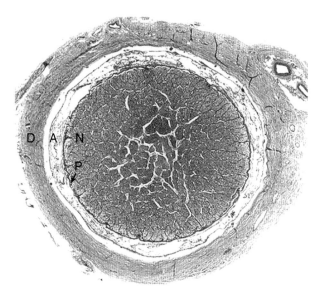

FIGURE 15.16 Optic nerve. A histologic cross section of the optic nerve (*N*) and surrounding leptomeninges, including the pia mater (*P*) and arachnoid (*A*) together with the enclosed cerebrospinal fluid-containing subarachnoid space. The leptomeninges and subarachnoid space are in turn covered by the densely fibrous dura mater (*D*), which, in this location, is often referred to as the optic nerve sheath. The dark red lines weaving through the optic nerve represent the fibrovascular pial septae (Modified from Mills SE. *Histology For Pathologists*. 3rd ed. Philadelphia, PA: Lippincott Williams & Wilkins; 2007.)

TABLE 15.1 Blood Supply to the Optic Nerve

Surface nerve fiber layer	Central retinal artery, cilioretinal artery (if present), small recurrent branches from long posterior ciliary arteries in some cases
Prelaminar optic nerve head	Centripetal branches from peripapillary choroidal arteries (not from choriocapillaris). Paroptic branches of short posterior ciliary arteries (SPCAs)
Lamina cribrosa	Centripetal branches from paroptic branches of short posterior ciliary arteries directly or through Circle of Zinn–Haller
Retrolaminar nerve	Centripetal branches of pial arteries (small branches) to periphery of nerve. Occasionally branches from central retinal artery to core of nerve
Intraconal nerve	CRA (axial), pia, recurrent branches of the SPCAs (paraxial)
Intracanalicular	Ophthalmic artery, small branches from CRA, pia
Intracranial and chiasm	Dorsal: Anterior cerebral artery, anterior communicating artery, branches of the internal carotid artery, superior hypophyseal artery Ventral: Posterior cerebral artery, posterior communicating artery, basilar artery
Lateral geniculate nucleus	Anterior choroidal artery, posterior choroidal artery
Optic tracts	Anterior choroidal artery, middle cerebral artery
Visual cortex	Posterior cerebral artery

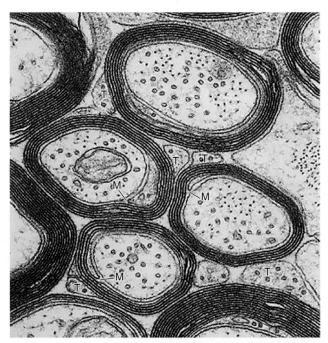

FIGURE 15.15 Myelinated sheaths (*M*) of optic nerve fibers, including outer tongue processes of oligodendrocytes (*T*), cut in cross section. (Courtesy of Dr. Alan Peters. In: Bear MF, Connors BW, Paradiso MA. *Neuroscience*. 4th ed. Philadelphia, PA: Wolters Kluwer; 2015.)

◉ Blood Supply to the Optic Nerve

The central retinal artery (CRA) pierces the meningeal covering of the optic nerve from below ~7 mm posterior to the globe. The artery passes to the center of the nerve, accompanied by its corresponding central retinal vein, to reach the superficial nerve fiber layer of the optic nerve head. Here the CRA and vein divide into smaller vessels supplying each retinal quadrant, which ramify in the nerve fiber layer of the retina. Despite its central position, the CRA does not contribute significantly to the blood supply to the nerve head itself, except for the superficial nerve fiber layer (Fig. 15.17).

The blood supplies for the various portions of the optic nerve and the visual pathway are summarized in Table 15.1. The main blood supply to the optic nerve head is provided by branches of the posterior ciliary arteries that arise from the ophthalmic artery. The posterior ciliary arteries give rise, in turn, to 10 to 20 paraoptic short posterior ciliary arteries that pierce the sclera in a partial ring around the exit point of the optic nerve.[20] In most cases, these paraoptic short posterior ciliary arteries anastomose to create a circumferential vascular bed within the peripapillary sclera, surrounding the laminar region of the optic nerve head.[21] When present, this anastomotic ring is termed the Circle of Zinn–Haller (Fig. 15.18). This "circle" is only partially complete in up to 55% of patients and is therefore a less

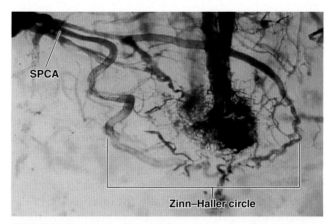

FIGURE 15.18   Circle of Zinn–Haller. Polymer cast of two short posterior ciliary arteries (SPCAs) forming the arterial circle of Zinn–Haller. SPCA, short posterior ciliary arteries. (Modified from Ramírez JM, Ramírez AI, Salazar JJ, et al. Triviño, Anatomofisiología de la úvea posterior: coroides. In: Monés J, Gómez-Ulla F, eds. *Degeneración macular asociada a la edad.* Barcelona: Prous Science; 2005:128.)

reliable source of collateral flow around the circumference of the optic nerve than its name would imply.[20]

THE SUPERFICIAL NERVE FIBER LAYER

The superficial nerve fiber layer of the optic nerve head is supplied by branches from the CRA. However, anatomic variants have been reported in which the temporal portion of the superficial nerve fiber layer may be additionally supplied by vessels originating from the short posterior ciliary arteries. In such cases, the short posterior ciliary arteries extend anteriorly from the prelaminar portion of the optic nerve head. It is also reported that in patients exhibiting a cilioretinal artery, this vessel may contribute to the blood supply of the temporal aspect of the superficial nerve fiber layer.

THE PRELAMINAR REGION

Most sources report that the prelaminar portion of the optic nerve head is served by small centripetal branches entering the optic nerve from the adjacent peripapillary choroid but not from the choriocapillaris. However, there is not unanimity on this point.[21–25] Where there is unanimity is in agreement that the CRA does not contribute to the blood supply of this portion of the optic nerve head (Fig. 15.17).

THE LAMINAR REGION

The laminar region of the optic nerve head is served by centripetal branches of the short posterior ciliary arteries, either directly or via the Circle of Zinn–Haller (Figs. 15.17 and 15.18).

THE RETROLAMINAR REGION

Finally, the retrolaminar region and the portion of the optic nerve extending posteriorly to the exit point of the central retinal vessel often have a dual blood supply. One

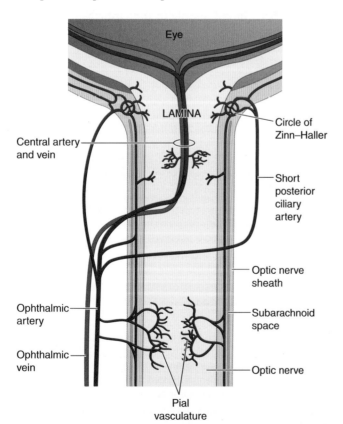

FIGURE 15.17   Blood supply to the intraocular and intraorbital optic nerve. Note three sources: choroidal feeder vessels, short posterior ciliary arteries, and the pial arterial network. (From Sadun AA. Anatomy and physiology. In: Yanoff M, Duker JS, eds. *Ophthalmology.* 2nd ed. St Louis: Mosby; 2004.)

Optic disc drusen are extra-axonal deposits of glycoasminoglycans that accumulate within the optic nerve head and can calcify over time. They are believed to arise from the remnants of RGCs that have degenerated during the process of optic nerve development. Optic disc drusen have a typical hard, mulberry appearance in adults (Fig. 15.19, A) but are often not visible in the optic disc of children, where they are buried deep within the nerve tissue. Instead, the optic disc just appears swollen (as with papilledema). With time, the drusen calcify, enlarge, and the overlying nerve fiber layer thins, revealing the classical appearance. A helpful method to confirm the diagnosis of optic disc drusen or to identify these lesions in the optic nerve head of children is to perform autofluorescence imaging (or occasionally ultrasound) (Fig. 15.19).[26,27]

 Anterior ischemic optic neuropathy (AION) is a common cause of vision loss in older age groups. It is characterized by optic disc swelling, often associated with flame-shaped (striate) hemorrhages, cotton-wool spots, and exudates (Fig. 15.20). AION is an ischemic process affecting the circulation of the optic nerve as it exits from the eye where the blood supply is more tenuous. It can be nonarteritic or arteritic in nature, the latter often being caused by giant cell arteritis. Patients with a small C/D ratio or no cup appear to have an anatomic predisposition to the nonarteritic form of the disease ("disc-at-risk").

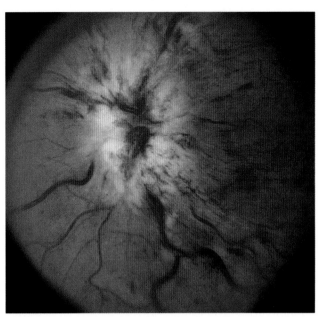

FIGURE 15.20 Anterior ischemic optic neuropathy. Clinically the optic nerve head appears swollen and hemorrhagic due to impaired axoplasmic flow from the ischemic injury. The large retinal veins are engorged due to impaired venous return through the swollen nerve head.

set of vessels arises from the surrounding pia mater and is carried centripetally within the pial septae. As the CRA passes anteriorly, it sometimes provides small centrifugal branches to the central core of the nerve (Fig. 15.17).

THE ORBITAL PORTION OF THE OPTIC NERVE

The orbital portion of the nerve receives its blood supply primarily from small branching arterioles of the pial

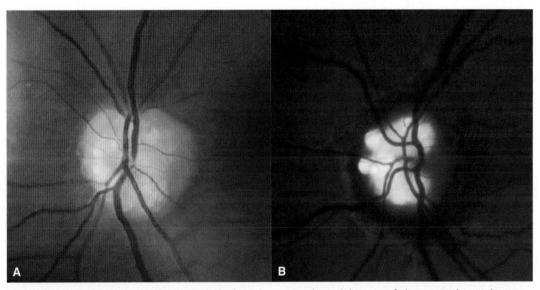

FIGURE 15.19 **A:** Optic disc drusen are mulberry-shaped, often glistening spherical deposits of glycosaminglycans that accumulate within the optic nerve head, and calcify over time. The drusen can simulate papilledema in children in whom they are less apparent than in this typical image from an adult. **B:** Optic disc drusen (in a different patient) are brightly autofluorescent and are easily identified using optical coherence tomography imaging.

plexus surrounding the nerve. These are derived from the ophthalmic artery and recurrent branches of the short posterior ciliary arteries and termed the paraxial circulation (**Fig. 15.17**). These vessels penetrate the nerve with the pial septae that provide structural support for the axons in the nerve. In addition, as the CRA passes through the center of the nerve, it provides small centrifugal branches as do the central collateral arteries which arise before the CRA pierces the nerve substance. This is referred to as the axial circulation. As noted earlier, however, most of the blood supply to the orbital portion of the nerve comes from pial branches forming the paraxial circulation.

THE INTRACANALICULAR PORTION OF THE OPTIC NERVE AND BEYOND

The intracanalicular portion of the optic nerve is supplied by medial collateral, lateral collateral, and ventral branches arising from the ophthalmic artery. Occasionally, an additional contribution is received from retrograde inferior branches from the CRA. The pial network of vessels (the major blood supply to the orbital portion of the nerve) is perfused by these vessels but is more limited in this region. The superior hypophyseal artery, and anterior cerebral and communicating arteries, branches of the internal carotid artery, are the main blood supply to the intracranial portion of the optic nerve and the chiasm, with the optic tracts being fed by the anterior choroidal and posterior communicating arteries.

The vessels feeding the optic nerve are similar in structure and function to the CRA and arterioles. Their endothelial cells form tight junctions and provide a blood–brain barrier to the optic nerve as is provided for both the brain and the retina. They demonstrate auto-regulation and thus are able to maintain stable perfusion to the nerve head under conditions of varying intraocular and perfusion pressures. Venous return from the pial and choroidal circulations is through local pial vessels and the vortex veins, respectively.

◉ Retinotopic Organization of Axons at the Optic Nerve Head

Beginning in the retina and continuing throughout the entire visual pathway, fibers carrying information from given locations in visual space maintain a strict anatomic relationship with fibers from other locations. This is referred to as retinotopic organization. The fibers forming the optic nerve are topographically organized within the nerve fiber layer and the nerve itself. This distributional pattern is shown in **Figure 15.21**. As one example, the ganglion cell axons from the peripheral retina run deeper within the nerve fiber layer and enter the optic nerve closer to its edge than its center. The large number of fibers that constitute the papillomacular bundle occupy the temporal edge of the optic disc (**Fig. 15.21**).

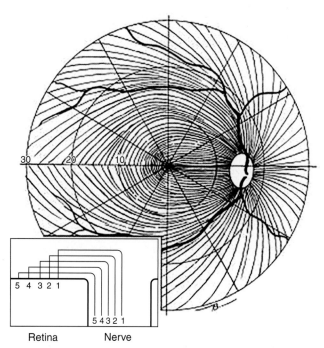

FIGURE 15.21 Distribution of retinal nerve fibers. Note arching of peripheral ganglion cell axons arching above and below the fibers running to the temporal side of the optic nerve head from the macular region (papillomacular bundle). *Inset* depicts cross-sectional arrangement of axons, with fibers originating from peripheral retina running closer to the choroid in the retina and then closer to the outside of the optic nerve, while fibers originating nearer to the nerve head are situated closer to the vitreous and occupy a more central portion of the nerve. (From Allingham RR, Damji KF, Freedman SF, et al. *Shields Textbook of Glaucoma*. 6th ed. Philadelphia, PA: Wolters Kluwer; 2010.)

This organizational architecture is preserved in the bundles of axons as they pass through the scleral canal. Thus, the visual field defects caused by damage at the optic nerve head (such as is seen in glaucoma) generally reflect the distribution of the atrophic nerve fibers and most commonly respect the horizontal raphe. The retinotopic packing of fibers becomes progressively reorganized into a different but consistent pattern as they track posteriorly within the orbital section of the nerve (**Fig. 15.22A**). The nerve fibers from the portion of the retina nasal to the fovea cross the midline to the opposite side of the brain at the optic chiasm, whereas the fibers from the portion of the retina temporal to the fovea do not cross the midline (**Fig. 15.22B**). This reorganization and separation of the ganglion cell axons into nasal and temporal groups, as they approach the chiasm is termed decussation and helps to distinguish disorders affecting the optic chiasm and posterior optic radiations in the brain. The result is that posterior to the chiasm rather than producing arcuate defects in the visual field that respect the horizontal raphe, vision loss generally produces defects that respect the vertical meridian, passing through the fovea, and separating the nasal and temporal hemifields (these are described in more detail below).

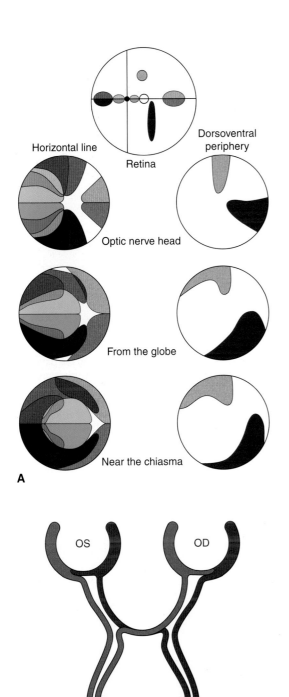

Overview of Visual Pathways Distal to the Optic Nerves

The intracranial portion of the optic nerve extends posteriorly from the optic canal approximately 15 mm to reach the optic chiasm above the cavernous sinus and overlying the pituitary fossa (sella turcica) (**Fig. 15.23**). Lateral to the chiasm on each side are the right and left internal carotid arteries as they emerge from the roof of the cavernous sinus and give off the ophthalmic artery and then the anterior cerebral artery on each side. Alteration of all of these, including the infundibulum of the pituitary gland, can produce predictable patterns of visual field loss because of the consistency of retinotopic projection within each part of the visual pathway.

As noted above, when the ganglion cell axons pass through the chiasm, fibers from the temporal retina pass ipsilaterally into the optic tract, whereas fibers from the nasal retina cross over to the contralateral side (**Fig. 15.22B**). The percentage of fibers that decussate is slightly greater than that remaining ipsilateral in the chiasm (53% to 47%). Importantly, there is no synapse at this location. RGC axons, whether decussating or not, continue uninterrupted to their synapses in the lateral geniculate nucleus of the thalamus. The generally accepted organization of RGC fibers in the chiasm is that the inferior and superior RGC fibers retain their inferior or superior organization, respectively; however, the inferonasal fibers pass more anteriorly in the chiasm whereas the superonasal fibers pass more posteriorly in the chiasm. As the inferior nasal fibers decussate to reach the contralateral optic tract, some first bow forward into the optic nerve on that side ("anterior knee of Wilbrand"). Previously it was thought that it was the presence of these knees of Wilbrand that give rise to the visual field defect known as a "junctional scotoma." Junctional scotomas are seen in some compressive lesions that affect the contralateral superotemporal hemifield and the ipsilateral central macula (macular scotoma). However, some more recent evidence suggests that Wilbrand's knee is an artifact of fixation.[28]

The Lateral Geniculate Nucleus

The visual information gathered and initially processed by the retinal neurons is secondarily processed through synaptic connections between the ganglion cell axons and the six neural layers of the lateral geniculate nucleus of the thalamus. This is the principal synaptic connection prior to reaching the primary visual cortex in the occipital lobe. Like the optic nerves and optic tracts, the lateral geniculate nucleus is retinotopically organized and is comprised of six layers (**Fig. 15.24**). The inferior layers, 1 and 2, are made up of large (magnocellular) cells. These magnocellular layers receive

FIGURE 15.22 **A:** Figures show preservation of retinotopic organization of retinal areas, with the location of the fibers representing these respective areas in the optic nerve head, posterior to the globe and near the optic chiasm (adult monkey optic nerve). The foveal region is at the intersection of the vertical and horizontal lines in the upper illustration of the retina. Foveal and perifoveal fibers initially occupy the lateral part of the nerve, but close to the chiasm these fibers come to be positioned more centrally. (From Naito J. Retinogeniculate projection fibers in the monkey optic nerve: a demonstration of the fiber pathways by retrograde axonal transport of WGA-HRP. *J Comp Neurol.* 1989;284:174–186.) **B:** Sketch of optic nerve fiber pathway from nasal and temporal hemiretina of right (*OD*) and left (*OS*) eye and decussation of fibers from nasal half of each retina at optic chiasm, en route to the lateral geniculate nucleus (LGN). (Modified from Chern KC, Saidel MA, eds. *Ophthalmology Review Manual.* 2nd ed. Philadelphia, PA: Wolters Kluwer; 2011.)

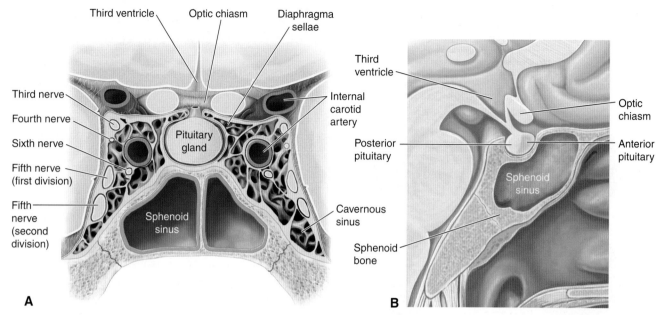

FIGURE 15.23   Coronal (**A**) and median (**B**) views of the normal anatomy in the region near the sella turcica surrounding the pituitary gland. The inferior nasal fibers of the optic nerve pass though the chiasm anteriorly and inferiorly and thus, are at greatest risk from expanding pituitary lesions arising from the pituitary fossa below the chiasm. Conversely, aneurysms of the internal carotids cause lateral compression of the optic nerves or chiasm. Temporal lesions would preferentially compress the uncrossed fibers from the temporal retinal hemifields. (From Di Ieva A, Rotondo F, Syro LV, et al. Aggressive pituitary adenomas—diagnosis and emerging treatments. *Nat Rev Endocrinol.* 2014;10:423–435.)

input from the parasol RGCs and comprise the ganglion cell "M-pathway." The M-pathway RGCs convey visual information from the rod photoreceptors about movement, depth, and small changes in brightness. These inputs are rapid and transient from the W- and Y-type ganglion cells (see **CHAPTER 14: THE NEUROSENSORY RETINA**).[29]

The overlying layers, 3, 4, 5, and 6, are made up of small (parvocellular) cells, which receive input from the midget RGCs and comprise the "P-pathway" (**Fig. 15.25A**). The P-pathway RGCs convey visual information from the red and green cone photoreceptors and convey visual information about color and fine visual discrimination. Its input is from the X-type ganglion cells and is slow and sustained. Beneath each M and P layer are small interlaminar cells, which form the koniocellular layers. The koniocellular layers receive their inputs from bistratified ganglion cells, the "K-pathway." The K-pathway RGCs primarily convey visual information from short wavelength "blue" cones. Continuing the retinotopic organization of the visual pathway, LGN layers 1, 4, and 6 receive their inputs from the contralateral retina, and layers 2, 3, and 5 receive inputs from the ipsilateral retina (**Fig. 15.25A**).[29]

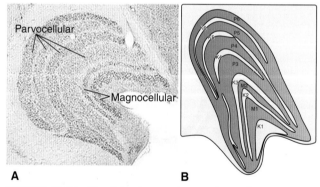

FIGURE 15.24   The lateral geniculate nucleus of the thalamus is retinotopically organized and is comprised of six layers. **A:** The inferior layers, 1 and 2 (*red*), are made up of large (magnocellular) cells that receive input from the parasol retinal ganglion cells. The overlying layers, 3, 4, 5, and 6 (*blue*), are made up of small (parvocellular) cells, which receive input from the midget retinal ganglion cells. (From Wagner T, Kline D. The sensorineural basis of color experience. University of Calgary, The Bases of Color Vision website. http://psych.ucalgary.ca/PACE/VA-Lab/Brian/neuralbases .htm. Accessed October 20, 2016.) **B:** Beneath each cellular layer (M1, M2, P3–P6), there are interlaminar cells of the koniocellular layers (K1–K6). These layers receive their input from bistratified ganglion cells that convey visual information from short wavelength "blue" cones. (From Pancrat. Lateral Geniculate Nucleus. Wikimedia Commons website. https://commons.wikimedia.org/wiki/File:Cgl_Nissl2 .svg. December 28, 2011. Accessed October 20, 2016.)

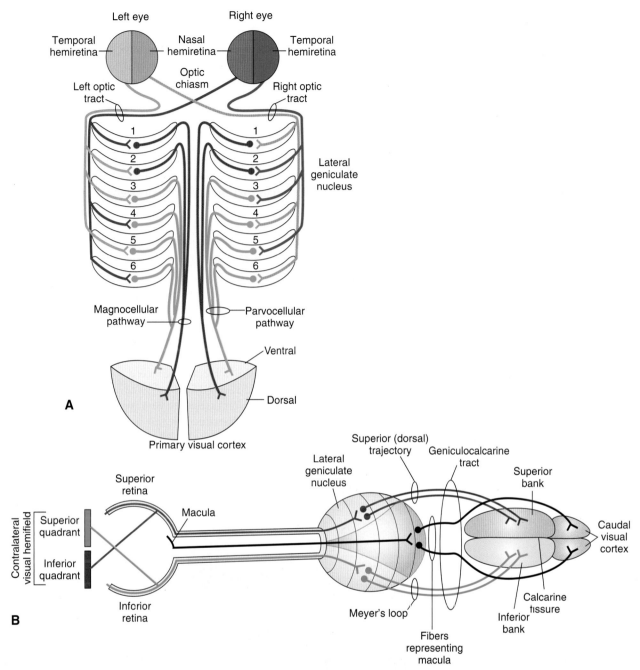

FIGURE 15.25 Course of axons from the nasal and temporal hemiretinae. **A:** On each side, the axons from the temporal hemiretinae remain ipsilateral in the optic tract and synapse in layers 2, 3, and 5 of the lateral geniculate nucleus. The axons from the nasal hemiretinae cross to the contralateral optic tract at the chiasm and synapse in layers 1, 4, and 6. The postsynaptic axons emerging from the lateral geniculate nucleus on each side project to the primary visual cortex. **B:** The axons from the superior retina and inferior retina project to the lateral geniculate nuclei. The postsynaptic neurons in the lateral geniculate nuclei receiving inputs from the inferior retinas form Meyer's loop through the cortex and project to the inferior bank of the calcarine fissure in the occipital lobe. The postsynaptic neurons in the lateral geniculate nuclei, receiving inputs from the superior retinas, form the superior trajectory and synapse on neurons in the superior bank of the calcarine fissure. The fibers conveying visual information from the macula synapse in the central regions of the lateral geniculate nucleus, and axons from the postsynaptic neurons in the lateral geniculate nucleus, project to the caudal pole of the occipital cortex. (Modified from Siegel A, Sapru HN. *Essential Neuroscience.* 3rd ed. Philadelphia, PA: Wolters Kluwer; 2014.)

Additional Neural Connections

A second major neural connection between the retina and the brain is faciliated by ganglion cell axons that project to the superior colliculus in the dorsal midbrain, a lamellar structure which is also retinotopically organized. The superior colliculus coordinates retinal and cortical control of ocular saccades and ocular fixation. Additional fibers to midbrain nuclei stabilize the retinal image during movement.

Bilateral (afferent) input from RGCs is also received by the pretectal nuclei in the midbrain. They are responsible for pupillary function and responses. Fibers from each nucleus project both ipsilaterally and contralaterally to the Edinger–Westphal nuclei of the third nerve nuclei. Parasympathetic axons return along the third nerve to the ciliary ganglion in the orbit, where they synapse. Postsynaptic parasympathetic fibers continue forward to reach the pupillary constrictor muscle, completing the pupillary light reflex. The bilateral projections from the retina to the pretectal nuclei and the Edinger–Westphal nuclei will normally induce equal constriction of both pupils in response to light stimulation. However, if the afferent pupillary input between the two optic nerves is substantially different, due to difference in the number of functional optic nerve axons, then the patient may manifest a relative afferent pupillary defect (also called a Marcus Gunn pupil) in which the pupillary constriction in response to light is asymmetric and there is paradoxical dilatation of the iris of the affected eye in response to light after the iris of the fellow (normal) eye is constricted.

Finally, a small number of optic nerve axons also pass via the retinohypothalamic tract to the suprachiasmatic nuclei and the paraventricular nucleus. These fibers participate in circadian rhythms and control of the sleep–wake cycle. A population of intrinsically photosensitive RGCs has also been identified, that utilize melanopsin as a photopigment. These cells project to the subthalamic nuclei and mediate circadian rhythm and pupillary light responses.[30,31]

The Optic Radiations and Occipital Cortex

After the RGCs synapse in the lateral geniculate nucleus of the thalamus, postsynaptic nerve fibers split into superior and inferior tracts and travel along the "optic radiations" in the parietal and temporal lobes of the brain to reach the striate "visual" cortex in the occipital lobes. The occipital cortex is located adjacent to the calcarine fissure (**Figs. 15.25B** and **15.26**). The upper and lower divisions of the postsynaptic nerve fibers are comprised of neuronal inputs from the superior and inferior retinal quadrants, respectively. Fibers projecting from the superior retina

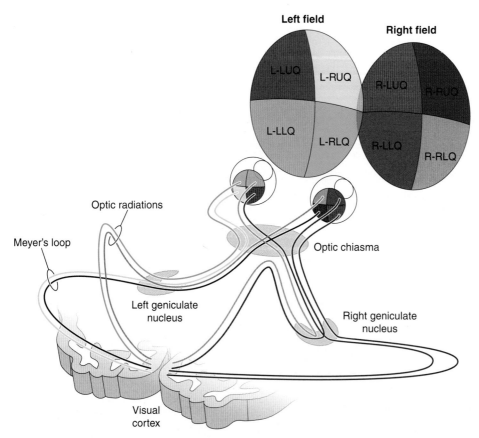

FIGURE 15.26 Retinotopic organization of the optic nerve, chiasm, and optic radiations. The impact of lesions at various sites in the course of the optic nerve and tracts from the eye to the brain depends upon where these fibers originate in the retina (and lateral geniculate nucleus [LGN]) and determine their impact upon visual perception. Color-coded diagram shows projections of quadrants in visual space onto the retina and posteriorly, through the optic nerve, chiasm, optic tracts, LGN. From the thalamus, cortical projections via Meyer's loop or the optic radiations can be followed to the visual cortex in the occipital lobe. (From Ratznium. Optic Cabling/Radiation. Wikimedia Commons website. https://commons.wikimedia.org/wiki/File:ERP_-_optic_cabling.jpg. September 12, 2015. Accessed October 20, 2016.)

travel more or less directly through the parietal lobe, along the internal capsule, to reach the superior portion of the occipital cortex, the cuneus (i.e., optic radiations) (**Fig. 15.26**). Conversely, fibers projecting from the inferior retina (Meyer's loop) track anteriorly after leaving the lateral geniculate nucleus and loop around the inferior horn of the lateral ventricle, passing through the temporal lobe, to synapse in the lingual gyrus, along the calcarine fissure (**Figs. 15.25B** and **15.26**).

There is a significant degree of topographical correlation between the visual input from the retina and its projections in the occipital cortex. These "retinotopic" maps are roughly correlated with the location of the visual input and the neuronal structure and organization of the retina (**Fig. 15.26**). The critical visual input from the fovea, which has a 1:1 neuronal input to the midget RGCs, provides the greatest degree of visual discrimination in the retina and is represented by a large area of the striate cortex. The peripheral visual field is perceived by the remaining anterior portion of the occipital cortex.

Functional Correlates of Injuries to the Optic Nerve and Radiations

Lesions affecting specific regions of the optic nerve, chiasm, and optic radiations present with characteristic visual field defects that mirror the topographical organization and retinotopic projections of the nerve fibers bringing vision from the retina to the brain (**Fig. 15.27**). Compressive lesions to the optic nerve give rise to unilateral scotomas that range from small central defects to complete loss of vision in the eye. Central chiasmal lesions (e.g., pituitary tumors) give rise to bitemporal visual field defects due to the crossing of the fibers from the nasal hemiretina in this region. Lesions between the chiasm and lateral geniculate nucleus, and those occurring more posteriorly in the optic radiations give rise to more homonymous (symmetric) hemianopic field defects.

The upper and lower divisions of the postsynaptic nerve fibers correspond to inferior visual field and superior visual field quadrants, respectively; thus, lesions affecting these

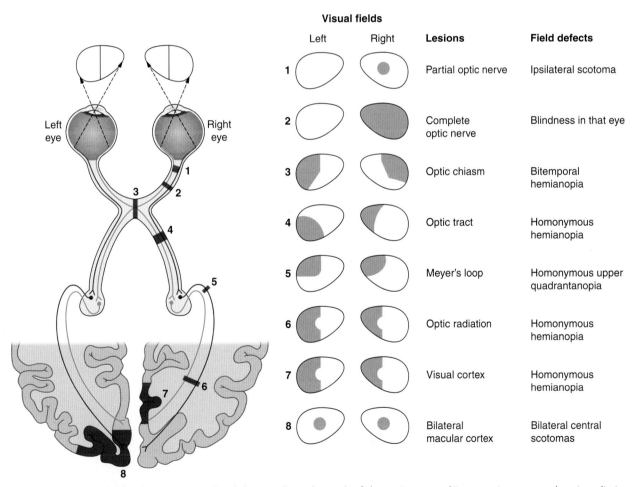

FIGURE 15.27 Visual field defects associated with lesions along the track of the optic nerve, chiasm, optic tracts, and optic radiations. Lesions anterior to the optic chiasm affect one eye. Lesions in the central chiasm affect the temporal hemifields of both eyes. Lesions posterior to the chiasm affect homonymous hemifields of both eyes, to a greater or lesser degree, with more posterior lesions being more congruent. Small occipital lesions can give rise to bilateral macular field defects. (Modified from Flood P, Rathtmell JP, Shafer S. *Stoelting's Pharmacology & Physiology in Anesthetic Practice.* 5th ed. Philadelphia, PA: Wolters Kluwer; 2014.)

tracts also present with characteristic visual field defects. Lesions affecting a single optic radiation (typically the inferior radiations via Meyer's loop which have a longer course in the brain), cause pie-shaped, superior quadrantanopic defects. Central sparing (the term used to describe preserved macular vision in the setting of visual pathway deficits like hemianopia) may occur in lesions that spare the central geniculocalcarine tract fibers (examples 6 and 7, **Fig. 15.27**).

REFERENCES

1. Harizman N, Oliviera C, Chang A, et al. The ISNT rule and differentiation of normal from glaucomatous eyes. *Arch Ophthalmol.* 2006;124:1579–1583.
2. Quigley HA, Brown AE, Morrison JD, et al. The size and shape of the optic disc in normal human eyes. *Arch Ophthalmol.* 1990;108:51–57.
3. Jonas JB. Clinical implications of peripapillary atrophy in glaucoma. *Curr Opin Ophthalmol.* 2005;16:84–88.
4. Jonas JB, Budde WM, Lang PJ. Parapapillary atrophy in the chronic open-angle glaucomas. *Graefes Arch Clin Exp Ophthalmol.* 1999;237:793–799.
5. Jonas JB, Nguyen XN, Gusek GC, et al. Parapapillary chorioretinal atrophy in normal and glaucoma eyes. I. Morphometric data. *Invest Ophthalmol Vis Sci.* 1989;30:908–918.
6. Jonas JB, Schmidt AM, Müller-Bergh JA, et al. Human optic nerve fiber count and optic disc size. *Invest Ophthalmol Vis Sci.* 1992;33:2012–2018.
7. Law SK, Choe R, Caprioli J. Optic disk characteristics before the occurrence of disk hemorrhage in glaucoma patients. *Am J Ophthalmol.* 2001;132:411–413.
8. Penfold PL, Madigan MC, Provis JM. Antibodies to human leucocyte antigens indicate subpopulations of microglia in human retina. *Vis Neurosci.* 1991;7:383–388.
9. Penfold PL, Provis JM, Liew SCK. Human retinal microglia express phenotypic characteristics in common with dendritic antigen-presenting cells. *J Neuroimmunol.* 1993;45:183–191.
10. Ye H, Hernandez MR. Heterogeneity of astrocytes in human optic nerve head. *J Comp Neurol.* 1995;362:441–452.
11. Skoff RP, Knapp PE, Bartlett WP. Astrocytic diversity in the optic nerve: a cytoarchitectural study. In: Fedoroff S, Vernadakis A, eds. *Astrocytes: Development, Morphology, and Regional Specialization of Astrocytes.* Vol. 1. Orlando: Academic Press; 1986:269.
12. Quigley HA, Addicks EM. Regional differences in the structure of the lamina cribrosa and their relation to glaucomatous optic nerve damage. *Arch Ophthalmol.* 1981;99:137–143.
13. Rehnberg M, Ammitzboll T, Tengroth B. Collagen distribution in the lamina cribrosa and the trabecular meshwork of the human eye. *Br J Ophthalmol.* 1987;71(12):886–892.
14. Rehnberg M, Ammitzböll T, Tengroth B. Ultrastructural immunocytochemical analysis of elastin in the human lamina cribrosa. Changes in elastic fibers in primary open-angle glaucoma. *Invest Ophthalmol Vis Sci.* 1992;33:2891–2903.
15. Rada JA, Johnson JM. Sclera. In: Krachmer J, Mannis M, Holland E, eds. *Cornea.* St. Louis: CV Mosby; 2004.
16. Sandberg-Lall M, Hagg PO, Wahlstrom I, et al. Type XIII collagen is widely expressed in the adult and developing human eye and accentuated in the ciliary muscle, the optic nerve and the neural retina. *Exp Eye Res.* 2000;70:775–787.
17. Wessel H, Anderson S, Fitae D, et al. Type XII collagen contributes to diversities in human corneal and limbal extracellular matrices. *Invest Ophthalmol Vis Sci.* 1997;38:2408–2422.
18. Watson PG, Young RD. Scleral structure, Organisation and disease. A Review. *Exp Eye Res.* 2004;78:609–623.
19. Keeley F, Morin J, Vesely S. Characterization of collagen from normal human sclera. *Exp Eye Res.* 1984;39:533–542.
20. Hayreh SS. Blood flow in the optic nerve head and factors that may influence it. *Prog Retin Eye Res.* 2001;20:595–624.
21. Olver JM, Spalton DJ, McCartney ACE. Microvascular study of the retrolaminar optic nerve in man: the possible significance in anterior ischemic optic neuropathy. *Eye.* 1990;4:7–24.
22. Francois J, Neetens A. Vascularization of the optic pathway. III. Study of intra-orbital and intracranial optic nerve by serial sections. *Br J Ophthalmol.* 1956;40:45–52.
23. Zhao Y, Li FM. Microangioarchitecture of optic papilla. *Jpn J Ophthalmol.* 1987;31:147–159.
24. Cioffi GA, Van Buskirk EM. Microvasculature of the anterior optic nerve. *Surv Ophthalmol.* 1994;38 suppl:S107–S116.
25. Onda E, Cioffi GA, Bacon DR, et al. Microvasculature of the human optic nerve. *Am J Ophthalmol.* 1995;120:92–102.
26. Friedman AH, Henkind P, Gartner S. Drusen of the optic disc. A histopathological study. *Trans Ophthalmol Soc UK.* 1975;95:4–9.
27. Tso MO. Pathology and pathogenesis of drusen of the optic nerve-head. *Ophthalmology.* 1981;88:1066–1080.
28. Horton JC. Wilbrand's knee of the primate optic chiasm is an artifact of monocular enucleation. *Trans Am Ophthalmol Soc.* 1997;95:579–609.
29. Wärntges S, Michelson G. Detailed illustration of the visual field representation along the visual pathway to the primary visual cortex: a graphical summary. *Ophthalmic Res.* 2014;51:37–41.
30. Hartwick AT, Bramley JR, Yu J, et al. Light-evoked calcium responses of isolated melanopsin-expressing retinal ganglion cells. *J Neurosci.* 2007;27:13468–13480.
31. Matynia A, Nguyen E, Sun X, et al. Peripheral sensory neurons expressing melanopsin respond to light. *Front Neural Circuits.* 2016;10:60.

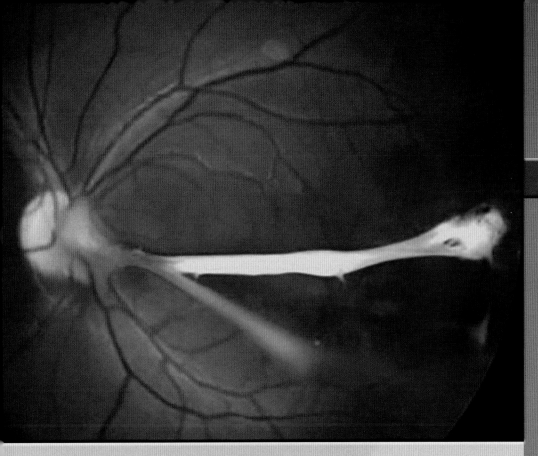

EMBRYOLOGY OF THE EYE AND ORBIT

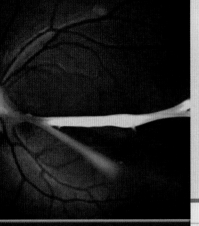

Embryology of the Eye and Orbit

CHAPTER 16

Overview

The embryologic development of the eye is by its very nature a highly ordered and complex process of tissue proliferation, differentiation, and organization. Though morphologically well characterized for over a century,[1,2] more recently we have begun to understand the molecular biology orchestrating these remarkable cellular processes and how genetic abnormalities may lead to many of the known congenital abnormalities seen in the eye. Although some of the molecular signaling that drives differentiation will be introduced in this chapter, our goal is not to present a comprehensive review of ocular embryology at the cellular and molecular level, or to provide a review of recent research on this topic. Rather, the purpose of this chapter is to give the reader an overview of the process of ocular differentiation and development at the tissue level, and in doing so to provide a foundation with which to understand the origins of the diverse spectrum of findings that present themselves in clinical practice. Mastering ocular development at the tissue level, however, is only a beginning. Because our knowledge of the molecular signaling pathways that drive these processes is rapidly changing, further reading of contemporary reviews will provide the reader with a better source for updated information than can be achieved in a textbook.[3,4]

The most critical period in ocular development is during the first trimester. It is during this period that perturbations of normal development have the most significant impact on ocular anatomy and function. This is the period in which the embryonic tissue types (neuroectoderm, surface ectoderm, neural crest cells and mesoderm) form the basic framework of the eye. By week 12, most of the structures of the eye and adnexa are recognizable. Therefore, this chapter is organized to first discuss development during weeks 1 to 12 in the context of the portions of each ocular tissue that are contributed by each of the respective embryonic tissue types. Further maturation of each formed ocular tissue, after the critical first 12 weeks, is then described.

Early Embryogenesis

By the second week of development, the human embryo is a bilaminar disc. The dorsal layer is referred to as the epiblast and the ventral layer (lying on the yolk sac) is the hypoblast. Epiblast cells proliferate in the dorsal midline, at the caudal end of the embryo, and form the primitive streak (which establishes the dorsal/ventral and right/left halves of the embryo [**Fig. 16.1A**]).[5] Appearance of the primitive streak marks the start of gastrulation and the formation of the three primary germ layers—the *ectoderm*, *mesoderm* and *endoderm*. As the primitive streak elongates by the addition of cells caudally, its cranial end thickens

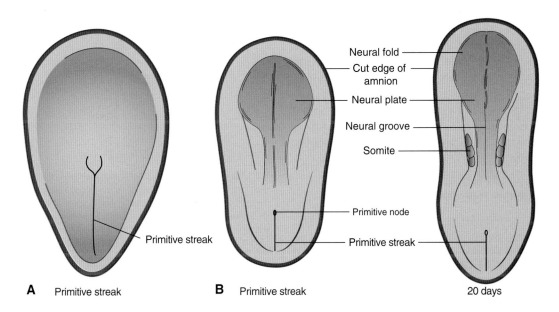

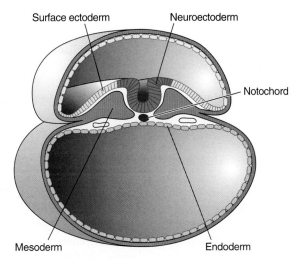

FIGURE 16.1 Early stages of gastrulation and neurulation in human embryogenesis. **A:** The primitive streak emerges as a groove at the caudal pole of the embryo, (dorsal view) with the primitive node at the cranial pole. **B:** Thickening of the ectoderm near the cranial pole forms the neural plate, whereas the primitive streak at the caudal end initiates gastrulation. By 20 days of gestation, the neural folds have elevated from the neural plate, and tips of the folds are closing. **C:** Cross-section of same embryo through the neural groove. Ectoderm in the area of the neural groove (*purple*) has differentiated into the neuroectoderm, whereas the remaining ectoderm on each side of the neural groove is the surface ectoderm overlying the mesoderm. (Redrawn and modified from Sadler TW. Embryology of neural tube development. *Am J Med Genet C Semin Med Genet*. 2005;135C:2–8 and Cook CS, Sulik KK, Wright KW. Embryology. In: Wright KW, ed. *Pediatric Ophthalmology and Strabismus*. St Louis: Mosby; 1995:3–43.)

to form the primitive node on day 19 (**Fig. 16.1B**). The primitive node serves to organize the embryonic axes cranially. Some epiblast cells migrate into the primitive streak and spread out between the epiblast and hypoblast creating a new middle layer, the mesoderm (**Fig. 16.1C**). Those mesodermal cells that migrate anteriorly along the midline, from the primitive node to the future mouth region (prochordal plate), will become the embryo's notochord. Other epiblast cells migrate inward and replace cells of the hypoblast, forming the endoderm. The epiblast cells that remain on the dorsal surface of the embryo form the ectoderm. Thus, the three major germ layers of the embryo, the ectoderm, mesoderm, and endoderm, are present by week 3.

The presence of the notochord induces the overlying surface ectoderm to form the neural tube via a process called neurulation (**Fig. 16.2**). In this process, the surface ectoderm overlying the notochord first thickens to form the neural plate, beginning just cranial to the primitive node. As the notochord elongates, the neural plate broadens and extends as far cranially as the prochordal plate. The ectoderm of the neural plate is referred to as the neuroectoderm to distinguish it from the remaining surface ectoderm.

FORMATION OF THE OPTIC SULCI

The primitive neural plate invaginates early in development. As invagination progresses, the neuroectoderm is pushed inward from the surface, forming the neural groove at around day 20 (**Fig. 16.2**, top/middle). As this occurs, the surface ectoderm that was originally lateral to the neuroectoderm is drawn toward the midline. The lateral walls of the neural groove (neural folds) then converge toward each other and fuse beginning in week 4. This fusion begins in the mid-region of the embryo and progresses anteriorly and posteriorly, creating the recognizable neural tube, the future central nervous system (CNS) of the developing embryo (**Fig. 16.2**, bottom). Failure of the neural tube to close posteriorly results in spina bifida. Failure of the neural tube to close anteriorly results in anencephaly.

At week 3 in neural development, there are three brain vesicles, the prosencephalon (forebrain), mesencephalon (midbrain), and rhombencephalon (hindbrain) (**Fig. 16.3**). Before final closure in the prosencephalon, two symmetric grooves appear in the neuroectoderm on each bank of the neural groove in this region. These are called the optic sulci (also optic grooves or pits). The optic sulci represent the first stage in development of the future eyes and they appear between days 21 and 22.[5,6] As such, the eye begins to form from the wall of the prosencephalon. By week 5, however, there are five brain vesicles, following subdivision of the prosencephalon into the telencephalon and diencephalon and the rhombencephalon into metencephalon and myencephalon. The portion of the

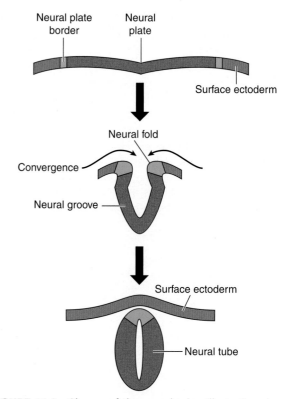

FIGURE 16.2 Closure of the neural tube. Illustration showing changes in the embryo during neurulation. The lateral edges of the neural folds come together and fuse at the dorsal midline. Progressive invagination of the neural groove forms the closed neural tube, which becomes the neuroectoderm. The remaining ectoderm on each side of the neural groove is termed the surface ectoderm. (Modified from Barkovich AJ, Raybaud C, eds. *Pediatric Neuroimaging*. 5th ed. Philadelphia, PA: Wolters Kluwer; 2011.)

prosencephalon to which the developing eye is attached thereafter is the diencephalon, near its junction with the telencephalon (**Fig. 16.3**).[6]

Upon closure of the neural tube, around day 24, its neuroectodermal wall separates from the overlying surface ectoderm (**Figs. 16.2** and **16.4**). The surface ectoderm then seals across the dorsal midline. With neural tube closure, a group of cells migrate from the neuroectoderm at the crest of the neural groove, into the underlying tissue mass (**Fig. 16.4**). These neural crest cells, named for their location of origin, transition from an epithelial to a migratory, mesenchymal cell type that initially resides just beneath the surface ectoderm, attached to the dorsal aspect of the closed neural tube. Ultimately, this central mass divides in the midline (**Fig. 16.4**).[7,8] In this way, the three major embryonic tissues from which the eye is derived are identified, the *neuroectoderm, surface ectoderm*, and the *neural crest cells*. An additional small but important contribution is also made by the *mesoderm*. The contributions of each of these embryonic tissues, through the first trimester of gestation, are discussed in succession below.

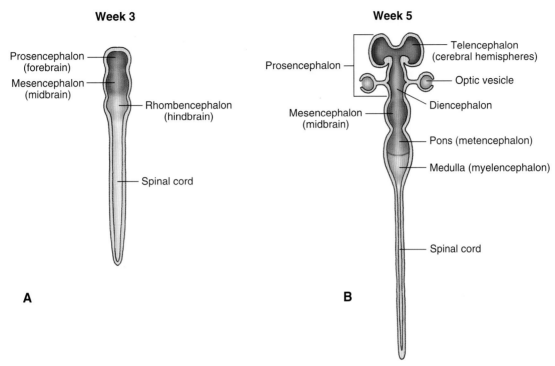

FIGURE 16.3 **A:** Three brain vesicles present at week 3 (prosencephalon, mesencephalon, and rhombencephalon). It is in the prosencephalon that the optic sulcus forms. **B:** Five brain vesicles present at week 5. The prosencephalon differentiates into the paired vesicles of the telencephalon and diencephalon. After this subdivision, it is to the wall of the diencephalon that the developing eye is attached. The mesencephalon forms the midbrain and the rhombencephalon (hindbrain) develops into the metencephalon (the pons and cerebellum) and the myelencephalon (the medulla oblongata and spinal cord). (Modified from Siegel A, Sapru HN. *Essential Neuroscience.* 3rd ed. Philadelphia, PA: Wolters Kluwer; 2014.)

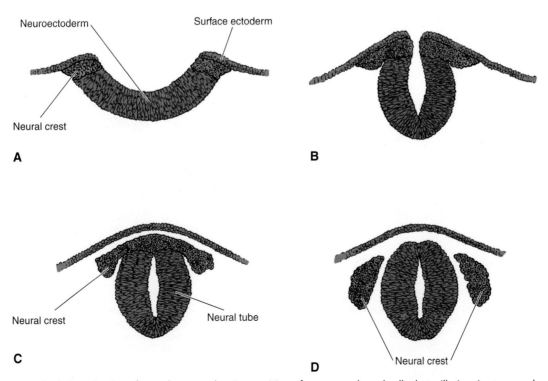

FIGURE 16.4 **A:** Early invagination of neural groove showing position of neuroectodermal cells that will give rise to neural crest mesenchyme. **B:** Position of future neural crest cells as the neural tube closes. **C:** Neural crest cells separate from the surface ectoderm at the dorsal (superior) margin of the closed neural tube. **D:** Separation of mesenchymal neural crest cells from the neural tube and subdivision into right and left. (Modified from Barkovich AJ. Congenital anomalies of the spine. In: Barkovich AJ, Raybaud C, eds. *Pediatric Neuroimaging.* 5th ed. Philadelphia, PA: Lippincott Williams & Wilkins; 2011:857–922.)

Early Development of Ocular Tissues from the Neuroectoderm

The tissues of the eye that arise from the neuroectoderm are shown in **Table 16.1**.

FORMATION OF THE OPTIC VESICLE AND OPTIC STALK

As the neuroectodermal optic sulci (grooves) lengthen laterally from the midline of the developing brain, the distal portions of these outpouchings expand to form hollow spheres, the optic vesicles, whereas the proximal portions constrict to form the optic stalks (**Fig. 16.5**).[9] The optic vesicle and optic stalk are each one cell layer in thickness. As the neuroectoderm is an epithelial tissue, its cells are polarized, having an apical and basal surface. It is important to appreciate that the apical surfaces of the cells lining the optic vesicle face inward and the outside of the vesicle are covered by the basement membrane of the neuroectoderm. The open space within the optic stalk maintains communication with the developing third ventricle of the brain. At this stage of ocular development, the eyes are laterally positioned in the head and ~180° apart. By 27 days, the optic vesicles reach the basal surface of the surface ectoderm and induce areas of focal proliferation and thickening on the sides of the head that are termed the lens placodes, which are discussed later (**Fig. 16.5**).[9,10]

TABLE 16.1 Derivatives of the Neuroectoderm

Retinal pigment epithelium
Neurosensory retina
Neuroglia of the optic nerve
Epithelia of the ciliary body and iris
Sphincter and dilator muscles of the iris
Secondary vitreous (discussed below with primary and tertiary vitreous)

 *Failure of the forebrain to develop normally or to divide into two hemispheres (and optic vesicles) causes major developmental defects of the eyes including anophthalmia, microphthalmia, and various forms of cyclopia (**Fig. 16.6**).[11] These conditions can occur in isolation, resulting from environmental and gestational causes. In a third of cases, however, they present as a feature of complex genetic syndromes that arise from chromosomal deletions, duplications, and translocations. Mutations in the transcription factor genes that direct ocular development have been identified as causing anophthalmia and microphthalmia, and are discussed briefly at the end of this chapter.*

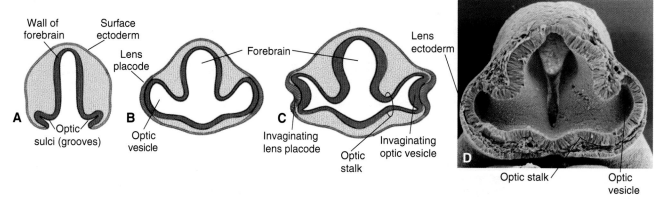

FIGURE 16.5 Schematic of formation of the optic grooves and conversion into optic vesicles and optic stalks. **A:** The optic grooves expand laterally, forming the optic vesicles distally and the optic stalks proximally. **B:** The vesicle reaches the basal surface of the surface ectoderm, which induces the formation of the lens placode. **C:** The lens placode and optic vesicle invaginate to begin formation of the lens and the optic cup, respectively. **D:** Scanning electron micrograph of coronal section through developing forebrain during the third week of gestation. ([A-C] From Sadler TW. *Langman's Medical Embryology.* 13th ed. Philadelphia, PA: Wolters Kluwer; 2014. [D] Courtesy of Dr. K. K. Sulik, Department of Cell Biology and Anatomy, University of North Carolina. From Sadler TW. *Langman's Medical Embryology.* 13th ed. Philadelphia, PA: Wolters Kluwer; 2014.)

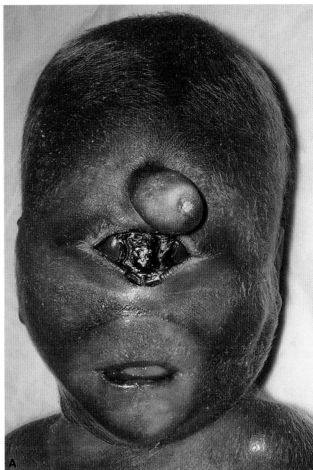

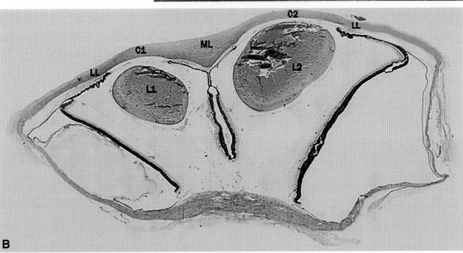

FIGURE 16.6   Holoprosencephaly, a spectrum of major developmental defects of the brain in which the embryonic forebrain fails to divide into right and left hemispheres, giving rise to midfacial developmental defects. **A:** Severe forms include cyclopia with midface proboscis, a single eye globe with varying degrees of doubling of intrinsic ocular structures (synophthalmia), and nasal agenesis with a proboscis above the midline eye. **B:** Light microscopic section through a cyclopic eye. Note how the specimen represents parts of a left and a right eye, fused along their medial walls. Two corneas (*C1, C2*) and two lenses (*L1, L2*) are evident, along with a fused medial limbus (ML), but with a lateral limbus (LL) on each side. There is corrugation of an incipient ciliary body with pigmentation only at the lateral aspects of the specimen, but no equivalent differentiation medially. ([A] from Sadler TW. *Langman's Medical Embryology.* 13th ed. Philadelphia, PA: Wolters Kluwer, 2014.)

FORMATION OF THE OPTIC CUP

Late in the fourth week of gestation, the optic vesicle begins a transformation that gives rise to the recognizable structures of the human eye. The spherical optic vesicle, formed by a single layer of neuroectodermal cells, invaginates to form the bilayered, hemispherical, optic cup. This process of invagination also includes the neuroectoderm of the optic stalk. Because the apical surfaces of all of these cells face inward, toward the center of the optic vesicle, this means that when the optic vesicle invaginates into a bilayered optic cup, the two cell layers of the hemispherical cup are brought into apposition at their apical surfaces on the inner wall of the cup (**Fig. 16.7**).[10,12] Apposition occurs earlier in the anterior portion of the cup than in the posterior portion. As the inner and outer layers of the optic cup come together in the posterior segment, fine ciliated attachments form between them. Notwithstanding these early connections, a potential space remains between the two layers thereafter and throughout life. This potential space becomes the plane of separation between the neurosensory retina and retinal pigment epithelium (RPE) in the various pathologic conditions that cause retinal detachment.

EARLY DEVELOPMENT OF THE INNER AND OUTER LAYERS OF THE OPTIC CUP

The inner and outer layers of the optic cup each make contributions to the retina, the ciliary body, and the iris. But the two layers of the cup give rise to distinct layers of these ocular tissues (**Fig. 16.8**).[12] The neuroectoderm of the inner layer of the invaginating cup differentiates into the various cell

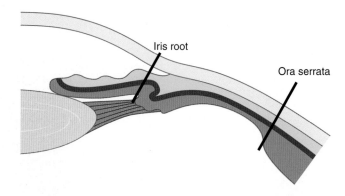

		Iris	Ciliary body	Retina
Outer layer		Anterior myoepithelium	Pigmented ciliary epithelium	Retinal pigment epithelium
Inner layer		Posterior pigmented epithelium	Non-pigmented ciliary epithelium	Neurosensory retina

FIGURE 16.8 Anatomic relationship between the adult tissue derivatives of the inner and outer layers of the optic cup. In the portion of the optic cup anterior to the ora serrata, the inner layer of the neuroectoderm gives rise to the nonpigmented ciliary epithelium that lines the inner surface of the ciliary body and the posterior pigmented epithelium lining the posterior surface of the iris. The outer layer of the cup, anterior to the ora serrata, gives rise to the pigmented ciliary epithelium and then, in turn, to the anterior myoepithelium of the iris. A bud from the putative anterior myoepithelium gives rise to the pupillary sphincter muscle early in the fourth month. Posterior to the ora serrata, the inner layer of the optic cup gives rise to the neurosensory retina and the outer layer gives rise to the retinal pigment epithelium. (Modified from Sadler TW. *Langman's Medical Embryology.* 12th ed. Philadelphia, PA: Wolters Kluwer; 2011.)

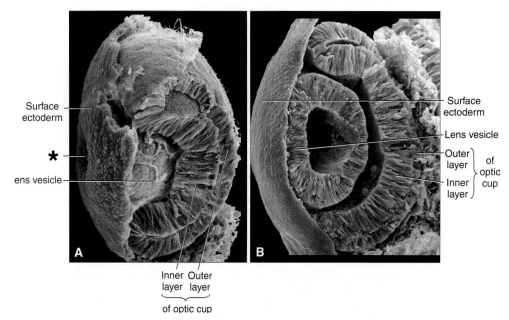

FIGURE 16.7 High-resolution scanning electron micrographs of the forming lens vesicle and optic cup. **A:** The lens vesicle and overlying lens pit (*asterisk*) have formed from the surface ectoderm. As the optic vesicle invaginates, the inner and outer layers of the optic cup are formed. The outer surface of the entire cup represents the basal surface of the neuroectodermal cells, whereas the apical surfaces of these cells face the cleft between the two layers. **B:** At this stage, the lens vesicle is completely detached from the surface ectoderm and will soon start to form lens fibers. The now resealed surface ectoderm will become the corneal epithelium. (From Sadler TW. *Langman's Medical Embryology.* 13th ed. Philadelphia, PA: Wolters Kluwer; 2014.)

types and cell layers of the neurosensory retina.[13] The axons of the ganglion cells that subsequently develop within the neurosensory retina will form the optic nerve. The neuroectoderm of the outer layer of the optic cup becomes the RPE. The anterior rim of the cup, where the inner and outer layers of the cup are continuous with one another, will become the pupillary margin (**Fig. 16.8**). The optic stalk provides a guide path for axons of the future retinal ganglion cells (RGCs) to form the optic nerve and the cells of the stalk also give rise the optic nerve-associated neuroglial elements.

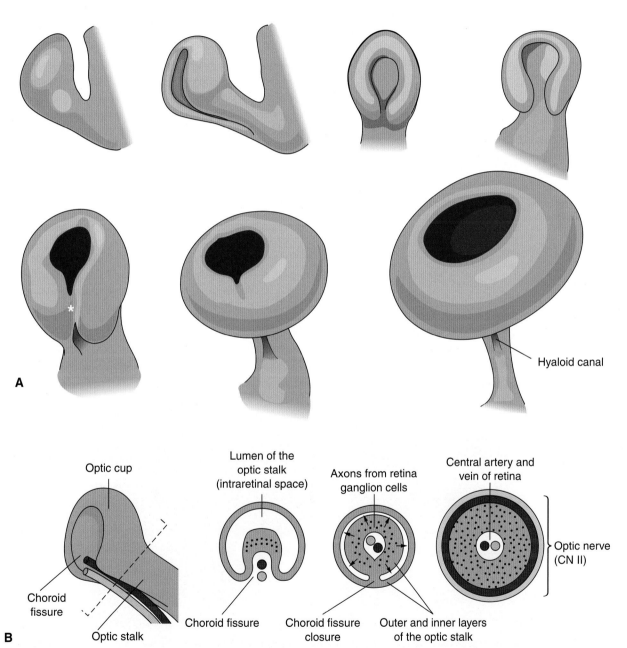

FIGURE 16.9 Formation of the optic cup and optic nerve from the optic stalk. **A:** Succession of images from top left to bottom right show progressive invagination of the optic cup and inferior location of the fetal (choroidal) fissure. Also shown is the process of closure of the fetal fissure in the optic cup and stalk, beginning at its midpoint (**asterisk, image, lower left**) and progressing both anteriorly and posteriorly from that point. **B:** The choroidal fissure, located on the undersurface of the optic stalk, permits access into the interior of the developing eye for the precursors of the hyaloid artery and vein. The choroidal fissure eventually closes to complete formation of the structural components of the optic nerve. As ganglion cells form in the retina, axons accumulate in the optic stalk, obliterating the lumen and forming the optic nerve. The embryologic legacy of the hyaloid artery and vein are the central retinal artery and vein. Closure of the fissure around the vessels explains the emergence of the central retinal artery and vein from the optic nerve head. ([A] modified from Development Stages in Human Embryos: Stage 18. The Endowment for Human Development website. https://www.ehd.org/developmental-stages/stage18.php. Accessed October 25, 2016. [B] modified from Dudek RW. *BRS Embryology.* 6th ed. Philadelphia, PA: Wolters Kluwer; 2014.)

Despite its name, the optic cup does not form a complete cup. As it invaginates, a cleft is present inferiorly (or inferomedially) that continues into the optic stalk (**Fig. 16.9A**). This cleft is termed the "choroidal," "embryonic," or "fetal" fissure. It is through this inferior cleft that the embryonic vasculature gains access to the interior of the developing eye (**Fig. 16.9B**). This transient set of arterial and venous vessels is the hyaloid vascular system. Late in the fifth week of gestation, the fetal fissure begins to close around this developing vasculature, thus enclosing these vessels within the cavity of the developing optic stalk and optic cup. Closure of the fetal fissure is usually complete by the end of the eighth week of gestation. The growth, distribution, and subsequent regression of this vascular system parallel the development of the vitreous.

The adult vestiges of the hyaloid artery and vein are the central retinal artery and central retinal vein. Closure of the fetal fissure in the region of the optic stalk accounts for the unique feature of the central retinal artery and vein emerging from the center of the optic nerve in the formed eye. Importantly, initial closure of the fetal fissure occurs at its midpoint, the approximate location of what will become the pars plicata region of the ciliary body. From this initiating point, the fissure closes in both anterior and posterior directions, just as occurred in closure of the neural tube.

The defining anatomic landmark of the ora serrata, the anterior termination of the neurosensory retina, is established early in the development of the inner layer of the optic cup and serves to distinguish the posterior segment

Incomplete or abnormal closure of the embryonic fissure gives rise to congenital abnormalities that are typically seen in the inferior or inferomedial portions of the affected tissues. These defects are referred to as colobomas, and they can affect any of the tissues to which the neuroectoderm contributes, including the retina, optic nerve, ciliary body, and iris (Fig. 16.10). These abnormalities can secondarily result in abnormalities of tissues whose development is guided by the neuroectoderm, such as the choroid and the lens.

There is a spectrum of natural variations when there is incomplete closure of the fetal fissure. These present as mild to major abnormalities of the affected tissues including the iris, ciliary body, optic nerve, and retina.[13,14] Among the most severe cases are those where fetal fissure closure has occurred only in the pars plicata region of the ciliary body and has not extended anteriorly or posteriorly from that point (Fig. 16.10A). In less severe cases, fetal fissure closure may be complete from the ciliary body back to the optic nerve, but a colobomatous defect remains in the inferior iris (Fig. 16.10B). The spectrum of fetal fissure closure defects in the posterior pole includes optic pits, morning glory syndrome, optic nerve colobomas, and combined optic nerve and retinal colobomas (Fig. 16.11). Severe fetal fissure closure defects in the posterior portion of the eye can preclude the establishment of an appropriate intraocular pressure. This deficiency in the internal pressure may contribute to impaired growth of the eye, a condition termed microphthalmia.

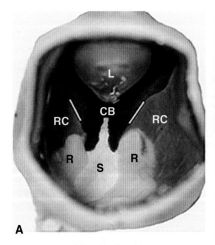

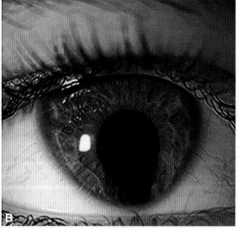

FIGURE 16.10 Colobomatous defects in the formation of anterior and posterior structures in the eye. **A:** View of a postmortem eye with superior calotte removed from an infant with numerous developmental defects including holoprosencephaly. Anterior portion of the eye is seen at the top of the image. Note inverted teardrop shape of the lens, rounded at the top and tapered inferiorly (L). The fetal fissure has fused only in the area of the developing pars plicata region of the ciliary body (CB). The developing pars plana region of the CB has not fused inferiorly, giving it the appearance of the posterior part of butterfly wings. The ora serrata is formed along the angled white lines. Immediately posterolateral to the two white lines there is relatively normal retina, including the RPE and underlying choroid (RC). Closer to the inferior midline, the retinal pigment epithelium (RPE) is not present and thus a choroid has not formed. This leaves just an abnormal sensory retina (R), overlying bare sclera (S). The optic nerve is not seen but was profoundly hypoplastic. RC, retina/choroid. **B:** Coloboma of the iris. ([B] from Iris Coloboma: Disfigured Eye Help. *Medcorp International Blog website.* http://medcorpint.com/blog /iris-coloboma/. Updated November 4, 2013. Accessed October 25, 2016.)

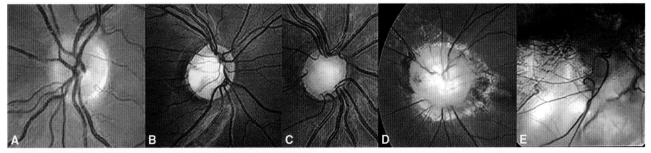

FIGURE 16.11   Clinical presentation of optic nerve variants and colobomas. **A:** Normal optic nerve. **B:** Optic nerve pit, usually temporal defect caused by imperfect closure of the superior edge of the embryonic fissure. **C:** Forme fruste colobomatous optic nerve defect with retinal vessels displaced to the margins of the optic nerve head. **D:** Typical appearance of a "morning glory" optic nerve and peripapillary retinal defect. **E:** Large coloboma of the optic nerve and retina. A large inferior defect in the formation of the retina and choroid is seen with an extensive area of bare sclera evident below the nerve.

of the eye from the anterior segment. Thus, further development of the layers of the optic cup that are anterior and posterior to this landmark are most easily interpreted when discussed separately.

Early Development of the Inner and Outer Layers of the Optic Cup Anterior to the Ora Serrata

During the third month of development, there is rapid growth of the anterior margin of the optic cup. Cells at this margin proliferate and the anterior rim of the optic cup begins to extend over the anterior surface of the developing lens. Evidence suggests that the presence of the lens is needed for normal development of the iris and ciliary body. (Lens development is discussed under Surface Ectodermal Derivatives.) As the anterior margin of the optic cup's neuroectoderm advances centrally, across the anterior surface of the lens, the outer layer of the optic cup in this region gives rise to the anterior myoepithelium of the iris and the inner layer of the optic cup gives rise to the posterior pigmented epithelium of the iris, both of which are pigmented.

Just anterior to the demarcation of the ora serrata, the inner layer of the optic cup's neuroectoderm gives rise to the nonpigmented ciliary epithelium that lines the inner surface of the ciliary body and continues anteriorly as the posterior pigmented epithelium lining the posterior surface of the iris. The outer layer of the optic cup gives rise to the pigmented ciliary epithelium and then, in turn, to the anterior myoepithelium of the iris. In this way, these two layers of epithelia, lining the ciliary body and iris, come to be arranged apex to apex in the adult iris and ciliary body. The anterior edge of the optic cup corresponds to the point of continuity between the anterior myoepithelium and the posterior pigmented epithelium of the iris, which coincides with the pupillary ruff (frill) in the formed eye (**Fig. 16.8**).

As the iris grows, a transient circumferential cleft appears between the two epithelial layers near the future pupillary margin (**Fig. 16.12**). This cleft, termed the "marginal sinus"

(also called the ring sinus of von Szily), disappears later in development. The sphincter pupillae muscle and dilator pupillae muscle are formed by the proliferation of the cell layer that will become the anterior myoepithelium of the iris. This myoepithelial layer differentiates from the outer layer of the optic cup. The sphincter pupillae muscle arises as buds of tissue from the putative antereior myoepithelium. Hence, the sphincter and dilator muscles of the iris are the only muscles in the human body that are derived from the neuroectoderm.[15] The differentiation of the sphincter and dilator muscles occurs later in development and is discussed below.

The rapid growth of the anterior margin of the optic cup additionally gives rise to ridges and folding of the neuroectodermal layers anterior to the ora serrata but posterolateral to the developing iris. This convoluted folding progresses to form ~75 radial folds and meridional ridges that increase in complexity and eventually become the

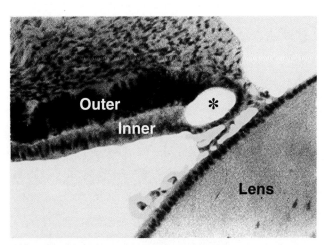

FIGURE 16.12   As the anterior margin of the optic cup neuroectoderm advances forward, across the anterior surface of the lens, it forms two distinct columnar epithelial layers, the anterior myoepithelium (*outer*) and the posterior pigmented epithelium (*inner*). As the iris grows, a transient circumferential cleft appears between these layers at the future pupillary margin, the "marginal sinus" (also called the ring sinus of von Szily—*asterisk*). (From Barber AN. *Embryology of the Human Eye.* St. Louis, MO: C.V. Mosby; 1955:136.)

epithelial layers covering the ciliary processes of the pars plicata region of the ciliary body. It is not until the fifth month that elongation of the ciliary body creates the region of the pars plana. The inner of the two epithelial layers, covering the inner surfaces of the pars plicata and pars plana, does not develop pigmentation. This layer becomes the nonpigmented ciliary epithelium, which is continuous with the neurosensory retina at the ora serrata. The outer of these two neuroectodermal layers does develop melanin pigment. It becomes the pigmented ciliary epithelium, which is continuous with the RPE at the ora serrata (**Fig. 16.8**). Although the RPE is the first epithelium in the body to be pigmented (during week 5), the posterior iris epithelium does not begin acquiring pigment until the 5th month of gestation, beginning at the pupillary margin and progressing toward the ciliary body.

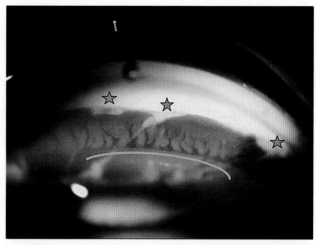

FIGURE 16.14 Goniophotograph of aniridia. If the rim of the optic cup does not migrate over the anterior surface of the lens, the iris does not form. In this case, the iris is represented by three residual pieces of tan tissue (*stars*), one of which extends a fine filamentous connection toward the lens. In this image, the lens and ciliary processes are clearly seen through the cornea because the iris is missing. The edge of the lens is highlighted (*yellow line*).

Iris anomalies: Cysts may develop at the pupillary margin in children prescribed miotics (e.g., pilocarpine) for the management of certain binocular vision problems. These cysts arise in the same location and in the same tissue plane as the marginal sinus (Fig. 16.13A).[16] Congenital malformations, such as the cystic elevation of the peripheral iris shown in Figure 16.13B, can also arise from defective axial migration of the neural crest cells and excessive atrophy of peripheral iris vascular arcades, causing separation between the iris stroma and neuroectodermally derived iris epithelia.[17–20]

If the rim of the optic cup does not proliferate and push forward over the anterior surface of the lens, the iris does not form, except for some residual tissue at the edge of the optic cup. This developmental anomaly is termed aniridia (Fig. 16.14). Aniridia is typically associated with severe iris hypoplasia, often with foveal hypoplasia and nystagmus.[21] It also has an important clinical association with Wilm's tumor (nephroblastoma) in a subset of patients.

Early Development of the Inner and Outer Layers of the Optic Cup Posterior to the Ora Serrata

The Inner Layer of the Optic Cup Posterior to the Ora Serrata

The cells of the inner neuroectodermal layer initially proliferate to form a thick layer of primitive "neuroblastic" cells (**Fig. 16.15**). The differentiation of the retinal neuroblasts (retinal stem cells) into different neuronal cell types, located at specific levels of the laminated retinal architecture, is a highly ordered, sequential, and well-described process at both the cellular and, more recently, the molecular level. The inner layer of the optic cup differentiates into the various cell types and cell layers of the neurosensory retina, and the axons of the RGCs that subsequently develop within

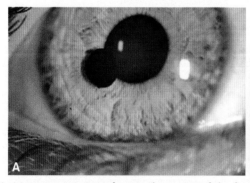
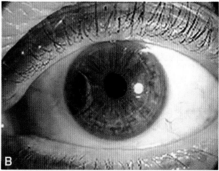

FIGURE 16.13 A: Iris cysts sometimes form in the region of the former marginal sinus following treatment with miotics. **B:** Failure of proper neural crest invasion and excessive atrophy of the peripheral vascular arcades causes separation between the neuroectodermal posterior epithelial layers of the iris and the neural crest-derived stromal component. This resulted in the formation of an atrophic cyst of the peripheral iris (9 o'clock). ([B] courtesy of Dr. William Morris, Hamilton Eye Institute, Memphis, TN.)

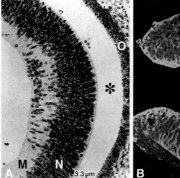
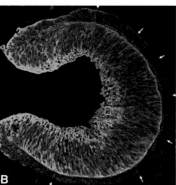

FIGURE 16.15 Formation of the optic cup. **A:** Light microscopic section showing early stage of retinal development. The inner layer of the optic cup is divided into a nuclear layer of neuroblasts (N) and a marginal zone (M) that is initially anucleate. Eventually, cells from the layer of neuroblasts begin to migrate into the marginal layer, a process that has already begun in this section (week 6). The outer layer of the optic cup (O) will become the retinal pigment epithelium. The outer and inner layers of the optic cup remain separated from each other at this stage (asterisk). **B:** Formation of an optic cup in vitro from human embryonic stem cells. The invaginating neuroectoderm of the optic vesicle empirically forms a bilayered optic cup in vitro. Grown in vitro without blood circulation, these "organ buds" reach a few millimeters in diameter. The developing retinal pigment epithelium, the outer layer of the optic cup (arrows), is initially a pseudostratified columnar epithelium. ([B] from Nakano T, Ando S, Takata N, et al. *Self-organized Formation of Optic Cups from hESCs. Cell Stem Cell.* 2012;10(6):771–785.)

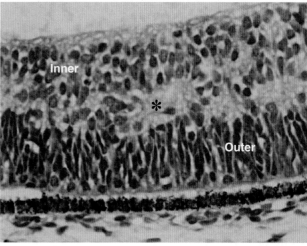

FIGURE 16.16 Micrograph showing the transient layer of Chievitz (asterisk) during the initial lamination of the retina into inner and outer neuroblastic layers. The layer of pigmented cells corresponds to the retinal pigment epithelium and is derived from the outer layer of the optic cup. (Courtesy of Dr. William Morris, Hamilton Eye Institute, Memphis, TN.)

the neurosensory retina will migrate into the embryonic optic stalk to form the optic nerve.

A simple way to view the process of differentiation of the retina is that the developing neurons first connect the retina to the brain and then the retinal neurons to each other as the retina forms and the cells differentiate. This occurs as waves of differentiation that begin from the inner retinal layers (near the developing vitreous) and progress to the outer retinal layers (near the RPE). Thus, the RGCs (that establish connections with the brain) will differentiate first and the photoreceptors will differentiate last. In this way, when the photoreceptors are ready to function, the entire visual pathway to the visual cortex already has its initial connections and is ready to function, even though additional maturation that improves visual acuity occurs postpartum.

Development of the neurosensory retina: Development of the neurosensory retina begins as early as week 4. As noted earlier, these cells proliferate to form a primitive "neuroblastic" layer, which, near the end of week 5 (32 to 33 days), is five to six cell layers thick. It is these cells that differentiate to become the various cell types of the neurosensory retina (**Fig. 16.15**).[22,23] With continued proliferation, early in week 6, the cells of this neuroblastic layer grow in thickness and number to about 10 to 12 cell layers. The inner layer of the optic cup is, at this point, organized into two zones: an outer "primary" or "nuclear"

zone of undifferentiated neuroblast cell bodies and an inner "marginal zone," which is entirely cytoplasmic in nature (**Fig. 16.15**). The basement membrane of the inner layer of the optic cup, which will delimit the future location of the internal limiting membrane (ILM) of the retina, separates the marginal zone from the future vitreous cavity.

Later in week 6, and over the next 2 months, the retinal neuroblasts continue to proliferate. Some of them begin to migrate into the marginal zone. With this migration, the cells of the nuclear zone separate into an *inner neuroblastic layer* and an *outer neuroblastic layer* (**Fig. 16.16**). After formation of the two neuroblastic layers, the major developmental events are primarily the differentiation of the retinal cell types, formation of the synapses and plexiform layers, and progressive lamination of the retina. The process of lamination and cell migration begins first in the region that becomes the posterior pole and thereafter spreads toward the periphery of the retina. Cell division in the retina is complete by about week 15, emphasizing the critical nature of the first trimester in ocular development.

Maturation of the retinal architecture and early development of the optic nerve: The cells arising in the inner neuroblastic layer differentiate into RGCs, amacrine cells, and Müller cells. The cells that remain in the outer portion of the nuclear zone form the outer neuroblastic layer and differentiate into photoreceptors, bipolar cells, and horizontal cells.[22] These are summarized in **Table 16.2**.

When the inner and outer neuroblastic layers separate from each other late in week 6, a nuclear-free zone is transiently present between them. This space between the two

TABLE 16.2   Derivatives of the Inner and Outer Neuroblastic Layers

Inner Layer	Outer Layer
Ganglion cells	Photoreceptor cells
Amacrine cells	Horizontal cells
Müller cells	Bipolar cells

separating layers of nuclei is termed the transient nerve fiber layer of Chievitz (**Fig. 16.16**). As the name implies, this transient layer is obliterated by further migration of retinal neurons later in development. The adult vestiges of this transient layer become incorporated into the inner plexiform layer.[24,25]

Retinal ganglion cells: The cells derived from the inner neuroblastic layer develop first. Indeed, the RGCs are the first neuronal cells of the retina to be recognized during development, beginning at about week 5. Beginning in the inner neuroblastic layer, the ganglion cells move toward the vitreous interface early in week 7. In week 8, these cell bodies establish the future ganglion cell layer of the retina. During this same week, the processes of the developing Müller cells begin to form the ILM of the retina, along the inner surface of the optic cup. Formation of the primitive ILM of the retina provides a definitive separation between the retina and primitive vitreous.[26]

Extension of ganglion cell axons to form the optic nerve: The path that the RGC axons take to reach the developing optic nerve lies along the inner surface of the developing layer of RGCs and beneath the primitive ILM. The ILM is formed by the end-foot processes of the Müller cells that are, in turn, overlain by the basement membrane of the inner layer of the optic cup, adjacent to the vitreous. The growth cones of the RGCs are guided by many molecular cues located primarily on the Müller cell end-feet and the vitreoretinal basement membrane. These cues are recognized by receptors on the surface of the growth cones. Upon contact with the end-feet of the Müller cells, the axons bend to travel toward the optic disc in the center of the posterior pole and undergo another shift in orientation to exit the retina by growing along the surface of the optic nerve head glial cells.[27] Because the inner layer of the optic stalk is continuous with the inner layer of the optic cup, the RGC axons can pass directly into the inner portion of the optic stalk. As ganglion cell axons grow into the optic stalk, some of the cells in the inner layer of the optic stalk undergo apoptosis (programmed cell death) to make room for these axons that are migrating into the developing optic nerve. By week 12, there are already nearly 2 million axons that have found their way to the optic stalk to continue their migratory path toward the developing lateral geniculate nucleus (LGN)

of the thalamus, minus a small portion that divert to other brainstem nuclei.

Interneurons: amacrine, horizontal and bipolar cells: During week 7, the first of the interneurons, the amacrine cells, begin to differentiate. Cell bodies of these cells and the future Müller cells initially remain localized in the inner neuroblastic layer. The axonal connections between developing amacrine cells and the RGCs (together with processes of the elongated Müller cells) later make up the acellular, inner plexiform layer, separating the RGC layer from the developing inner nuclear layer.

Although immature at this point in time, the inner retina has been shown to generate spontaneous cascades of electrical activity that propagate in a wave-like fashion across the retina prior to differentiation of the photoreceptors.[28,29] These action potentials are endogenously generated by the ganglion cells (and adjacent amacrine cells) and are believed to be required for normal retinal development and the formation of proper topographical connections between the different cell layers within the retina. They are also essential to organizing retinal communication with the LGN and patterning spatiotemporal activity between the retina and the brain.

The cells destined to become bipolar cells will begin migrating from the middle portion of the outer neuroblastic layer and join the amacrine and Müller cell bodies, whereas the horizontal cells and photoreceptors differentiate in the outer portion of the outer neuroblastic layer. Horizontal cells will then also migrate to join the bipolar, amacrine, and Müller cell bodies and, in this way, the inner nuclear layer of the retina starts to form during weeks 8 to 9. The interneurons of the retina become separated from the developing photoreceptors with the formation of the outer plexiform layer at about 10 to 12 weeks.

Photoreceptor cells: The various cellular migrations described above complete the separation of the populations of interneurons (amacrine, horizontal, and bipolar cells) from those of the photoreceptors. This separation of interneurons from the developing photoreceptors establishes the outer nuclear layer of the retina, which is comprised solely of photoreceptor cell bodies.

The nucleus-free zone that intervenes between the two populations of cell nuclei (those of the photoreceptors and those of the interneurons and Müller cells in the newly established inner nuclear layer) becomes the outer plexiform layer by about the 12th week. It is within this layer that the connections of the rods and cones to the bipolar and horizontal cells develop. Although the cells are still immature, the synapses between the photoreceptors and bipolar cells begin forming in the fourth month. At this time, the horizontal cells can be recognized as an irregular layer of cells in the outer portion of the inner nuclear layer.

As noted above, the photoreceptor cell bodies arise from the outer portion of the outer neuroblastic layer. The outer nuclear layer quickly becomes six to seven cells thick, with the outermost nuclei being primarily those of the cones. The inner segments of the developing photoreceptors form early in week 10 and are derived from the cilia of the outer cells of the original nuclear zone. The cell membranes of the cilia eventually involute, envelop the cilia, and form cytoplasmic processes that face the apices of the RPE cells. The photoreceptor outer segments are thought to arise as separate developmental units from these cytoplasmic processes. Development of the photoreceptor outer segments begins for cones at about the fifth month and for rods much later in the seventh month. Details of retinal differentiation beyond the first trimester are discussed later in the chapter.

Because each photoreceptor cell will be wired to represent a specific portion of visual space relative to its surrounding cells, it is imperative that these cells not shift their relative positions as they mature and complete their neural connections. Not surprisingly then, the external limiting membrane of the retina, the system of zonula adherens junctions that holds the photoreceptor cells into this critical, fixed mosaic, develops early and is seen by week 5.[30]

Evolutionary Concepts Relating to the Birth Order of Retinal Neurons

As mentioned earlier, the cells of the two neuroblastic layers begin as proliferating, homogeneous cell layers of retinal progenitor cells (RPCs), and ultimately differentiate into three classes of neurons (input cells [photoreceptors], output cells [RGCs], and interneurons) connecting and integrating the signal from input to output (horizontal, bipolar, and amacrine), plus one class of glial (Müller) cells. However, within these broad classes of cells, over 60 different subclasses are currently known, exhibiting different morphologies, neurotransmitters, and roles in visual processing in the retinal circuit.

The work describing the differentiation of the RPCs and the birth order of the retinal cells has been examined in detail in diverse species from fruit flies and frogs, to mice and humans. Although species-specific aspects of retinal development are evident, there are clearly common organizing processes that are shared by all species at both the cellular and the molecular level. These mechanisms driving retinal differentiation have been shown to be derived from both intrinsic cellular and genetic programming as well as extrinsic cues in the retinal milieu that appear to play a role in cell fate. The exact roles of these intrinsic and extrinsic processes in developing specific retinal neurons, as well as where, why, and when they appear, are not fully understood. However, an overview of what is known, and potential mechanisms by which the RPCs differentiate, is presented.

All retinal cells arising from the two neuroblastic layers are derived from a population of multipotent stem cells called RPCs. The daughter progeny of the RPCs are also stem cells as the inner and outer neuroblastic cell layers proliferate, but at specific points in the process they produce daughter cells with a more restricted lineage potential, eventually giving rise to terminally differentiated neuronal cells or Müller cells. In the mammalian retina, the earliest retinal neurons to differentiate are the RGCs, the cone photoreceptors, and the horizontal cells. Conceptually, these represent the earliest phylogenic cell types of the most primitive light detection systems in animal species. The most primitive visual systems include a light-sensitive input (cones), a visual output to the brain (RGCs), and a modulating interneuron (horizontal cell) (**Fig. 16.17**).[31] Within specific cell subtypes, there are defined birth orders. For example, cone opsins evolved prior to rod opsins and thus it is not surprising that the cones of the human visual system develop before rods during embryogenesis. In turn, cone bipolar cells develop before rod bipolar cells, as would be expected.

Amacrine cell subtypes also emerge at different times. Starburst amacrine cells appear very early, and glycinergic amacrine cells arise late in development (**Fig. 16.18**).[32] It has been proposed that the early differentiation of the starburst amacrine cells reflects their evolutionary importance as mediators of sensory detection of motion and direction (e.g., a predator or prey). The last retinal cells to differentiate are the rod photoreceptors, bipolar cells, and the Müller cells.[32] The photoreceptors and bipolar cells share a number of morphologic features and molecular expression profiles and may be developmentally related. It has been proposed that the Müller cells arose to provide structural and trophic support for the increasingly complex retina as the evolutionary hierarchy progressed.

A number of different models have been proposed to explain the process by which multipotential RPCs differentiate into the many retinal cell types.[32–34] These include the concepts of both intrinsic programming and extrinsic (environmental) interactions to yield ultimate cell fates. Basic concepts for which there is evidence include (1) intrinsic (but progressively restricted) competency of RPCs to produce specific types of daughter cells, (2) intrinsic competency, but early RPC patterning that leads to biased production of specific retinal lineages, (3) extrinsic modulation of RPC daughter progeny that then directs cell fate determination, and (4) stochastic models in which variations in the molecular signals that determine cell fate are present within RPCs, which are then biased toward generating certain daughter progeny.[31,35–38]

Müller Cells: The Müller cells are the glial support cells of the retina.[39] As noted earlier, the multiple end-feet of the Müller cells form a mosaic representing the ILM of the retina. From the retinal surface, these cells extend processes deeply into the retina, but not all the way to the RPE. The Müller cells reach just external to the external

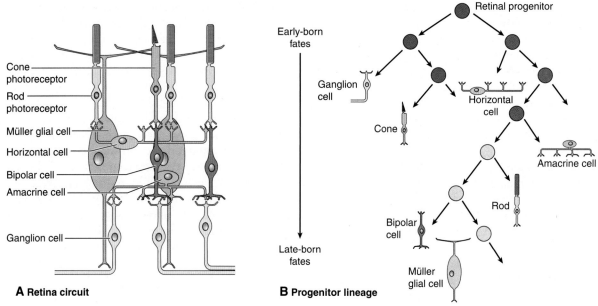

FIGURE 16.17   Temporal fate specification in mammalian retina. **A:** Schematic illustration of the main cell types in the retina and their organization within the retinal circuit. The retina is comprised of six major classes of neurons and one type of integral glial cell (the Müller cell). **B:** Retinal progenitors give rise to these distinct cell types in an overlapping but sequential order. Ganglion cells are generated first by early retinal progenitors and bipolar cells, and photoreceptors are born last, from late progenitors. (Redrawn from Kohwi M, Doe CQ. Temporal fate specification and neural progenitor competence during development. *Nat Rev Neurosci.* 2013;14:823–838.)

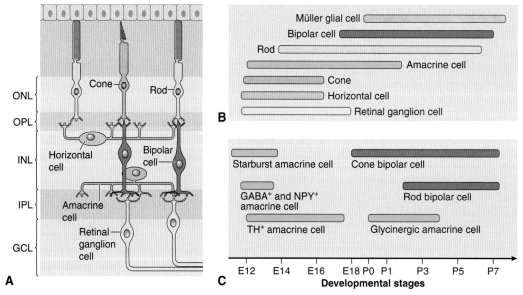

FIGURE 16.18   Temporal birth order of retinal cell types. **A:** The retina is organized into three layers of cell bodies (the outer nuclear layer [ONL], inner nuclear layer [INL], and the ganglion cell layer [GCL]) and two layers of neuropil (the outer plexiform layer [OPL] and inner plexiform layer [IPL]). The entire retina has the full complement of cell types and each subtype is evenly spaced or tiled across the retina. **B:** The birth dates of each of the major cell types in the rodent retina are indicated and are similar across many species. Birth dating has shown that amacrine and bipolar cell subtypes are born in a specific order. Amacrine cells that use GABA (γ-aminobutyric acid) as a neurotransmitter are born earlier than those that use glycine. **C:** Starburst amacrine cells use GABA as well as acetylcholine and are born very early, whereas GABAergic amacrine cells that also express neuropeptide (NPY) are born later, and tyrosine hydroxylase (TH)-expressing amacrine cells are born later still. Glycinergic amacrine cells are born primarily in the postnatal period. Cone bipolar cells are born throughout the period of bipolar cell genesis, and rod bipolar cells are born only in the later part of this period. (From Cepko C. Intrinsically different retinal progenitor cells produce specific types of progeny. *Nat Rev Neurosci.* 2014;15(9):615–627.)

limiting membrane of the retina and become joined to the surrounding photoreceptor cells by zonula adherens junctions (the principal structural element of the external limiting membrane). In this way, the Müller cells are integrated into the matrix that fixes the position of the photoreceptors with respect to each other.

The optic nerve: The formation of the optic nerve occurs from the migration of the ganglion cell axons into and proliferation of glial elements within the optic stalk. The meninges (dura, arachnoid, pia) that surround the optic nerve are of neural crest origin. Recall that as the optic vesicle invaginates into a bilayered optic cup early, the optic stalk likewise undergoes invagination and the two cell layers in the optic cup and stalk come to be in apposition to each other. With the exception of the hyaloid vessels enclosed within the cavity of the developing optic stalk, all the structures that develop from the optic stalk's inner and outer layers are of neuroectodermal origin, as are the RGC axons passing through it.

The Outer Layer of the Optic Cup Posterior to the Ora Serrata

The retinal pigment epithelium: The proliferation of cells of the inner layer of the optic cup into a multilayered tissue is in contrast to the proliferation of the RPE cells of the outer layer of the optic cup. These cells proliferate, but do so in a single plane as an epithelial cell monolayer, increasing in total area with the growth of the eye but not in volume. The cells at the anterior region of the invaginating optic cup are intimately associated with the differentiation of the mesenchyme into the ciliary body and iris. The RPE is the first tissue in the body to form melanosome pigment and melanogenesis in the RPE is continuous throughout fetal life. The developing RPE layer of the optic cup is initially a pseudostratified columnar epithelium. Beginning at about 5 weeks, with the onset of pigmentation, the pigment epithelium morphology becomes more cuboidal (**Fig. 16.16**). The RPE cell layer is confluent and postmitotic (under normal conditions) after birth, with the RPE cells in the periphery increasing in area to cover the residual growth of the eye. Although RPE cells do not normally divide in situ, in the fully formed eye they can be activated to proliferate in the setting of retinal injury.

◉ Early Development of Ocular Tissues from the Surface Ectoderm

The tissues of the eye that arise from the surface ectoderm are shown in **Table 16.3**.

FORMATION OF THE LENS PLACODE, LENS VESICLE, AND EMBRYONIC LENS NUCLEUS

As the optic vesicle expands laterally from the developing forebrain, during weeks 3 to 4, the neuroectoderm comes to lie directly beneath the surface ectoderm (**Fig. 16.7**). This apposition is critical to the induction of the invagination of the optic cup and induction of development of the lens

TABLE 16.3   Derivatives of the Surface Ectoderm

Lens
Primary and tertiary vitreous (also associated with neuroectoderm)
Epithelium of the cornea
Epithelium of the lids, conjunctiva, and nasolacrimal drainage apparatus, including goblet cells
Epithelial derivatives: eyelash follicles, Meibomian glands, glands of Zeis and Moll, lacrimal gland, Glands of Krause and Wolfring

from the overlying surface ectoderm.[40,41] The first sign of impending lens development is the appearance of a focal plaque of proliferating surface ectoderm on the lateral surface of developing head. This focal area is termed the optic or lens placode and it first appears in the fourth week of development (**Figs. 16.19** and **16.20**).

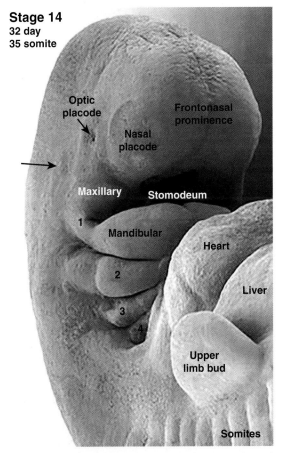

FIGURE 16.19 Anterolateral view of 32-day human embryo shows frontonasal prominence, the upper maxillary and lower mandibular processes of the first branchial arch, and the numbered positions of branchial arches 2 to 4. Three pre-otic somites develop posterior to the optic (lens) placode and anterior to the developing ear (otic placode—*arrow*). Each is innervated by one of the three cranial nerves that serve the extraocular muscles. The muscles develop from the mesoderm of these pre-otic somites. Note more visible thoracic somites at the bottom of the photograph. (From Hill MA. Embryology Stage14. UNSW Embryology website. https://embryology.med.unsw.edu.au/embryology/index.php/File:Stage14_sem2.jpg. Updated June 9, 2011. Accessed November 30, 2016.)

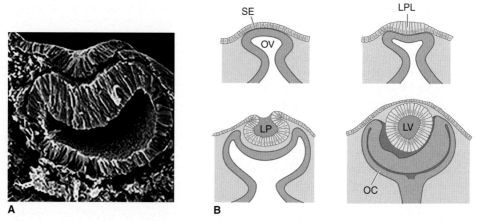

FIGURE 16.20   The first sign of impending lens development is the appearance of a focal plaque of proliferating surface ectoderm on the lateral surface of the developing head. This focal area is termed the lens (or optic) placode. It first appears in the fourth week of development. **A:** Scanning electron micrograph shows cross-section of early invagination of lens placode (*red*) and anterior surface of developing optic cup (*purple*). **B:** Sketches depicting progressive thickening and invagination of the surface ectoderm (SE), producing, in turn, the lens placode (LPL), lens pit (LP), and lens vesicle (LV). Neuroectoderm shown in purple. Note how invagination of the optic vesicle (OV) into the optic cup (OC) parallels invagination of the lens cup into the lens vesicle. ([A] modified from Wilson ME, Trivedi RH, eds. *Pediatric Cataract Surgery*. 2nd ed. Philadelphia, PA: Wolters Kluwer; 2014.)

Later in week 4, the lens placode begins to invaginate in parallel with the formation of the optic cup. Invagination first creates a shallow depression on the lateral surface of the head that is termed the lens pit (**Figs. 16.19** and **16.20**). As invagination continues, the lens pit deepens and enlarges in parallel with the invaginating optic cup. As invagination deepens, the ring of continuity between the cells lining the lens cup and the ectoderm remaining at the surface, "purse-strings" closed, sealing the lens cup into a lens vesicle (**Fig. 16.20B**).[42,43] During week 5, after the lens cup closes upon itself, the resulting lens vesicle separates from the overlying surface ectoderm. The now resealed surface ectoderm will go on to form the early corneal epithelium, later in week 5 (**Fig. 16.20**). Note that as the hollow ball of surface ectoderm closes upon itself and pulls beneath the surface, the apical surfaces of these cells face the inside of the lens vesicle and the basal surfaces, with their basement membrane, face the outside of the lens vesicle. It is from this hollow ball of surface ectodermal cells that now fills much of the space within the invaginated optic cup that the lens will develop. The basement membrane on the outside of the lens vesicle will become the lens capsule.[44]

The cells lining the lens vesicle rapidly divide and continue to synthesize and secrete new basement membrane, thus thickening the lens capsule. As the lens develops, the cells in the anterior portion of the lens vesicle retain their epithelial morphology and become the anterior lens epithelium. But the neuroectoderm of the developing optic cup induces the cells in the posterior portion of the lens vesicle to differentiate, elongating to form the primary lens fibers.[45–47] These fibers extend anteriorly and grow to fill the cavity of the lens vesicle. As the fibers grow anteriorly, filling the void of the lens vesicle, the cell nuclei also migrate anteriorly within the cells and form a transient, arcuate crescent of cell nuclei across the interior of the lens (**Fig. 16.21**). As

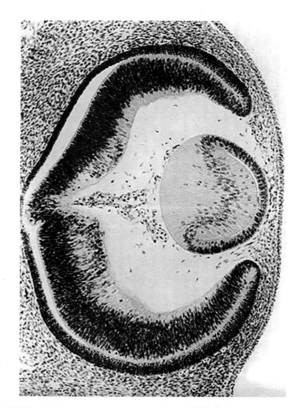

FIGURE 16.21   Light micrograph of human embryonic lens: Primary lens fibers. The neuroectoderm of the developing optic cup induces the cells in the posterior portion of the lens to elongate and form the primary lens fibers. These fibers extend anteriorly and grow to fill the cavity of the lens vesicle. As the fibers grow anteriorly, the cell nuclei migrate anteriorly within the cells and form a transient, arcuate distribution of nuclei within the lens. Note that the darkly stained epithelial cell nuclei remain present along the anterior surface of the lens but have been depleted from the posterior surface of the lens during development of primary lens fibers. (From Development Stages in Human Embryos: Stage 18. The Endowment for Human Development website. https://www.ehd.org/developmental-stages /stage18.php. Accessed October 25, 2016. Copyright © 1987 Carnegie Institution of Washington.)

the lens enlarges, beyond this earliest stage, the lens fibers become progressively longer (up to 12 mm) more concave and bow outward toward the equator, growing as concentric laminae of fibers (**Fig. 16.22**).[48] Note that as these fibers grow anteriorly, from their point of attachment to the basement membrane (i.e., lens capsule), the apical surfaces of the primary lens fibers are brought into contact with the inward-facing apical surfaces of the anterior epithelial cells, creating another apex-to-apex configuration like that seen between the neuroectodermal cells of the inner and outer layers of the optic cup (**Fig. 16.21**).

PRIMARY LENS FIBERS

Most of the growth of the lens during this earliest period is due to the differentiation and elongation of cells lining the posterior portion of the lens vesicle. By the end of week 6, the primary lens fibers derived from these posterior epithelial cells have completed their growth. The original cavity of the lens vesicle is filled by these fibers, thus forming the *embryonic nucleus* of the lens (**Figs. 16.21** and **16.22**).

Because mitotic replenishment of the posterior epithelial cell population does not occur during development of the primary lens fibers, this process fully depletes the population of posterior epithelial cells, leaving the posterior aspect of the lens devoid of an epithelium thereafter. The absence of a posterior epithelium from such an early stage in development makes it unsurprising that the thinnest portion of the lens capsule in the adult eye is at the posterior pole.

SECONDARY LENS FIBERS

Once the embryonic nucleus is formed by the primary lens fibers, continued growth of the lens occurs by the addition of new secondary lens fibers. Secondary lens fibers are derived from the anterior epithelium of the lens through a process that involves cell division.[48,49]

The anterior epithelial cells in the central 80% of the anterior lens surface, beneath the lens capsule, constitute what is termed the central zone (**Fig. 16.23A**). These cells are cell cycle arrested. Concentric to this central zone is a pre-germinative zone in which cells divide to provide additional anterior epithelial cells as the surface of the lens increases in size with age (**Fig. 16.23A**). Beyond the ring of the pre-germinative zone is the germinative zone in which cells undergo active mitosis but then migrate closer to the equator of the lens (**Fig. 16.23A**). Note that the pre-germinative and germinative zones of the anterior lens epithelium, in which mitosis occurs throughout life, are protected from the DNA-damaging effects of incoming

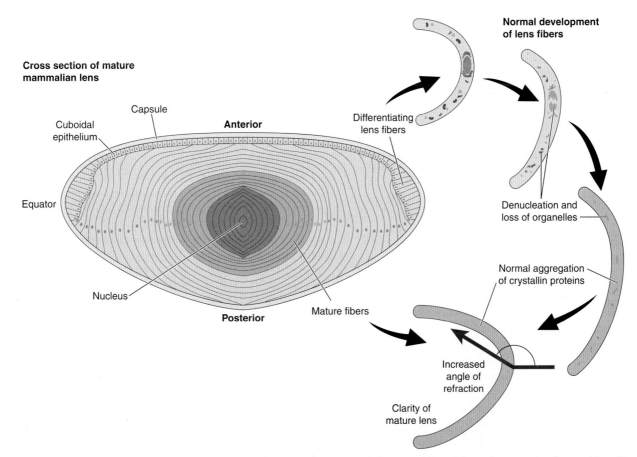

FIGURE 16.22 Formation of the lens: Secondary lens fibers. Cross-section of the normal lens (**left**). Differentiation of normal lens fibers leads to denucleation and loss of organelles. Mature lens fibers filled with crystallin proteins provide a clear lens with a refractive index above that of water to facilitate vision (**bottom**).

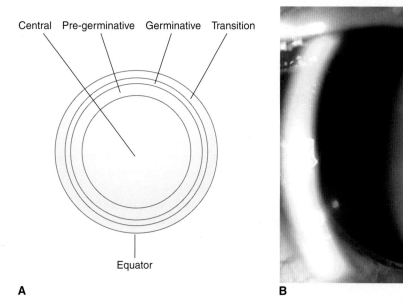

Central   Pre-germinative   Germinative   Transition

Equator

A
B

FIGURE 16.23   **A:** Sketch depicts the concentric zones of the anterior epithelium of the developing lens. **B:** Clinical photograph shows anterior Y-suture in a young eye. The posterior Y-suture (not shown) is inverted. (Courtesy of Dr. Daniel Roberts.)

light by being positioned behind the iris, leaving only the cell cycle–arrested cells of the central zone exposed to incoming light within the pupillary aperture.

Once cells divide in the germinative zone, they differentiate in the transition zone to form the secondary lens fibers. These fibers are added to the lens fiber mass at the equator and each new layer overlays previous layers, creating growth shells around the original group of primary lens fibers.[49] The process of fiber formation employed in creating the secondary lens fibers is the same process responsible for all of the lens growth thereafter.

Formation of secondary lens fibers begins late in week 6. As lens fiber layers are added, the cells become crowded together. The terminals of these fibers are not long enough to span the now greater distance between the posterior and anterior poles of the lens. Instead, they terminate peripheral to each pole along a seam. The fibers form interdigitating seams with adjacent fibers near the anterior and posterior poles of the lens. These seams are visible in the postnatal eye as the anterior and posterior "Y-sutures" (**Fig. 16.23B**). These "sutures" are inverted relative to each other. They begin as a horizontal suture at the anterior pole of the lens and a vertical suture posteriorly, but quickly, both form tri-radial structures, that are Y-shaped, upright in front and inverted in back. This region of the developing lens, whose many growth shells are bounded by the Y-sutures, is termed the *fetal nucleus*.

As the lens fibers continue to mature and differentiate, they continue to synthesize and accumulate large amounts of crystalline proteins, known as crystallins, within their cytoplasm and ultimately extrude their cell nuclei and other organelles (**Fig. 16.22**). These clear proteins act to refract light (the primary function of the lens) and minimize light scattering in the mature lens cells.[49]

The developing lens fibers are prone to injury and opacification from a number of insults including biochemical (e.g., galactosemia), infectious and inflammatory (e.g., congenital rubella infection), and genetic causes. Lens fibers may fail to form, may degenerate after formation, or may form aberrant layering, leading to light scattering and opacification. The timing of the insult can be inferred by observing which layers within the lens develop a defect, be it the embryonic or fetal nucleus, or later on in gestation. Note how in **Figure 16.24A** *the central portion of lens is opaque, including both the embryonic and fetal nuclei, as evidenced by the vague outline of the inverted, posterior Y-suture. One can see the outline of the abnormal area, but these opaque fibers do not represent the outer margin of the lens. After this early stage, in which abnormal lens fibers were formed, lens fiber formation continued normally. As such, there is normal transparent lens surrounding the opaque central region.*

*Focal developmental defects of the ciliary body from incomplete closure of the fetal fissure (coloboma) result in the absence of lens zonule deployment in the affected region as the zonules originate largely from the nonpigmented ciliary epithelial cells. Because it is the zonules that pull the equatorial region of the lens out to its normal rounded contour, the lack of zonules in the affected areas of the ciliary body is the proximate cause of the indentation in the edge of the lens (*Fig. 16.24B*). In such cases, the lens itself is normal.*

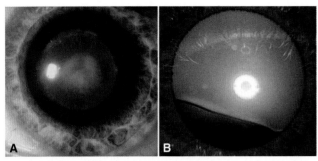

Defects in the formation of the lens capsule can give rise to anterior or posterior polar defects termed lenticonus or posterior globular defects, termed lentiglobus. Lenticonus is associated with genetic syndromes including Alport's (anterior lenticonus)[51] and Lowe's syndrome (posterior lenticonus) and others. Note the focal, teardrop bulges on the anterior (A) and posterior (B) surfaces of the lens (Fig. 16.25).

FIGURE 16.24 A: Abnormal growth of lens fibers early in development has given rise to central opacities limited to the embryonic and fetal nuclei of the lens. The posterior lens suture of the fetal nucleus, exhibiting an inverted Y shape, is vaguely outlined in the center of the lens. Of importance, the edge of the opaque region does not represent the periphery of the lens. After an early period of abnormal growth, lens development continued normally and produced transparent lens fibers. Hence, there is normal clear lens extending to the normal lens diameter. **B:** Coloboma of the inferior (inferonasal) lens. Failure to form portions of the inferior ciliary body due to a coloboma leads to the absence of zonular fibers in this region that would normally pull the equator of the lens out to its usual round contour. The lens itself is normal. ([A] courtesy of Drs. Edward Chaum and William Morris, Hamilton Eye Institute, Memphis, TN. [B] from Lens Columba. MCPHS Anterior Seg: Lens Quizlet website. 2016. https://quizlet.com/108728043 /mcphs-anterior-seg-lens-flash-cards. Accessed October 25, 2016.)

THE LENS CAPSULE

As the lens matures, the anterior epithelial layer continues to lay down a basement membrane, adding to the thickness of the anterior capsule of the lens. The lens capsule is highly elastic in nature. This elasticity permits enlargement of the lens as the ongoing formation of lens fibers continues throughout life, while permitting deformation of the fiber mass by the lens zonules, to permit changing focus from far to near (i.e., accommodation).

The early formation of the posterior lens capsule by the posterior epithelial cells sequesters the lens fiber mass from the primary vitreous. The presence of the lens is essential for proper vitreous development. The lens capsule also becomes the substrate on which the incipient hyaloid arterial system grows to transiently nourish the lens through these early and metabolically most active phases of growth.[50] Once the supply of posterior epithelial cells is exhausted, growth of the posterior lens capsule is reduced. Some maintenance of the posterior lens capsule likely occurs through contributions of additional basement membrane made from the basal surfaces of the continually developing lens fibers, before they detach from the posterior lens capsule and are enveloped by yet newer lens fibers.[44] However, the posterior pole remains the thinnest portion of the lens capsule throughout life.

THE VITREOUS AND THE HYALOID VASCULATURE

The vitreous develops in three phases. It is formed by contributions from both neuroectoderm and surface ectoderm. These intertwine in an inextricable way during the three phases of vitreous development. As such, the contributions of both embryonic tissues to vitreous development are discussed together.

The formation of the lens capsule posteriorly sequesters the lens fibers from the primary vitreous, completing the role of the lens in vitreous production. The lens capsule becomes the substrate on which the incipient hyaloid arterial system grows to transiently nourish the lens through this active phase of growth.[50] These vessels, the tunica vasculosa lentis, arise from a fibrovascular capsule posterior to the lens, the capsula perilenticularis fibrosa. At about 10 weeks, the lens has completed its major developmental phase and the hyaloid vasculature and its network of vessels within the vitreous begins to regress.[52]

The Primary Vitreous

Formation of the vitreous is related to development of the hyaloid vasculature that enters the developing eye through the fetal fissure. Both begin to develop during the fifth week of gestation. The primary vitreous begins to form

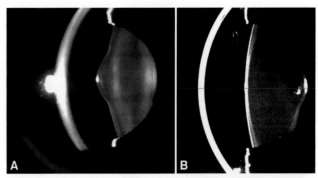

FIGURE 16.25 Lenticonus. **A:** Anterior lenticonus, a cone-shaped elevation of the crystalline lens in a patient with Alport's syndrome. **B:** Optical coherence tomography (OCT) image of posterior lenticonus showing a similar defect of the posterior capsule in a pediatric patient. OCT, optical coherence tomography. (From Bastola P, Joshi SN, Chaudhary M, et al. Alport's syndrome. *Kathmandu Univ Med J.* 2010;8(30):238–240.)

from thin fibrils that originally connected the invaginating lens vesicle with the inner surface of the developing optic cup (although some cell processes may be present earlier). Hence, there are contributions from both surface ectoderm and neuroectoderm. Some historical theories about the origin and structure of the vitreous also hypothesize a possible mesodermal component.[53,54]

The primary vitreous is a syncytium through which mesodermal cells migrate via the choroidal fissure. These mesodermal cells condense to form the endothelial linings of the hyaloid vasculature (**Fig. 16.26**). The hyaloid artery is a terminal branch of the dorsal ophthalmic artery. When the choroidal fissure closes, the mesodermal cells remain within the cavity of the developing optic cup and optic stalk and differentiate into the hyaloid artery and its branches within the primary vitreous. The adventitial tissue surrounding these vessels contains mononuclear phagocytes and fibroblasts that synthesize collagen and by 8 weeks, the primary vitreous is fully formed. The hyaloid artery and its branches form a transient embryonic vascular bed to support the rapid growth and metabolic requirements of the lens and growth of the developing optic cup until the adult ocular vasculature is established.

The hyaloid artery forms ramifying vascular beds within the primary vitreous that are termed the vasa hyaloidea propria (**Fig. 16.27**). Serving the rapidly developing lens are the capsula perilenticularis fibrosa and posterior tunica vasculosa lentis (a dense network of fine vessels surrounding the posterior lens capsule) (**Fig. 16.27**). Other branches of the hyaloid artery follow the optic cup margin anteriorly and anastomose as an annular artery near the anterior rim of the optic cup. Pupillary vessels from the capsula perilenticularis fibrosa continue anteriorly to join with vessels of the developing anterior segment. By week 6, branches of the annular artery will send vascular loops centrally over the anterior lens capsule, forming the anterior tunica vasculosa lentis.

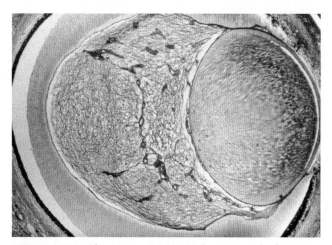

FIGURE 16.26 The primary vitreous. Light micrograph of a section through the eye of a 13-mm human fetus. The fine, fibrillar structure of the primary vitreous is evident. Note the well-developed network of vascular structures (*dark brown*) within the vitreous body (vasa hyaloidea propria) and on the posterior surface of the lens. (From Spalton DJ, Hitchings RA, Hunter PA, eds. *Atlas of Clinical Ophthalmology.* 3rd ed. Philadelphia, PA: Mosby; 2004.)

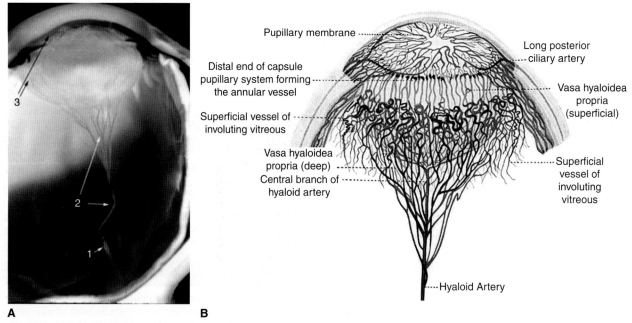

FIGURE 16.27 **A:** Macrophotograph of the hyaloid vascular system spanning the developing vitreous to reach the lens. (*1*) Main trunk of the hyaloid artery; (*2*) Multiple branches that constitute the vasa hyaloidea propria; (*3*) Anterior connections to the anterior tunica vasculosa lentis and the pupillary membrane. **B:** Schematic diagram of entire hyaloid vascular system. ([A] from Hartnett ME, ed. *Pediatric Retina.* 2nd ed. Philadelphia, PA: Wolters Kluwer; 2013. [B] from Duke-Elder S. *System of Ophthalmology. Part 1: Embryology Plate III.* Vol 3. London, UK and St Louis, MO: Henry Kimpton and The C. V. Mosby Co; 1970:201.)

Unlike the primary vitreous, the secondary vitreous is not of surface ectodermal origin. It is, instead, secreted from the neuroectodermal derivatives in the retina.

The Secondary Vitreous

The secondary vitreous begins to form after closure of the choroidal fissure in week 8. It is secreted from the surface of the retina and, as it grows, it compresses the primary vitreous inward to the central axis of the vitreous body. The secondary vitreous is almost completely formed by the third month of development. Unlike the primary vitreous, it is avascular and is comprised of both collagen and a hyaluronate ground substance.[54] It also contains the first true cells of the vitreous, primitive hyalocytes, with attributes of both fibroblasts and macrophages. These cells are found at highest density in the vitreous cortex and vitreous base. They are responsible for hyaluronic acid, glycoprotein, and collagen synthesis in the vitreous thereafter.

Secretion of secondary vitreous continues into the third month of development and accumulation of vitreous appears to be essential for normal growth of the eye. The ground substance of the vitreous is continuously secreted and, together with subsequent secretion of aqueous humor from the developing pars plicata region of the ciliary body, is accompanied by an increase in globe volume. Failure to close the eye wall and establish appropriate intraocular pressure (e.g., as can result from choroidal fissure defects) is associated with impaired growth of the eye, termed microphthalmia.

Initial Regression of the Hyaloid Vascular System

By early in the 10th week, the lens has completed its major developmental phase and the hyaloid vasculature and its network of vessels within the vitreous begins to regress. The regression proceeds from anterior to posterior, with sequential atrophy of the vasa hyaloidea propria, followed by the tunica vasculosa lentis, and then the hyaloid artery itself. The process is believed to be facilitated by the activity of hyalocytes, macrophages that induce occlusion and apoptosis of the capillary vessels. This process of vascular regression is normally completed by the seventh month. After regression of the hyaloid vasculature, hyalocytes come to lie in the vitreous cortex where they will begin to secrete hyaluronic acid.

The Tertiary Vitreous

The anterior portion of the secondary vitreous occupying the region near the ora serrata, between the ciliary body and the equator of the lens, begins to condense toward the end of the third month, forming the marginal bundle of Druault, which is firmly attached to the inner layer of the optic cup and is the embryonic precursor to the vitreous

base and zonules (**Fig. 16.28**).[55] As the eye grows, condensed fibrils of the secondary vitreous lying anterior to the marginal bundle of Druault elongate and become the lens zonules, also called the suspensory ligament of the lens or "tertiary vitreous." These fibers pull on the lens capsule, reshaping the lens to control focus and accommodation. The cells that produce the zonular fibers are believed to be the nonpigmented ciliary epithelium, although the equatorial lens epithelium (derived from surface ectoderm) may also play a small role. Over time, the secondary vitreous atrophies anteriorly and becomes posteriorly displaced to the region of the pars plicata and vitreous base, leaving the zonules structurally distinct. As it recedes, it maintains a ring of attachment to the posterior surface of the lens capsule termed the ligamentum hyaloidea capsulare or Wieger's ligament.

EARLY DEVELOPMENT OF THE CORNEAL EPITHELIUM

For development of the cornea to proceed normally, the lens must be present.[56] As noted earlier, the lens vesicle begins to separate from the surface ectoderm during week 5. The presence of an intact lens vesicle beneath the surface ectoderm from which it arose triggers the surface ectoderm

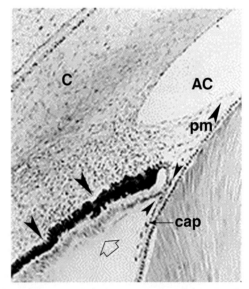

FIGURE 16.28   Portion of anterior segment of the eye at 3 months. Blood vessels (*large arrowheads*) are adjacent to the indented portions of the pigment epithelium. The nonpigmented epithelium of the inner layer also starts to buckle (*hollow arrow*). Fiber strands (faisceau isthmique of Druault) or "marginal bundle" connect the vitreous with the mesoderm around the rim of the optic cup (*small arrowheads*). AC, anterior chamber; cap, capsulopupillary vessel of the hyaloid system; C, cornea; pm, pupillary membrane. (From Cook CS, Ozanics V, Jakobiec FA. Prenatal development of the eye and its adnexa. In: Tasman W, Jaeger EA, eds. *Duane's Ophthalmology on CD-Rom, 2006 Edition*. Philadelphia, PA: Lippincott Williams & Wilkins; 2006.)

overlying the lens vesicle to differentiate into the corneal epithelium. Initially, the corneal epithelium consists of two layers of cells. The detachment of the lens vesicle from the corneal epithelium induces the basal layer of corneal epithelial cells to secrete a primitive corneal stroma, which consists of a few filaments, amorphous substrate, and a few collagen fibrils that extend beneath the epithelium. By 3 months, the corneal epithelium is a more stratified epithelium, four cell layers thick, which then produces a basement membrane. The remaining layers of the cornea are formed by mesenchymal cells of neural crest cell origin. These are discussed below under the heading Development of Ocular Tissues from the Neural Crest Cells.

EARLY DEVELOPMENT OF THE EYELIDS, CONJUNCTIVAL EPITHELIUM, AND ADNEXAL STRUCTURES

The Eyelids and Adnexa

As early as week 4, the future location of the eyelids is determined based on the presence of the optic vesicle. The upper eyelids form from mesenchymal condensations called the frontonasal processes, whereas the lower eyelids form from mesenchymal condensations called the maxillary processes that develop in the region of the first branchial arches of the embryo (**Fig. 16.19**). After the surface ectoderm begins differentiating into the corneal epithelium, two horizontal folds develop in the ectoderm above and below the cornea on the surface of the head. Around day 40 (sixth week), these folds become the epidermis of the eyelid skin (**Fig. 16.29A**). This epithelium continues on the undersurface of these folds as the palpebral conjunctival epithelium and then onto the surface of the eye as the bulbar conjunctival epithelium, reaching the demarcation of the limbus and continuity with the corneal epithelium. The lid folds become more pronounced as undifferentiated mesenchyme fills their interior. There is an ingrowth of mesenchyme of neural crest cell origin beneath the surface epithelium, which brings with it fibrovascular collagen supporting tissue, blood vessels, and nerve fibers. Later, mesoderm originating from the second branchial arch (innervated by cranial nerve [CN] VII) will invade the lids and differentiate into the orbicularis oculi palpebral musculature.

The lid folds grow toward each other and meet to fuse along a horizontal plane over the center of the cornea starting during week 8 (**Fig. 16.29**). Once the lids are completely fused, between weeks 9 and 10, the eyelash follicles and glandular structures of the lids and conjunctiva begin to differentiate within the lid margins and goblet cells first appear in the conjunctival epithelium. (**Fig. 16.30**).[57] In week 10, ingrowths of surface ectoderm create buds and columns of cells from the surface ectoderm into the underlying mesenchyme. These begin to differentiate into the eyelash follicles within the fused

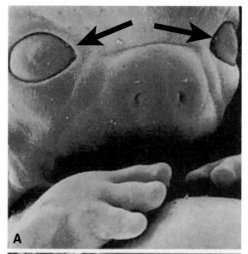

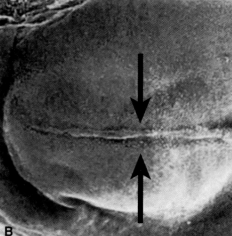

FIGURE 16.29 Scanning electron micrographs of developing eyelids in the human embryo. **A:** At 8 weeks of gestation, the facial prominences have fused and the lid folds are present (*arrows*). **B:** At 10 weeks of gestation, fusion is complete, and the epithelial proliferation associated with formation of the seam can be seen (*arrows*). (From Cook CS, Ozanics V, Jakobiec FA. Prenatal development of the eye and its adnexa. In: Tasman W, Jaeger EA, eds. *Duane's Ophthalmology on CD-ROM, 2006 Edition*. Philadelphia, PA: Lippincott Williams & Wilkins; 2006.)

margins of both the upper and lower lids. The glands of Zeis and Moll differentiate from the walls of the eyelash follicles beginning in the fourth month.[58] The Meibomian glands will develop in a similar manner by driving solid columns of surface ectodermal cells into the underlying mesenchyme, where they will proliferate and differentiate into acini of sebaceous glands and resorb a hollow duct leading to the surface from which initial development of the gland began. At the same time, there is condensation of the mesenchyme around the Meibomian glands, which gives rise to the tarsal plates. Separately, the levator palpebrae superioris muscle develops from a delamination of the superior rectus beginning at 10 weeks and will share its innervation from CN III. This separation is complete by the fourth month.

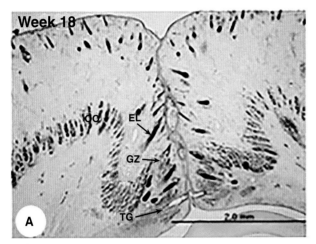

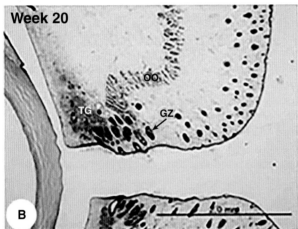

FIGURE 16.30 The developing upper eyelid in 18-week **(A)** and 20-week **(B)** human fetuses: **(A)** Gomori's trichrome stain and **(B)** Masson's trichrome stain. A: The tarsal (Meibomian) glands (TG) have grown toward the tarsal plate in the 18th-week fetus and the eyelashes (EL) are evident. B: Although from the outside the eyes of the 20th week fetus may appear closed, clearly the eyelids have already begun to separate. GZ, glands of Zeis; OO, orbicularis oculi muscle. (From Byun TH, Kim JT, Park HW, et al. Timetable for upper eyelid development in staged human embryos and fetuses. *Anat Rec.* 2011;294;789–796.)

Initial fusion of the lids serves an important function. The fusion of the lids, mediated through the formation of desmosomes in the adjoined layers of surface ectoderm, sequesters the underlying ectoderm that will give rise to the corneal and conjunctival epithelia, from the external surface of the embryo. This protects the corneal and conjunctival epithelia from the influence of the amnion during the period of development in which the process of keratinization of exposed surface ectodermal derivatives is initiated in the skin. Recent evidence suggests that fusion may also play a role in the normal formation of components of the ocular adnexa.[59]

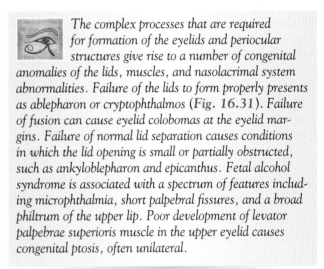

The complex processes that are required for formation of the eyelids and periocular structures give rise to a number of congenital anomalies of the lids, muscles, and nasolacrimal system abnormalities. Failure of the lids to form properly presents as ablepharon or cryptophthalmos (Fig. 16.31). Failure of fusion can cause eyelid colobomas at the eyelid margins. Failure of normal lid separation causes conditions in which the lid opening is small or partially obstructed, such as ankyloblepharon and epicanthus. Fetal alcohol syndrome is associated with a spectrum of features including microphthalmia, short palpebral fissures, and a broad philtrum of the upper lip. Poor development of levator palpebrae superioris muscle in the upper eyelid causes congenital ptosis, often unilateral.

The Conjunctival Epithelium

The nonkeratinized epithelium posterior to the lid margin lines the inner surface of the eyelid and reflects onto the surface of the developing eye to its continuation with the corneal epithelium. The portion of the epithelium lining the undersurface of the developing lid becomes the

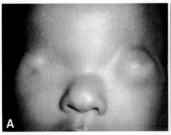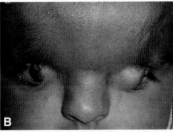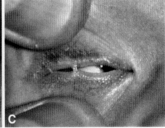

FIGURE 16.31 Cryptophthalmos. **A:** Failure of the lids to properly form can present as ablepharon or cryptophthalmos, seen here. It is characterized by the absence of a palpebral fissure and failure of differentiation of eyelid structures. **B:** The overlying skin blends with the cornea beneath. Partial forms of cryptophthalmos are also seen. **C:** Failure of the eyelids to completely separate after otherwise normal formation of the globe and lids is termed ankyloblepharon. (A, From Answers: January 15, 2013. Cybersight website. https://cybersight.org/. January 15, 2013. Accessed October 25, 2016. B, modified from Annie BMB Weeks 3/4 at University of Cincinnati College of Medicine. StudyBlue website. https://www.studyblue.com/notes/note/n/annie-bmb-weeks-3-4/deck/7211537. August 26, 2013. Accessed October 25, 2016. C, from Ankyloblepharon. *Rui's Optomblog website.* http://optometrui.tumblr.com/post/99443685385/ankyloblepharon-is-when-small-strands-of-tissue. Updated October 7, 2014. Accessed October 25, 2015.)

palpebral conjunctival epithelium and that which reflects onto the surface of the developing eye to join the corneal epithelium is the bulbar conjunctival epithelium. Unlike the corneal epithelium, the conjunctival epithelium develops a complement of unicellular glands called goblet cells. These first appear between weeks 10 and 11. The accessory lacrimal glands of Krause and Wolfring develop by inward budding from the palpebral conjunctival epithelium, in a manner similar to the formation of the Meibomian glands and the glands of Zeis and Moll from the epidermis of the fused lid margins.

The Lacrimal Gland

The lacrimal gland develops as six to eight epithelial buds that arise from the basal cells of the superior temporal conjunctival epithelium in the upper fornix, early in the ninth week of development. As such, most investigators believe the lacrimal gland to be principally of surface ectodermal origin, the same origin as the accessory lacrimal glands. However, some investigators suggest that the lacrimal gland acini develop from neural crest cells.[60]

The original ectodermal buds divide to form solid cords of cells, around which the mesenchyme of neural crest cell origin condenses and proliferates. The ectodermal cords differentiate into ducts by apoptotic vacuolization that create a lumen. The associated neural crest cells develop into cell clusters that also begin to appear at 3 months of gestation. These clusters of cells differentiate into the secretory acini of the gland. The lacrimal gland is still small at birth and does not produce tears until about 6 weeks after birth.

The Nasolacrimal Drainage System

During the fifth week of gestation, development of the nasolacrimal drainage system begins within the fold of surface ectoderm created between the adjacent margins of the lateral nasal process and the maxillary process of the first branchial arch. This fold extends from the lateral edge of the future nasal cavity to the point that will become the medial canthal region of the developing eyelids (**Fig. 16.32**).

The surface ectoderm covering the processes is thicker over the grooved interface separating the processes. As the maxillary process grows forward, upward, and over the thickened ectodermal groove to fuse with the lateral nasal processes around days 32 and 33, the cord of ectodermal cells becomes encased in the fissure called the nasolacrimal groove (**Fig. 16.32**, *black arrows* in right-hand image). The ectoderm in the floor of the groove detaches from the surface ectoderm, forms a solid cord or several shorter

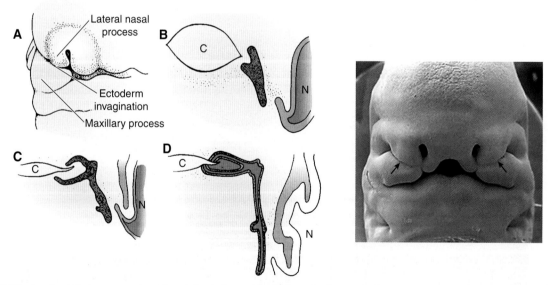

FIGURE 16.32 Lacrimal drainage system embryology. **A:** During the fifth week of gestation, an ectodermal invagination forms between the lateral nasal process and maxillary process of the first branchial arch. Near the surface, these two processes fuse along the line of contact (the nasolacrimal groove), leaving the buried trough of surface ectoderm beneath the surface. (Also see *arrows* in frontal view of embryo in the scanning electron microscopy image at right). This buried rod of surface ectoderm pinches off from the surface. **B:** At 6 weeks of gestation, this solid cord of ectoderm extending from the medial canthus to the nasal cavity begins to differentiate into the elements of the nasolacrimal system. **C:** At 12 weeks of gestation, proliferation of the cord occurs laterally toward the medial canthus and inferiorly toward the inferior portion of the developing nasal cavity. The cell columns are continuous, and the future canaliculi, lacrimal sac, and nasolacrimal duct are all recognizable; in addition, a lumen has begun to form in the lacrimal sac. **D:** By 7 months, canalization is nearly complete. Perforation of the puncta usually occurs before birth. C, cornea; N, nasal cavity. (Left image from Doxanas MT, Anderson RL. *Clinical Orbital Anatomy.* Baltimore, MD: Williams & Wilkins; 1984:9. Right image from Clinicalgate website. Head and Neck. In: Human Embryology and Developmental Biology. Clinical gate website. http://clinicalgate.com/head-and-neck-6/. June 13, 2015. Accessed October 25, 2016.)

cords that later fuse and comes to lie in the underlying mesenchyme. This ectodermal cord is located between the future medial canthus and the nasal cavity at week 6 of gestation. As the cells of the cord proliferate, the upper end of the ectodermal cord widens to form the lacrimal sac, whereas projections are sent laterally toward the medial canthus to form the canaliculi and inferiorly toward the inferior turbinate process of the nasal cavity to form the nasolacrimal duct (**Fig. 16.32C**). The canaliculi may also develop from separate cords that eventually fuse with the main cord. On the surface, the edges of the nasolacrimal groove fuse, providing a smooth contour to the epidermis of the skin overlying this region.[61]

Formation of a patent lumen begins at the lacrimal sac and proceeds toward both the canaliculi and the nasolacrimal duct starting at 12 to 13 weeks of development. The solid cords hollow out through apoptotic vacuolization, rendering the ectodermal-derived linings of the canaliculi, lacrimal sac, and the nasolacrimal duct. Initially, the superior end of the canalized nasolacrimal apparatus is closed by a membrane composed of canalicular and conjunctival epithelium. The inferior end is closed by a membrane composed of nasolacrimal duct and nasal epithelium. The superior membranes of the puncta are usually completely canalized when the eyelids separate, so the puncta are patent at birth. However, delays can occur in these processes, primarily at the distal end of the nasolacrimal duct near the valve of Hasner. This results in a nasolacrimal system that is not patent at birth. Such cases are usually managed conservatively when possible, allowing the duct to eventually open on its own.

Although there is general agreement as to when development of the nasolacrimal apparatus begins (fifth week) and when canalization is normally completed (by the seventh month of gestation), opinions differ as to the order of formation of the component parts once a solid ectodermal cord forms. The presentation above represents the most prevalent opinion; however, an alternative interpretation suggests that the entire nasolacrimal apparatus develops contemporaneously, followed by canalization occurring simultaneously throughout the nasolacrimal system.[62]

Early Development of Ocular Tissues from the Neural Crest Cells

Much of the connective tissue, all of the stromal pigmented cells, and some of the smooth muscle of the eye develops from mesenchymal tissues. The sources of these mesenchymal cells vary in different species but usually include neural crest cells and sometimes contributions from cranial paraxial mesoderm-derived cells.[63] For simplicity, we will discuss these contributions as being principally of neural crest origin. The tissues of the eye that arise from neural crest cells are shown in **Table 16.4**.

TABLE 16.4 Derivatives of the Neural Crest

Stroma of cornea, iris, ciliary body, choroid, and sclera
Corneal endothelium
Trabecular meshwork
Ciliary muscle
Sheaths and septae of the optic nerve and Tenon's capsule
Adipose tissue, ligaments, and connective tissues of the upper and lower eyelids
Orbital cartilage, bone, adipose and connective tissues
Stromal melanocytes of the iris, ciliary body, and choroid

OVERVIEW

Neural crest cells surround the outside of the optic cup during week 4. These cells will give rise to the choroidal stroma and its vessel walls, except for the endothelium, which is derived from the mesoderm. An additional outer layer of neural crest cells gives rise to the sclera. Still greater numbers of neural crest cells contribute to formation of the orbital walls.

By the sixth week of gestation, waves of neural crest cells enter the initially undifferentiated tissue mass between the basal surface of the corneal epithelium and the plane that includes the anterior surface of the lens and the anterior margin of the optic cup.[64,65] The initial wave will give rise to the corneal endothelium (**Fig. 16.33**). Subsequent waves

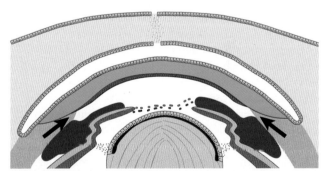

FIGURE 16.33 Derivatives of neural crest cells. Early in development, neural crest cells surround the developing optic cup (*dark pink*). In the posterior segment, these neural crest cells will condense into the choroidal stroma and the surrounding sclera, up to the scleral spur (*arrows*). A first wave of neural crest cells then transects the future anterior chamber to establish the plane of the corneal endothelium and the future Descemet's membrane (*dark orange*). The peripheral terminus of Descemet's membrane is Schwalbe's line. Another wave then splits as it enters. The cells that pass anterior to the edge of the corneal endothelium (*light green*) become the corneal stroma. The cells that pass posterior to the edge of the corneal endothelium (*dark green*) become the iris stroma, ciliary body stroma, and ciliary muscle, plus the trabecular meshwork. The neural crest cells forming the sclera meet those giving rise to the stromas of the iris and ciliary body, plus the ciliary muscle and trabecular meshwork, at the scleral spur (*arrows*). *Gray* represents light neuroectodermal derivatives of the outer wall of the optic cup and light orange represents neuroectodermal derivatives of the inner wall of the optic cup. Light blue elements are derived from the surface ectoderm, including the lens and the epithelia of the eyelids and conjunctiva, plus the adnexal glands and lashes.

during the next 2 weeks will give rise to the stroma of the cornea and iris and both the stroma and smooth muscle of the ciliary body during the first trimester. Certain of the intraocular structures that are formed in large part by the neural crest cells will not even begin to form until after the first 3 months of development, including the tissues of the aqueous humor outflow pathway. As such these structures, including the trabecular meshwork (TM), are detailed later in the chapter.

As mentioned above, waves of neural crest cells enter the cleft between the corneal epithelium and the anterior margins of the optic cup between weeks 6 and 8. Various sources disagree on how many waves of neural crest cells come through. Some of this variability is due to the fact that our understanding of these processes comes from an array of species, especially avian species. For simplicity, we will describe two main waves of neural crest invasion. The first of these waves cuts across the tissue mass between the corneal epithelium and the anterior margin of the optic cup, anterior to the lens, and establishes a dividing line that will guide further development. The cells along this plane will become the corneal endothelium and the endothelium will secrete its basement membrane, Descemet's membrane (**Fig. 16.33**).

As the second wave of neural crest cells moves into the space between the corneal epithelium and the anterior margin of the optic cup, these cells are confronted with a pylon, the edge of the first wave of neural crest invasion. Some of these cells will pass anterior to the tissue plane established by the first wave and become the corneal stroma. A portion of this wave will pass posterior to the tissue plane established by the first wave and become the stroma of the iris and ciliary body, the ciliary muscle, and the TM (**Fig. 16.33**). Subsequent dissolution of tissue between the developing corneal endothelium and the developing iris stroma will give rise to the anterior chamber.

As noted earlier, the neural crest cells that envelop the outside of the optic cup posteriorly become the choroidal stroma and, in turn, the surrounding sclera and Tenon's capsule. The neural crest cells of the developing sclera and the mass of neural crest cells contributing to the development of the anterior uveal tissues and aqueous outflow pathways all converge at the scleral spur (**Fig. 16.33**).

FORMATION OF THE CORNEAL ENDOTHELIUM, DESCEMET'S MEMBRANE, AND CORNEAL STROMA

As described above, the corneal endothelium develops primarily from the first wave of neural crest cell entry. The subsequent wave of neural crest cells that invades the space between the plane of the corneal endothelium and the surface ectoderm–derived corneal epithelium (with its primary stroma), gives rise to keratocytes of the future corneal stroma.[65] Thus, by the end of week 6, the cornea consists of a two-layered epithelium—a primordial stroma and a double layer of flattened endothelial cells.

Descemet's membrane is secreted by the endothelium and is first seen in week 8 of gestation as a discontinuous disorganized accumulation of basement membrane material. This initially incomplete basement membrane becomes confluent and thickens over time.[64,66] During embryogenesis, Descemet's membrane demonstrates striations at the ultrastructural level. These striations are not found in the progressive thickening of Descemet's membrane that occurs postpartum (**SEE CHAPTER 4: THE CORNEA**). The lateral margins of this first wave of neural crest invasion will establish the placement of the peripheral edge of Descemet's membrane, known as Schwalbe's line.

Proper placement of Schwalbe's line is critical to the proper development and differentiation of the anterior chamber angle and the tissues of the aqueous outflow system. A hierarchy of increasingly complex malformations can arise if Schwalbe's line is anteriorly displaced. The most benign of these is posterior embryotoxon in which anterior displacement of Schwalbe's line is the sole abnormality (SEE CHAPTER 9: ANATOMY OF THE AQUEOUS OUTFLOW PATHWAYS). Moderate dysgenesis is seen in cases of Axenfeld–Rieger's syndrome, which cause abnormal formation of the angle structures and iris and is commonly associated with congenital glaucoma (Fig. 16.34A). More severe dysgenesis of the angle, iris, and cornea is seen with Peter's anomaly and sclerocornea (Fig. 16.34B). The Axenfeld–Rieger's syndromes are inherited in an autosomal dominant fashion in most cases. Peter's anomaly is usually sporadic but genetic mutations do occur. These syndromes are caused by mutations in various homeobox genes, the transcription factor genes controlling the developmental program of the eye. These include the PAX6 gene (aniridia, Peter's), PITX2, FOXC1, PAX6, and FOXO1A (Axenfeld–Rieger's, genetically heterogeneous), and FOXE3 (sclerocornea).[21,67] These are discussed again at the end of this chapter.

During week 8, the cells between the corneal epithelium and the endothelium begin to deposit a secondary corneal stroma composed of type I collagen and proteoglycans/glycosaminoglycans. This gives rise to an initial thickening of the corneal stroma that becomes organized into regularly arranged lamellae from posterior to anterior. By 3 months of age, the epithelium has thickened into a multilayered, stratified squamous epithelium. At this time, the corneal epithelium is four cell layers thick, the stroma contains 25 to 30 layers of keratocytes, and the corneal endothelium is reduced to a single layer of cells overlying the now continuous Descemet's membrane. At this same time, nerve fibers, arising from the ophthalmic division of CN V, are evident within the corneal stroma. By the 5th month, they reach the epithelium.

THE IRIS AND ANGLE STRUCTURES

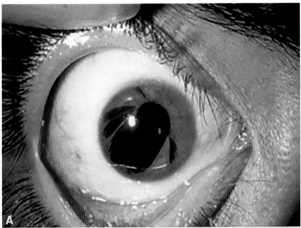

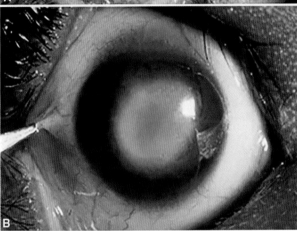

FIGURE 16.34 Other developmental abnormalities of the anterior segment. Anterior segment dysgenesis syndromes are also associated with abnormal neural crest cell migration during the formation of the anterior segment structures including the iris and the aqueous outflow pathways. **A:** The features of anterior segment dysgenesis may be mild and without clinical consequences, or more severe as seen in Axenfeld–Rieger's syndrome, which causes abnormal formation of the angle structures and iris (note the stretched appearance of the iris and multiple openings, polycoria). This syndrome is commonly associated with glaucoma. **B:** Very severe dysgenesis of the angle, iris, and cornea is seen with Peter's anomaly and sclerocornea. Peter's anomaly usually results from delayed or incomplete separation of the lens vesicle from the surface, leaving a central corneal opacity due to a defect in the continuity of Descemet's membrane and the corneal endothelium, leading to stromal edema centrally (as shown in B). Behind such an opacity, there may be an opaque, malformed lens still attached to the posterior surface of the cornea and to which iris tissue is often attached. ([A] from Rieger Syndrome Axenfeld. *Clinica Valle website.* http://www.clinicavalle.com/galeria-alteraciones-oculares/glaucoma/sindrome-axenfeld-rieger.html. Accessed October 25, 2016. [B] from Review, glaucoma: conditions with increased risk of glaucoma. *Ophthalmology Review website.* http://www.ophthalmologyreview.org/test-preparation/review-increased-risk-glaucoma. March 23, 2016. Accessed October 25, 2016.)

Thus, all of the layers of the cornea, with the exception of Bowman's layer, are present by the end of the third month of gestation. At the fourth month of gestation, Bowman's layer is a thin lamina, but it thickens by the fifth month to be visible at the light microscopic level.[64,65]

As noted earlier, the epithelial layers of both the iris and ciliary body, as well as the muscles of the iris, develop from the neuroectoderm of the optic cup. In the seventh to eighth week, the iris stroma arises from the wave of neural crest cells that entered posterior to the developing corneal endothelium. This matrix of neural crest cells coalesces anterior to the two layers of neuroectodermally derived iris epithelia and makes attachments to the convoluted basal processes of the differentiating anterior myoepithelial cells. Ultimately, the fibroblasts and melanocytes of the future iris stroma and anterior border layer of the iris emerge. Pigmentation of these melanocytes begins at about the 10th week. It is primarily the fibroblasts that produce the collagenous matrix of the stroma.

In addition to the initial formation of an iris stroma, a thin, vascularized membrane of neural crest cells migrates over the anterior surface of the lens to form the transient, pupillary membrane in week 8.[68] Despite its name, the pupillary membrane takes origin from the midpoint of the developing iris stroma and not the pupillary margin. The pupillary membrane instead vaults over the actual pupillary margin formed by the iris epithelia making connections to the underlying anterior tunica vasculosa lentis.

The vascular supply of the iris and the pupillary membrane also develops during the eighth week, from branches of the long posterior ciliary arteries (LPCAs). The LPCAs help form the major arterial circle and provide vascular supply to the developing anterior segment, the pupillary membrane, and the ciliary body via recurrent branches.

As with the rest of the intraocular vasculature, the endothelial linings of these vessels are mesodermal in origin, whereas the remainder of the vessel wall is of neural crest origin. The pupillary membrane vessels become continuous with the anterior vessels of the tunica vasculosa lentis and provide continuous blood flow to these vessels after the hyaloid artery begins to regress. With closure and resorption of the hyaloid vascular system, including the blood supply for the pupillary membrane, the pupillary membrane resorbs back to its connections with the midpoint of the iris surface, completing resorption in the eighth month of gestation.[68,69] This ring of tissue connections at the midpoint of the anterior surface of the iris remains visible as the collarette of the adult iris.

 Remnants of the pupillary membrane are commonly seen in patients at the slit lamp and are invariably present in premature infants. Conversely, excessive atrophy of the vessels of the pupillary membrane, affecting the larger vessels of the peripheral iris arcades, may adversely impact the development of the iris stroma, leading to separation of the anterior and posterior layers of the iris with formation of an atrophic cyst (**Fig. 16.13B**).

TRABECULAR MESHWORK AND THE ANTERIOR CHAMBER

Some of the neural crest cells from the first wave that migrate into the anterior segment of the eye will come to lie at the confluence of several tissues including the developing iris stroma, the anterior margin of the ciliary body stroma, the anterior margin of the ciliary muscle, and the peripheral termination of Descemet's membrane (Schwalbe's line). These cells will differentiate into trabecular endothelial cells.[70,71] As noted earlier, proper positioning of Schwalbe's line seems to be critical to proper formation of the angle structures. During weeks 7 and 8, the undifferentiated mesenchymal tissue between the corneal endothelium and the anterior surface of the developing iris stroma begins to resorb, creating larger and larger spaces that ultimately become confluent as the anterior chamber. This process begins in the center of what will become the anterior chamber and progresses toward what will become the anterior chamber angle. Remarkably, this entire process is completed merely by remodeling the tissues. Neither apoptosis nor phagocytic resorption by macrophages appears to play a role in the process.[72]

Once the anterior chamber becomes confluent, it is not uncommon for residual strands of pigmented connective tissue to remain evident spanning the far periphery of the anterior chamber angle. These remain into adulthood as slender stalks of pigmented connective tissue arising from the peripheral iris surface and terminating in the TM. They are a common clinical finding termed iris processes. Unless found in large numbers, or in conjunction with an anteriorly displaced Schwalbe's line, these iris processes are considered to be a normal anatomical variant.

Prior to the third month of development and even into the fourth month, the area destined to become the TM is a wedge-shaped structure filled with loosely organized, undifferentiated mesenchymal cells. At this stage, some investigators have claimed that the inner surface of the anterior chamber angle is covered by a single layer of endothelial cells that are continuous with the corneal endothelium. This continuous endothelial covering over the developing outflow pathway has been termed Barkan's membrane, after the person who first claimed its existence.[73]

However, there is by no means consensus on the existence of such a continuous layer of endothelium over the outflow pathway at any stage of development. Several prominent investigators were subsequently unable to confirm the existence of this membrane by either light or electron microscopy.[74,75]

Differentiation of the TM into uveal and corneoscleral portions begins only after the first trimester, sometime in the fourth month of gestation.[76,77] Some of these neural crest cells lying at the chamber angle will differentiate into trabecular endothelial cells. These will, in turn, elaborate the connective tissue elements of the meshwork. Note that Schlemm's canal makes an appearance in the deepest part of the anterior chamber angle still later in the fourth month of development.[74,77]

Development of the outflow structures after the third month is presented in more detail later in this chapter.

THE CILIARY BODY STROMA AND MUSCLE

The wave of of neural crest cells that invades posterior to the developing corneal endothelium gives rise to the iris stroma, the ciliary body stroma, and the ciliary muscle. As the neuroectodermal layers of the optic cup begin folding the layers of the ciliary epithelium into the ciliary processes, as noted earlier, neural crest cells external to the outer layer of the optic cup (the future pigmented ciliary epithelium of the ciliary body) begin to organize the initial ciliary body stroma. To this early stroma, the first ciliary muscle fibers are added but not until the fourth month.[78]

As noted, the layer of neural crest cells arising outside of the optic cup and the tissue derived from the waves of neural crest invasion, which enter the eye between the corneal epithelium and the anterior margin of the optic cup, finally reunite at the scleral spur, to which the ciliary muscle becomes attached in the fourth month. Tenon's capsule begins to form in the region of the equator around weeks 10-11. Further development of the ciliary muscle after the first trimester is discussed later in this chapter.

THE CHOROIDAL STROMA AND VASCULATURE

The choroid is derived from two embryonic tissues, both of which are influenced by contact with the developing RPE. The stromal fibrocytes and stromal melanocytes, plus the pericytes forming the tunica media of the choroidal vasculature, are derived from periocular mesenchyme of neural crest cell origin that is initially deposited around the developing optic cup as early as week 4. This layer of neural crest cells envelops the developing eye from anterior to posterior, finally reaching the optic stalk. The endothelial lining of the vessels, as with all blood vessels of the eye, is derived from mesoderm.

After the optic cup invaginates and the outer layer of the cup (destined to become the RPE) begins to develop its pigmentation in the fifth week, the primordial vasculature of the choroid begins to form as a loose network of fine vessels adjacent to the outer surface of the developing optic cup adjacent to the RPE.[79] Initially, in week 6, these endothelial lined tubes that will become the choriocapillaris lack a defined stromal matrix around them. Beginning late in the 3rd month, however, there is progressive condensation of a loose structural syncytium that becomes the choroidal stroma and overlying, denser scleral mesenchyme.[80,81]

The RPE plays a critical role in both the development and the maintenance of the vessels of the choriocapillaris, through the secretion of pro-angiogenic growth factors. The tunica intima of these vessels arise only from the mesoderm that has been in direct contact with the RPE, and loss of overlying RPE cells leads to chorioretinal atrophy and degeneration of the underlying capillary bed, the chorio-capillaris. If the tunica intima fails to form, the remainder of the vessel wall, derived from neural crest, also fails to form.

Initially, the border between Bruch's membrane and the choroid is made up of collagen fibrils from the choroidal stroma. Eventually, the endothelium of the choriocapil-laris lays down its basement membrane, which becomes the outer layer of Bruch's membrane. The appearance of this earliest portion of Bruch's membrane, in week 6, is the most visible landmark separating the RPE and the choriocapillaris at this early stage of development.[82]

The primitive network of larger choroidal vessels is ini-tially continuous with two vascular networks: annular vessels at the anterior rim of the optic cup that anastomose with small branches from the hyaloid artery, and vessels that are continuous with supraorbital and infraorbital plexi within the orbit. As these small vascular channels grow in size and number, they form a vascular bed posterior to the equator, with maturing connections to the short posterior ciliary arteries. Vessels consolidate into larger channels and vascular sinuses to form the rudimentary vortex veins (typically 4 to 7 per eye). This large, primarily venous network of vessels lies beneath the choriocapillaris and, together with the larger arterial vessels, gives rise to the vascular elements of the outer choroidal vascular layers of Sattler and Haller. It has been proposed that the choriocapillaris is the only choroidal vasculature seen through the third month of development.[83] It is not until shortly after the first trimester of gestation that the choroidal stroma and the vascular network of large to medium-sized blood vessels begins to develop, with the appearance of arterioles and venules located outside the choriocapillaris in week 15. Development of the choroid beyond the first trimester is discussed later in this chapter.

THE SCLERA

The sclera is derived from periocular mesenchyme of both neural crest cell origin and mesodermal origin. The neural crest cells contribute to all of the sclera except for the sclera's temporal aspect, which develops from mesenchymal cells of mesodermal origin. Like the choroidal primordium, all of these mesenchymal cells coalesce around the developing optic cup beginning as early as week 4. Organization of this mesenchyme into the earliest recognizable primordium of the sclera does not begin until week 7. As with the choroid, the presence of RPE cells appears to be required to initiate the process of scleral development. Unlike the choroid, however, it appears that the presence of the RPE is not re-quired to complete the formation of the sclera. Even in cases where there is near total failure of the fetal fissure to close, and neither an RPE nor a choroid is present inferiorly, the process of scleral formation continues and still provides the eye with a complete, fully enclosed envelope, in most cases.

The anterior sclera forms first, through condensation of the mesenchyme of neural crest cell origin at the limbus and at the future site of insertion of the rectus muscles.[84]

The anterior sclera is continuous with the corneal stroma. Condensation of neural crest cells proceeds posteriorly until the 11th week of development, at which time the sclera, though thin, is now recognizable surrounding the devel-oping optic nerve and forming the posterior scleral canal. This process of condensation is augmented by secretion of collagen and elastin in a concentric manner by resident scleral fibroblasts. Note, however, that deposition of the sclera's collagen and elastin occurs not only from anterior to posterior but also from inside to outside.[85] So, although the neural crest mesenchyme initially reaches the optic nerve by the end of the third month, there will be further deposition of collagen and elastin throughout the second trimester, which will further thicken the sclera.[86]

Although the sclera forms the outer, structural coat of the eye, it appears to play little, if any, role in directing the shape of the eye, its growth, or the differentiation of the internal ocular structures during development. This role is played by the optic cup, the lens, the retina, the RPE, and the choroid. Recently, the choroid has been recognized as playing a key role in the growth of the eye which is as-sociated with progressive refractive myopia.[87] This further demonstrates that scleral development is largely controlled by intraocular tissues and the intraocular pressure, once aqueous humor formation begins.

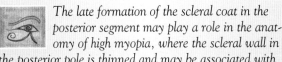

The late formation of the scleral coat in the posterior segment may play a role in the anat-omy of high myopia, where the scleral wall in the posterior pole is thinned and may be associated with pathologic thinning, termed a staphyloma (Fig. 16.35).

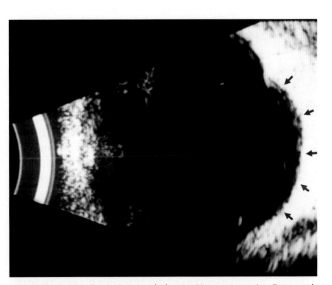

FIGURE 16.35 Posterior staphyloma. Anteroposterior B-scan ul-trasonic image of highly myopic eye, with anterior segment at left, showing dramatic thinning and posterior bowing of the posterior scleral wall, termed a staphyloma (*red arrows*). This finding is more commonly seen in patients with high myopia.

THE ORBIT

The orbital bones are derived from the cranial neural crest cells that migrate into the head, surround the developing eye, and form the frontonasal and maxillary processes. The lateral wall and floor of the orbit form from the maxillary process, and the lacrimal and ethmoid bones form from the nasal process. Except for the lesser wing of the sphenoid bone, which derives from cartilage, the orbital bones form through the process of intramembranous bone formation rather than endochondral ossification. The earliest of the orbital bones to begin the process of ossification is the ethmoid bone, which can be seen at the end of the 6th week of gestation. Ossification of all of the orbital bones is underway by the third month, a process that is completed between the sixth and seventh months.

Early Development of Ocular and Periocular Tissues from Mesoderm

Most of the striated muscles of the body develop segmentally from mesodermal somites; however, there are no somites in the head. Rather, the paraxial mesoderm in this region contains seven regions, termed somitomeres, which appear as furrowed ridges on the surface of the embryo (**Fig. 16.19**). They are the embryologic origin of the muscles and connective tissues of the head.[88]

The tissues of the eye and adnexa that arise from the mesoderm are listed in **Table 16.5**.

THE ENDOTHELIUM OF THE INTRAOCULAR VASCULATURE

For virtually all of the intraocular vasculature, the endothelial lining of these vessels (tunica intima) is derived from mesoderm. For vessels large enough to have a tunica media and adventitia, these layers of the vessel wall are derived from cells of neural crest origin.

THE EXTRAOCULAR MUSCLES

The tissues and structures in the orbit, including the orbital bones, muscle tendons, intermuscular septae, connective tissue components of the extraocular muscles (EOMs), and orbital adipose tissue are of neural crest origin. However, the striated EOMs of the orbit are of mesodermal origin.[89]

TABLE 16.5   Derivatives of the Mesoderm

Vascular endothelium
Temporal portion of the sclera
Extraocular muscles
Skeletal muscles of the eyelids (orbicularis oculi muscle and levator palpebrae superioris)

The neural crest cell precursors surrounding the eye are believed to play a significant role in spatial organization of the orbital structures, including playing a role in migration, differentiation, and morphogenesis of primitive myoblasts in the periocular region as precursors of the striated EOMs. This occurs through the laying down of an extracellular matrix, which stimulates myoblast proliferation and differentiation.

The EOMs develop from three mesodermal condensations located on each side of the head—one "premandibular" condensation and two "maxillomandibular" condensations (**Fig. 16.19**).[90,91] On day 26, an axial pair of premandibular mesodermal condensations are seen that give rise to the EOMs that become innervated by CN III (i.e., the superior rectus, inferior rectus, medial rectus, and inferior oblique). Shortly thereafter, two maxillomandibular condensations give rise to the lateral rectus and superior oblique, innervated by CN VI and CN IV, respectively. The condensations that give rise to the lateral rectus are seen on day 27, and those for the superior oblique on day 29. Thus, the EOMs are derived from head mesoderm (associated with either CN III, IV, or VI) that migrate into the region surrounding the developing eye. These immature myoblasts migrate to the proper region of the eye before they differentiate to form striated muscle fibers. The muscles themselves form secondarily from interactions with the mesenchymal condensations in the area.[92,93]

In the region of the superior mesenchymal condensation, the superior rectus, superior oblique, and the upper halves of the medial and lateral rectus muscles form. The levator palpebrae superioris arises through delamination from the superior rectus beginning in the 8th week. The inferior mesenchymal condensation gives rise to the inferior rectus, inferior oblique, and the lower halves of the medial and lateral rectus muscles. There are thus two stages of myogenesis.[94] In the first, primitive myoblasts are guided to the site by the neural crest–derived connective tissue in the area. Thereafter, normal differentiation and formation of striated muscle fibers require an interaction between the appropriate cranial nerves and the developing muscle.[95] Whether the muscle differentiates from the apex forward along the length of the muscle or the reverse remains unresolved.[95,96] The attachment of the muscles to the globe occurs in the middle of the third month with the fusion of the tendons of the EOMs to the sclera near the equator. Concurrently there is condensation of Tenon's capsule.

Summary of Development in the First Trimester

By the end of the third month of gestation, the eye has reached a stage at which a majority of the tissues that constitute the adult eye are recognizable (**Fig. 16.36**). Initial formation of the eyelids has occurred and the lids are fused. The adnexal glands of Zeis and Moll, and the Meibomian glands have begun to form, along with the

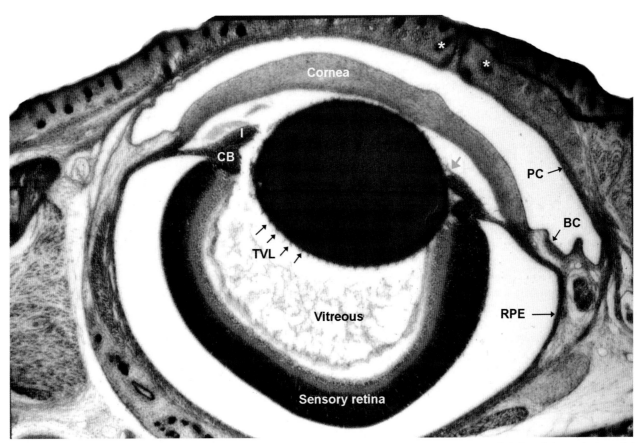

FIGURE 16.36 Eye and anterior orbit of a 12-week old embryo. Note lid margins are fused between the follicles of the eyelashes of the upper and lower lids (*asterisks*). The inner surface of the eyelid is clearly lined by the palpebral conjunctival epithelium (PC), which can be traced to the conjunctival fornix and its continuation toward the cornea as the bulbar conjunctiva (BC). A primitive iris (I) and ciliary body (CB) are evident. Note the delicate fibrovascular connection from the collarette region of the iris (*gray arrow*) and fibrovascular network of the tunica vasculosa lentis (TVL) that envelops the entire lens. At this stage, a prominent cleft remains between the differentiating cell mass of the sensory retina and the retinal pigment epithelium (RPE). Note that this is the same plane of separation that occurs in a retinal detachment. A well-defined sclera is not present and only a rudimentary choroid is seen.

eyelashes. The conjunctival epithelium and its underlying stroma are in place and goblet cells have begun to appear. The layers of the cornea, except for Bowman's layer, are discernable and the anterior chamber is well defined. The lens is still growing rapidly and remnants of the resorbing tunica vasculosa lentis are still present on its surface. The iris and ciliary body are distinguishable, but differentiation of the aqueous outflow structures in the anterior chamber angle is only about to begin. The vitreous cavity is readily apparent. Differentiation of all of the sensory retinal layers is incomplete as is fusion of the sensory retina and the RPE. The tissues of the early choroid and sclera are evident as well.

Maturation of the Eye after the Third Month

By the end of the first trimester, the embryonic sources of the eye and adnexa (neuroectoderm, surface ectoderm, neural crest, and mesoderm) have combined to form at least rudimentary forms of the adult tissues. From this point in development, the contributions of the embryonic tissues become less distinct as further somatic maturation integrates these contributions into the anatomically recognized tissues of the adult eye. Further maturation of the ocular and adnexal tissues, through the end of gestation and into the early postpartum period, is discussed in this section.

MATURATION OF THE CORNEA

After the third month, there is progressive maturation of the corneal epithelial layers, with the formation of identifiable "wing cells." The corneal epithelium does not reach its adult thickness until 6 months after birth. The endothelium is a single layer of cells by the end of the 11th week. Descemet's membrane develops into a continuous membrane during the fourth month and the corneal endothelial cells develop tight junctions, which appear with the onset of aqueous humor secretion, also in the fourth month. Deposition of the acellular Bowman's membrane, beneath the epithelial basal lamina, begins in the fourth month and by the end of the fifth month, Bowman's layer is fully formed. Initially, the corneal stroma is much thicker than in its adult configuration, but hyaluronidase begins to appear in the stroma in the fifth to sixth month. Enzymatic removal of hyaluronic acid in the stromal substrate causes progressive dehydration (deturgescence) of the connective tissue components, beginning posteriorly and proceeding anteriorly, so that the cornea becomes thinner and importantly, more transparent. The primitive mesenchymal cells originating at the margins of the optic cup, which migrate anteriorly to form the corneal layers, will also migrate posteriorly and give rise to the iris stroma and the scleral condensation that ultimately encapsulates the globe. As these populations of cells diverge anatomically, they also begin to differ in the secretion of collagen and noncollagen proteins, the lamination of the cornea being more regular and thus more transparent to light.[97]

By 7 months of age, the cornea is anatomically mature, but continues to grow in diameter through the first year of life. Because the diameter of the cornea is determined by the size of the optic cup, if the eye fails to grow to normal size, the cornea will be qualitatively normal but comparably smaller (microcornea—SEE CHAPTER 4: THE CORNEA). Corneal nerves which first entered the developing cornea around the third month continue to grow through the stroma to reach the epithelium by the fifth month.[97] From then until birth, nerves increase and branch, thereby forming a diffuse whorl network in the stroma and subepithelial layers. By the time the lids open, in the fifth month, the cornea is highly innervated.

MATURATION OF THE IRIS

The vascularization of the iris stroma continues during the fifth month, forming arteriovenous loops of vessels centrally in the tissue, the iris collarette. By the sixth month, the portion overlying the future pupil begins to atrophy and the pupillary membrane disappears by the eighth month. The more peripheral, mesenchymal portions of the pupillary membrane remain to act as a substrate for the growing iris stroma. Their adult legacy will be the visible collarette on the anterior surface of the iris.

In the fifth month, the muscle bundles of the pupillary sphincter muscle are invaded by small capillaries and connective tissue septae, running parallel to the stromal axis. By the eighth month, the sphincter muscle separates from the underlying iris epithelia except at the pupil margin and comes to lie in the iris stroma, giving the sphincter pupillae muscle its mature appearance as smooth muscle. A few strands continue to connect the sphincter to the developing anterior myoepithelium. These are sometimes referred to as Michel's spur.

The dilator pupillae muscle of the iris actually begins developing after the sphincter muscle, late in the fifth month and into the sixth month. The first sign of its differentiation is the appearance of fine fibrils in the base of the anterior epithelial cells of the iris just peripheral to Michel's spur. Fibril development then proceeds toward the iris root. The myofibrils accumulate in the cytoplasm of the basal part of the cells, whereas the nuclei and pigment granules are displaced apically. These myofibrils represent the "myo" component of the anterior myoepithelium of the iris and first appear in the sixth month. Unlike the sphincter muscle, the myofibrils of the dilator pupillae remain within the cytoplasm of the epithelial cell layer, thus it is a "myoepithelium" rather than a true smooth muscle like the sphincter. The dilator pupillae myofibrils only mature after birth, which is why it is difficult to dilate an infant's eyes.

Although the RPE is the first epithelium to be pigmented in the body (fifth week), the posterior iris epithelium does not begin acquiring pigment until the 3rd month, beginning at the pupillary margin and progressing toward the ciliary body. Pigmentation of the posterior pigmented and anterior myoepithelial layers of the iris is completed during the seventh month of gestation.[41]

MATURATION OF THE AQUEOUS OUTFLOW PATHWAY

Trabecular Meshwork

Up until the third month, the developing eye is more or less spherical; the corneal and scleral coats of the eye share the same radius of curvature. Thereafter, as the anterior segment develops, the curvature of the cornea increases relative to the sclera, giving rise to the anterior chamber. Initially the anterior chamber is shallow, but it increases in depth as the structures of the angle differentiate and as aqueous humor formation begins. Late in the third and into the fourth month the differentiated structures of the anterior chamber angle begin to appear.[98] It is during this period that the issue arises whether there is a continuous membrane extending from the corneal endothelium and separating the anterior chamber from the developing TM. Whether this membrane is truly continuous, as originally described by Barkan, remains a matter for debate.[73,99–101] This stage of development is shown in **Fig. 16.37**.

During the fourth month, the structures of the iridocorneal angle begin to differentiate. The primitive TM begins as a triangular mass of undifferentiated mesenchymal cells. The apex of this tissue mass tapers anteriorly, making connections with the peripheral edge of the future Descemet's membrane (Schwalbe's line) and the most posterior elements of the corneal stroma (**Fig. 16.37**). The cores of the trabecular beams will become continuous with the most posterior lamellae of the corneal stroma, whereas the neural crest-derived corneal endothelium becomes continuous with the differentiating trabecular endothelial cells, also of neural crest origin.[102]

In the earliest phase of trabecular beam development, the corneal endothelium and Descemet's membrane initially overlap the most anterior portions of the future meshwork. This area of overlap is referred to as the operculum. With further differentiation, this operculum disappears, but it remains present in the adult outflow pathway in the rhesus monkey eye (**Fig. 16.38**).

Most of the cells in the developing TM begin to take on an epithelial morphology, exhibiting an apical and basal surface. From their basal surface, these cells begin to secrete collagen fibers and proteoglycans to create the avascular cores of the endothelial cell-wrapped trabecular beams of the future uveal and corneoscleral TM. The remaining cells maintain a stellate, connective tissue cell phenotype and accumulate between the outermost trabecular beams and the developing lumen of Schlemm's canal. These cells make connections with both the endothelium of Schlemm's canal and with the trabecular beams to form the juxtacanalicular or cribriform meshwork.

At this early stage, clear separation of the TM, iris stroma, ciliary body stroma, and ciliary muscle begins. There is, as yet, no scleral spur and the mesenchymal cells that are differentiating into the TM lie slightly posterior to this junction. Thus, the TM is not fully open to the anterior chamber angle; rather, it is overlaid by ciliary body muscle and ciliary processes.

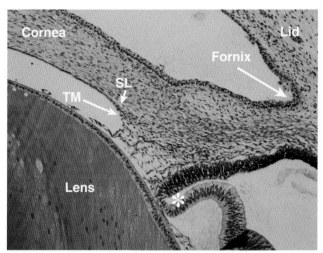

FIGURE 16.37 Immature angle. Micrograph from a 21-week fetus showing the development of the angle. The primitive trabecular meshwork (TM) begins as a triangular mass of undifferentiated mesenchymal cells. The apex of this tissue makes connections with the peripheral edge of the future Descemet's membrane (Schwalbe's line-SL). The cores of the trabecular beams will become continuous with the posterior lamellae of the corneal stroma, whereas the neural crest-derived corneal endothelium will become continuous with the trabecular endothelial cells, also of neural crest origin. The future pupillary margin is shown by an *asterisk*. Also shown is the conjunctival fornix. (Courtesy of Dr. Bill Morris, Hamilton Eye Institute, Memphis, TN.)

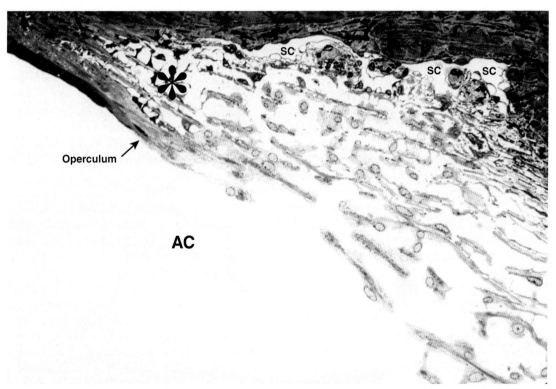

FIGURE 16.38 Light micrograph of trabecular meshwork of the adult rhesus monkey eye. Note how the operculum extends posteriorly, separating the anterior meshwork (*asterisk*) from the anterior chamber (AC). SC, Schlemm's Canal.

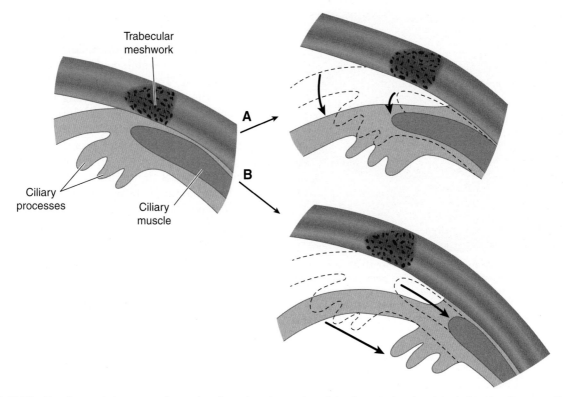

FIGURE 16.39 Developmental process of exposing the trabecular meshwork to the anterior chamber during development. If the uveal tract simply splits away by cleavage or by atrophy of tissue (*A*), the result would be an angle configuration in which the ciliary muscle extends into the iris and the ciliary processes are on the back of the iris. However, with slippage of the layers (*B*) due to differential growth rate, the ciliary muscle and the ciliary processes that initially overlapped the surface of the trabecular meshwork come to lie posteriorly. (Adapted from Anderson DR. The development of the trabecular meshwork and its abnormality in primary infantile glaucoma. *Trans Am Ophthalmol Soc.* 1981;79:458–485.)

A critical phase of anterior chamber angle development ensues when differential growth of the anterior uvea, relative to the corneosclera, rapidly occurs (**Fig. 16.39**). In this process, the differentiating tissues of the anterior uvea (iris stroma, ciliary body stroma, and ciliary muscle) shift posteriorly, relative to the edge of the first wave of neural crest invasion at Schwalbe's line.[62] In this process of posterior migration, the anterior chamber angle opens more deeply and shifts posteriorly. As the root of the iris shifts posteriorly, there is also an expansion of the ciliary body in which an emerging pars plana region extends posteriorly from the posterior margin of the pars plicata to the ora serrata. It is also during this process that the ciliary muscle develops, the scleral spur becomes clearly discernable and the longitudinal bundle of the ciliary muscle makes its attachments to the spur (**Fig. 16.39**). Failure to complete this process leaves Schwalbe's line anterior to its normal proper position. When Schwalbe's line fails to shift posteriorly, it becomes visible through the peripheral cornea. This abnormality is termed posterior embryotoxon. This abnormality may occur as an isolated finding of little clinical consequence or it may be a sign of more complex abnormalities that fall under the spectrum of Axenfeld–Rieger's syndrome, discussed earlier (**SEE CHAPTER 9: ANATOMY OF THE AQUEOUS OUTFLOW PATHWAYS**).

By the end of the sixth month, the trabecular endothelial cells have enveloped the now separating layers of trabecular beams. These beams increase in size as more collagen is synthesized within their cores. By the seventh month, the layering of trabecular beams is quite evident. It is around this time that aqueous humor outflow begins.[99,100]

Aqueous production is believed to begin late in the fourth month of gestation. So it may be that between the time of the earliest production of aqueous humor, and the establishment of aqueous outflow, the risk of a damaging elevated intraocular pressure is mitigated by enlargement of the eye. Outflow facility of fetal eyes under constant pressure reveals that there is a progressive increase in outflow facility during gestation. Outflow facility increases from an average of 0.09 μL/min/mm Hg before 7 months to 0.3 μL/min/mm Hg by 8 months.[99,100] This increase in outflow facility may result from the development of increasingly large lacunae between developing layers of trabecular beams that are referred to as spaces of Fontana.[101,102]

Posterior shifting of the anterior uveal tissues continues through the ninth month of gestation. At term, the iris root and the attachment of the ciliary body and ciliary muscle have receded to the level of the scleral spur. At birth, the TM is open and drains into Schlemm's canal, where giant vacuoles are clearly evident. At this stage, the outflow pathway is functional. The anterior chamber angle continues to grow as the eye enlarges and the limbal circumference increases. By 6 months after birth, the angle achieves its adult appearance.

Schlemm's Canal

The embryologic development of Schlemm's canal has recently been the subject of intense study. Although the canal is clearly continuous with episcleral veins of the vascular system in the fully formed eye, it conveys a clear fluid across its endothelium and into its lumen in a manner more similar to a lymphatic channel.[101,103–105] It now appears that the endothelium of Schlemm's canal shares certain molecular markers (e.g., PROX 1) with lymphatic endothelia, but differences exist as well.[106] Current consensus suggests that differentiation of the endothelial cells lining Schlemm's canal results in transdifferentiation of venous endothelial cells in the eye into lymphatic-like endothelial cells. As such, they are presumed to be of mesodermal origin.[106] There is also evidence that classic lymphatic channels arise from additional tissue sources that are yet to be identified.[107]

Most studies at the tissue level suggest that Schlemm's canal derives from a multifocal origin around the circumference of the developing anterior chamber angle.[108] As the anterior segment increases in size, Schlemm's canal develops from small plexi of venous canaliculi that may arise from the deep scleral venous plexus as an identifiable circumferential channel late in the fifth month.[109] Also, in the fifth month, giant vacuoles and tight junctions appear in the endothelium.[109] From the end of the sixth month of gestation onward, the frequency of giant endothelial vacuoles and pores increases, along with frequent discontinuities in the basement membrane. All of these features are related to the increase in aqueous flow that occurs during this period.[110]

MATURATION OF THE CILIARY BODY AND CILIARY MUSCLE

The ciliary processes grow in length to reach the lens equator during the fourth month. As they make contact, fine fibrils condense from the rifts between the radial folds of the ciliary processes, perpendicular to the marginal bundle of Druault of the secondary vitreous, to form the long, thick, zonular fibers connecting the ciliary body to the lens capsule. Between the two layers of the ciliary epithelium and the developing sclera, the ciliary processes become invested with mesenchymal cells of neural crest origin, forming the stromal component of each process. Each process has its own anterior and posterior arterial vessels, derived from the major circle of the iris. The anterior artery gives rise to fenestrated capillaries near the tips of the processes and the posterior artery gives rise to nonfenestrated capillaries in the core of each process. Both sets drain into the choroidal circulation. Growth of the eye as a whole during and after the fifth month causes the ciliary processes to retract away from the lens equator. This occurs in conjunction with the formation and elongation of the pars plana region of the ciliary body. This same action translocates the tissues of the outflow pathways posteriorly as well. Enlargements of the intercellular spaces between the apposed surfaces of the pigmented and nonpigmented epithelial cells of the ciliary processes are seen beginning in the fourth month and are believed to correlate with the onset of aqueous humor secretion.

The ciliary muscle forms from a triangular condensation of mesenchymal cells of neural crest cell origin lying between the developing scleral spur and the ciliary epithelium. This process begins in the region of the anterior margin of the optic cup. The ciliary muscle requires the presence of the ciliary epithelium to form, suggesting that the ciliary epithelium induces formation of the muscle during the fourth month of gestation.[78] The outer longitudinal (meridional) fibers form first, whereas the innermost circular fibers form last. The longitudinal fibers are readily visible by the seventh month, extending from the inner surface of the sclera near the ora serrata, to the scleral spur, which was in place in the fourth month. The oblique fibers appear thereafter and in turn, the circular fibers appear in the eighth month. The circular fibers and the ciliary muscle continue to increase in size for several years after birth as the eye grows.

MATURATION OF THE VITREOUS

The hyaloid artery and its vascular network within the vitreous normally regresses completely by about the seventh month, with the anterior vessels of the pupillary membrane regressing somewhat later, in the eighth month. The process of hyaloid regression is thought to be facilitated by the activity of hyalocytes and macrophages, which induce occlusion and apoptosis of the capillary vessels. The regression proceeds from anterior to posterior, with sequential atrophy of the tunica vasculosa lentis, vasa hyaloidea propria, and then the hyaloid artery itself.[51]

During the period before regression of the hyaloid system starts, branches have begun to ramify within the inner layer of the optic cup to form the intraretinal vasculature. The hyaloid vasculature regresses to the surface of the optic nerve. Its legacy in the fully formed eye is the central retinal artery and vein and the microvasculature of the inner retina.

A pinpoint remnant of the distal end of the hyaloid artery sometimes remains attached to the posterior lens capsule inferonasally. This remnant is referred to as a Mittendorf dot. It appears as a small punctate opacity on the back surface of the lens (white in direct illumination, black when illuminated using reflected light) (Fig. 16.40A). Pupillary remnants of the fetal vasculature are seen in a small percentage of full term infants but are seen in almost all premature infants, as might be expected. This persistent pupillary membrane is evident clinically in very early premature infants (Fig. 16.40B) and can impair visualization and laser treatment of the peripheral retina in infants with retinopathy of prematurity (ROP).

*Epicapsular stars are common remnants of the anterior tunica vasculosa lentis (also **SEE CHAPTER 10: CRYSTALLINE LENS AND ZONULES**). They are light brown or tan star-shaped deposits on the anterior lens capsule. Their star-shaped appearance distinguishes them from more irregular and clumped pigment deposits due to trauma or inflammation (Fig. 16.40C). Glial tissue surrounding the bases of the hyaloid vessels, as they emerge from the formed optic nerve head, may persist. Some may be dramatic, even extending like stalks from the optic nerve head into the vitreous. This developmental anomaly in its various appearances is called a Bergmeister's papilla (Fig. 16.40D-F).*

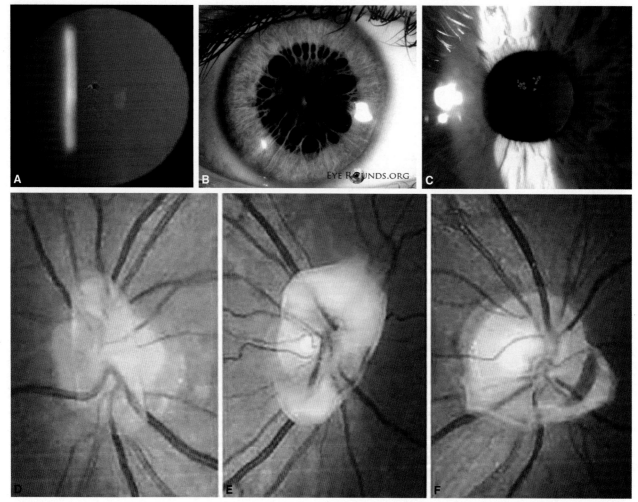

FIGURE 16.40 Commonly seen remnants of the hyaloid arterial system in the eye. **A:** Mittendorf dot shows focal dark opacity on posterior lens surface using retroillumination, backlit by the red reflex. **B:** Remnants of the pupillary membrane are commonly seen on the iris. Most are less significant than shown in this example. **C:** Epicapsular stars on the anterior lens capsule are light brown or tan star-shaped pigmented cells that were associated with the anterior tunica vasculosa lentis. **D to F:** Fibroglial remnants termed Bergmeister's papilla are seen projecting from the optic nerve head into the vitreous cavity. ([A] from Weed M. *Mittendorf dot: Ophthalmic Atlas Images.* Eyerounds University of Iowa Health Care Ophthalmology and Visual Sciences website. http://www.eyerounds.org/atlas/pages/mittendorf-dots.htm. 2013. Accessed October 25, 2016. [B] from Vislisel J. *Persistent Pupillary Membrane: Ophthalmic Atlas Images.* Eye Rounds University of Iowa Health Care Ophthalmology and Visual Sciences website. http://webeye.ophth.uiowa.edu/eyeforum/atlas/pages/persistent-pupillary-membrane.htm. 2013. Accessed October 25, 2016. [C] from Vislisel J. *Epicapsular Stars: Ophthalmic Atlas Images.* Eyerounds University of Iowa Health Care Ophthalmology and Visual Sciences website. http://webeye.ophth.uiowa.edu/eyeforum/atlas/pages/epicapsular-stars.htm. 2013. Accessed October 25, 2016. D to F, from Makino S. Prevalence of Bergmeister papilla. *Sch J Appl Med Sci.* 2015;3(2C):682–683.)

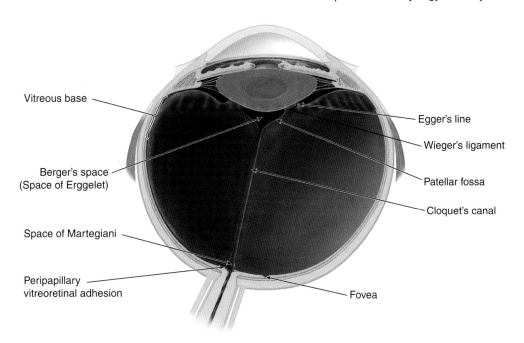

Vitreous base

Berger's space
(Space of Erggelet)

Space of Martegiani

Peripapillary
vitreoretinal adhesion

Egger's line

Wieger's ligament

Patellar fossa

Cloquet's canal

Fovea

FIGURE 16.41 The major anatomic landmarks and points of attachment of the mature vitreous include Wieger's ligament (anterior hyaloid membrane to posterior lens capsule), the vitreous base (overlying the region of the ora serrata), and peripapillary attachments around the optic nerve head. Firm attachments can also occur in the region of the fovea and surrounding macula. The secondary vitreous progressively collapses the primary vitreous centrally to form Cloquet's canal, a residual tract that extends from the optic nerve to the posterior lens capsule. The spaces of Berger/Erggelet and Martegiani define the anterior and posterior limits of Cloquet's canal, respectively. (From Tank PW, Gest TR. *Lippincott Williams & Wilkins Atlas of Anatomy.* Philadelphia, PA: Wolters Kluwer; 2008.)

As the hyaloid vasculature regresses, the secondary vitreous progressively collapses the primary vitreous centrally around the resorbing hyaloid vasculature to form the wall of Cloquet's canal, a residual S-shaped tract that extends from the optic nerve to the posterior lens capsule in the adult eye (**Fig. 16.41**). As such, Cloquet's canal is formed by remnants of the primary vitreous and tunica media and adventitia of the atrophic hyaloid vessels.

 Failure of the hyaloid artery to regress fully causes a spectrum of posterior segment disease originally called persistent hyperplastic primary vitreous, now termed persistent fetal vasculature (PFV).[111] The condition is usually unilateral (90%) and sporadic (Fig. 16.42). However, its association with mutations in a number of transcription factor genes and genes that play a role in cell cycle control and proliferation have been identified in patients and in animal models, suggesting a genetic component to the condition.[112] Vitreous cysts are sometimes seen in eyes with PFV and have been reported to contain remnants of the hyaloid vasculature.[113]

A primarily anterior form of PFV presents as a plaque of residual fibrovascular tissue, which is densely adherent to the posterior lens capsule. In some cases,

this disorganized white fibrous mass may even invade the posterior lens capsule, giving rise to secondary cataract formation (Fig. 16.43A). Elongated and centrally displaced ciliary processes may also accompany this process (Fig. 16.43A). Anterior displacement of the entire lens-iris diaphragm may also produce a secondary form of glaucoma. There may be persistence of the hyaloid artery, which is occasionally perfused, but retinal development in the anterior form of PFV is typically normal. The hallmark of posterior PFV is the formation of retinal folds, retinal dysplasia, and tractional retinal detachments that can also produce "leukocoria." Additional complications of the syndrome can include cataract, secondary angle-closure glaucoma, and microphthalmia.[111]

Leukocoria refers to an abnormal "white" reflex seen in the pupil (unlike the usual dark pupil or a "red" reflex seen in flash photographs caused by light reflecting off of the vascular choroid, Fig. 16.44). Leukocoria is a clinical sign of intraocular disease. It is seen in several developmental conditions including congenital cataracts, PFV, Coat's disease and other developmental abnormalities of the retina. Importantly, leukocoria can also be the presenting sign of retinoblastoma, the most common intraocular malignancy seen in children.

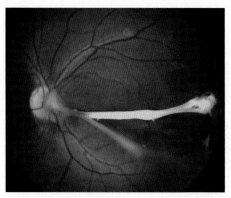

FIGURE 16.42   Persistent fetal vasculature presents as a failure of the hyaloid artery to regress fully. It causes a spectrum of posterior segment and anterior segment conditions. A non-perfused central arterial hyaloid trunk is seen coursing from the optic nerve toward the posterior lens capsule. The retina appears otherwise normal. The condition is usually unilateral and sporadic in nature and was formerly termed persistent hyperplastic primary vitreous.

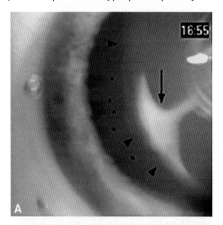

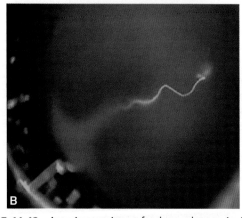

FIGURE 16.43   Anterior persistent fetal vasculature. **A:** Anterior view of lens capsule through a dilated pupil. A fibrotic plaque is seen on the anterior lens capsule (*arrow*). Medial subluxation (i.e., partial dislocation) of the lens and an irregular shape to the margin to the capsule are also evident (*arrowheads*). Medial dragging of ciliary body processes is evidenced by the large black triangular-shaped processes (*black dots*) extending toward the lens capsule from the edge of the gray iris. **B:** Fluorescein angiogram shows fluorescein in patent hyaloid arterial tree as it reaches the lens. Annular iris vessels are dragged to the pupillary margin and residual vessels of the tunica vasculosa lentis adherent to the anterior lens capsule are seen (**lower left corner**). (From Chaum E, Kerr NC, Kaste SC, et al. A 5 year old girl who failed her school vision screening. *Digital J Ophthalmol.* 2004;10(5).)

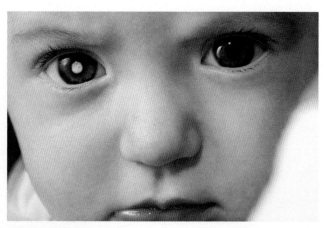

FIGURE 16.44   Leukocoria. A white pupillary reflex is seen in the right eye of a child with an intraocular retinoblastoma. (From Retinoblastoma. Childhood Cancer Trust website. 2015. https://chect .org.uk/retinoblastoma-2/. Accessed October 25, 2016.)

MATURATION OF THE RETINA

By the end of the third month of gestation, retinal development is well underway, the major cell types have all begun to differentiate; however, substantial integration of the neural circuity remains to be completed. In this process of integration, by the third month, the following retinal layers have already been established: ILM, nerve fiber layer, ganglion cell layer, inner plexiform layer, and the external limiting membrane. By the end of the third month, separation of the bipolar and horizontal cell interneuron cell bodies from the cell bodies of the photoreceptors has been completed. The separation of the bipolar and horizontal cells from the primitive photoreceptors establishes the outer nuclear layer (photoreceptor nuclei) and the inner nuclear layer (horizontal, bipolar, amacrine, and Müller cell nuclei). The separation created between them reveals the outer plexiform layer, containing the connections of the rods and cones to the bipolar and horizontal cells in the retinal circuit.[114] Although the cells are still immature, the synapses between the photoreceptors and bipolar cells, and their synaptic complexes connecting the signals from the outer retina to the amacrine cells, begin forming in the fourth month. At this time, the horizontal cells can be recognized as an irregular layer of cells in the outer portion of the inner nuclear layer.

As noted above, the photoreceptor cell bodies arise from the outer portion of the outer neuroblastic layer. The photoreceptor nuclear layer is six to seven cells thick early in the second trimester, with the outermost nuclei being primarily the cones. The photoreceptor outer segments are thought to arise as separate developmental units from the cytoplasmic processes that replace the cilia of the original external limiting membrane. Development of the outer segments of cones begins in the fifth month and those of the rods in the seventh month. These project toward the RPE from the level of the external limiting membrane and interdigitate with the microvilli on the apical side of the maturing RPE.

Macular and Foveal Development

Until the fifth month of development, the RGCs are seen as a multilayered cell strata in the posterior pole in the region of the future macula. In the sixth month, the region of the macula is noticeably thicker (~8 to 9 rows of RGC nuclei). However, starting at around the seventh month, these ganglion cells begin to migrate away from the central fovea, giving rise to the foveal pit (and eliminating the last vestiges of the layer of Chievitz), exposing the underlying photoreceptors in the fovea, virtually all of which are cones at this time (**Fig. 16.45**). To accommodate this centrifugal movement of neurons in the inner nuclear layer and retinal ganglion cell layer (a process which continues after birth), the cones, the cones develop long basal axons and their outer segments elongate to resemble the slender rod cells. This thinning of the foveal cones also permits an increase in the density of foveal cones in this region. The fovea continues its maturation for up to 4 months after birth.[115–118] It is during this time that the fixation reflex, a critical functional component of the development of normal vision, is established.

Although there are early signs of the foveal depression in the fifth month, there are still two layers of ganglion over the forming fovea; however, RGC migration reduces this to a single layer at term. The overlying neurons and supportive Müller cells of the inner nuclear layer also migrate laterally and become displaced away from the center

As the fovea matures, development of fine visual perception ("20/20" acuity) occurs through the process of active communication between the retina and the visual cortex of the brain. Anatomic or pathologic processes that interfere with the ability to deliver a clear image to the brain, e.g., cataract and high refractive errors (blurred image), or strabismus (different images from each eye causing cortical suppression of one image), and anatomic conditions that impair foveal maturation (e.g., albinism, ocular albinism, Fig. 16.45) will impair the acquisition of fine acuity in one or occasionally both eyes, resulting in a reduction in the best corrected visual acuity. This condition is termed amblyopia. Conditions that are severe enough to impair the acquisition of the fixation reflex in both eyes are associated with the development of nystagmus.

of the macula and fovea. As the cell bodies of the inner nuclear layer become displaced laterally, the fibers of the outer plexiform layer connecting the foveal cones to their laterally displaced interneurons must change direction. The result is that, in the macular region, the orientation of the fibers in the outer plexiform layer becomes more parallel with the retinal surface instead of being perpendicular. This parafoveal region of the outer plexiform layer is termed *Henle's nerve fiber layer* and can be inferred in conditions

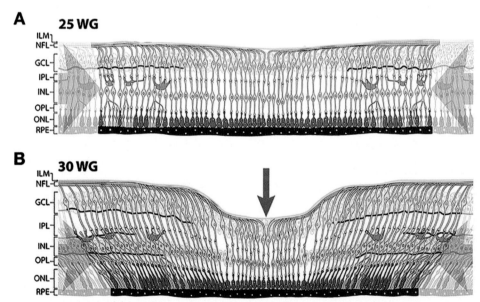

FIGURE 16.45 Diagrammatic representation of four stages in development of the fovea. Ages (WG—weeks of gestation) are an approximate indication of stages of human development. Cones are shown in *red*, rods in *gray*, bipolar cells in *blue*, amacrine cells in *pink*, and ganglion cells in *yellow*. The relationships between cells in the different layers approximate the midget circuits in the retina. *Red lines* represent the approximate arrangements of the retinal vessels. **A:** Indicating the appearance of the central macula just prior to the early appearance of the fovea. Retinal vessels are present only in the GCL. At this stage, cells in all layers tend to crowd toward the incipient fovea (centripetal displacement), as indicated by the *large gray arrows*. Photoreceptors on the edge of the foveal cone mosaic are more elongated than those in the center. **B:** Once the FAZ is defined, the inner surface of the retina within the FAZ is deformed, forming a shallow depression, which is the first indication of formation of the fovea. Centripetal displacement of cells in the outer layers of the retina continues, as indicated by the *large gray arrows*. Cones outside the fovea are narrower and more elongated than those within the developing fovea. *(continued)*

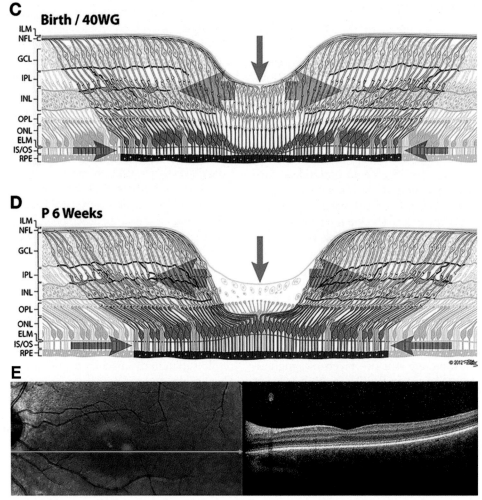

FIGURE 16.45 *(continued)* **C:** By birth, the GCL is significantly reduced in thickness because of the centrifugal displacement of ganglion cells (indicated by *arrows* in the inner retina). However, all cell layers are present within the fovea at birth. Cones in the fovea remain in a monolayer, are less elongated, and have only rudimentary inner and outer segments. **D:** In the first few weeks postnatal, cones in the central fovea differentiate rapidly so that by 1 to 2 months the central cones are more elongated than those on the edge of the fovea. Ganglion cells, bipolar cells, and the synaptic pedicles of cones have been displaced from the central fovea. The mature form of the fovea continues to develop over a period of many months, and includes further centripetal displacement of photoreceptors, increasing photoreceptor density in the foveola, continued centrifugal displacement of bipolar and ganglion cells, and morphologic remodeling of the shape of the depression. INL, inner nuclear layer; ILM, inner limiting membrane; IPL, inner plexiform layer; IS/OS, inner and outer segments; ELM, external limiting membrane; GCL, ganglion cell layer; FAZ, foveal avascular zone; NFL, nerve fiber layer; ONL, outer nuclear layer; OPL, outer plexiform layer; P, postnatal; RPE, retinal pigmented epithelium; WG, weeks of gestation. **E:** Retinal photograph with green line showing position of optical coherence tomography cross-section shown at right. Note failure of the fovea to fully mature and displace inner retinal layers in a child with ocular albinism. (**A** to **D**, from Provis JM, Dubis AM, Maddess T, et al. Adaptation of the central retina for high acuity vision: cones, the fovea and the avascular zone. *Prog Retin Eye Res.* 2013;35:63–81.)

like neuroretinitis, where retinal exudates highlight the underlying architecture of the nerve fibers in this area. Its radial orientation explains why hard exudates accumulating the macular region demonstrate a radiating star figure in their distribution (**Fig. 16.46**).

The Peripheral Retina

Retinal maturation progresses from inner to outer retina and from the posterior pole anteriorly to the ora serrata, the anterior border of the neural retina. The demarcation of the ora serrata forms with the earliest stages of ciliary

body development. Its location relative to the ciliary muscle changes and migrates posteriorly as the eye and anterior segment grow later in development. It is only in the process of this posterior migration that the pars plana region of the ciliary body emerges. This region grows during the first 2 years of life and is the point of access to the vitreous cavity for posterior segment surgery by the retinal surgeon; it is posterior to the vascular ciliary body and anterior to the neural retina. The cellular anatomy of the peripheral retina also differs from the retina of the posterior pole. The retinal cell layers and nerve fiber layer become progressively thinner as one moves toward the periphery,

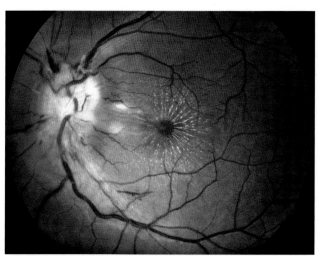

FIGURE 16.46 Macular exudates in a patient with neuroretinitis with retinal exudates accumulated in a pattern governed by the radial orientation of Henle's nerve fiber layer in the central macula. Optic disc swelling and hemorrhage is also present and commonly seen in this typically self-limited condition.

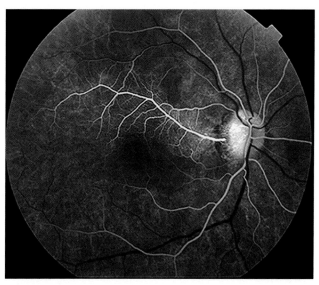

FIGURE 16.47 Cilioretinal artery. Arterial phase fluorescein angiogram showing early filling of a cilioretinal artery from the choroidal circulation in this right eye image. This vessel can be seen to provide the majority of the blood flow to the superior macula, having replaced the usual superior arcade derived from the central retinal artery.

with microcystic degenerative changes commonly seen beyond the terminal arcade of the retinal vessels in almost all eyes over the age of 20 years.

Retinal Vascularization

The vascularization of the inner retina does not begin to develop until the hyaloid artery system begins its regression. As described in the Vitreous section, the hyaloid artery supplies the lens and retina until the fourth month. In the fourth month of development, the central retinal artery and vein will arise as vascular buds from the hyaloid vessels where they emerge from the optic disc. These vascular buds begin as a primitive bed of mesenchymal cells and endothelial cords which start to invade the nerve fiber layer from the optic disc to form the retinal vascular tree.[119–121] This vascular system expands slowly outward from the optic nerve, advancing small branches into the laminating retina, ultimately as deep as the outer border of the inner nuclear layer, but not deeper. Thus, the retinal vessels supply oxygen and nutrients only to the inner retina.

The central retinal artery and vein divide into superior and inferior branches, and each of these divides again into the temporal and nasal arcades seen in the retina. Up to 18% of people have a cilioretinal artery that perfuses a portion of the macula (**Fig. 16.47**). This "aberrant" vessel is derived from the choroidal circulation and emerges immediately adjacent to or from the temporal margin of the optic disc. Progressive branching of the retinal vasculature continues to just posterior to the ora serrata (which is not fed by the retinal vessels) where the terminal capillary beds are found.

There are two distinct capillary beds within the inner retinal circulation, both arising from the central retinal artery. The superficial capillary plexus (at the level of the ganglion cells) provides nutrition and oxygen to the RGC layer (and nerve fiber layer). By contrast, the deep capillary plexus (at the junction between the inner nuclear and outer plexiform layers) does the same for the inner nuclear cell layer, with some diffusion into the outer plexiform layer.[122,123] Hence, all of the retinal layers deeper than the inner nuclear–outer plexiform layer junction are avascular and will come to depend upon the underlying choriocapillaris for their oxygen and nutrition.

During the late second and early third trimesters, the retinal vessels grow outward toward the retinal periphery.[123] The retinal capillary beds are present throughout most of the retina, but are absent in specific places. These include (1) the foveal avascular zone, (2) a capillary-free zone immediately surrounding the larger retinal arterioles (but not the venules), and (3) the most peripheral retina near the ora serrata. By the eighth month, the retina is fully vascularized nasally but only to the region of the equator temporally. Retinal vasculogenesis completes its maturation with the appearance of pericytes after birth. The angiogenic signals that drive vasculogenesis are regulated by the spatiotemporal secretion of vascular endothelial growth factor (VEGF) by microglia and astrocytes in the developing retina in response to the hypoxic environment. The budding endothelial cells, of mesodermal origin, follow a VEGF gradient and proliferate, filling in the avascular tissue until they reach the retinal periphery.

Infants born very early are at risk of the development of ROP because of the incomplete vascularization of the retina at the time of delivery, which normally proceeds to completion in the low oxygen tension environment in utero. Because of the immaturity of the lungs, many premature babies require oxygen supplementation (the earlier the delivery, the greater the severity of lung disease in general). Under the conditions of enhanced oxygen delivery, the retinal blood vessels growing toward the retinal periphery close off, because the tissues are oxygenated without additional blood vessel growth.[124,125] *When the supplemental oxygen is no longer required, the blood vessels begin forming again in response to the sharp reduction in oxygen levels, but they grow abnormally as fibrovascular tissue into the vitreous at the margin of perfused and non-perfused tissue (Fig. 16.48). Risk factors for the development of ROP include gestational age, birth weight, oxygen supplementation, and tissue hypoxia, among others. This growth of abnormal new vessels can be associated with vascular engorgement (referred to as "plus disease"), a disease feature that is an indication for treatment of the hypoxic tissue of the peripheral retina. Treatment regimens for ROP include cryopexy, which has been mostly replaced by laser retinopexy, and more recently, anti-VEGF drugs injected into the vitreous cavity. When first recognized in the 1940s,*[126,127] *the disease often led to tractional retinal detachments and blindness in these infants and was termed "retrolental fibroplasia" for the contractile membranes which formed, drawing the detached retina up behind the lens.*

Other developmental abnormalities of retinal vascularization are known. Some are primarily sporadic, such as Coat's disease, which is a telangiectasis of the peripheral vasculature that causes exudative detachments of the retina (Fig. 16.49A and B). Some are genetic (autosomal dominant) such as familial exudative vitreoretinopathy and von Hippel–Lindau disease, which is associated with the formation of hemangioblastomas throughout the CNS and body, including the retina (Fig. 16.49C).

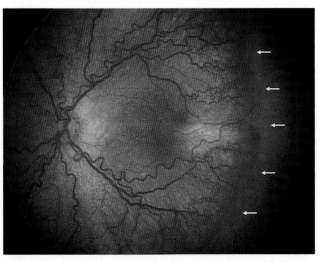

FIGURE 16.48 Retinopathy of prematurity. The vessels are tortuous and do not reach the temporal retinal periphery. They terminate prematurely, forming an elevated ridge of vascular shunts (*arrows*). The peripheral retina beyond the ridge is ischemic and secretes pro-angiogenic growth factors that can contribute to the neovascularization and progression of the disease.

MATURATION OF THE OPTIC NERVE

The number of RGC axons in the developing optic nerve changes greatly over time. At 10 to 12 weeks, the optic nerve contains ~1.9 million axons and this number increases to ~3.7 million axons by 16 weeks. However, by 33 weeks, the number of ganglion cell axons in the optic nerve is reduced to only ~1.1 million. This reduction in cell number is due in part to apoptosis of ganglion cells in the developing retina that have not made functional connections in the brain. Myelination of the optic nerve begins near the chiasm around the seventh month and progresses toward the eye. It is complete to the level of the lamina cribrosa shortly after birth.[128] However, myelination is not uncommonly seen in the retina as opaque yellow/white fibers emanating from the optic nerve head and occasionally as tracts of fibers isolated in the retina. Myelinated retinal nerve fibers are seen in ~1% of patients and are bilateral in 7.7% of affected patients (**Fig. 16.50**). They are nonspecifically seen in a variety of anterior and posterior segment abnormalities.

The inner layer of the optic stalk is continuous with the inner layer of the optic cup so that RGC axons can pass directly into the inner portion of the optic stalk. As ganglion cell axons grow into the stalk, some of the cells in the inner layer of the stalk undergo apoptosis to make room for RGC axons that are migrating into the developing nerve.[129] As the RGC axons enter the optic stalk, they split off a cone-shaped mass of glial cells at the surface of the optic disc that surrounds the base of the hyaloid vessels. During the seventh month, the glial sheath begins to atrophy and the degree to which it regresses determines the extent of natural cupping of the optic disc.

In addition to providing a critical guide path for ganglion cell axons, the layers of the optic stalk make additional contributions to the developing optic nerve. Cells of the outer layer of the optic stalk give rise to the border layer of Jacoby and intermediary tissue of Kuhnt that surround the optic nerve, plus astrocytes of the lamina cribrosa. Cells that remain in the inner layer of the optic stalk will become the astrocytes and oligodendroglia cells of the nerve.[130]

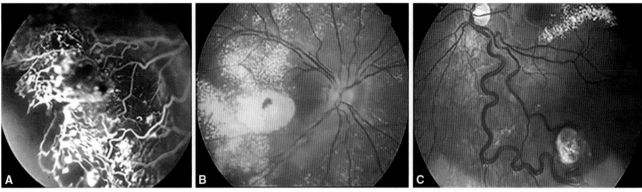

FIGURE 16.49 Fundus images of the retinal vascular anomalies: Coat's disease, and von Hippel–Lindau disease. Coat's disease is a congenital peripheral retinal telangiectasis in which abnormally dilated vessels in the retinal periphery leak serum leading to exudative retinal detachment. These abnormal vessels are seen in the angiogram **(A)**. Chronic exudates often consolidate in the region of the macula following treatment (laser or cryopexy), limiting visual outcomes in most patients **(B)**. Fortunately, Coat's disease is almost always unilateral. von Hippel–Lindau disease is characterized by the formation of hemangioblastomas in the retina, the central nervous system, and other organs. A large hemangioblastoma with a dilated feeding and draining vessel is seen in the inferior retina (with macular exudates, **C**).

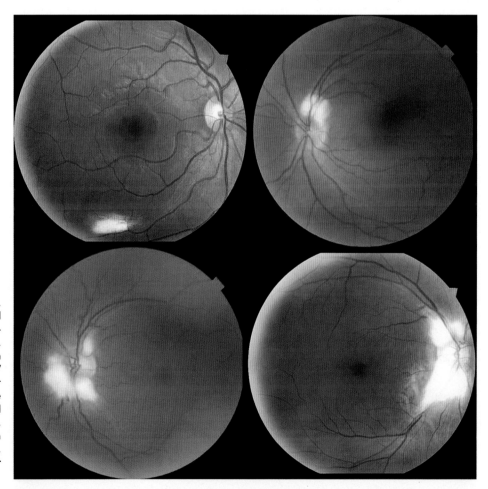

FIGURE 16.50 Myelin in the retina. Myelination of the retinal ganglion cell axons in the optic nerve typically terminates abruptly at the lamina cribrosa. However, myelin is occasionally seen in the retina as a feathery, yellow/white opacification of the nerve fiber layer, most often contiguous with the optic nerve head **(upper right and both lower images)**. Occasionally, isolated tracts of myelin are seen in the retina at isolated locations, remote from the nerve head **(upper left image)**.

MATURATION OF THE CHOROID

At 3 months, the choroid is represented almost exclusively by the choriocapillaris. However, in the fourth month, a primarily arterial network of large to medium-sized blood vessels arising from the short posterior ciliary arteries migrates beneath the lamina suprachoroidea. Their tunica intima is derived from mesodermal cells, and their tunica media and tunica adventitia arise from neural crest cells. These larger vessels give rise to the adult choroidal anatomy of Haller's layer (during the fourth month) and Sattler's layer (during the fifth month). The medium-sized Sattler's layer vessels branch extensively, anastomosing with the choriocapillaris. The anterior choroidal circulation is primarily venous and is comprised of a network of anastomoses in the region of the developing ciliary body. Thus, with growth and development of the choroid, the more posterior arterial circulation comes to anastomose with the more anterior venous drainage.

 Starting in about the fifth month, the chromatophores in the outer layers of the choroidal stroma begin to pigment, and pigmentation progresses inward, toward the RPE. Uveal melanocytes of the choroid originate from neural crest cells (as do dermal melanocytes), and pigmented choroidal nevi are seen commonly in clinical practice (Fig. 16.51A). Rarely, they undergo malignant transformation to become ocular melanomas (transformation rate being very low, ~1:9,000). However, choroidal melanomas that form in the retinal periphery can grow to be quite large before they become visually symptomatic (Fig. 16.51B).

MATURATION OF THE SCLERA

The scleral coat thickens progressively during development, progressing from the anterior segment to the posterior segment. As noted earlier, the scleral spur becomes visible as a distinct structure by the fourth month. Fibrous condensation of the sclera continues in the region of the posterior scleral foramen with deposition of collagen and elastin connective tissue lamellae traversing the axons in the optic nerve. Thus, the lamina cribrosa is laid down after the ganglion cell axons have passed through the posterior scleral foramen. The lamina cribrosa is fully formed by the seventh month of development.

MATURATION OF THE EYELIDS

The apocrine sweat glands of Moll and sebaceous glands of Zeis develop around the fourth month from the walls of the lid lash follicles as epidermal cells invaginate into the underlying mesenchyme. The muscles of the eyelids and face are derived from the second branchial arch mesoderm. The orbicularis oculi, corrugator supercilii, and procerus muscles arise from the infraorbital lamina, of the second branchial arch, and the frontalis muscle comes from the temporal lamina. Aponeurotic fibers of the galea envelop the developing frontalis muscle to reach the anterior muscle sheath of the frontalis, orbicularis, and the eyelid as the posterior orbicularis fascia. The previously fused eyelid margins begin to separate anterior to posterior usually starting from the nasal side during the fifth month. This occurs through a combination of desmosome breakdown, keratinization of the eyelid margins, lid muscle contraction, and secretion of sebum by the Meibomian glands (Fig. 16.30). The eyelashes begin to protrude from the follicles as the adhesions between the lid margins break down, a process that is typically completed by about 20 weeks of age.

Reopening of the eyelids begins in the fifth month and is completed by the seventh month of gestation. Opening of the fused lids after this period of development ensures that keratinization of the corneal and conjunctival epithelia does not occur.

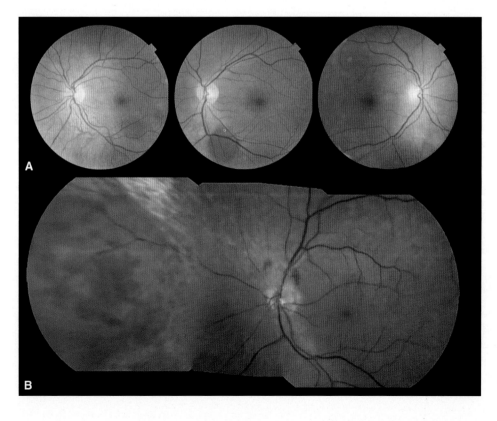

FIGURE 16.51 Choroidal nevi and melanoma. **A:** Fundus photographs of pigmented choroidal nevi of different sizes. Small lesions are typically flat (**left and middle**) whereas larger nevi may elevate the retina as they grow inward and elevate the retinal vessels (**right**). **B:** A large choroidal melanoma in the nasal peripheral retina. Detection of large tumors in this location may be delayed because of the absence of visual symptoms. (Courtesy of Matthew Wilson, Hamilton Eye Institute, Memphis, TN.)

MATURATION OF THE LACRIMAL GLAND AND NASOLACRIMAL DRAINAGE SYSTEM

The lacrimal gland is still vestigial at birth and does not function fully for about 6 weeks. It is for this reason that during the first 6 weeks of life, newborn infants do not produce tears when they cry. Lacrimation from the gland appears at around 2 months and the gland is fully developed by around 3 years of age. Formation of a patent lumen begins at the lacrimal sac and proceeds toward the canaliculi and nasolacrimal duct starting at ~12 weeks of development. The solid ectodermal cords hollow out and the canaliculi, lacrimal sac, and nasolacrimal duct become lined with ectoderm. By 4 months, the cord of cells is canalized leaving a residual superior membrane composed of canalicular and conjunctival epithelium, and an inferior membrane of nasolacrimal and nasal epithelium. The lacrimal puncta open after the eyelids separate and the entire nasolcarimal system is usually patent, including the Valve of Hasner, by the 7th month.

Although the lumen of the entire nasolcarimal system is usually patent by the seventh month of development, incomplete canalization at the inferior end of the duct is a common cause of nasolacrimal duct obstructions in infants. This manifests as epiphora (tearing, often monocular) and occasionally formation of a dacryocele (swollen lacrimal sac) or dacryoadenitis (infection of the lacrimal sac) (**Fig. 16.52**).

MATURATION OF THE ORBITS

The orbital bones begin to ossify during the third month, a process that is completed between the sixth and seventh months. As the orbits form, there is a progressive decrease in the angle of the orbital axes, which begins at almost 180° in the early embryo. This occurs because of the differential growth of the tissues behind and lateral to the eyes. The angle between the orbital axes decreases to 105° at the third month, and further decreases to ~71° at birth. The angle approximates 68° in the adult. The orbital limits are determined by the optic cup, which is present before the bony orbit is laid down. If the eye does not grow, the orbit will remain small. Of clinical importance, the portion of the frontal bone forming the orbital roof has not reached its full thickness at birth. Hence in infants and young children blunt trauma to the orbit that would normally cause a fracture of the orbital floor in an adult, may cause a fracture of the orbital roof instead.

Genetic Programming of Eye Development

It is important to appreciate that the orchestration and integration of the various embryonic tissues is achieved following a genetic blueprint that is implemented through

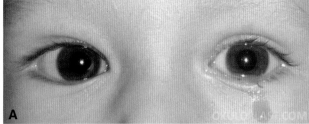
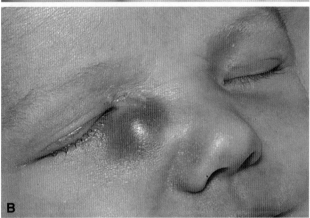

FIGURE 16.52 Incomplete canalization of the nasolacrimal duct. **A:** Failure to open the nasolacrimal system prior to the postpartum onset of tearing initially results in spilling of tears over the lid margin (epiphora, fluorescein-stained in this image). Obstruction of the nasolacrimal duct in infants is often monocular. **B:** If the punctum is open, but the valve of Hasner has not yet perforated, tears can become stagnant, resulting in infection within the nasolacrimal system (dacryocystitis). ([A] from Tasman W, Jaeger EA, eds. *Duane's Ophthalmology on CD-Rom, 2006 Edition.* Philadelphia, PA: Lippincott Williams & Wilkins; 2006. [B] from Gauger EH, Longmuir SQ. *Epicapsular Stars: Ophthalmic Atlas Images.* Eyerounds University of Iowa Health Care Ophthalmology and Visual Sciences website. http://www.eyerounds.org/cases/166-dacryocystocele.htm. Updated March 7, 2013. Accessed October 25, 2016.)

gene-specific cell signaling in a highly ordered sequence of events that is phylogenetically conserved. Much of ocular differentiation occurs through the action of "homeobox" genes and some of the abnormal clinical manifestations that can occur, especially early in the formation of the eye, are caused by mutations of these important regulatory genes. Although the molecular and cellular events that direct the differentiation of the embryonic tissue layers into the formation of the eyes are by their very nature an early and continuous process, we have chosen to place it at the end of this chapter on ocular embryology. The genetics of eye development and the molecular mechanisms that induce differentiation of the ocular structures are highly complex and beyond the scope of this book; however, interested readers are encouraged to seek out excellent review articles, from which some of the figures in this chapter are taken.[131,132]

The structural complexity of the eye is not unique to humans, vertebrate animals, or even multicellular organisms. The eye evolved as a complex sensory organ prior to the development of that portion of the brain which functions to process visual information in higher order species. In fact, the intrinsic retinal circuitry provides a significant amount of information processing before visual

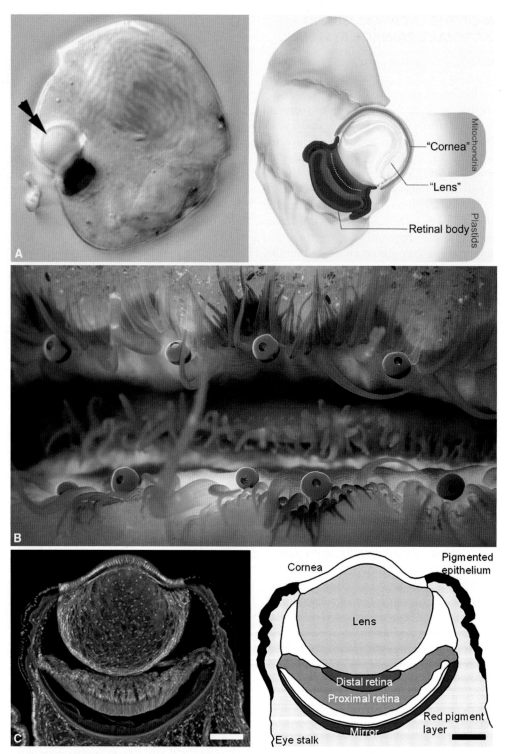

FIGURE 16.53 Phylogenetically primitive but complex eyes. **A:** The ocellus (ocular organ) of a dinoflagellate is comprised of a cornea, lens (*arrow*), and retinal body, which transduce light and provide a form of vision for this unicellular organism. **B:** The eyes of the sea scallop, *Placopecten magellanicus*, are arrayed along the shell mantle margins. **C:** Cross-section of a scallop eye, which contains a cornea, lens, and vitreous, with retina and retinal pigment epithelium in a parabolic configuration. Bar represents 100 μm. ([A], from Gavelis GS, Hayakawa S, White III RA, et al. Eye-like ocelloids are built from different endosymbiotically acquired components. *Nature.* 2015;523(7559):204–207, with permission. [C] from Speiser DI, Loew ER, Johnsen S. Spectral sensitivity of the concave mirror eyes of scallops: potential influences of habitat, self-screening and longitudinal chromatic aberration. *J Exp Biol.* 2011;214(pt 3):422–431.)

signals are even exported to the brain. The finding of highly developed eyes with a lens, vitreous, retina, and pigment is seen from primitive *unicellular* dinoflagellates (in the form of its ocular organelle, the ocellus) to mollusks and many other more primitive species (**Fig. 16.53**).[133,134]

These findings demonstrate that the cellular and molecular processes for making a sophisticated eye are phylogenetically ancient. Over the past two decades, the molecular mechanisms that control the process of development of the eye and CNS have begun to be elucidated. There is a family of master control genes termed homeobox genes that direct the early development of the eye in all species studied. These genes encode key transcription factors (proteins that turn on the expression of other genes) that direct the expression of specific genes that play a critical role in the early patterning and formation of the eye and CNS. The transcription factor products of these homeobox genes target the promoter region and, together with other transcription factor complexes, activate signaling cascades of genes that establish the body axes and formation of the CNS during embryogenesis.[135]

The canonical master control gene for eye (and also brain) development is *Pax6*, a transcription factor that is required to initiate eye development in species from fruit flies to humans.[136,137] Sonic hedgehog (*SHH*) acts indirectly by regulating *Pax6* expression. Mutations in *Pax6* and *SHH* manifest as a spectrum of developmental ocular anomalies, from defective anterior segment morphogenesis in humans (aniridia and Peter's syndrome) to complete absence of formation of ocular structures in the fruit fly ("eyeless") (**Fig. 16.54**).[138] Other genes acting to control early development of the CNS and eye, mutations of which cause anophthalmia and microphthalmia, include *Rx*, *Sox2*, *Mitf*, *Chx10*, and *Six3*.[139–141]

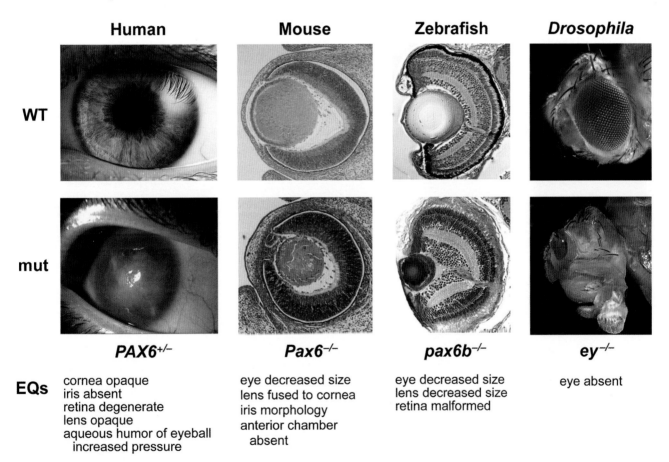

FIGURE 16.54   The canonical master control gene for eye development—Pax6. Pax6 homologue mutations show similar ocular developmental abnormalities across species. Phenotypes of wild-type (WT) **(top)** and PAX6 ortholog mutations (mut) **(bottom)** in human, mouse, zebrafish, and fruit fly can be described with the Entity-Quality (EQ) method. In the EQ method, the affected entity (E) and how it is affected (Q) are recorded using terms from a variety of ontologies. EQ annotations of the abnormal phenotypes are listed below each set of images per organism. These PAX6 phenotypes have been described as follows. Human mutations may result in aniridia (absence of iris), corneal opacity (aniridia-related keratopathy), cataract (lens clouding), glaucoma, and long-term retinal degeneration. For mouse, the mutants exhibit extreme microphthalmia with lens/corneal opacity and iris abnormality, and there is a large plug of persistent epithelial cells that remains attached between the cornea and the lens. For zebrafish, the mutants express a variable and modifiable phenotype that consists of decreased eye size, reduced lens size, and malformation of the retina. Drosophila eye (a PAX6 ortholog mutation) causes loss of eye development. The genotypes shown are E15 mouse Pax614Neu/14Neu, 5-day zebrafish pax6btq253a/tq253a, human PAX6+/−, and Drosophila ey−/−. (From Washington NL, Haendel MA, Mungall CJ, Ashburner M, Westerfield M, Lewis SE—Figure 1 of Washington NL, Haendel MA, Mungall CJ, et al. Linking human diseases to animal models using ontology-based phenotype annotation. *PLoS Biol.* 2009:7(11):e1000247.)

Numerous other transcription factors, plus structural and functional proteins, act later during embryologic development of the eye and play a role in the later formation and function of specific ocular structures. Mutations in these genes are associated with more restricted developmental abnormalities in the target tissues. Examples include *PITX* family, *MAF* family, and *FOX* family genes (in anterior segment dysgenesis syndromes, cataract), crystallin family genes, gap junction connexin and various other membrane proteins (cataract), and many that are restricted to retinal dystrophies and retinal dysfunction, e.g., *RPE65*, *CRX*, and others.[142]

The power of these homeobox genes to direct the formation of the eye across species and as an evolutionary mechanism can be seen in both experimental manipulation of their expression to produce vestigial or accessory organs in various genetic models and in presumed natural variations seen in the wild. A remarkable example of the latter is the spookfish (*Bathylychnops*), which possesses a second completely formed eye that has evolved as a form of parasitic twin conjoined with its primary globe (**Fig. 16.55**). One can imagine how being able to see predators and prey both above and below, simultaneously, might confer a natural selective advantage to a fish possessing such an unusual set of eyes.

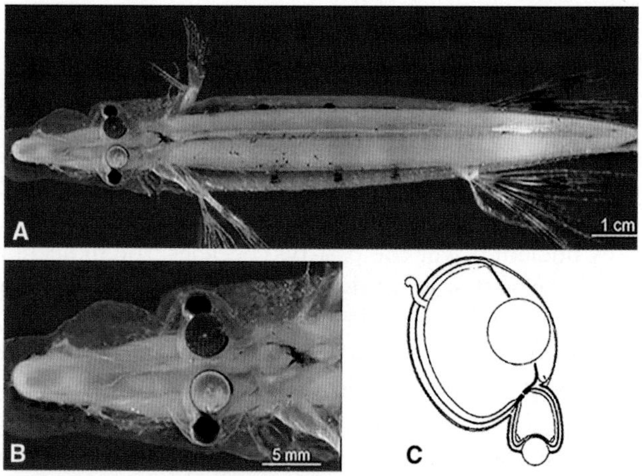

FIGURE 16.55 A remarkable presumptive example of homeobox genes directing the formation of the eye is the spookfish (*Bathylychnops*, **A, B**), which possesses a second, completely formed eye that has evolved as a form of parasitic twin attached to its primary globe. (Courtesy of Hans-Joachim Wagner, Tammy Frank, Harbor Branch Oceanographic Institution, Florida Atlantic University, Boca Raton, FL.) A drawing of the twinned eye in crosssection (**C**). (From Dawkins R. *Climbing Mount Improbable*. New York, NY: W. W. Norton & Company, 1997:19.)

TABLE 16.6 Timeline of Major Events in Ocular Development

Term						
Month	**Week**	**Day**	**Neuroectoderm**	**Surface Ectoderm**	**Neural Crest**	**Mesoderm**
1	3	20	Neural plate thickens—neuroectoderm arises and neurulation forms neural groove	Derived from dorsal epiblast cells (week 3)		Derived from epiblast cells (week 3)
	End of week 3	21–22	Optic sulci appear in forebrain			
	4	24	Neural tube closure in forebrain		Neural crest cells arise	
		25 26	Optic vesicle and stalk formed		Neural crest mesenchyme migrates to surround optic vesicle	Premandibular condensations for EOMs served by CN III arise
		27	Optic vesicle reaches surface ectoderm	Induction of lens placode		Maxillomandibular condensations for lateral recti, served by CN VI arise
2	5	29	Late week 4 or early week 5—invagination of optic cup and optic fissure begin Differentiation of neurosensory retina begins	Invagination of lens placode to lens pit and then lens vesicle begins Primary vitreous formation commences	Hyaloid artery enters optic vesicle through the optic fissure—tunica media and adventitia from neural crest	Maxillomandibular condensations for superior obliques, served by CN IV, arise Hyaloid artery enters optic vesicle through the optic fissure—tunica intima from mesoderm

TABLE 16.6 **Timeline of Major Events in Ocular Development (*continued*)**

Month	Term Week	Day	Neuroectoderm	Surface Ectoderm	Neural Crest	Mesoderm
	5	32–33	Choroidal fissure begins to close Oculomotor nerve present Abducens and Trochlear nerves arrive at target muscles Pigmentation of RPE begins late in week 5 External limiting membrane of retina forming Earliest retinal ganglion cells appear	Lens cup pinches from surface, forming lens vesicle surrounded by basement membrane (lens capsule) Corneal epithelium begins formation Cord of surface ectoderm buried within nasolacrimal groove between frontonasal process and maxillary process of first branchial arch		
	6		Fetal fissure of optic cup closed from midpoint toward pupil and optic nerve early in this week. Cleft of optic stalk still open Inner layer of optic cup exhibits outer nuclear zone and inner, anucleate marginal zone	Primary lens fibers fill lens vesicle forming embryonic nucleus Conjunctival epithelium begins to develop Acellular primordial corneal stroma present	First wave of neural crest invasion begins in anterior segment—establishing plane of corneal endothelium/future Descemet's RPE induces choriocapillaris to form around the optic cup—tunica adventitia from neural crest	RPE induces choriocapillaris to form around the optic cup—tunica intima from mesoderm Earliest signs of Bruch's membrane Tunica intima of anterior tunica vasculosa lentis present
		40	Migration of nuclei into marginal zone. Transient layer of Chievitz appears Inner and outer neuroblastic layers emerge	Secondary lens fibers form Beginning of lid folds present	Bilayered corneal endothelium present First orbital bone formation (ethmoid)	
	7	43–45	Ganglion cells form ganglion cell layer. Amacrine and Müller cells differentiated in inner neuroblastic layer.		Early sclera formation (medial superior and inferior)—progresses anterior to posterior	
	8	46–49	Müller cells produce internal limiting membrane of the retina Ganglion cell axons give rise to nerve fiber layer and axons reach optic stalk, guided by ILM		Lacunae coalescing to form anterior chamber Optic nerve meningeal sheath begins formation	Early temporal sclera formation
	8	50–56	Closure of fetal fissure in optic stalk. Optic stalk cavity obliterated by optic nerve fibers which now reach the thalamus Future bipolar and horizontal cell migration from outer neuroblastic layer Secondary vitreous begins to form	Eyelid fusion begins Primary vitreous complete	Earliest signs of Descemet's membrane Second wave of anterior segment neural crest invasion—early iris stroma/pupillary membrane Vascular beds of the hyaloid artery ramify throughout the primary vitreous—tunica media and adventitia from neural crest	Orbicularis oculi muscle emerges Levator muscle begins delamination from superior rectus Tunica intima of early vessels of iris, including major circle of the iris Vascular beds of the hyaloid artery ramify throughout the primary vitreous—tunica intima from mesoderm

(*continued*)

TABLE 16.6   Timeline of Major Events in Ocular Development (*continued*)

Term			Neuroectoderm	Surface Ectoderm	Neural Crest	Mesoderm
Month	Week	Day				
3	9	57–63	Transient fiber layer of Chievitz disappears, except in macula Earliest indication of inner plexiform layer	Epithelial buds of lacrimal ducts begin to form	Cellular corneal stroma expanding (5–7 layers) Descemet's membrane present (not continuous) Scleral condensation present	Hyaloid vascular system regression begins (mesoderm and neural crest origins)
	10	64–70	Inner segment of photoreceptors appears Rapid growth of anterior optic cup across lens Early pigmentation of iris epithelia	Fusion of eyelids complete Lash follicles begin to form First goblet cells in conjunctiva	Tenon's capsule evident Acini of lacrimal gland begin to form around ducts	Fusion of EOMs with sclera Delamination of levator palpebrae superioris from superior rectus completed
	11	71–77	Cilia within developing inner segments Approximately 1.9 million axons in developing optic nerve		Corneal endothelium single layer	
	12	78–90	Outer plexiform layer separates horizontal and bipolar nuclei from rudimentary rods and cones Synapses develop between photoreceptors, ganglion cells, and bipolar cells in central retina First indication of ciliary processes Secondary vitreous complete	Proliferation of nasolacrimal cords Marginal bundle of Druault/vitreous base present	Earliest indications of trabecular meshwork formation Sclera reaches optic nerve	Rectus muscle tendons fuse with sclera
4			Cell division in developing retina ceases Emergence of sphincter pupillae muscle Tight junctions in ciliary epithelium Aqueous humor production begins Tertiary vitreous begins to form Approximately 3.7 million axons in developing optic nerve	Meibomian glands developed Lash follicles develop along with Glands of Zeis and Moll Canalization of nasolacrimal system begins	Early differentiation of trabecular meshwork Corneal endothelial tight junctions and continuous Descemet's membrane formed Choroidal stroma, plus tunica media and adventitia of choroidal vessels—Haller's layer of the choroid develops Scleral spur and ciliary muscle arise and are connected	Tight junctions in iris blood vessels Early vascularization of the sensory retina begins from resorbing hyaloid system (tunica intima from mesoderm)
5			Pigmentation of iris epithelia complete Differentiation of dilator pupillae myofilaments Pars plana arises Cone outer segment formation Earliest signs of macula Branches of CN V reach corneal epithelium Optic nerve axons reduced to approximately 1.1 million	Eyelids begin to reopen Eyelashes present	Bowman's layer fully formed Cloquet's canal evident Choroidal layers complete, including Sattler's layer Schlemm's canal present	Canalization of retinal vessels begins
6			Full differentiation of dilator muscle		Resorption of pupillary membrane begins	Canalization of retinal vessels completed

TABLE 16.6   Timeline of Major Events in Ocular Development (*continued*)

Term			Neuroectoderm	Surface Ectoderm	Neural Crest	Mesoderm
Month	Week	Day				
7			Rod outer segment formation begins Foveal pit visible Complete disappearance of transient layer of Chievitz	Canalization of nasolacrimal system completed Completion of lid separation	Myelination optic nerve begins at chiasm Lamina cribrosa formation complete Hyaloid arterial system regression typically complete Completion of orbital bones late in the 7th month Iris stromal and uveal pigmentation Maturation of ciliary muscle fibers	
8			Adult number of axons in optic nerve		Complete resorption of pupillary membrane	Retina fully vascularized nasally (mesoderm and neural crest)
9				Nasolacrimal drainage system fully open	Completion of myelination of optic nerve to lamina cribrosa	Early in the 9th month, retinal vessels complete terminal arcades in periphery

It is important to appreciate that these times represent a consensus from numerous sources that differ slightly. Some sources use days, some use crown-rump length, etc., and the conversions between them are not all the same. Complicating these times further, some of the data are based upon sources that have projected from nonhuman species to equivalent times in human development.

EOM, extraocular muscle; CN, cranial nerve; RPE, retinal pigment epithelium; ILM, internal limiting membrane.

REFERENCES

1. Mann I. *The Development of the Human Eye.* 3rd ed. New York, NY: Grune & Stratton; 1969.
2. Oyster CW. *The Human Eye: Structure and Function.* Sunderland, MA: Sinauer Associates; 1999.
3. Cvekl A, Tamm ER. Anterior eye development and ocular mesenchyme: New insights from mouse models and human diseases. *Bioessays.* 2004;26(4):374–386.
4. Gould DB, Smith RS, John SW. Anterior segment development relevant to glaucoma. *Int J Dev Biol.* 2004:48(8–9):1015–1029.
5. Sadler T. Embryology of neural tube development. *Am J Med Genet C Semin Med Gene.* 2005;135(1):2–8.
6. O'Rahilly R. The early development of the eye in staged human embryos. *Contrib Embryol.* 1966:38:1.
7. Bartelmez GW. The formation of neural crest from the primary optic vesicle in man. *Contrib Embryol.* 1954;35:55–71.
8. Meier S. The distribution of cranial neural crest cells during ocular morphogenesis. *Prog Clin Biol Res.* 1982;82:1–15.
9. Cook C, Sulik K, Wright K. Embryology. In: Wright KW, Spiegel PH, Hengst T, eds. *Pediatric Ophthalmology and Strabismus.* St Louis, MO: Springer Science & Business Media; 2013:1–61.
10. Barber A. *Embryology of the Human Eye.* St Louis, MO: Mosby; 1955.
11. Torczynski E, Jacobiec FA, Johnston MC, et al. Synophthalmia and cyclopia: a histopathologic, radiographic, and organogenetic analysis. *Doc Ophthalmol.* 1977;44(2):311–378.
12. Schook P. A review of data on cell actions and cell interaction during the morphogenesis of the embryonic eye. *Acta Morphol Neerl Scand.* 1978;16(4):267–286.
13. Hollenberg MJ, Spira AW. Early development of the human retina. *Can J Ophthalmol.* 1972;7(4):472–491.
14. Acers TE. *Congenital Abnormalities of the Optic Nerve and Related Forebrain.* Philadelphia, PA: Lea & Febiger; 1983.
15. Tamura T, Smelser GK. Development of the sphincter and dilator muscles of the iris. *Arch Ophthalmol.* 1973;89(4):332–339.
16. Naumann G, Green WR. Spontaneous nonpigmented iris cysts. *Arch Ophthalmol.* 1967;78:496–500.
17. Cook CS. Embryogenesis of congenital eye malformations. *Vet Comp Ophthalmol (USA).* 1995;5(2):109–123.
18. Graw J. Genetic aspects of embryonic eye development in vertebrates. *Dev Genet.* 1996;18:181–197.
19. Anderson DR. The development of the trabecular meshwork and its abnormality in primary infantile glaucoma. *Trans Am Ophthalmol Soc.* 1981;79:458–485.
20. Cook CS. Experimental models of anterior segment dysgenesis. *Ophthalmic Paediatr Genet.* 1989;10(1):33–46.
21. Moore MH, Aniridia A. In Pagon RA, Adam MP, Ardinger HH, et al (eds.). *GeneReviews.* Seattle, WA:University of Washington; 2013; 1–61. Online journal.
22. Stenkamp DL. Development of the vertebrate eye and retina. *Prog Mol Biol Transl Sci.* 2015;134:397–414.
23. Brachet J. *Advances in Morphogenesis.* New York, NY: Academic Press Inc; 1961.
24. Smelser GK, Ozanics V, Rayborn M, et al. The fine structure of the retinal transient layer of chievitz. *Invest Ophthalmol Vis Sci.* 1973;12(7):504–512.
25. Keefe J, Ordy J, Samorajski T. Prenatal development of the retina in a diurnal primate (macaca mulatta). *Anat Rec.* 1966;154(4):759–783.
26. Fuhrmann S. Eye morphogenesis and patterning of the optic vesicle. *Curr Top Dev Biol.* 2010;93:61–84.
27. Stuermer CAO, Bastmeyer M. The retinal axon's pathfinding to the optic disk. *Prog Neurobiol.* 2000;62:197–214.
28. Shatz CJ. Emergence of order in visual system development. *Proc Natl Acad Sci USA.* 1996;3(2):602–608.
29. Wong ROL. Retinal waves and visual system development. *Annu Rev Neurosci.* 1999;22:29–47.

30. Barishak YR. *Embryology of the Eye and Its Adnexa*. Basel, Switzerland: Karger; 2001.

31. Cepko C. Intrinsically different retinal progenitor cells produce specific types of progeny. *Nat Rev Neurosci*. 2014;15(9):615–627.

32. Cepko CL, Austin CP, Yang X, et al. Cell fate determination in the vertebrate retina. *Proc Natl Acad Sci USA*. 1996;93(2):589–595.

33. Lamb TD. Evolution of phototransduction, vertebrate photoreceptors and retina. *Prog Retin Eye Res*. 2013;36:52–119.

34. Arendt D. Evolution of eyes and photoreceptor cell types. *Int J Dev Biol*. 2003;47(7/8):563–572.

35. Cayouette M, Barres BA, Raff M. Importance of intrinsic mechanisms in cell fate decisions in the developing rat retina. *Neuron*. 2003;40(5):897–904.

36. Livesey FJ, Young TL, Cepko CL. An analysis of the gene expression program of mammalian neural progenitor cells. *Proc Natl Acad Sci USA*. 2004;101(5):1374–1379.

37. Watanabe T, Raff MC. Diffusible rod-promoting signals in the developing rat retina. *Development*. 1992;114(4):899–906.

38. Johnston RJ Jr, Desplan C. Stochastic mechanisms of cell fate specification that yield random or robust outcomes. *Annu Rev Cell Dev Biol*. 2010;26:689–719.

39. Bhattacharjee J, Sanyal S. Developmental origin and early differentiation of retinal Müller cells in mice. *J Anat*. 1975;120(pt 2):367–372.

40. Karkinen-Jaaskelainen M. Permissive and directive interactions in lens induction. *J Embryol Exp Morphol*. 1978;44:167–179.

41. Mund ML, Rodrigues MM, Fine BS. Light and electron microscopic observations on the pigmented layers of the developing human eye. *Am J Ophthalmol*. 1972;73(2):167–182.

42. Grainger RM, Herry JJ, Henderson RA. Reinvestigation of the role of the optic vesicle in embryonic lens induction. *Development*. 1988;102(3):517–526.

43. Smelser GK. Embryology and morphology of the lens. *Invest Ophthalmol Vis Sci*. 1965;4(4):398–410.

44. Parmigiani CM, McAvoy JW. The roles of laminin and fibronectin in the development of the lens capsule. *Curr Eye Res*. 1991;10:501–511.

45. Woerdeman M. The differentiation of the crystalline lens. *Development*. 1953;1(3):301–305.

46. Beebe DC, Compart PJ, Johnson MC, et al. The mechanism of cell elongation during lens fiber cell differentiation. *Dev Biol*. 1982;92(1):54–59.

47. Hendrix R, Zwaan J. Cell shape regulation and cell cycle in embryonic lens cells. *Nature*. 1974;247:145–147.

48. Zwaan J. Fine structure of the developing lens. *Int Ophthalmol Clin*. 1975;15(1):39–52.

49. Kuwabara T. The maturation of the lens cell: a morphologic study. *Exp Eye Res*. 1975;20(5):427–443.

50. Mutlu F, Leopold IH. The structure of fetal hyaloid system and tunica vasculosa lentis. *Arch Ophthalmol*. 1964;71(1):102–110.

51. Bastola P, Joshi SN, Chaudhary M, et al. Alport's syndrome. *KUMJ*. 2010;8(30):238–240.

52. Jack RL. Regression of the hyaloid vascular system: an ultrastructural analysis. *Am J Ophthalmol*. 1972;74(2):261–272.

53. Balazs EA. Fine structure of the developing vitreous. *Int Ophthalmol Clin*. 1975;15(1):53–63.

54. Balazs E, Toth L, Ozanics V. Cytological studies on the developing vitreous as related to the hyaloid vessel system. *Albrecht Von Graefes Arch Klin Exp Ophthalmol*. 1980;213(2):71–85.

55. Hogan MJ, Alvarado JA, Weddell J. *Histology of the Human Eye: An Atlas and Textbook*. Philadelphia, PA: Saunders; 1971.

56. Genis-Galvez J. Role of the lens in the morphogenesis of the iris and cornea. *Nature*. 1966;210:209–210.

57. Byun TH, Kim JT, Park HW, et al. Timetable for upper eyelid development in staged human embryos and fetuses. *Anat Rec*. 2011;294(5):789–796.

58. Sevel D. A reappraisal of the development of the eyelids. *Eye*. 1988;2:123–129.

59. Meng Q, Mongan M, Carreira V, et al. Eyelid closure in embryogenesis is required for ocular adnexa development. *Invest Ophthalmol Vis Sci*. 2014;55(11):7652–7661.

60. Jakobiec F, Iwamoto T. Ocular adnexae: introduction to lids, conjunctiva, and orbit. In: Jakobiec FA, ed. *Ocular Anatomy, Embryology, and Teratology*. Philadelphia, PA: Harpercollins; 1982.

61. Hurwitz JJ. Embryology of the lacrimal drainage system. In: Hurwitz JJ, ed. *The Lacrimal System*. Philadelphia, PA: Lippincott-Raven; 1996:9–13.

62. Sevel D. Development and congenital abnormalities of the nasolacrimal apparatus. *J Pediatr Ophthalmol Strabismus*. 1981;18(5):13–19.

63. Cook CS, Ozanics V, Jakobiec FA. Prenatal development of the eye and its adnexa. In: Tasman W, Jaeger EA, eds. *Duane's Foundations of Ophthalmology on CD-ROM*. Philadelphia, PA: Lippincott; 2006:chap 2.

64. Zinn KM, Mockel-Pohl S. Fine structure of the developing cornea. *Int Ophthalmol Clin*. 1975;15(1):19–37.

65. Pei Y, Rhodin J. Electron microscopic study of the development of the mouse corneal epithelium. *Invest Ophthalmol Vis Sci*. 1971;10(11):811–825.

66. Hay ED. Development of the vertebrate cornea. *Int Rev Cytol*. 1980;63:263–322.

67. Berry FB, Lines MA, Oas JM, et al. Functional interactions between FOXC1 and PITX2 underlie the sensitivity to FOXC1 gene dose in Axenfeld-Rieger syndrome and anterior segment dysgenesis. *Hum Mol Genet*. 2006;15(6):905–919.

68. Ito M, Yoshioka M. Regression of the hyaloid vessels and pupillary membrane of the mouse. *Anat Embryol*. 1999;200(4):403–411.

69. Matsuo N, Smelser GK. Electron microscopic studies on the pupillary membrane: the fine structure of the white strands of the disappearing stage of this membrane. *Invest Ophthalmol Vis Sci*. 1971;10(2):108–119.

70. Wulle KG. Electron microscopic observations of the development of Schlemm's canal in the human eye. *Trans Am Acad Ophthalmol Otolaryngol*. 1968;72(5):765–773.

71. Reme C, d'Epinay SL. Periods of development of the normal human chamber angle. *Doc Ophthalmol*. 1981;51(3):241–268.

72. Meghpara B, Li X, Nakamura H, et al. Human anterior chamber angle development without cell death or macrophage involvement. *Mol Vis*. 2008;14:2492–2498.

73. Barkan O. Pathogenesis of congenital glaucoma: gonioscopic and anatomic observation of the angle of the anterior chamber in the normal eye and in congenital glaucoma. *Am J Ophthalmol*. 1955;40:1–11.

74. Tawara A, Inomata H. Developmental immaturity of the trabecular meshwork in congenital glaucoma. *Am J Ophthalmol*. 1981;92(4):508–525.

75. deLuise VP, Anderson DR. Primary infantile glaucoma (congenital glaucoma). *Surv Ophthalmol*. 1983;28(1):1–19.

76. McMenamin PG. A morphological study of the inner surface of the anterior chamber angle in pre and postnatal human eyes. *Curr Eye Res*. 1989;8(7):727–739.

77. Wulle K. Development of productive and draining system of the aqueous humor in human eye-light and electron-microscopic study on formation and beginning of function of ciliary processes, trabecular meshwork and Schlemm's canal. *Adv Ophthalmol*. 1972;26:296.

78. Bard JB, Ross AS. The morphogenesis of the ciliary body of the avian eye: I. Lateral cell detachment facilitates epithelial folding. *Dev Biol*. 1982;92(1):73–86.

79. Heimann K. The development of the choroid in man. *Ophthalmic Res*. 1972;3(5):257–273.

80. Ozanics V, Rayborn M, Sagun D. Observations of the ultrastructure of the developing primate choroid coat. *Exp Eye Res*. 1978;26(1):25–45.

81. Berson D. The development of the choroid and sclera in the eye of the foetal rat with particular reference to their developmental interrelationship. *Exp Eye Res*. 1965;4(2):102IN3–103IN9.

82. Takei Y, Ozanics V. Origin and development of Bruch's membrane in monkey fetuses: an electron microscopic study. *Invest Ophthalmol Vis Sci.* 1975;14(12):903–916.

83. Sellheyer K. Development of the choroid and related structures. *Eye.* 1990;4:255–261.

84. Ozanics V, Rayborn M, Sagun D. Some aspects of corneal and scleral differentiation in the primate. *Exp Eye Res.* 1976;22(4):305–327.

85. Sellheyer K, Spitznas M. Development of the human sclera. A morphological study. *Graefe's Arch Clin Exp Ophthalmol.* 1988;226:89–100.

86. Sainz De La Maza M, Foster CS. Chapter 23—Sclera. In: Tasman W, Jaeger EA, eds. *Duane's Foundations of Clinical Ophthalmology. Vol. 1, Ocular Anatomy, Embryology, and Teratology.* Philadelphia, PA: Lippincott; 1994.

87. Zhang Y, Wildsoet CF. RPE and choroid mechanisms underlying ocular growth and myopia. *Prog Mol Biol Transl Sci.* 2015;134:221–240.

88. Meier SP. The development of segmentation in the cranial region of vertebrate embryos. *Scan Electron Microsc.* 1982;(pt 3):1269–1282.

89. Gilbert P. *The Origin and Development of the Human Extrinsic Ocular Muscles.* Vol 246. 59th ed. Baltimore, MA: Carnegie Institution of Washington Publication; 1957.

90. Noden DM. The role of the neural crest in patterning of avian cranial skeletal, connective, and muscle tissues. *Dev Biol.* 1983;96(1):144–165.

91. Jacobson AG. Somitomeres: mesodermal segments of vertebrate embryos. *Development.* 1988;104(suppl):209–220.

92. Sevel D. The origins and insertions of the extraocular muscles: development, histologic features, and clinical significance. *Trans Am Ophthalmol Soc.* 1986;84:488–526.

93. Sevel D. A reappraisal of the origin of human extraocular muscles. *Ophthalmology.* 1981;88(12):1330–1338.

94. Porter J, Baker R. Prenatal morphogenesis of primate extraocular muscle: neuromuscular junction formation and fiber type differentiation. *Invest Ophthalmol Vis Sci.* 1992;33(3):657–670.

95. Sohal G, Holt R. Role of innervation on the embryonic development of skeletal muscle. *Cell Tissue Res.* 1980;210(3):383–393.

96. Fink WH. The development of the extrinsic muscles of the eye. *Am J Ophthalmol.* 1953:36:10–23.

97. Smelser G, Ozanics V. Morphological and functional development of the cornea. In: Duke-Elder S, Perkins ES, eds. *The Transparency of the Cornea.* Oxford, UK: Blackwell Scientific; 1960:23.

98. Smelser GK, Ozanics V. The development of the trabecular meshwork in primate eyes. *Am J Ophthalmol.* 1971;71(1):366–385.

99. Kupfer C, Ross K. The development of outflow facility in human eyes. *Invest Ophthalmol Vis Sci.* 1971;10(7):513–517.

100. Pandolfi M, Åstedt B. Outflow resistance in the foetal eye. *Acta Ophthalmol.* 1971;49(2):344–350.

101. Gong H, Tripathi RC, Tripathi BJ. Morphology of the aqueous outflow pathway. *Microsc Res Tech.* 1996;33:336–367.

102. Hansson H, Jerndal T. Scanning electron microscopic studies on the development of the iridocorneal angle in human eyes. *Invest Ophthalmol Vis Sci.* 1971;10(4):252–265.

103. Kwon YH, Fingert JH, Kuehn MH, et al. Primary open-angle glaucoma. *N Engl J Med.* 2009;360:1113–1124.

104. Ramos RF, Hoying JB, Witte MH, et al. Schlemm's canal endothelia, lymphatic, or blood vasculature? *J Glaucoma.* 2007;16:391–405.

105. Hamanaka T, Bill A, Ichinohasama R, et al. Aspects of the development of Schlemm's canal. *Exp Eye Res.* 1992;55:479–488.

106. Kizhatil K, Ryan M, Marchant JK, et al. Schlemm's canal is a unique vessel with a combination of blood vascular and lymphatic phenotypes that forms by a novel developmental process. *PLoS Biol.* 2014;12:e1001912. doi:10.1371/journal.pbio.1001912.

107. Keener AB. Rethinking lymphatic development. *The Scientist.* August 1, 2015.

108. Dvorak-Theobald G. Further studies on the canal of Schlemm; its anastomoses and anatomic relations. *Am J Ophthalmol.* 1955;39(4 Pt 2):65–89.

109. Ramírez JM, Ramírez AI, Salazar JJ, et al. Schlemm's canal and the collector channels at different developmental stages in the human eye. *Cells Tissues Organs.* 2004;178:180–185.

110. Sugiura T, Mizokami K, Yamamoto M. The development of the Schlemm's canal in human eyes [in Japanese]. *Nippon Ganka Gakkai Zasshi.* 1991;95:650–656.

111. Sang D. Embryology of the vitreous. Congenital and developmental abnormalities. In: Schepens CL, Neetens A, eds. *The Vitreous and Vitreoretinal Interface.* New York, NY: Springer; 1987:11–35.

112. Martin AC, Thornton JD, Liu J, et al. Pathogenesis of persistent hyperplastic primary vitreous in mice lacking the arf tumor suppressor gene. *Invest Ophthalmol Vis Sci.* 2004;45(10):3387–3396.

113. Chaum E, Kerr N, Kaste S, et al. A 5 year old girl who failed her school vision screening. *Digit J Ophthalmol.* 2004;10(5). http://www.djo.harvard.edu/site.php?url=/physicians/gr/615&page=GR_HY. Accessed February 6, 2017.

114. Hollenberg MJ, Spira AW. Human retinal development: ultrastructure of the outer retina. *Am J Anat.* 1973;137(4):357–385.

115. Maldonado RS, O'Connell RV, Sarin N, et al. Dynamics of human foveal development after premature birth. *Ophthalmology.* 2011;118(12):2315–2325.

116. Weidman TA. Fine structure of the developing retina. *Int Ophthalmol Clin.* 1975;15(1):65–84.

117. Yuodelis C, Hendrickson A. A qualitative and quantitative analysis of the human fovea during development. *Vision Res.* 1986;26(6):847–855.

118. Provis JM, Dubis AM, Maddess T, et al. Adaptation of the central retina for high acuity vision: cones, the fovea and the avascular zone. *Prog Retin Eye Res.* 2013;35:63–81.

119. Cogan D. Development and senescence of the human retinal vasculature. *Trans Ophthalmol Soc U K.* 1963;83:465–489.

120. Shakib M, De Oliveira LF, Henkind P. Development of retinal vessels. II. Earliest stages of vessel formation. *Invest Ophthalmol Vis Sci.* 1968;7(6):689–700.

121. Wise G, Dollery C, Henkind P. *The Retinal Circulation.* New York, NY: Harper & Row; 1971.

122. Engerman RL. Development of the macular circulation. *Invest Ophthalmol Vis Sci.* 1976;15(10):835–840.

123. Mutlu F, Leopold IH. The structure of retinal vascular system of the human fetus eye. *Arch Ophthalmol.* 1964;71(4):531–536.

124. Ashton N. Retinal angiogenesis in the human embryo. *Br Med Bull.* 1970;26(2):103–106.

125. Ashton N. Oxygen and the growth and development of retinal vessels: in vivo and in vitro studies: the XX Francis I. Proctor lecture. *Am J Ophthalmol.* 1966;62(3):412–435.

126. Terry TL. Extreme prematurity and fibroblastic overgrowth of persistent vascular sheath behind each crystalline lens: I. Preliminary report. *Am J Ophthalmol.* 1942;25(2):203–204.

127. Ashton N, Ward B, Serpell G. Effect of oxygen on developing retinal vessels with particular reference to the problem of retrolental fibroplasia. *Br J Ophthalmol.* 1954;38(7):397–432.

128. Kanazawa S. Electron microscopic study of the human fetal optic nerve. *Nippon Ganka Gakkai Zasshi.* 1969;73(8):1330–1353.

129. Silver J, Hughes A. The role of cell death during morphogenesis of the mammalian eye. *J Morphol.* 1973;140(2):159–170.

130. Sturrock RR. A light and electron microscopic study of proliferation and maturation of fibrous astrocytes in the optic nerve of the human embryo. *J Anat.* 1975;119(pt 2):223–234.

131. Gehring WJ. The genetic control of eye development and its implications for the evolution of the various eye-types. *Int J Dev Biol.* 2002;46(1):65–74.

132. Graw J. The genetic and molecular basis of congenital eye defects. *Nat Rev Genet.* 2003;4(11):876–888.

133. Gavelis GS, Hayakawa S, White III RA, et al. Eye-like ocelloids are built from different endosymbiotically acquired components. *Nature.* 2015;523(7559):204–207.

134. Speiser DI, Loew ER, Johnsen S. Spectral sensitivity of the concave mirror eyes of scallops: potential influences of habitat, self-screening and longitudinal chromatic aberration. *J Exp Biol.* 2011;214(pt 3):422–431.

135. Gehring WJ. The homeobox in perspective. *Trends Biochem Sci.* 1992;17(8):277–280.

136. van Heyningen V, Williamson KA. PAX6 in sensory development. *Hum Mol Genet.* 2002;11(10):1161–1167.

137. Xu PX, Zhang X, Heaney S, et al. Regulation of Pax6 expression is conserved between mice and flies. *Development.* 1999;126(2):383–395.

138. Washington NL, Haendel MA, Mungall CJ, et al. Linking human diseases to animal models using ontology-based phenotype annotation. *PLoS Biol.* 2009;7(11):e1000247.

139. Mathers PH, Grinberg A, Mahon KA, et al. The Rx homeobox gene is essential for vertebrate eye development. *Nature.* 1997;387(6633):603–607.

140. Wallis DE, Roessler E, Hehr U, et al. Mutations in the homeodomain of the human SIX3 gene cause holoprosencephaly. *Nat Genet.* 1999;22(2):196–198.

141. Fantes J, Ragge NK, Lynch S, et al. Mutations in SOX2 cause anophthalmia. *Nat Genet.* 2003;33(4):462–463.

142. Fazzi E, Signorini SG, Scelsa B, et al. Leber's congenital amaurosis: an update. *Eur J Paediatr Neurol.* 2003;7(1):13–22.

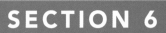

OCULAR ANATOMY BY OPTICAL COHERENCE TOMOGRAPHY

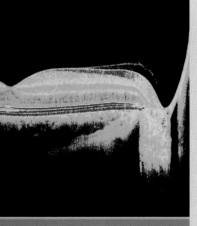

Ocular Anatomy by Optical Coherence Tomography

CHAPTER 17

General Principles of Optical Coherence Tomography (OCT)

Optical coherence tomography (OCT) is a technology that uses the echo time delay of light to uncover cross-sectional tissue structure.[1-4] Its incorporation into the field of eye care has augmented the clinician's ability to resolve anatomic features of the eye, at the histologic level, in everyday practice. OCT is a technology analogous to ultrasound that images tissue with depth. Whereas ultrasound uses acoustic waves with frequencies of several megahertz,[5] OCT records backscattered near-infrared light to infer optical properties of underlying tissue. Although this permits a ~10- to 100-fold resolution improvement over ultrasound, imaging is restricted to superficial features, with depths up to a few millimeters (though endoscopes and other tools allow for the imaging of internal structures from accessible surfaces). These features have made this technology ideal for ocular imaging, and so it becomes imperative that the clinician be able to appreciate the anatomy and histology of ocular tissues as seen using this technology.

The basic apparatus used in OCT is a Michelson interferometer, which consists of a light source, a sample arm, a reference arm, and a detector (**Fig. 17.1**). Unlike a traditional Michelson interferometer, the light source used in OCT is not a laser and is only partially coherent, meaning interference occurs only at the detector when the path length difference between the two arms of the interferometer is short: less than a distance termed "the coherence length." The coherence length represents the resolution depth of OCT and is typically a few microns. This is accomplished with a broad-spectrum light source (such as a superluminescent diode). The light from the source is divided into the two component beams using a beam splitter or partially reflecting mirror. One beam is directed toward the tissue of interest, while the other is sent along a reference arm pathway, where it travels a set distance before reflecting off a mirror and retracing its path. The back-reflected or backscattered light from the tissue of interest is collected and recombined with light from the reference arm. The resulting interference pattern is recorded at the detector. This is used to glean information about the depth reflectivity profile of the tissue probed by the sample arm.

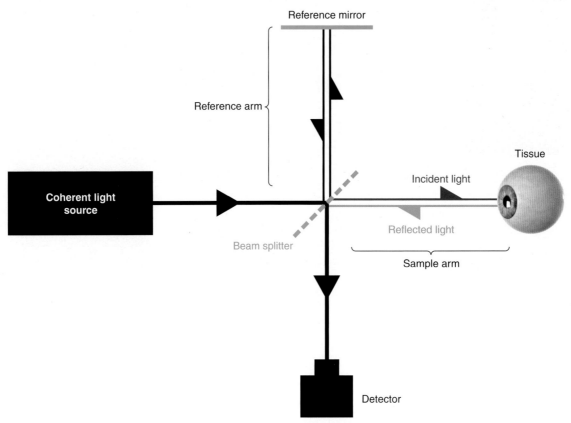

FIGURE 17.1   Diagram of Michelson interferometer apparatus used for OCT. Light for imaging originates at a low-coherence source and is divided into two beams with a beam splitter. One beam is directed toward the tissue sample, and the remaining light is sent toward a reference mirror. After reflection/backscattering, the beams are recombined and interference is recorded at a photodetector element.

Although clinicians use OCT to infer information about the health of imaged tissue, OCT merely records the optical properties of the tissue in question. Light passing through any medium is either absorbed or transmitted or scattered.[6,7] Absorption occurs when the energy of incident light equals transitional energies for component chromophores in the tissue. Because water has an absorption spectrum as well, the wavelength of light used for OCT is chosen such that minimal water absorption occurs en route to the region of interest. The incident beam of the sample arm is attenuated by absorption and scattering while traveling through the eye. Transmitted light propagates until it is absorbed or scattered deeper in the tissue. Eventually, some of the light is back-reflected or backscattered by structures along the optical path. The returning light is further attenuated, and only a small portion is eventually collected for measurement.

Incident light focused onto the retina traverses a vertical column measuring the reflectivity of structures at different depths. This is referred to as an A-scan. Repeating A-scans in a transverse sweep across the tissue is used to compile a cross-sectional image of tissue structure. These compilations are termed "B-scans." By taking a series of adjacent B-scans, a full 3D tissue volume may be rendered, permitting in vivo qualitative and quantitative analysis of tissue architecture. From the 3D data cube, the structure

at a particular coronal plane (i.e., the photoreceptors, choroid, etc.) can be digitally isolated in postprocessing, and this is termed "C-mode" (**Fig. 17.2**). Depending on the region of interest, any one of these scanning modes can be used to evaluate the health of the tissue.

There are two principal variants of OCT, time domain (TD) and Fourier or spectral domain (SD). In TD-OCT, the length of the reference arm is mechanically adjusted to sample the tissue at different depths. Conversely, SD-OCT has a fixed reference mirror and makes use of a Fourier transform to demodulate the depth reflectivity profile. The stationary mirror makes SD-OCT significantly faster with higher resolution than TD-OCT, and thus it is currently used in a majority of clinical devices. A third type of OCT, swept source OCT (SS-OCT), has more recently been implemented in experimental and clinical devices. It operates on the same premise as SD-OCT, but whereas SD-OCT uses a broad-spectrum light source, SS-OCT has a tunable, narrow bandwidth light source that sweeps through a range of frequencies. These systems also differ on the detection side; SD-OCT utilizes a spectrometer and a camera to detect the interference pattern from reflected tissue, whereas SS-OCT has a single detector, which picks up interference fringes as a function of time. SS-OCT has the added advantage of deeper penetration and thus is used to visualize deeper posterior structures.

OCT Device Evolution

OCT was developed in 1991 and produced the first ever seen noninvasive, in vivo, near-histologic level cross-sectional images of the retina. The Massachusetts Institute of Technology (MIT) prototype was introduced to the clinic in 1994, and the first commercial device was launched in 1996 with a rapid evolution of new devices that followed. Each iterative device had a demonstrable improvement in scan speed with resulting higher resolution. A major generational leap took place in 2006 with the development of SD-OCT. The emergent properties of the higher speed and resolution allowed for topographical mapping, microstructural identification, 3D image rendering, and the capability to evaluate flow of fluid. It is imperative to understand that direct comparisons for clinical decisions should not be made between different generations of OCT devices.

The clinician should refrain from making assessments of disease progression when comparing longitudinal changes across generations of devices. However, in the absence of other objective data, prior generation images can give the clinician an overall impression of the disease state at that point in time.

OCT Clinical Acumen and Sources of Misinterpretation

Diagnostic and treatment decisions are now routinely made on the basis of OCT scans. OCT interpretation requires understanding artifacts and sources of misinterpretation that can mislead the clinician.

1. Media opacities - Since OCT utilizes light waves, any interfering opacity can hinder optimal imaging.

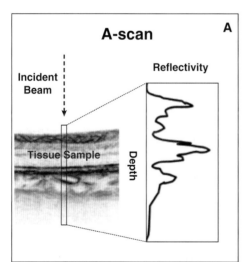

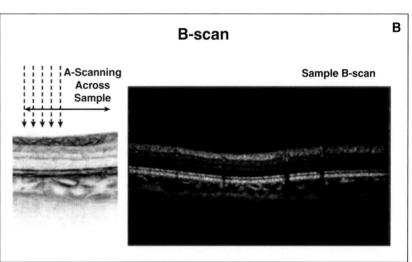

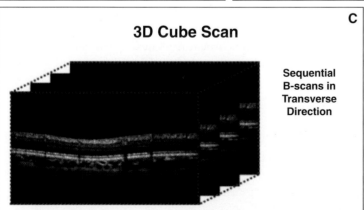

FIGURE 17.2 Using OCT, the reflectivity of ocular tissue can be measured as a function of depth. In a single location this is termed an "A-scan" **(A)**, and by taking sequential A-scans in a horizontal sweep of the tissue, a cross section or B-scan can be formed **(B)**. Compiling multiple, adjacent B-scans permits a 3D view (cube scan) of tissue structure **(C)**.

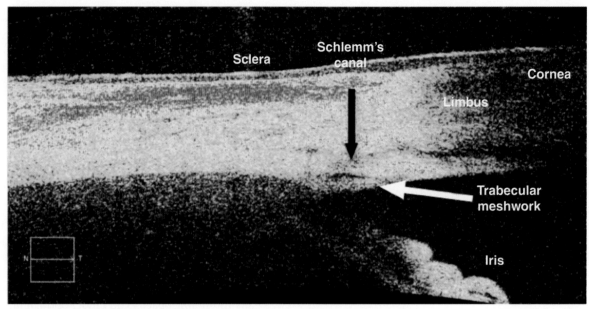

FIGURE 17.3   False-color OCT image of the anterior chamber angle. Schlemm's canal is the dark, horizontal slit below the tip of the black arrow. (Obtained with Cirrus HD-OCT; Carl Zeiss Meditec, Dublin, CA, USA.)

As such, OCT is limited in the setting of corneal opacities, dense cataracts, and vitreous hemorrhage.

2. Signal quality - Once a scan is acquired, it is critical to assess the adequacy by reviewing the signal strength before making clinical judgments. Every device has a standard acceptable and best quality indicator.

3. Blink and saccades - Eye movement can interfere with scan alignment and result in missing data that are represented by black on the image printout.

4. Segmentation error - OCT software can quantify tissue thickness with image segmentation algorithms by detecting tissue boundaries and measuring the distance between respective end points. It is important to assess that the automated segmentation protocol is detecting the appropriate boundaries for clinically meaningful measurements.

OCT Ocular Anatomy and Histology

OCT can visualize the anterior and posterior segments of the eye. Anteriorly, OCT can identify the cornea, sclera, iris, trabecular meshwork, Schlemm's canal, and the corneoscleral limbus (**Fig. 17.3**). Posteriorly, the macula, peripapillary retina, and optic nerve head (ONH) region can be visualized at what amounts to the histologic level (**Fig. 17.4**).

ANTERIOR SEGMENT OCT

Clinically relevant parameters can be quantitatively assessed from anterior segment OCT (ASOCT) images, including corneal thickness and curvature as well as anterior chamber depth and thickness. Using higher resolution OCT imaging of the cornea, it is possible to distinguish the epithelium, Bowman's layer, the stroma, Descemet's membrane, and the endothelium (**Fig. 17.5**). ASOCT can be used to detect and measure anterior and posterior corneal boundaries and curvature on cross-sectional images. Based on this imaging data, corneal maps are created, and an automated software algorithm measures the corneal thickness (pachymetry) and curvature (keratometry) (**Fig. 17.6**).

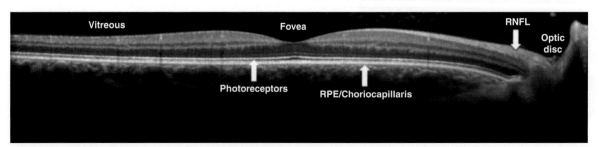

FIGURE 17.4   OCT image of papillomacular region. RNFL, retinal nerve fiber layer; RPE, retinal pigment epithelium. (Obtained with Spectralis HRA+OCT; Heidelberg Engineering, Heidelberg, Germany.)

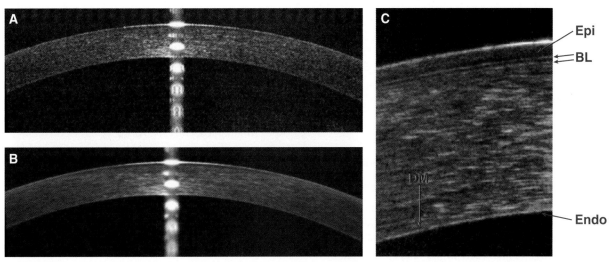

FIGURE 17.5 High-definition OCT image of normal human cornea. **A:** Single frame. **B:** Average of 16 registered frames. **C:** Enlarged section of the frame-averaged image labeling epithelium (Epi). Bowman's layer (BL), Descemet's membrane (DM); and endothelium (Endo).

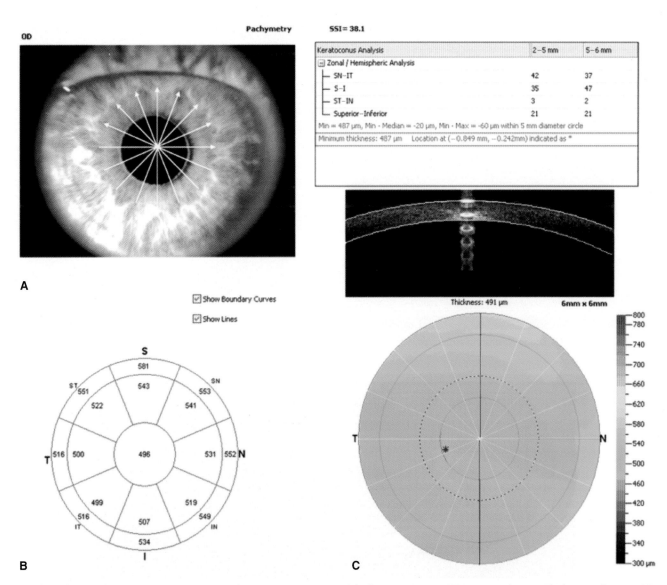

FIGURE 17.6 Pachymetry scan pattern **(A)** and sector average corneal thickness in microns **(B)** in scanned areas. Thickness color map **(C)**. Image of apical cross section of the cornea appears above color map. (Obtained with RTVue; Optovue, Fremont, CA, USA.)

Conventional keratometry measures anterior curvature and extrapolates posterior corneal power based on a keratometric index.[8] OCT corneal power measurements are likely more accurate than conventional keratometry because they directly measure both anterior and posterior curvature.

ASOCT can also be used to image the anterior chamber angle, including the scleral spur, ciliary body band, angle recess, and iris root (**Fig. 17.7**). Using the scleral spur as an anatomic landmark, the following quantitative parameters can be measured: angle opening distance, angle recess area, trabecular iris space area, iris thickness, anterior chamber width, and lens vault (**Figs. 17.8** and **17.9**). A narrow

anterior chamber angle between the trabecular meshwork and iris is an anatomic variant that can be imaged with ASOCT; however, not all narrow angles are potentially and pathologically occludable (**Fig. 17.10**).

*ASOCT can be used to visualize postoperative anatomic changes. The trabecular cleft can be identified after ab interno trabeculectomy with the Trabectome (NeoMedix Corp, San Juan Capistrano, CA, USA) that was used to ablate trabecular meshwork tissue (**Fig. 17.11**). Anterior chamber angle widening can be noted when comparing pre and post laser peripheral iridotomy (**Fig. 17.12**).*

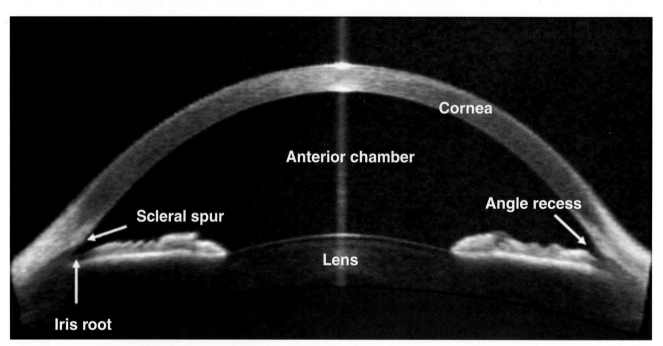

FIGURE 17.7   ASOCT image illustrating structures in the anterior segment.

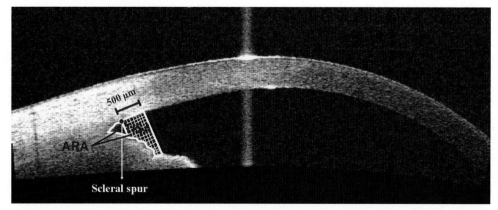

FIGURE 17.8   ASOCT image of the anterior chamber angle illustrating the angle opening distance by the scleral spur (AOD-SS), angle recess area (ARA), and trabecular iris space area (TISA; *cross-hatched in white*). (Obtained with Visante OCT; Carl Zeiss Meditec, Dublin, CA, USA.)

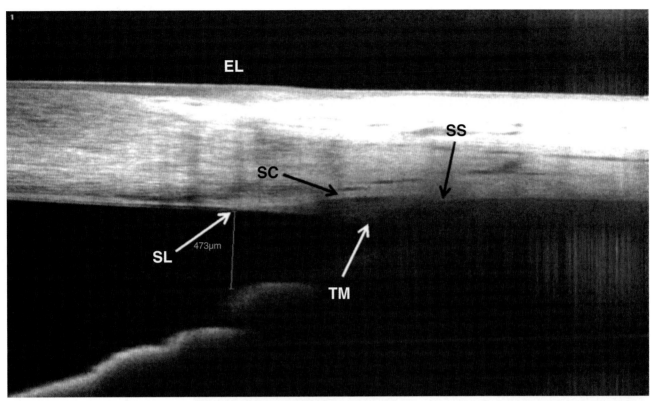

FIGURE 17.9 ASOCT image of nasal angle in normal subject illustrating the termination of the endothelium and Descemet's membrane (Schwalbe's line, SL). Also visible are the external limbus (EL), trabecular meshwork (TM), the scleral spur (SS), and the location of Schlemm's canal (SC). The angle recess, iris root, and ciliary body are not visible owing to blocking by the sclera. The angle opening distance between SL and the anterior surface of the iris (angle opening distance [AOD]-SL, vertical, *yellow caliper line*) was large, measuring 473 μm, indicating that the angle was open.

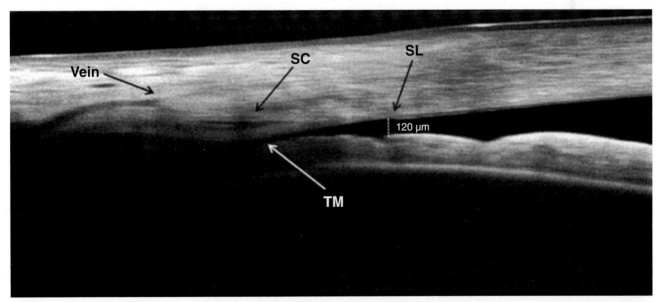

FIGURE 17.10 ASOCT image of the nasal angle in an eye with narrow angles. Note the small distance between the trabecular meshwork (TM) and the iris root, indicating a narrow, potentially occluded angle. The angle opening distance (AOD)-SL (*dotted line* extending to Schwalbe's line [SL]) was narrow, measuring 120 μm. Also visible are Schlemm's canal (SC) and an aqueous vein.

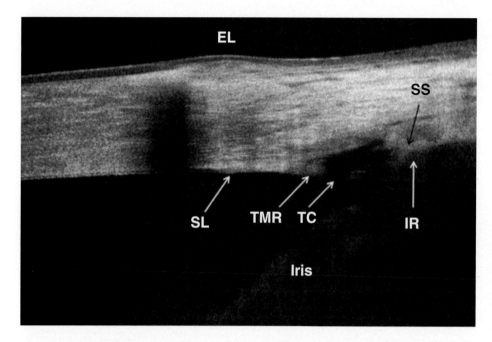

FIGURE 17.11 ASOCT image of nasal angle in glaucomatous eye after trabectome surgery to ablate the trabecular meshwork, leaving a trabecular cleft (TC) and trabecular meshwork remnant (TMR). EL, external limbus; SL, Schwalbe's line; SS, scleral spur; IR, iris root.

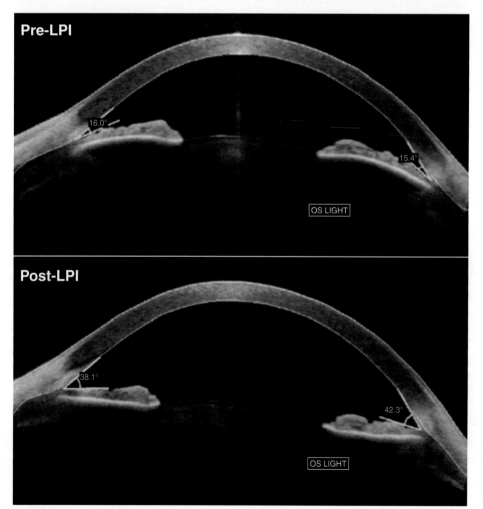

FIGURE 17.12 ASOCT image of eye with narrow angles upon clinical presentation. Images show this eye before and after a laser peripheral iridotomy (LPI). Note the widening of the anterior chamber angle after the procedure.

POSTERIOR SEGMENT OCT

The cross-sectional structure of the retina and optic disc, as well as their respective microstructures, can be visualized with OCT. A large field of view OCT image along the papillomacular bundle (spanning from the fovea to the optic disc) is shown in **Figure 17.4**. Major anatomic features of the retina, including the fovea, optic disc, retinal profile, and curvature, are identifiable by their characteristic morphology. The vitreoretinal interface can be identified beyond the surface of the inner retina by the increased backscatter between the retina and transparent vitreous. The foveal pit in the center of the macula is identified by a characteristic depression associated with thinning of the retina owing to the absence of the inner retinal layers but with continuity of the internal limiting membrane. The optic disc is evident by its unique features. The highly scattering retinal pigment epithelium (RPE) and choriocapillaris layer delineate the posterior retinal boundary. Anteriorly, a closely spaced, second, highly scattering layer is observed owing to the reflection between the inner and outer segments of the photoreceptors. These two posterior layers (RPE/choriocapillaris and inner segment [IS]/outer segment [OS] junction) terminate at the margin of the optic disc, coincident with the termination of choroid at the lamina cribrosa (LC). The details of optic disc anatomy visible with OCT will be discussed further in the respective section later. Posterior to the choriocapillaris, a variable, weak signal can be detected from the deep choroid and sclera, limited by the light attenuation of the retina, RPE, and choriocapillaris. The nerve fiber layer (NFL) is a highly scattering layer and of variable thickness at the inner margin of the retina. The NFL thickness variability can be appreciated by observing the progressive thickening of this layer toward the ONH. The other inner retinal layers thin out approaching the fovea, with only the outer nuclear layer (ONL) and photoreceptors remaining in the foveal region.

As noted earlier, there is not perfect correspondence between the layers of the retina as seen in histologic sections and the layers of the retina identifiable by OCT. This is because the appearance and prominence of a given structure in an OCT image depends on its reflectivity, not its staining characteristics. This lack of correspondence led to initial uncertainties regarding OCT nomenclature within the sensory retina and ONH. To address this issue, an international group of experts was convened to produce a consensus on nomenclature to be used when reviewing normal posterior segment SD-OCT images.[9] The two principal figures from that publication are shown

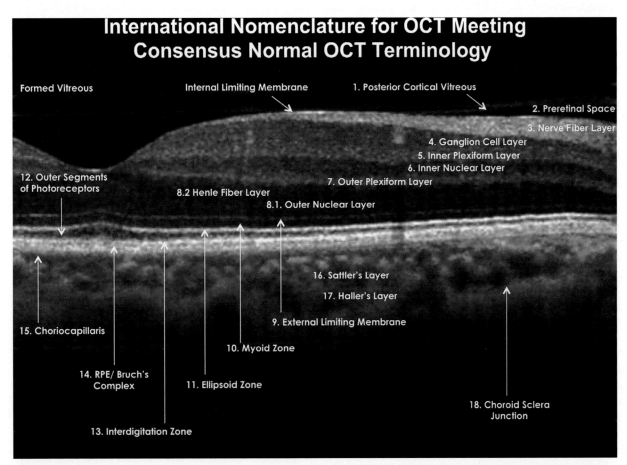

FIGURE 17.13 Adopted nomenclature for anatomic landmarks of normal retina and choroid as seen with spectral-domain OCT imaging. RPE, retinal pigment epithelium. (From Staurenghi G, Sadda S, Chakravarthy U, et al. Proposed Lexicon for anatomic landmarks in normal posterior segment spectral-domain optical coherence tomography: The In-OCT Consensus. *Ophthalmology*. 2014;121:1572–1578.)

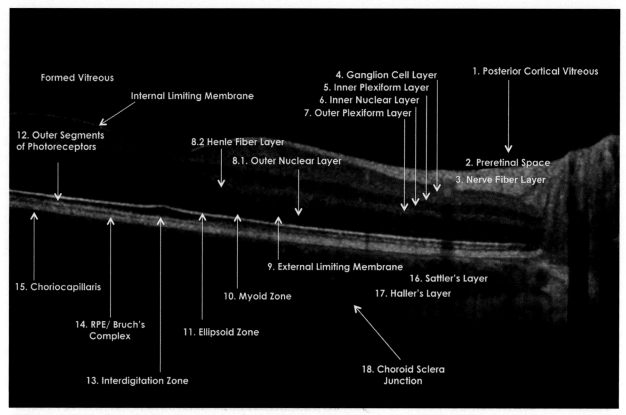

FIGURE 17.14 Lower magnification image providing adopted nomenclature for anatomic landmarks of normal retina, choroid, and peripapillary region as seen with spectral-domain OCT imaging. RPE, retinal pigment epithelium. (From Staurenghi G, Sadda S, Chakravarthy U, et al. Proposed Lexicon for anatomic landmarks in normal posterior segment spectral-domain optical coherence tomography: The In-OCT Consensus. *Ophthalmology*. 2014;121:1572–1578.)

in **Figures 17.13** and **17.14**, representing the consensus labeling of the structures seen in the retina and optic nerve using SD-OCT. Compare that labeling with the histologically defined layers depicted in **Figure 17.15**.

Retinal Microstructure

Microstructural anatomy of various retinal layers can be differentiated with OCT on the basis of backscattering intensities of various tissues in the context of well-known morphology.[10–12] **Figure 17.16** shows a normal macular OCT scan in grayscale with labeled layers. **Figure 17.17** shows the same image represented with false-color analysis indicating retinal layers with different reflectivities that can be correlated with established morphology of the histologically defined retinal layers shown in **Figure 17.15**. In these false-color scans, warmer colors (more red) indicate retinal structures with higher reflectivity. As such, OCT enables the resolution of the distinct retinal layers and has been compared, confirmed, and validated with histologic findings.[3,13–15]

With onboard imaging software, OCT can create 3D representations of portions of the retina from known specific locations, allowing for remarkable precision in analyzing either normal or diseased tissue at what amounts to histologic detail.

Note the contrast between the highly backscattering (red) axonal structures in the NFL and plexiform layers compared with the weakly backscattering (blue-green) structures in the nuclear layers on the false-color OCT image (**Fig. 17.17**). The three, weakly backscattering layers are the ganglion cell layer (GCL), inner nuclear layer (INL), and ONL. Unlike the NFL, the GCL increases in thickness in the parafoveal region, toward the center of the macula. The moderately backscattering inner plexiform layer is adjacent to the GCL and INL. The outer plexiform layer is located between the INL and the ONL (**Fig. 17.16**).

OCT does not directly visualize anatomic structures but rather their optical tissue interaction. This is most notable in visualizing the obliquely running photoreceptor axons, Henle's fiber layer (HFL), within the OPL. HFL is highly backscattering but has been noted to be dependent on directional reflectance.[16] Figure 17.18 demonstrates how the detection of HFL within the OPL is dependent on the angle of the incident light. Thus, any abnormality that distorts the anatomy in a way that impacts the angle at which the light is reflected will have an impact on the presence and extent of visualization of HFL.

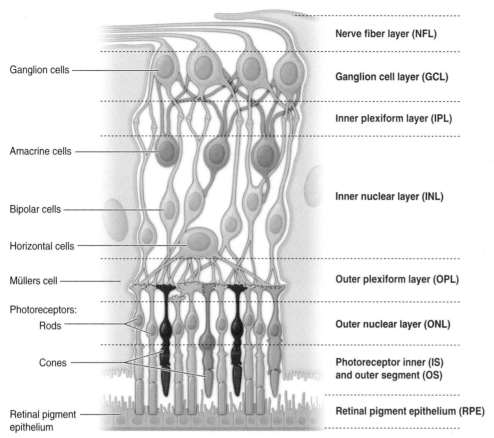

FIGURE 17.15   Histologically defined layers of the retina. GCL, ganglion cell layer; INL, inner nuclear layer; IPL, inner plexiform layer; IS-OS, inner and outer segments of photoreceptor layer; NFL, nerve fiber layer; ONL, outer nuclear layer; OPL, outer plexiform layer; RPE, retinal pigment epithelium.

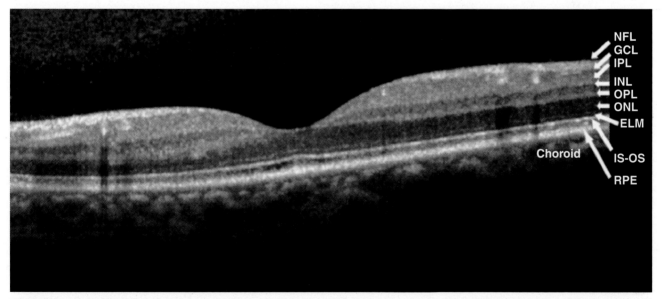

FIGURE 17.16   OCT image of macular scan in grayscale showing layers of the retina. ELM, external limiting membrane; GCL, ganglion cell layer; INL, inner nuclear layer; IPL, inner plexiform layer; IS-OS, inner and outer segments of photoreceptor layer; NFL, nerve fiber layer; OCT, optical coherence tomography; ONL, outer nuclear layer; OPL, outer plexiform layer; RPE, retinal pigment epithelium. (Obtained with Spectralis HRA+OCT; Heidelberg Engineering, Heidelberg, Germany.)

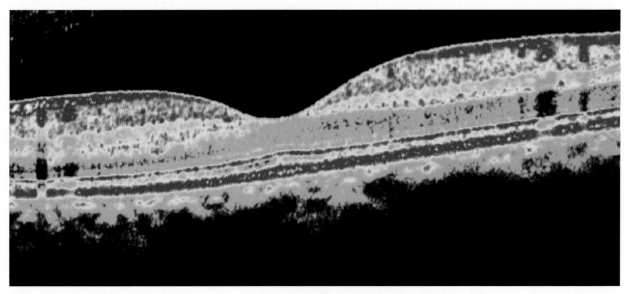

FIGURE 17.17 OCT image of a macular scan in false color showing layers of the retina. Correlate colors with labeled layers in Figure 17.16. (Obtained with Spectralis HRA+OCT; Heidelberg Engineering, Heidelberg, Germany.)

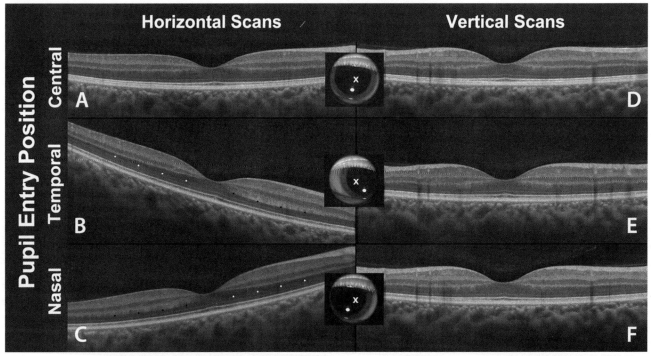

FIGURE 17.18 The effects of horizontally varying pupil entry position on horizontal and vertical B-scans in a right eye. Pupil entry position for each set of OCT images is marked with a *white* (x) in the three photographs of the cornea at the center of the figure. This entry point is different from the corneal reflection (Purkinje image), which is the round, inferior corneal reflection denoted by the small white dot in each picture. **A:** Central entry position with flat B-scans and poor visualization of Henle's fiber layer (HFL—the macular equivalent of the outer plexiform layer). **B:** Temporal displacement of the entry beam. Although the foveal anatomy has not changed, there is an apparent tilt to the horizontal B-scan because of unequal optical path lengths (see Fig. 17.1). A temporal entry position results in hyperreflectivity of HFL relative to the ONL on the nasal side of the fovea (*black dots*) and hyporeflectivity of HFL temporal to the fovea (*white dots*), where distinct demarcations among the outer nuclear layer, HFL, and the inner plexiform layer are apparent. **C:** Nasal displacement of the entry beam showing the opposite effects of (B). **D to F:** Vertical scans at each pupil entry position show only minimal HFL reflectivity changes and no tilt because vertically, the optical path lengths remain equal despite horizontal translation.

Photoreceptors, RPE, and Choroid

The photoreceptor IS/OS junction is a highly backscattering thin band that is anterior to the RPE. The photoreceptor IS/OS junction thickens in the foveal region, owing to the increase in the length of the cone OS in this region. The IS/OS junction has also been referred to as the ellipsoid portion of inner segments, the portion of the inner segments known to be enriched with mitochondria. Anterior to the IS/OS junction and posterior to the ONL, the external limiting membrane (ELM) can be visualized as a thin backscattering layer. The ELM is an alignment of zonulae adherentes junctions between the photoreceptors and the Müller cells that is visualized as another example of an optical tissue interaction.

The RPE is also highly backscattering owing to its content of melanin. By contrast, Bruch's membrane, the compound basement membrane of the RPE and choriocapillary endothelium, cannot be visualized as an independent structure with OCT. Continuing posteriorly, past the RPE and Bruch's membrane, is the choriocapillaris, which is another strongly backscattering structure. Because the RPE and choriocapillaris are separated only by Bruch's membrane, they are often not distinguishable as separate layers on OCT. Using OCT, it is evident that the choroid is thickest under the fovea. The densely vascular composition of the choriocapillaris and choroid are highly optically backscattering, thus producing vertical shadow effects that limit the OCT imaging depth. The most pronounced larger blood vessels of the choroid can be identified by their increased backscatter and shadowing of deeper structures (**Fig. 17.19**). Larger retinal vessels, such as the major branches of the central retinal artery and vein that are present near the ONH, also produce vertical shadowing of deeper structures.

Structurally and functionally, the normal choroidal vasculature is vital to retinal function. Detecting changes in known choroidal parameters can be used to diagnose and guide treatment in chorioretinal diseases. OCT allows the clinician to appreciate normal choroidal thickness compared with the notably increased thickness of the choroid in central serous chorioretinopathy (Figs. 17.20 and 17.21) and decreased choroidal thickness in macular degeneration (Fig. 17.22).

Optic Disc

OCT can visualize the contour of the optic disc in a two-dimensional cross-sectional scan (**Fig. 17.23**) and 3D volumetric scans, even merging them with a scanning laser ophthalmoscopic image of the corresponding retinal surface (**Fig. 17.24**). Note that the normal cupping of the optic disc is apparent and the contour is demarcated by the boundary between the low backscattering vitreous and the highly backscattering NFL. As the NFL approaches the rim of the optic nerve, it increases in thickness. Similar to the NFL of Henle in the macular region shown in **Figure 17.18**, the NFL also exhibits directional reflectance. The reflected signal intensity from the NFL decreases at the optic disc rim as the fibers bend into the ONH and are no longer perpendicular to the incident OCT optical beam.

As noted earlier, the RPE/choriocapillaris is a highly backscattering layer, making its termination at the edge of the optic nerve readily apparent. Concurrently, the

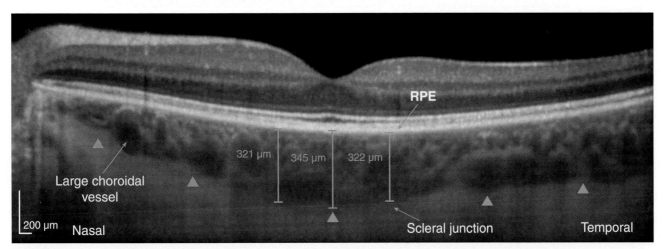

FIGURE 17.19   OCT with enhanced depth imaging of normal choroid illustrating choroidal thickness (*green lines*), choroid–sclera junction (*green arrows*), and presence of large choroidal vessels. Note how the shadows of the larger vessels produce vertically oriented shadows (*darker stripes*) in the deeper layers, extending even into the sclera. RPE, retinal pigment epithelium. (Obtained with Spectralis HRA+OCT; Heidelberg Engineering, Heidelberg, Germany.)

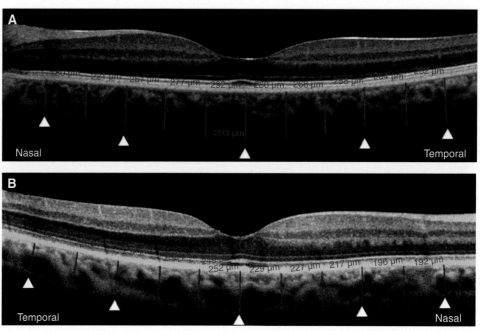

FIGURE 17.20 OCT images of normal choroid. **A:** Scan from a normal 24-year-old subject. **B:** Scan from a normal 76-year-old subject. Choroid–sclera junction is denoted by *white arrowheads*. Note that the choroid is thinner in the older subject. (Obtained with Cirrus HD-OCT; Carl Zeiss Meditec, Dublin, CA, USA.)

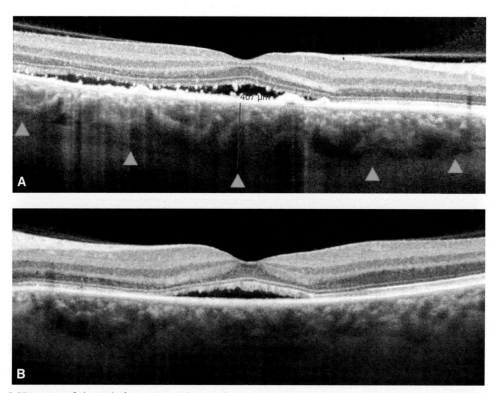

FIGURE 17.21 OCT images of choroid of a patient with central serous chorioretinopathy. **A:** Note that the choroid is thicker than normal (*vertical red line*). Choroid–sclera junction is denoted by *green arrowheads*. **B:** Note that it is not possible to visualize the choroid–sclera junction because the choroid is so thick that it limits signal penetration. (Obtained with Cirrus HD-OCT; Carl Zeiss Meditec, Dublin, CA, USA.)

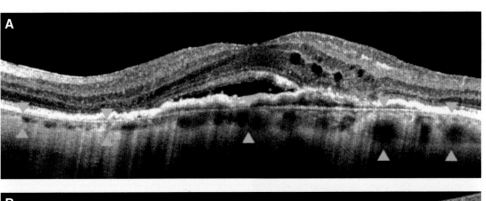

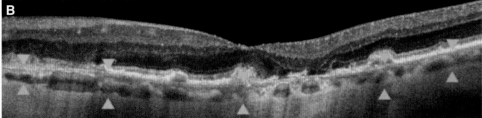

FIGURE 17.22   A: OCT image of the choroid of a patient with exudative ("wet"), age-related macular degeneration. Note that the choroid is thinner than normal and can be visualized under the choroidal neovascularization. *Blue arrowheads* denote the outer edge of the hyper-reflective RPE, and the *green arrowheads* denote the choroid–sclera junction in both **A** and **B**. **B:** OCT image of the choroid of a patient with dry age-related macular degeneration. Note that the choroid is similarly thinner than normal and hyperreflective areas of choroid can be visualized owing to the areas of RPE atrophy. (Obtained with Cirrus HD-OCT; Carl Zeiss Meditec, Dublin, CA, USA.)

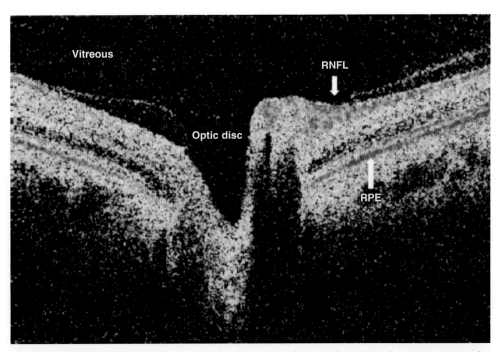

FIGURE 17.23   OCT image of optic nerve head presented as cross-sectional B-scan illustrating the vitreous, optic disc, retinal pigment epithelium (RPE), and retinal nerve fiber layer (RNFL). Note the detachment of the posterior vitreous face (arcuate, stippled green line on retinal surface for a short distance, along the sloping retina to the left of the optic disc). (Obtained with RTVue; Optovue, Fremont, CA, USA.)

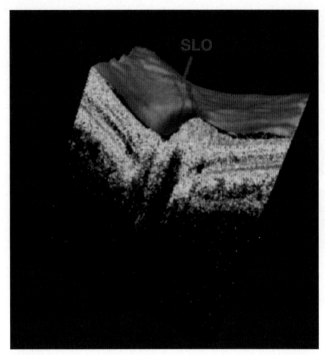

FIGURE 17.24 3D OCT cross-sectional image of optic nerve head and peripapillary retina with scanning laser ophthalmoscope (SLO) image overlaid on retinal and optic nerve surfaces. (Obtained with RTVue; Optovue, Fremont, CA, USA.)

 OCT imaging of the optic nerve and neuroretinal rim is valuable in assessing glaucoma and neuro-ophthalmic diseases. Notably, OCT is capable of differentiating glaucomatous from nonglaucomatous optic nerve cupping with identification of preferential superior/inferior quadrant retinal NFL loss and diffuse loss, respectively.[17] In cases where the ONH looks elevated with blurred margins, OCT allows for differentiation of ONH drusen as well (Fig. 17.25).[18]

Peripapillary Region

The NFL of the retina, representing the axons of the retina ganglion cells, is highly visible as a well-demarcated, highly backscattering layer in the OCT image. The retinal NFL can be detected automatically using segmentation algorithms with boundary detection, and its thickness can be quantitatively measured. The measurement of NFL thickness with OCT was one of the earliest technologic applications in the field of eye care.[19,20] The ability to quantify NFL thickness in the peripapillary region is essential to glaucoma diagnosis and treatment, because loss of NFL thickness is a cardinal finding in glaucoma. Note that direct evaluation of ganglion cell loss would be very useful as well, but recall that the GCL is, unfortunately, not well resolved with this technology.

photoreceptor IS/OS junction is a thin, highly backscattering layer that can be identified immediately anterior to the RPE/choriocapillaris layer. Because the photoreceptor IS/OS junction layer and RPE both terminate at the edge of the optic disc, they can be used as a landmark to define the optic disc margin.

OCT is not limited to obtaining linear cross sections through the retina. One can also create circular scans around the optic disc or cube scans in the circumpapillary

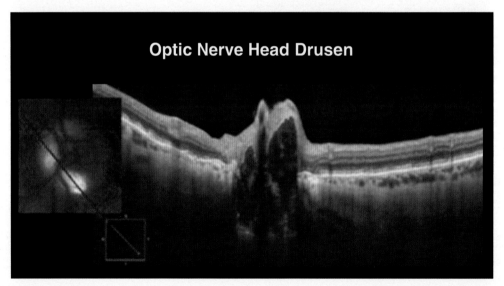

FIGURE 17.25 OCT image of linear, cross-sectional scan of optic nerve head demonstrating optic nerve drusen. Optic nerve drusen show a distinct "lumpy-bumpy" internal contour. *Inset:* Clinical photograph of optic nerve head, with bright drusen of the optic nerve, showing plane of section for main image along red line. (Image acquired on Cirrus HD-OCT; Carl Zeiss Meditec, Dublin, CA, USA.)

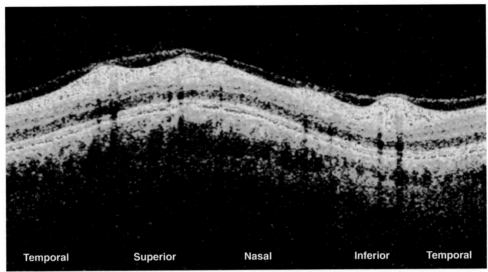

FIGURE 17.26   OCT image of circumpapillary scan illustrating the unwrapped peripapillary quadrants. Note also the blue-green line just above the retinal surface, which corresponds to the posterior vitreous face. (Obtained with Cirrus HD-OCT; Carl Zeiss Meditec, Dublin, CA, USA.)

region to optically capture all nerves emanating toward nerve head for a truly comprehensive sample of the retinal NFL. **Figure 17.26** shows a circumpapillary OCT scan centered on the ONH. The circle sampled in the cube scan is marked in red in the fundus photograph in **Figure 17.27**. **Figure 17.26** is displayed "unwrapped," as though the circle in **Figure 17.27** was cut and the cross-sectional image of the retina obtained along that circle was presented as a straight line. The superior, inferior, temporal, and nasal quadrants around the ONH are labeled. It is well known that in the normal eye, the thickness of the NFL follows what is termed the "ISNT rule."[21] The ISNT rule states that in a normal eye, the NFL thickness changes from thickest to thinnest in the following order: inferior, superior, nasal, and temporal.

 Of clinical importance, when there is NFL loss resulting from glaucoma, these losses are selective and not uniform around the circumference of the ONH. These uneven losses in NFL thickness eventually change the relative thicknesses around the circumference of the optic nerve in a way that the ISNT rule is violated, and this has been shown to be an important and reliable indicator of glaucomatous damage.[21]

New Frontiers in OCT Ocular Anatomy

OCT is widely recognized as the most powerful ophthalmic imaging technique and is continuing to evolve in a variety of ways. Faster scanning speeds and higher resolution have extended the use of OCT beyond the major anterior and posterior eye structures. In addition, novel image processing algorithms and combining alternate imaging modalities with OCT have allowed investigators to visualize anatomic structures that have never previously been resolved in vivo. All of these, and future developments, serve to emphasize the need for clinicians in the field of eye care to have an exceptionally good grasp of the histology of the various parts of the eye.

In this final section, we will briefly discuss new frontiers in OCT ocular anatomy. The details of these technologies and methods are beyond the scope of this chapter. These approaches have not yet been validated for clinical decision-making, but we wish to conclude this text on the anatomy of the eye by introducing these upcoming frontiers.

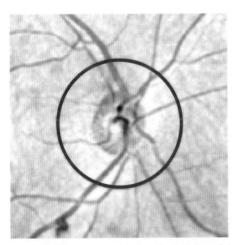

FIGURE 17.27   Fundus image indicating the location of the circumpapillary scan shown in **Figure 17.27**. (Obtained with Cirrus HD-OCT; Carl Zeiss Meditec, Dublin, CA, USA.)

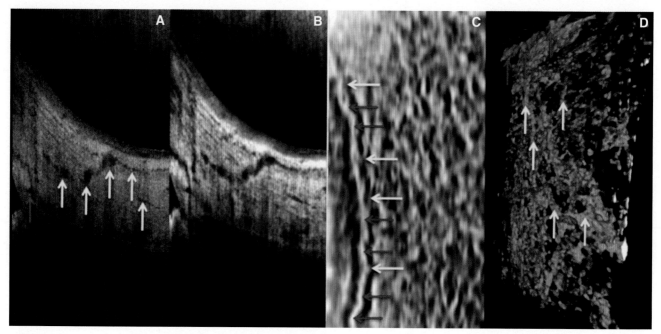

FIGURE 17.28   A: Raw OCT scan of limbus allows for visualization of Schlemm's canal (*red arrow*) and reveals dark, nonreflective regions within reflective tissue (*yellow arrows*), likely representing aqueous humor within its draining channels. **B:** Postimaging processing (averaging, resampling, contrast enhancement filter) allows for improved visualization of the AH outflow system. **C:** Inverting the image (*white to black*) and isolating a slab of tissue at the level of Schlemm's canal allows for extended visualization of Schlemm's canal (*red arrow*), collector channels (*yellow arrows*), and distal outflow vasculature throughout the limbus (white tubular interconnecting vessels). **D:** An alternative approach to visualize the aqueous humor (AH) outflow system by isolating the outflow structures and rendering a 3D view of the morphology of the outflow system (Schlemm's canal = *red arrows*, distal outflow channels leading toward episcleral veins = *yellow arrows*). (Obtained with Cirrus HD-OCT; Carl Zeiss Meditec, Dublin, CA, USA.)

IMAGING AQUEOUS HUMOR OUTFLOW PATHWAYS WITH OCT CANALOGRAPHY

Research OCT protocols have been used to image human aqueous humor (AH) outflow pathways, including Schlemm's canal and collector channels.[22] The human AH outflow system has been visualized in 3D using physical corrosion casting as well as OCT virtual casting using a morphometric analysis.[23] Commercially available OCT devices have been used to scan the limbus of living human subjects and create volumetric data to visualize the AH outflow system, specifically Schlemm's canal, the collector channels, and blood vessels (**Fig. 17.28**). Realizing that Schlemm's canal is not continuous and often bifid or segmental has been a critical OCT-driven anatomic insight. As 3D volumetric data processing improves, it may allow for the development of OCT canalography to provide clinically relevant localization data of areas of increased outflow resistance in the AH outflow system. This may allow for more precisely targeted intraocular pressure (IOP)-lowering interventions, such as placement of shunts, valves, and stents, in glaucoma patients.

IMAGING BLOOD VESSEL AND BLOOD FLOW WITH OCT ANGIOGRAPHY

Abnormal circulation is a contributing factor in some of the leading causes of irreversible blindness, including glaucoma, diabetic retinopathy, and macular degeneration.

OCT angiography is a dye-less, infection-free, 3D imaging modality providing the ability to visualize ocular vascular circulation using an ultra-high speed OCT. OCT angiography was first attempted using Doppler OCT but faced difficulties because the ocular vasculature is often oriented perpendicular to the OCT beam. Using novel techniques more recently developed, it has become possible to do OCT angiography. One such method is optical microangiography, which can resolve the microvasculature in retinal, choroidal, and ONH structures by separating scattering signals from stationary and moving particles (such as red blood cells).[24,25]

Phase variance and Doppler variance also use SD-OCT to visualize retinal and choroidal microvascular networks.[26,27] More recent advancements have centered on SS-OCT technology and amplitude-based approaches (as opposed to spectral-based with SD-OCT). These include speckle variance OCT and a split-spectrum amplitude-decorrelation algorithm.[28] With these advanced methods, one can achieve remarkable images of the microvasculature in the choroid, optic disc, and retina, including the foveal avascular zone (**Fig. 17.29**). Unlike traditional dye-based angiography, however, OCT angiography cannot visualize fluid leakage and perivascular staining.

Preliminary work suggests that this technology can detect reduced optic disc perfusion correlated with visual field progression in glaucoma (**Fig. 17.30**).[29,30] Recently, OCT angiography has been applied to visualize drusen on Bruch's membrane and geographic atrophy in non-neovascular

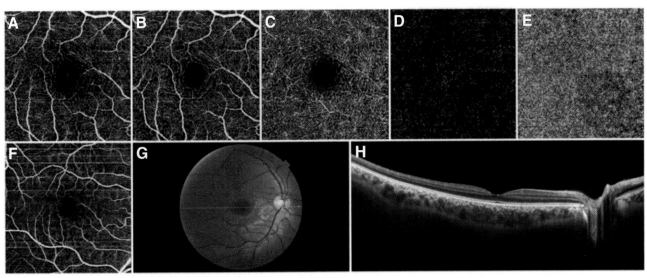

FIGURE 17.29 OCT angiogram fields of view and segmentation layers of a healthy human eye acquired using the SS OCT Angio software on the Swept Source OCT DRI OCT-1 Triton (Topcon Corporation, Tokyo, Japan). **A:** *En face* composite of entire retinal thickness (internal limiting membrane to Bruch's membrane) 3 × 3 mm OCT angiogram. **B:** 3 × 3 OCT angiogram of the "superficial" inner retina. **C:** 3 × 3 mm OCT angiogram of the "deep" inner retina. **D:** 3 × 3 OCT angiogram of the outer retina. **E:** 3 × 3 mm OCT angiogram of the choriocapillaris. **F:** Full-thickness 6 × 6 mm OCT angiogram. **G:** Red-free fundus image. Light horizontal line corresponds to B-scan in (**H**). **H:** Highly sampled B-scan image.

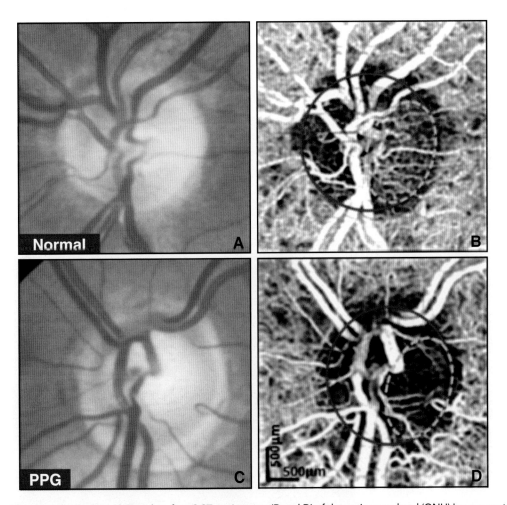

FIGURE 17.30 Disc photographs (**A** and **C**) and *en face* OCT angiograms (**B** and **D**) of the optic nerve head (ONH) in representative normal (**A** and **B**) and preperimetric glaucoma subjects (PPG—i.e., before clear signs of visual field loss have occurred in visual field obtained by perimetry) (**C** and **D**). Both examples are from left eyes. In (**B**) and (**D**), the *solid red circles* indicate the edge of the disc, and the *dashed gold ellipses* indicate the temporal ellipses. A dense microvascular network is visible on the OCT angiogram of the normal disc (**B**). This network is greatly attenuated in the glaucomatous disc (**D**). Compare images within the *dashed gold ellipses* in (**B**) and (**D**). OCT, optical coherence tomography; ONH, optic nerve head.

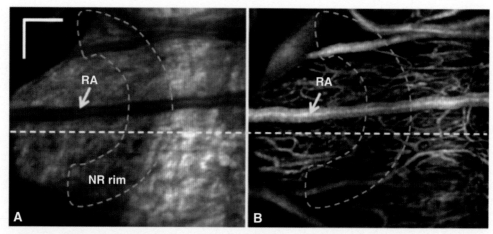

FIGURE 17.31 **A:** A high-magnification OCT fundus image of the temporal region of the optic nerve head (ONH). **B:** Enhanced resolution in the projection image of corresponding 3D (RA, retinal artery). The *dashed yellow line* is a location landmark for comparison of the two images, and the arcuate *dashed orange lines* designate the neuroretinal rim of the optic nerve.

age-related macular degeneration (AMD), choroidal neovascularization in neovascular AMD, macular ischemia, and neovascularization in diabetic retinopathy, as well as vascular occlusions.[31–33]

IMAGING LAMINA CRIBROSA MICROARCHITECTURE WITH MULTIMODAL OCT AND SS-OCT

The LC is a sieve-like elastic structure within the ONH at the level of the sclera, through which all retinal ganglion cell axons pass en route to the brain. The LC has been implicated as an important player in the pathogenesis of glaucoma. The mechanism resulting in cell death in glaucoma is not well understood, but the LC's role in a healthy eye is to provide structural support to axons and their blood supply within the portion of the ONH within

the scleral canal. Recent OCT studies have permitted the visualization of this structure and its associated vasculature, hoping to elucidate its role in the pathogenesis of glaucoma. The thickness and anterior–posterior displacement of the LC has been considered, as well as the microarchitecture and microvasculature of the LC[25,34–36] (Figs. 17.31 and 17.32).

Imaging microarchitecture and thickness of the lamina has been augmented by innovations in OCT technology. One such improvement is SS-OCT, which permits the visualization of deeper structures such as the LC.[37,38] Adaptive optics is another optical enhancement strategy taken from astronomy that corrects for aberrations in the imaging path and improves lateral resolution to sizes on the order of a few microns. When combined with OCT, individual beams of the LC can be seen and analyzed (Fig. 17.32).[38]

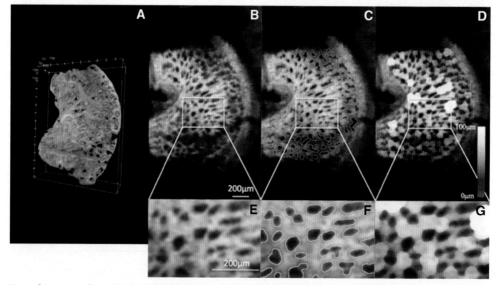

FIGURE 17.32 3D *en face* view of roughly half of the lamina cribrosa (**A**) and C-scan (**B** and **E**) visualization showing woven matrix of lamina cribrosa. **C** and **F:** C-mode slices permitting the quantification of structural parameters such as area of dimensions of openings for axons and measurements of beam thickness (**D** and **G**), where thicker beams are shown in *yellow* and thinner beams in *purple*.

◉ Summary

OCT in its various iterations has quickly become an essential tool in everyday clinical practice, and the level of resolution can only be expected to improve. To optimally use this tool and the array of other imaging technologies available, it is critical for contemporary clinicians to have a strong foundational understanding of the anatomy of the tissues of the eye in histologic detail. These new and deeper levels of understanding of ocular anatomy are now "The Clinical Essentials" required in everyday practice.

REFERENCES

1. Huang, D, Swanson EA, Lin CP, et al. Optical coherence tomography. *Science.* 1991;254:1178–1181.
2. Hee MR, Izatt JA, Swanson EA, et al. Optical coherence tomography of the human retina. *Arch Ophthalmol.* 1995;113:325–332.
3. Toth CA, Narayan DG, Boppart SA, et al. A comparison of retinal morphology viewed by optical coherence tomography and by light microscopy. *Arch Ophthalmol.* 1997;115:1425–1428.
4. Fujimoto JG, Pitris C, Boppart SA, et al. Optical coherence tomography: an emerging technology for biomedical imaging and optical biopsy. *Neoplasia.* 2000;2:9–25.
5. Szabo TL. *Diagnostic Ultrasound Imaging: Inside Out.* New York: Academic Press; 2004.
6. Patterson MS, Chance B, Wilson BC. Time resolved reflectance and transmittance for the non-invasive measurement of tissue optical properties. *Appl Opt.* 1989;28:2331–2336.
7. Boustany NN, Boppart SA, Backman V. Microscopic imaging and spectroscopy with scattered light. *Annu Rev Biomed Eng.* 2010;12:285–314.
8. Ag B. *Bennett and Rabbetts' Clinical Visual Optics.* Edinburg: Butterworth-Heinemann; 1998.
9. Staurenghi G, Sadda S, Chakravarthy U, et al. for the In-OCT Panel. Proposed lexicon for anatomic landmarks in normal posterior segment spectral-domain optical coherence tomography: the In-OCT Consensus. *Ophthalmology.* 2014;121:1572–1578.
10. Hogan MJ, Alvarado JA, Weddell JE. *Histology of the Human Eye.* Philadelphia, PA: WB Saunders, 1971.
11. Gass JDM. *Stereoscopic Atlas of Macular Diseases: Diagnosis and Treatment.* St Louis: Mosby, 1997.
12. Spalton DJ, Hitchings RA, Hunter P. *Atlas of Clinical Ophthalmology.* Edinburgh: Elsevier Health Sciences, 2013.
13. Strouthidis NG, Grimm J, Williams GA, et al. A comparison of optic nerve head morphology viewed by spectral domain optical coherence tomography and by serial histology. *Invest Ophthalmol Vis Sci.* 2010;51:1464–1474.
14. Huang Y, Cideciyan AV, Papastergiou GI, et al. Relation of optical coherence tomography to microanatomy in normal and rd chickens. *Invest Ophthalmol Vis Sci.* 1998;39:2405–2416.
15. Chen TC, Cense B, Miller JW, et al. Histologic correlation of in vivo optical coherence tomography images of the human retina. *Am J Ophthalmol.* 2006;141:1165–1168.
16. Lujan BJ, Roorda A, Knighton RW, et al. Revealing Henle's fiber layer using spectral domain optical coherence tomography. *Invest Ophthalmol Vis Sci.* 2011;52:1486–1492.
17. Gupta PK, Asrani S, Freedman SF, et al. Differentiating glaucomatous from non-glaucomatous optic nerve cupping by optical coherence tomography. *Open Neurol J.* 2011;5:1–7.
18. Johnson LN, Diehl ML, Hamm CW, et al. Differentiating optic disc edema from optic nerve head drusen on optical coherence tomography. *Arch Ophthalmol.* 2009;127:45–49.
19. Schuman JS, Hee MR, Puliafito CA, et al. Quantification of nerve fiber layer thickness in normal and glaucomatous eyes using optical coherence tomography. *Arch Ophthalmol.* 1995;113:586–596.
20. Chong GT, Lee RK. Glaucoma versus red disease: imaging and glaucoma diagnosis. *Curr. Opin. Ophthalmol.* 2012;23:79–88.
21. Harizman N, Oliveira C, Chiang A, et al. The ISNT rule and differentiation of normal from glaucomatous eyes. *Arch Ophthalmol.* 2006;124:1579–1583.
22. Kagemann L, Wollstein G, Ishikawa H, et al. Identification and assessment of Schlemm's canal by spectral-domain optical coherence tomography. *Invest Ophthalmol Vis Sci.* 2010;51:4054–4059.
23. Francis AW, Kagemann L, Wollstein G, et al. Morphometric analysis of aqueous humor outflow structures with spectral-domain optical coherence tomography. *Invest Ophthalmol Vis Sci.* 2012;53:5198–5207.
24. Wang RK. Optical microangiography: a label free 3D imaging technology to visualize and quantify blood circulations within tissue beds in vivo. *IEEE J Sel Top Quantum Electron.* 2010;16:545–554.
25. An L. Optical microangiography provides correlation between microstructure and microvasculature of optic nerve head in human subjects. *J Biomed Opt.* 2012;17:116018.
26. Fingler J, Zawadzki RJ, Werner JS, et al. Volumetric microvascular imaging of human retina using optical coherence tomography with a novel motion contrast technique. *Opt Express.* 2009;17:22190–22200.
27. Yu L, Chen Z. Doppler variance imaging for three-dimensional retina and choroid angiography. *J Biomed Opt.* 2010;15:016029.
28. Jia Y, Tan O, Tokayer J, et al. Split-spectrum amplitude-decorrelation angiography with optical coherence tomography. *Opt Express.* 2012;20:4710–4725.
29. Jia Y, Morrison JC, Tokayer J, et al. Quantitative OCT angiography of optic nerve head blood flow. *Biomed Opt Express.* 2012;3:3127–3137.
30. Jia Y, Wei E, Wang X, et al. Optical coherence tomography angiography of optic disc perfusion in glaucoma. *Ophthalmology.* 2014;121:1322–1332.
31. Jia Y, Bailey ST, Hwang TS, et al. Quantitative optical coherence tomography angiography of vascular abnormalities in the living human eye. *Proc Natl Acad Sci USA.* 2015;112:E2395–402. doi:10.1073/pnas.1500185112.
32. Jia Y, Bailey ST, Wilson DJ, et al. Quantitative optical coherence tomography angiography of choroidal neovascularization in age-related macular degeneration. *Ophthalmology* 2014;121:1435–1444.
33. De Carlo TE, Romano A, Waheed NK, et al. A review of optical coherence tomography angiography (OCTA). *Int J Retin Vitr.* 2015;1:14354.
34. Lee EJ, Kim TW, Weinreb RN, et al. Three-dimensional evaluation of the lamina cribrosa using spectral-domain optical coherence tomography in glaucoma. *Invest Ophthalmol Vis Sci.* 2012;53:198–204.
35. Agoumi Y, Sharpe GP, Hutchison DM, et al. Laminar and prelaminar tissue displacement during intraocular pressure elevation in glaucoma patients and healthy controls. *Ophthalmology.* 2011;118:52–59.
36. Wang B, Nevins JE, Nadler Z, et al. In vivo lamina cribrosa micro-architecture in healthy and glaucomatous eyes as assessed by optical coherence tomography. *Invest Ophthalmol Vis Sci.* 2013;54:8270–8274.
37. Omodaka K, Horii T, Takahashi S, et al. 3D evaluation of the lamina cribrosa with swept-source optical coherence tomography in normal tension glaucoma. *PLoS One.* 2015;10:e0122347.
38. Nadler Z, Wang B, Wollstein G, et al. Repeatability of in vivo 3D lamina cribrosa microarchitecture using adaptive optics spectral domain optical coherence tomography. *Biomed Opt Express.* 2014;5:1114–1123.

Index